MUSCULOSKELETAL MRI

SECOND EDITION

CLYDE A. HELMS, MD

Professor
Radiology and Surgery
Director
Division of Musculoskeletal Imaging
Duke University Medical Center
Durham, North Carolina

NANCY M. MAJOR, MD

Associate Professor
Radiology, Surgery, Biological Anthropology and Anatomy
Division of Musculoskeletal Imaging
Director
Medical Student Radiology Education
Duke University Medical Center
Durham, North Carolina

MARK W. ANDERSON, MD

Associate Professor
Radiology and Orthopaedic Surgery
Chief
Division of Musculoskeletal Radiology
University of Virginia
Charlottesville, Virginia

PHOEBE A. KAPLAN, MD

Musculoskeletal Radiologist
Réso Concorde and Réso Carrefour MRI Centers
Laval, Quebec, Canada
Musculoskeletal Radiologist
Laennec Radiology Clinic
Montreal, Quebec, Canada

ROBERT DUSSAULT, MD

Musculoskeletal Radiologist
Réso Concorde and Réso Carrefour MRI Centers
Laval, Quebec, Canada
Musculoskeletal Radiologist
Laennec Radiology Clinic
Montreal, Quebec, Canada

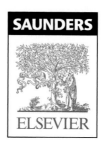

SAUNDERS

ELSEVIER

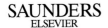

1600 John F. Kennedy Blvd.
Ste 1800
Philadelphia, PA 19103-2899

MUSCULOSKELETAL MRI   ISBN: 978-1-4160-5534-1

Copyright © 2009, 2001 by Saunders, an imprint of Elsevier Inc.

Library of Congress Cataloging-in-Publication Data
Musculoskeletal MRI / Clyde A. Helms . . . [et al.].—2nd ed.
      p. ; cm.
  Includes bibliographical references and index.
  ISBN 978-1-4160-5534-1
  1. Musculoskeletal system—Magnetic resonance imaging.   I. Helms, Clyde A.
  [DNLM: 1. Musculoskeletal Diseases—diagnosis.   2. Magnetic Resonance Imaging—methods.
3. Musculoskeletal System—anatomy & histology. WE 141 M98581 2009]

  RC925.7.M874 2009
  616.7′07548—dc22   2008029887

Senior Acquisitions Editor: Rebecca Schmidt Gaertner
Associate Developmental Editor: Joanie Milnes
Publishing Services Manager: Tina Rebane
Senior Project Manager: Amy L. Cannon
Design Director: Ellen Zanolle
Illustration Coordinator: Kari Wszolek
Marketing Manager: Catalina Nolte

Printed in the United States of America.

Last digit is the print number: 9   8   7   6   5   4   3   2

To Austin Michael. Teaching you is the greatest joy in our lives.
NMM and CAH

To the residents and fellows who have made me a better radiologist and my job worth doing.
MWA

Once again, to each other. In our varied roles in life, which include being professional colleagues, business partners, life partners, best friends, chef/sous chef, driver/backseat driver, etc, we remain one hell of a team.
PAK and RD

Preface

Since the first edition of *Musculoskeletal MRI* was published in 2001, much has changed in the realm of musculoskeletal MRI. Scores of new articles have been published on every anatomic area, and new imaging techniques have been developed, including 3T magnets. Although we have attempted to incorporate these advances in the current edition, we stand firm in our original maxim that "less is more" when it comes to a text explaining the basics. Therefore, we resolved to not let the size of this work increase dramatically. Almost every chapter has been significantly updated. Many new figures have been added and many of the original figures have been replaced by better examples using more current techniques.

All five of the authors have contributed to each chapter; therefore, the chapters themselves are not identified with the author who was primarily responsible for the writing. This adds to the uniformity of the text and gave each of us an opportunity to challenge one another when we disagreed over something (which, surprisingly, was not that often).

Working on the second edition of *Musculoskeletal MRI* made each of us a little better at what we do, which is to practice and teach musculoskeletal MRI, and we are certain it also will help improve the skills of every reader of this book.

Contents

Basic Principles of Musculoskeletal MRI

1

Although a detailed understanding of nuclear physics is not necessary to interpret magnetic resonance imaging (MRI) studies, it also is unacceptable to read passively whatever images you are given without concern for how the images are acquired, or how they might be improved. Radiologists should have a solid understanding of the basic principles involved in acquiring excellent images. This chapter describes the various components that go into producing high-quality images, stressing the fundamental principles shared by all MRI scanners.

Every machine is different. Clinical scanners are now available at strengths ranging from 0.2 Tesla (T) to 3.0T. Additionally, each vendor has its own language for describing its hardware, software, and scanning parameters, and an entire chapter could be devoted to deciphering the terms used by different manufacturers. Time spent learning the details of your machine with your technologists or physicists would be time well spent. If you are interested, read one of the excellent discussions of MRI physics in articles or other textbooks[1-5] because, for the most part, in this book we leave the physics to the physicists.

What Makes a Good Image?

LACK OF MOTION

Motion is one of the greatest enemies of MRI (Fig. 1-1). It can arise from a variety of sources, such as cardiac motion, bowel peristalsis, and respiratory movement. For most musculoskeletal applications, motion usually stems from body movement related to patient discomfort. Patient comfort is of paramount importance because even if all the other imaging parameters are optimized, any movement would ruin the entire image.

Patient comfort begins with positioning. Every effort should be made to make the patient comfortable, such as placing a pillow beneath the knees when the patient is supine to reduce the stress on the back or providing padding at pressure points. When the patient is in a comfortable position, passive restraints, such as tape, foam rubber, or sandbags, can be used for maximal immobilization. Music via headphones can help alleviate anxiety; oral sedation may be required for claustrophobic patients.

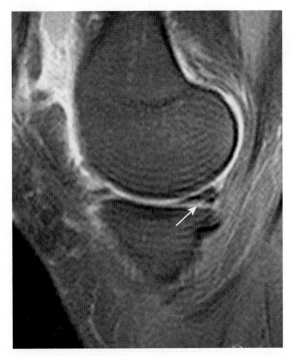

Figure 1-1 **Motion artifact. A,** FSE–proton density image of the knee. The image is markedly degraded by patient motion artifact. Increased signal intensity in the posterior horn of the meniscus *(arrow)* may represent artifact versus a true tear.

Another cause of patient motion is a prolonged examination, which is one reason why set imaging protocols are useful. By designing streamlined imaging sequences, the necessary scans are obtained in as short a time as possible, resulting in better patient compliance, improved technologist efficiency, and maximal scanner throughput. Standardized protocols also reduce the need for direct physician oversight during the scan and allow for improved image interpretation because the radiologist views the same anatomy in the same imaging planes and using the same sequences each time.

SIGNAL AND RESOLUTION (Table 1-1)

Signal is the amount of information on an image. Other factors are important, but if the image is signal-poor (ie, "noisy"), even the best radiologist would be unable to interpret it (Fig. 1-2).

Each image is composed of *voxels* (volume elements) that correspond to small portions of tissue within the patient. One dimension of the voxel is defined by the *slice thickness*. The other dimensions are determined by the *field of view* and *imaging matrix* (number of squares in the imaging grid) (Fig. 1-3). Because the signal is proportional to the number of protons resonating within each voxel, anything that increases the size of the voxel would increase the signal (Fig. 1-4). Increasing slice thickness or field of view or, alternatively, decreasing the matrix (spreading the imaging volume over fewer but larger boxes), would increase the signal.

Another factor that affects the signal is the number of *signal acquisitions* (also known as the number of *signal averages*). A signal average of 2 means that the signal arising from the protons in each voxel is collected twice, resulting

Table 1-1 SIGNAL AND RESOLUTION: LIFE'S TRADEOFFS

↑ Signal/↓ Resolution	↑ Resolution/↓ Signal
↑ Slice thickness	↓ Slice thickness
↑ Field of view	↓ Field of view
↓ Imaging matrix	↑ Imaging matrix

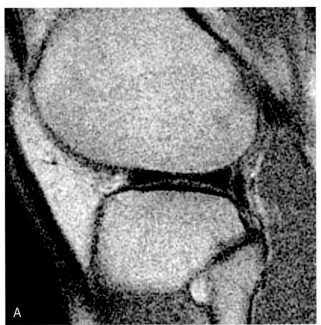

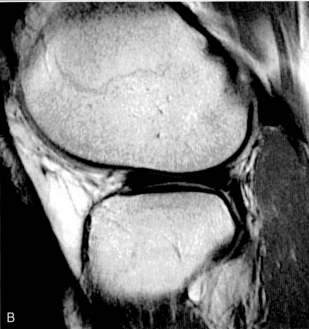

Figure 1-2 **Image noise and effect of surface coil. A,** FSE–proton density sagittal image of the knee. This image was obtained with the body coil. Note the marked image noise and poor delineation of anatomic structures. **B,** FSE–proton density sagittal image of the knee. The scanning parameters used for this image were identical to those used in **A,** but this was obtained with a dedicated knee coil. Note the markedly improved signal-to-noise ratio and depiction of the anatomic structures compared with **A.**

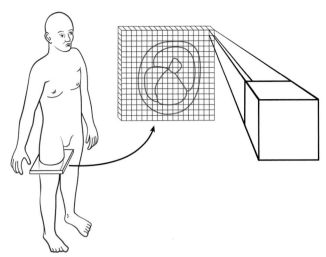

Figure 1-3 Imaging voxel. Schematic diagram illustrating the imaging matrix and an individual voxel from an axial MR image of the proximal thigh.

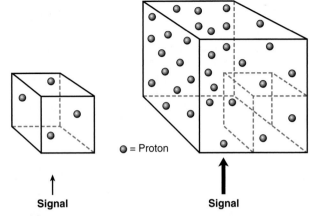

Figure 1-4 Voxel size versus signal. Signal is directly proportional to the number of protons within the voxel. Note the larger number of protons and the resulting increased signal in the larger imaging voxel.

in a doubling of the overall signal, but this also doubles the imaging time.

Finally, signal may be adversely affected if the slices are obtained too close together because of the phenomenon of "cross talk." When adjacent slices are acquired, some interference from one slice may spill over into the adjacent slice, resulting in increased noise. This is especially true for T2-weighted sequences. This effect is lessened by interposing a "gap" between the slices (a small portion of tissue that is not imaged), resulting in decreased noise and increased signal. Typical gaps range from 10% to 25% of the slice thickness. The larger the gap, the greater the amount of unimaged tissue, and the greater the possibility of missing a small lesion.

Now that we have discussed several ways to improve the signal of the image (also known as *increasing the signal-to-noise ratio*), we need to look at the second major factor that makes for a good image: *resolution*. Resolution is the ability to distinguish small objects. It is absolutely critical in most musculoskeletal applications.

As in life, there is no such thing as a free lunch in MRI, and any changes designed to improve resolution negatively affect the signal. Decreasing the size of the voxel (by decreasing slice thickness, decreasing the field of view, or increasing the imaging matrix) not only would improve resolution but also would decrease the number of protons in each voxel and decrease the signal. Consequently, when designing imaging protocols, there is always a compromise between (1) maximizing signal and (2) optimizing resolution. Another factor, (3) coil selection, can help to minimize this tradeoff.

The image in MR is created using the signal that returns from resonating protons within tissue. Just as it is easier to hear a speaker's voice the closer he or she is to you, the closer the receiver coil is to the tissues of interest, the better the signal and the lower the noise.

In MRI, every attempt should be made to use the smallest coil possible to produce the maximum signal. Coils that can be placed on or close to the body part of interest are called *surface coils* and result in markedly improved signal compared with the *body coil*. A factor that must be considered

when selecting a coil relates to its size. A coil must be able to detect signal from the entire length and depth of the tissues of interest; for a flat surface coil, the depth of penetration equals roughly half of the coil's diameter or width. Beyond this distance, the signal begins to drop off, as evidenced by decreasing signal in that region of the image (Fig. 1-5). To avoid this problem, so-called volume coils often are used in the extremities. These encircle the arm or leg, providing uniform signal throughout the tissues of interest. Most newer coils also are constructed with a phased array design. A phased array coil is composed of several smaller coils placed in a series, resulting in maximal signal from each small coil and from each segment of tissue covered by the coils. The use of a surface coil usually provides more than adequate signal and allows for the use of high-resolution imaging parameters.

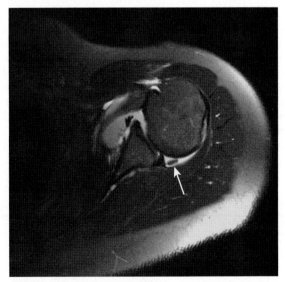

Figure 1-5 Coil size and signal drop-off. T1 axial image of the shoulder after intra-articular injection of a dilute Gd-DTPA solution. The use of a dedicated shoulder surface coil results in excellent signal in the region of interest; however, note the relatively rapid drop-off in signal intensity in the deeper tissues of the axilla and chest wall. (*Arrow* indicates loose body.)

TISSUE CONTRAST

Both computed tomography (CT) and MRI are capable of producing high-resolution scans, but the superior soft tissue contrast of MRI (the ability to differentiate different types of tissue based on their signal intensities) sets it apart. A CT image is based on the x-ray attenuation properties of tissues, whereas soft tissue contrast in MRI is related to differences in proton resonance within the tissues. The protons within fat resonate differently than the protons in fluid, and by changing the imaging parameters at the MRI console, differences in these tissue-specific properties can be emphasized. This is known as *weighting* the image. Tissues can be differentiated based on their signal intensities on various sequences. The signal intensity of a tissue on MRI should be described in relative terms (eg, hyperintense relative to muscle) because the gray scale values of the image are not assigned in a quantitative fashion as with CT but are scaled relative to the brightest voxel on the image.

Pulse Sequences (Tables 1-2 and 1-3)

The collection of specific imaging parameters selected for a single scan are called a *pulse sequence*. A typical musculoskeletal examination includes three to six sequences obtained in various anatomic planes. There are many different kinds of sequences and each has specific strengths and weaknesses. We do not want to get bogged down in technical details at this point; in the following discussion, typical imaging parameters for each pulse sequence are provided in parentheses. These are summarized in Table 1-3, and there is a glossary at the end of the chapter to help with understanding any unfamiliar terms.

Spin Echo. Conventional spin echo pulse sequences include T1-weighted (T1W), T2-weighted (T2W), and proton density–weighted sequences (Table 1-4).

T1. T1 (TR <800 msec; TE <30 msec) is considered a "short TR, short TE" sequence. Fat and subacute hemorrhage are bright on these images (Fig. 1-6). Proteinaceous fluid (as in an abscess or ganglion cyst) may be of intermediate or high signal intensity owing to the protein content. Most other soft tissues are of intermediate to low signal intensity on T1W images, and fluid is especially low (hypointense relative to muscle) (Fig. 1-7). T1W images are useful for delineating anatomic planes, marrow architecture, fat content within masses, and subacute hemorrhage. T1W sequences also are used to evaluate tissue enhancement after intravenous (IV)

Table 1-2 PULSE SEQUENCES: STRENGTHS AND WEAKNESSES

Sequence	Strength	Weakness
Spin Echo		
T1	Anatomic detail Fat, subacute hemorrhage Meniscal pathology Gd-DTPA enhancement (with fat saturation) Marrow pathology	Poor detection of soft tissue edema and other T2-sensitive pathology Not as sensitive as STIR or FSE-T2 with fat saturation for marrow pathology
Proton density	Anatomic detail Meniscal pathology	Poor detection of fluid and marrow pathology
T2	Detection of fluid and many pathologic processes	Long imaging times—as a result, no longer used
Fast Spin Echo		
Proton density T2	Anatomic detail T2 contrast obtained with shorter imaging times Excellent detection of marrow pathology when combined with fat saturation Good in patients with metal hardware (↓ susceptibility effects)	Potential blurring artifact can lead to missing meniscal tears Poor detection of marrow pathology when not combined with fat saturation
Gradient Echo		
T2*	Fibrocartilage (meniscus, labrum) Loose bodies and hemorrhage (↑ susceptibility effects) 3D imaging	Poor detection of marrow pathology at high field strengths Metallic hardware (↑↑ artifacts due to susceptibility effects)
STIR	Marrow and soft tissue pathology	Should not be used with Gd-DTPA

Gd-DTPA, gadolinium-DTPA; STIR, short tau inversion recovery.

administration of gadolinium-DTPA (Gd-DTPA) (see later in this chapter).

T2. T2 (TR >2000 msec; TE >60 msec) is considered a "long TR, long TE" sequence. Fluid is bright on T2W images (see Fig. 1-7). An easy way to remember this is that fluid (H_2O) is bright on T2W images. Likewise, most pathologic processes (eg, tumor, infection, injury) often are highlighted on

Table 1-3 PULSE SEQUENCES: IMAGING PARAMETERS (OR "HOW TO RECOGNIZE A SEQUENCE BY THE NUMBERS")

Sequence	TR (msec)	TE (msec)	TI (msec)	Flip Angle (°)	ETL
T1	≤1000	≤30	N/A	90	N/A
Proton density	≥1000	≤30	N/A	90	N/A
T2	≥2000	≥60	N/A	90	N/A
FSE T2	≥2000	≥60	N/A	90	2-16
GRE T1	Variable	≤30	N/A	70-110	N/A
GRE T2*	Variable	≤30	N/A	5-20	N/A
FSE STIR	≥2000	≥60	120-150	180→90	2-16

ETL, echo train length; FSE, fast spin echo; GRE, gradient echo; TE, echo time; TI, inversion time; TR, repetition time.

Table 1-4 TISSUE SIGNAL INTENSITY: T1 AND T2

	T1	T2
Fat	↑↑	↑
Subacute hemorrhage	↑↑	↑↑
Proteinaceous fluid	↑	↑↑
Fluid	↓	↑↑
Fibrous tissue/scar	↓	↓ or ↑
Cortical bone	↓↓	↓↓
Chronic hemorrhage/hemosiderin	↓↓	↓↓
Air	↓↓	↓↓

↑, brighter than muscle; ↓, darker than muscle.

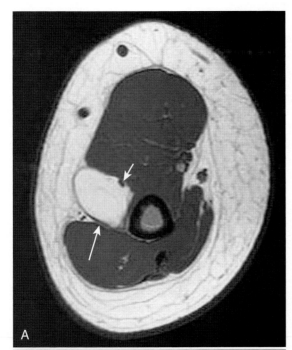

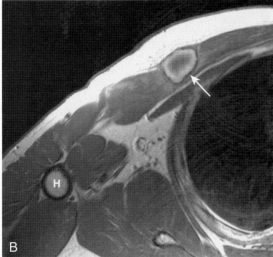

Figure 1-6 **T1-weighted images: high signal intensity tissues. A,** T1 axial image of the upper arm. Note the high signal intensity subcutaneous fat and intermuscular lipoma (*large arrow*) between the biceps and triceps muscles. The mass partially surrounds the radial nerve (*small arrow*). **B,** T1 axial image of the right axilla. There is a well-circumscribed mass within the right pectoralis major muscle in this 55-year-old man, who felt a "pop" while playing Frisbee golf. Note the high signal intensity rim along the periphery of this subacute hematoma (*arrow*). H, humerus.

T2W images because of their increased fluid content. Fat is less bright than on T1W images, and muscles remain of intermediate signal intensity. Conventional T2W spin echo sequences have been a part of most imaging protocols in the past but now are used much less frequently because of their relatively long imaging times.

Proton Density. Proton density (TR >1000 msec; TE <30 msec) is considered an "intermediate TR, short TE" sequence. Also known as *spin density,* these images represent a mixture of T1 and T2 weighting, with contrast being primarily a function of the number of protons within each tissue. This sequence also provides good anatomic detail but relatively little overall tissue contrast because of its intermediate weighting (see Fig. 1-7).

Fast Spin Echo. Fast spin echo (FSE; also known as *turbo spin echo*) allows for much more rapid acquisition of images than the conventional spin echo method. Several samples are acquired in the time one sample is obtained with a conventional spin echo technique (Fig. 1-8). The time saved is directly proportional to the number of samples (also designated as the *echo train length*). An FSE sequence with an echo train length of 4 would acquire the same amount of information as a conventional spin echo sequence in one fourth the time. Decreased overall imaging time lessens the potential for patient motion. Alternatively, the time saved can be used for obtaining additional signal averages to improve signal. FSE sequences commonly are used in musculoskeletal imaging.

This technique has some drawbacks. First, the signal intensity of fat remains quite bright on FSE-T2W images. Consequently, pathology in subcutaneous fat or marrow may be obscured on these images because of the similar signal intensity of fat and fluid (Fig. 1-9). This problem can be overcome by combining this technique with fat saturation (see later in this chapter).

Second, the FSE technique can result in blurring along tissue margins, especially when proton density–weighted images are acquired using long echo train lengths (>4). Although it is tempting to use a longer echo train length to decrease imaging time, the associated increase in blurring may result in missing some types of pathology, such as meniscal tears in the knee (Fig. 1-10).

Inversion Recovery. Historically known as *short tau inversion recovery* (STIR) imaging, inversion recovery (TR >2000 msec; TE >30 msec; TI = 120-150 msec) is a fat-saturation technique that results in markedly decreased signal intensity from fat and strikingly increased signal from fluid and edema (Fig. 1-11; see Fig. 1-10). As a result, inversion recovery is an extremely sensitive tool for detecting most types of soft tissue and marrow pathology. We use an FSE-STIR sequence with most of our musculoskeletal protocols. The FSE-STIR sequence does not suffer from the long imaging times, limited number of slices, and poor signal that plagued older, conventional STIR sequences. For the remainder of this book, when the term *STIR* is used, it refers to the FSE-STIR technique, unless otherwise indicated. On a practical note, FSE-STIR imaging is, in many respects, equivalent to an FSE-T2W sequence

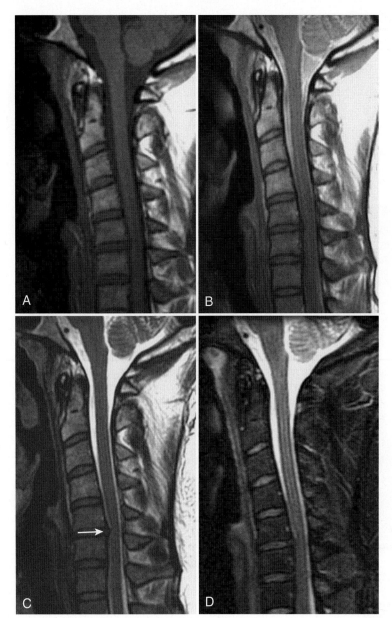

Figure 1-7   Fluid signal intensity. A, T1 sagittal image of the cervical spine. The cerebrospinal fluid shows lower signal intensity relative to the intervertebral disks. **B,** Proton density sagittal image of the cervical spine. The fluid is slightly hyperintense to disk. **C,** FSE-T2 sagittal image of the cervical spine. The signal intensity of the fluid is strikingly hyperintense to disk. Note also the disk protrusion deforming the cord at the C5-6 level (*arrow*). **D,** Sagittal STIR image of the cervical spine. The cerebrospinal fluid remains hyperintense relative to disk, but note the diffuse suppression of signal from fat.

with fat saturation, and many clinicians use these sequences interchangeably.

Gradient Echo. The gradient echo (TR variable; TE <30 msec; flip angle = 10-80 degrees) family of pulse sequences was originally developed to produce T2W images in less time than was possible with a conventional spin echo technique. As their names imply, gradient echo and spin echo pulse sequences acquire images in different ways. Consequently, although fluid appears bright on gradient echo T2W images (designated T2*W) and spin echo–T2W images, the appearance of other tissues differs on the two sequences. Ligaments and articular cartilage are particularly well shown with gradient echo sequences, as are fibrocartilaginous structures such as the knee menisci and glenoid labrum. Contrast between other soft tissues is relatively poor, however, on gradient echo images.

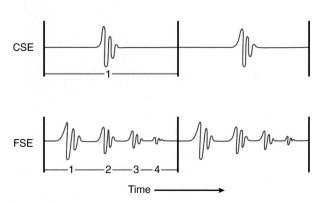

Figure 1-8   Conventional versus FSE pulse sequences. Diagram showing the efficiency of an FSE sequence in which four echoes are obtained within a single repetition time compared with one echo using a conventional spin echo (CSE) technique.

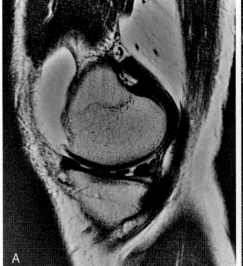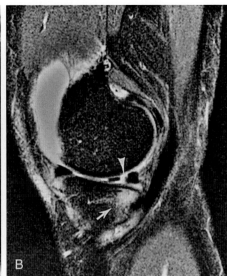

Figure 1-9 Pitfall of FSE imaging. **A,** FSE-T2 sagittal image of the knee. There is a bone contusion of the posterior medial tibial plateau. The contusion is difficult to detect because it is isointense with the relatively bright marrow fat. **B,** STIR sagittal image of the knee in the same patient. The contusion (*arrow*) is much more conspicuous against the dark, saturated fat. Note also the vertical tear in the posterior horn of the medial meniscus (*arrowhead*).

Gradient echo imaging can be performed using a two-dimensional technique (in which slices are obtained individually) or a three-dimensional (3D) "volume" technique. In 3D imaging, the signal from an entire volume of tissue is obtained at one time, and these data can be partitioned into extremely thin (<1 mm) slices such that the voxel dimensions are nearly isotropic (equal in all dimensions) (Fig. 1-12). This technique allows for high-resolution imaging and is especially useful when evaluating extremely small structures, such as ligaments in the wrist. These 3D sequences also provide the ability to create reformatted images in virtually any plane without a significant loss of resolution (Fig. 1-13). Although most 3D sequences require relatively long imaging times, if the reformatted images are of adequate quality, other sequences may be omitted from the protocol, minimizing this effect.

One feature of gradient echo sequences is a heightened sensitivity to *susceptibility effects.* This refers to artifactual signal loss at the interface between tissues of widely different magnetic properties, such as metal and soft tissue. This feature can be advantageous when searching for subtle areas of hemorrhage because these would be highlighted on gradient echo images owing to susceptibility effects of the hemoglobin breakdown products within the tissue (Fig. 1-14). Similarly, these sequences are useful for detecting loose bodies and soft tissue gas because of susceptibility effects.

Conversely, drawbacks of these susceptibility effects include overestimating the size of osteophytes in spine

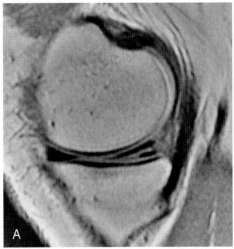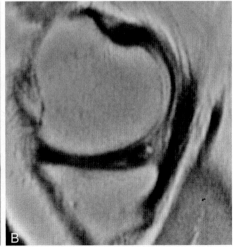

Figure 1-10 Blurring artifact, FSE sequence. **A,** Conventional spin echo–proton density sagittal image of the knee. An oblique tear in the posterior horn of the medial meniscus is well shown. **B,** FSE–proton density sagittal image of the knee (echo train length = 16). Note the decreased conspicuity of the meniscal tear and blurring of all tissue margins.

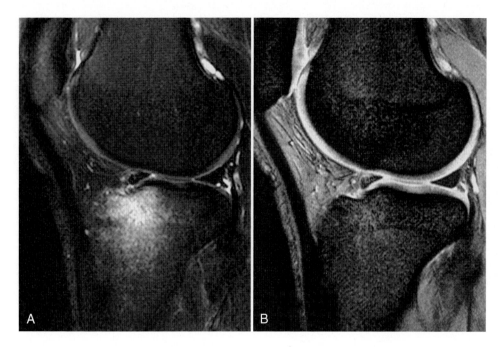

Figure 1-11 Fat-saturated T2 versus gradient echo sequences for marrow pathology. A, FSE-T2 sagittal image of the knee. There is a focal marrow contusion involving the anterior portion of the tibial plateau. Note the conspicuity of the contusion relative to the dark, suppressed marrow fat. **B,** Gradient echo T2* sagittal image of the knee. The contusion is much less apparent because of susceptibility effects of the trabecular bone in the tibial plateau.

imaging and missing marrow pathology when trabecular bone is not destroyed, because of susceptibility artifact at the interfaces between trabecular bone and marrow fat (see Fig. 1-11). Susceptibility effects also can be problematic when imaging patients with metallic hardware because of obscuring of adjacent normal tissue by the susceptibility artifacts. FSE sequences tend to minimize susceptibility artifacts and are useful when imaging patients with a history of prior surgery, especially if it is known that metallic hardware is present (Fig. 1-15).

Fat Saturation

There are certain clinical situations in which it is advantageous to suppress the high signal intensity of fat. Two main techniques are used to accomplish this: frequency-selective (chemical) fat saturation and STIR imaging.

Frequency-Selective. The frequency-selective technique exploits the differences in resonant frequencies between fat and water by applying a "spoiler" pulse at the frequency of fat. This pulse wipes out the signal from fat without affecting the signal from water. Likewise, the signal from Gd-DTPA (either IV or intra-articular) is preserved.

This technique can be used with T1W imaging to confirm the fatty nature of a mass (Fig. 1-16), to distinguish between fat and hemorrhage (both of which would be bright on non–fat-saturated T1W images), and to make tissue enhancement more conspicuous after the IV administration of Gd-DTPA contrast material (Fig. 1-17). Fat-saturated T1W images also are used with Gd-DTPA arthrography. FSE-T2W imaging often is combined with frequency-selective fat saturation to highlight areas of soft tissue and marrow pathology because the high signal intensity of fluid and edema is extremely conspicuous against the dark background of suppressed fat. A major problem with frequency-selective fat saturation is the potential for inhomogeneous suppression of fat signal. Because the technique is sensitive to mag-

netic field inhomogeneities and susceptibility effects, the fat saturation may be incomplete across an imaging volume; this may even result in inadvertent suppression of water signal in these areas. This suppression is especially common along curved surfaces, such as the shoulder and ankle, and may result in spurious signal intensity that mimics pathology. This problem often can be identified by noticing the lack of suppression of the overlying subcutaneous fat signal in these regions, but it can be difficult to recognize and may result in diagnostic errors (Fig. 1-18).

Frequency-selective fat saturation relies on adequate separation of the fat and water peaks, which occurs only at high field strengths (≥1.0T). Consequently, another drawback of this technique is that it is not available on mid and low field strength machines.

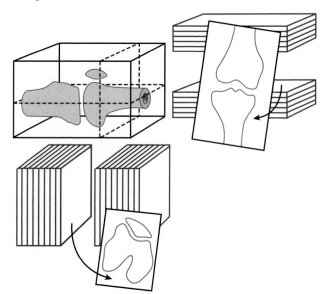

Figure 1-12 3D imaging. Diagram showing axial and coronal reconstructions from a single acquisition 3D volume sequence.

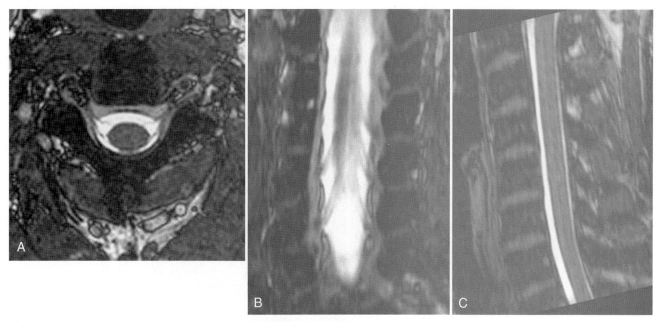

Figure 1-13   3D volume imaging. **A,** T2* gradient echo axial image of the cervical spine (obtained with a 3D technique). There is excellent contrast between the high signal intensity cerebrospinal fluid and low signal intensity spinal cord and exiting nerve roots. **B,** Coronal reformatted image of the cervical spine (from the axial dataset). The cord and nerve roots are well shown within the bright cerebrospinal fluid. **C,** Sagittal reformatted image of the cervical spine (from the axial dataset). The myelographic effect of the bright cerebrospinal fluid reveals no disk bulge or protrusion.

Inversion Recovery. The STIR technique also results in fat saturation, but it is based on the relaxation properties of fat protons, rather than their resonant frequency, as is the case with frequency-selective fat saturation. Many clinicians use a FSE-T2W sequence with fat saturation rather than STIR imaging, and although these appear similar in terms of image contrast, there are some differences because the two techniques are based on different mecha-nisms. First, the STIR technique tends to produce more homogeneous fat suppression because it is not as sensitive to field inhomogeneity as the frequency-selective technique. Second, a STIR sequence should not be used with IV or intra-articular Gd-DTPA because the contrast agent has similar relaxation properties to fat protons, and its signal intensity would be saturated along with fat on the STIR images.

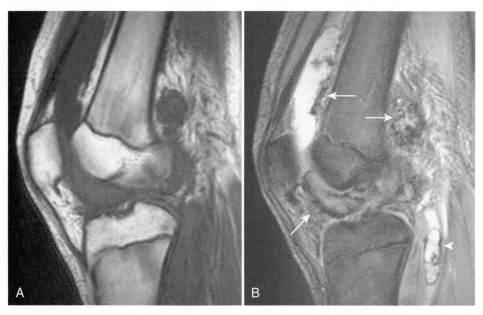

Figure 1-14   Gradient echo imaging: susceptibility effect. **A,** T1 sagittal image of the knee. There is a large joint effusion showing intermediate signal intensity. **B,** T2* gradient echo sagittal image of the knee. Note the extensive low signal intensity foci throughout the joint (*arrows*) and Baker's cyst (*arrowhead*), which are related to the susceptibility artifacts arising from the hemosiderin within these areas of pigmented villonodular synovitis.

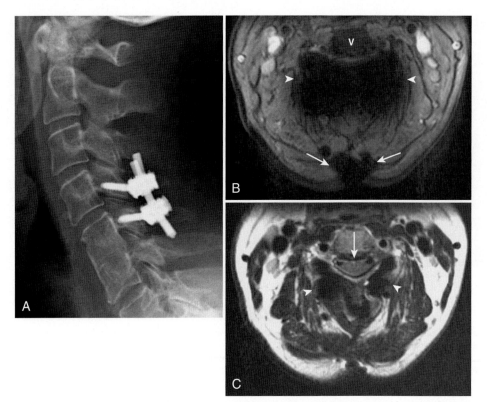

Figure 1-15   **FSE imaging: decreased susceptibility artifacts. A,** Lateral radiograph of the cervical spine. Posterior hardware is present from a prior cervical fusion. **B,** Prominent susceptibility artifact from the hardware obscures adjacent structures, including the spinal canal and cord (*arrowheads*). Additional artifact related to other postoperative changes is evident in the more superficial tissues (*arrows*). V, vertebral body. **C,** FSE-T2 axial image of the cervical spine (same level as in **B**). Note the decreased artifact related to the metal hardware (*arrowheads*) and the improved depiction of the spinal canal and contents (*arrow*).

Gadolinium (Box 1-1)

Gd-DTPA is a paramagnetic compound that shows increased signal intensity on T1W images. It has two major routes of administration: IV and intra-articular. Intra-articular use of Gd-DTPA in MR arthrography is discussed in the next section. IV Gd-DTPA should be used only for certain indications, especially in light of more recent reports of an apparent link between Gd-DTPA agents and a rare, but potentially devastating, condition, nephrogenic systemic fibrosis. This condition is most commonly seen in patients with poor renal function.[6]

When administered via IV, Gd-DTPA is analogous to iodinated radiographic contrast agents and results in enhancement proportional to soft tissue vascularity. Contrast enhancement is best evaluated on T1W–fat saturated images. By administering Gd-DTPA *and* applying fat saturation, however, two variables affecting tissue contrast have been changed, and care must be taken to avoid diagnostic errors. When pre–Gd-DTPA T1W images are obtained *without* fat saturation, a hematoma may show apparent enhancement on T1W–fat saturated, postcontrast images, not because of true tissue enhancement, but because the subacute blood products within the hematoma may *appear* brighter because of the suppression of adjacent fat.

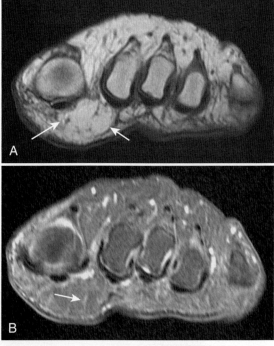

Figure 1-16   **Frequency-selective fat saturation. A,** T1 short-axis image of the forefoot. There is an irregular lipoma within the plantar fat at the level of the first and second metatarsophalangeal joints (*arrows*). **B,** T1 short-axis image with fat saturation of the forefoot, after IV injection of Gd-DTPA. There is complete suppression of the signal arising from this mass, with the exception of a thin intralesional septum (*arrow*), confirming its lipomatous nature.

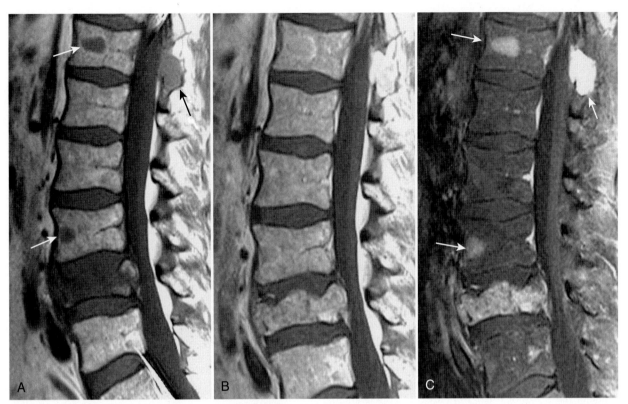

Figure 1-17 **Frequency-selective fat saturation and Gd-DTPA enhancement. A,** T1 sagittal image of the lumbar spine. A pathologic burst fracture of the L4 vertebra is evident in this patient with myeloma. Note the low signal edema or tumor, or both, within the fractured vertebra and the other neoplastic foci at the T12 and L3 levels (*arrows*). **B,** T1 sagittal image of the lumbar spine, with IV contrast. Note the diffuse enhancement of the fractured vertebra and metastatic foci that are now hard to distinguish from adjacent marrow. **C,** T1 sagittal image of the lumbar spine, with IV contrast and fat suppression. There is strikingly increased conspicuity of the enhancing metastatic foci (*arrows*) and fractured vertebra when the fat is suppressed.

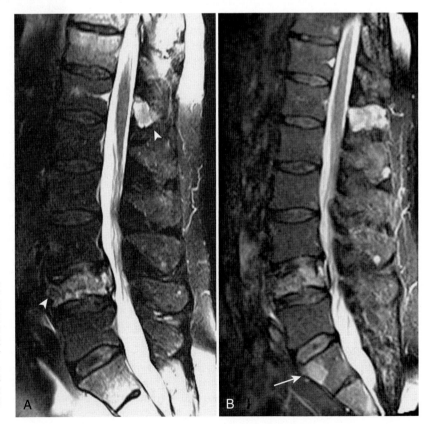

Figure 1-18 **Pitfall: heterogeneous fat saturation.** **A,** FSE-T2 sagittal image with fat saturation of the lumbar spine (same patient as in Fig. 1-17). The high signal intensity within the pathologic burst fracture at L4 and the myelomatous focus in the spinous process of T12 (*arrowheads*) are well shown against the suppressed fat in those regions. Tissues at the superior and inferior margins of the image are not well evaluated, however, owing to poor fat saturation in these regions. **B,** STIR sagittal image of the lumbar spine. An additional lesion is detected at S1 as a result of the improved fat saturation obtained with this technique (*arrow*).

IV Gd-DTPA is not administered for most musculoskeletal MRI examinations, but it is indicated in certain situations, as follows.

Cystic Versus Solid. Gd-DTPA is useful for distinguishing cystic lesions from cystic-appearing solid masses. A true cyst shows thin peripheral enhancement without enhancement of the cyst fluid centrally (Fig. 1-19). A solid mass shows diffuse enhancement or at least large areas of enhancement.

Tumor. We do not use Gd-DTPA routinely in the evaluation of soft tissue or osseous tumors, with the exception of differentiating cystic from solid lesions. Gd-DTPA can be helpful in directing a biopsy by differentiating enhancing, viable tumor tissue from areas of nonenhancing necrosis.

Infection. In cases of soft tissue infection, Gd-DTPA enhancement can assist in differentiating soft tissue edema or phlegmon from a focal abscess, which can be difficult on T2W or STIR images alone. An abscess shows a thick enhancing wall and lack of central enhancement. Similarly, small sinus tracts are detected more easily on enhanced images. Marrow enhancement is a nonspecific finding because it can result from osteomyelitis and areas of noninfected, reactive marrow edema with hyperemia.

Spine. Gd-DTPA is useful in a postoperative patient for differentiating enhancing scar tissue from nonenhancing disk material. Gd-DTPA also is helpful for evaluating cord lesions (eg, tumor, demyelinating disease) and intradural/extramedullary lesions (eg, metastases, nerve sheath tumors).

MR Arthrography

Distention of a joint with a solution containing dilute Gd-DTPA is extremely useful for detecting certain types of pathology, such as labral tears in the shoulder and hip. MR arthrography of the knee also is useful in patients with a history of prior surgery because it allows for differentiating between a meniscal tear (contrast extends into the tear) and scar within a healed meniscal tear.

We mix 10 mL of sterile saline with 3 mL of iodinated radiographic contrast agent to confirm the intra-articular needle position under fluoroscopy; to this mixture, we add 0.1 mL of Gd-DTPA immediately before joint puncture.

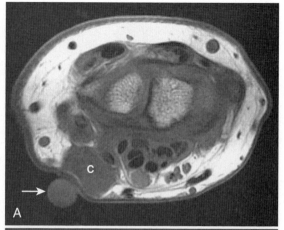

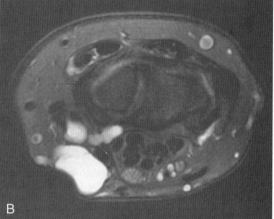

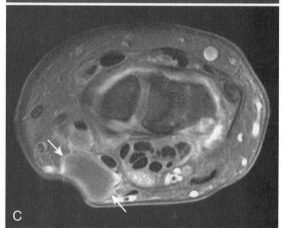

Figure 1-19   Gd-DTPA: cyst versus solid mass. A, T1 axial image of the wrist. There is a low signal intensity mass (C) along the radial aspect of the wrist (*arrow* indicates skin marker). **B,** Fat-saturated T2 coronal image of the wrist. The well-circumscribed mass shows homogeneous, bright signal intensity. **C,** T1 axial image of the wrist, after the administration of IV Gd-DTPA. The cystic nature of this ganglion is confirmed by its thin peripheral enhancement (*arrows*) and lack of enhancement centrally.

Only this small amount of Gd-DTPA is administered because if the Gd-DTPA is too concentrated, it will result in a loss of signal from the fluid.

T1W images are sufficient for arthrographic imaging, and fat saturation often is employed to distinguish Gd-DTPA from fat (eg, in the subacromial/subdeltoid bursa in the

Table 1-5 MUSCULOSKELETAL TISSUES: BEST SEQUENCES

Bone	STIR	Fast T2 with fat saturation	T1
Cartilage	STIR	Fast T2 with fat saturation	GRE (especially with fat saturation)
Meniscus	Spin echo proton density (± fat saturation)	GRE T2*	T1
Labrum	T1 after intra-articular Gd-DTPA injection	GRE T2*	
Tendons/ ligaments	Fast T2 (± fat saturation)	STIR	
Muscle	STIR	T1	

GRE, gradient echo; STIR, short tau inversion recovery.

shoulder). A T2W sequence in at least one plane also is necessary to detect edema, cysts, or other T2-sensitive abnormalities in the soft tissues or marrow.

Musculoskeletal Tissues

This section is a summary of the appearance of various musculoskeletal tissues on MRI and the sequences we have found most helpful in their evaluation (Table 1-5).

BONE

Normal Appearance

Cortical bone is black on all imaging sequences because protons within the mineralized matrix are unable to resonate and produce signal. Within the medullary cavity, fat and hematopoietic marrow are identified. Hematopoietic marrow is slightly hypointense to fat on T1W images and mildly hyperintense to muscle on all sequences (Fig. 1-20).

Most Useful Sequences

1. *STIR:* Extremely sensitive for detecting subtle marrow pathology
2. *FSE-T2 with fat saturation:* Sensitivity similar to STIR but may show heterogeneous fat suppression
3. *T1:* Good for detecting tumors and prominent marrow edema. It is not as sensitive as STIR for more subtle pathology, but it is very helpful for further characterizing abnormalities observed on STIR or FSE-T2 with fat saturation.
4. *Gradient echo T2*:* On mid and low field strength machines, some gradient echo sequences are useful for detecting marrow pathology. Also, when trabecular or cortical bone has been destroyed, this is a sensitive sequence for detecting lesions.

Pitfalls

1. Marrow pathology may be obscured on FSE-T2W images without fat suppression because of the similar

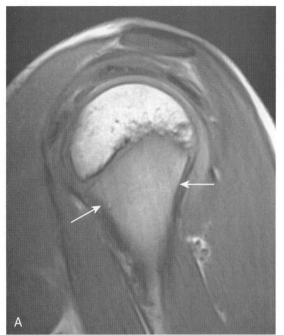

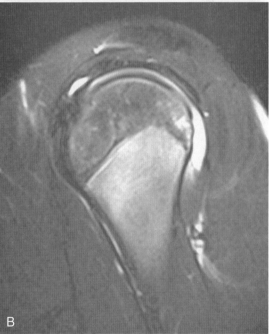

Figure 1-20 Normal marrow. A, T1 oblique-sagittal image of the proximal humerus. There is intermediate signal intensity within the proximal humeral shaft and metaphysis (*arrows*) that is slightly brighter than skeletal muscle. **B,** STIR sagittal image of the proximal humerus. The hematopoietic marrow is even more conspicuous because of its high signal intensity (related to its cellularity and fluid content) and suppression of the adjacent marrow fat.

high signal intensity of fat and pathologic lesions on these images.

2. Marrow pathology is easily missed on gradient echo images (on high field strength machines) because of the susceptibility effects of trabecular bone, as described earlier.

ARTICULAR CARTILAGE

Normal Appearance

The normal appearance of articular cartilage varies, depending on sequence.

Most Useful Sequences

1. *STIR or fat-saturated FSE-T2:* Cartilage is dark gray and easily distinguished from joint fluid, making focal defects quite conspicuous (Fig. 1-21). The cartilage is difficult to separate from underlying subchondral bone, but this distinction is less important than identifying abnormalities of the articular surface.
2. *3D–T1W gradient echo with fat saturation:* Cartilage is very bright and easily distinguished from subchondral bone and fluid. Because this sequence is quite time-consuming and must be added to the standard imaging sequences (in contrast to a STIR sequence), it is impractical for most uses.

FIBROCARTILAGE

Normal Appearance

Fibrocartilage normally appears dark on all sequences.

Useful Sequences: Meniscus

Meniscal tears are best shown with short TE sequences.
1. Spin echo proton density (with or without fat saturation)
2. Gradient echo T2*
3. T1

Pitfalls

1. Most tears are not well seen with long TE (T2W) images.
2. The inherent blurring artifact of FSE–proton density sequences obscures some meniscal tears.

Useful Sequences: Glenoid or Acetabular Labrum (Fig. 1-22)

1. T1W images after intra-articular Gd-DTPA injection (with or without fat suppression)
2. Gradient echo T2*

TENDONS AND LIGAMENTS

Normal Appearance

Tendons and ligaments are generally dark on all sequences, with the exception of the anterior cruciate ligament, which shows a striated appearance owing to the thickness and orientation of its collagen bundles. The quadriceps and triceps tendons normally have longitudinal striations as well. Some tendons, such as the posterior tibial, show increased signal near their insertions as a result of multiple osseous attachments.

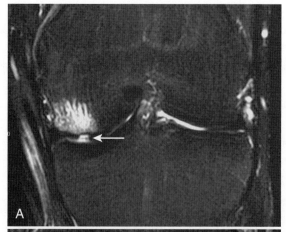

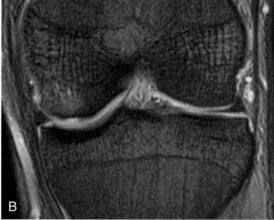

Figure 1-21   **Focal cartilage defect. A,** STIR coronal image of the knee. There is a small focal defect within the articular cartilage of the medial femoral condyle (*arrow*) with an adjacent subchondral contusion. Note the excellent contrast between the low signal intensity of the articular cartilage and the high signal joint fluid. **B,** T2* gradient echo sagittal image of the knee. The cartilage defect is difficult to identify because of the relative isointensity of joint fluid and articular cartilage.

Most Useful Sequences (Fig. 1-23)

1. STIR/FSE-T2 with or without fat saturation
2. Gradient echo T2* (thin section; 3D imaging useful for small ligaments)
3. T1

Pitfalls

Magic angle refers to spuriously increased signal intensity that may occur within any tissue containing highly structured collagen fibers (tendon, ligament, meniscus, labrum), depending on its position within the magnetic field (Fig. 1-24). This magic angle effect is due to the orientation of the collagen bundles and occurs when the structure lies at an angle near 55 degrees to the main magnetic field.[7] The resulting increased signal is seen on images obtained with a short TE (T1, proton density, and most gradient echo sequences), but disappears on long TE (T2W) images. This latter feature allows for differentiation from true tendon pathology. Other supportive signs include a lack of tendon enlargement or peritendinous edema.

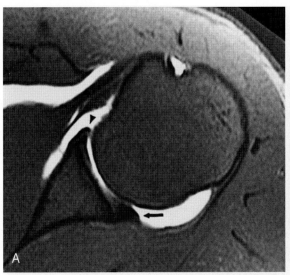

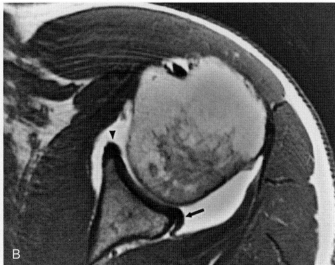

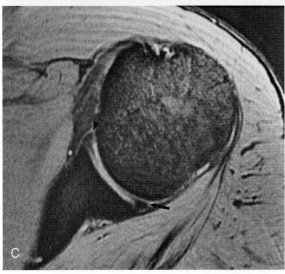

Figure 1-22 **Fibrocartilage: glenoid labrum. A,** T1 axial image, with fat suppression, of the left shoulder after intra-articular administration of dilute Gd-DTPA solution. The anterior labrum (*arrowhead*) and posterior labrum (*arrow*) are well shown, primarily owing to the excellent joint distention and contrast between the Gd-DTPA solution and low signal intensity labral tissue. Fibrocartilage is normally low signal on all pulse sequences. **B,** T1 axial image of the left shoulder after the intra-articular administration of dilute Gd-DTPA solution. There is better contrast between the low signal anterior labrum (*arrowhead*) and posterior labrum (*arrow*) underlying bone when fat suppression is not performed. **C,** T2* gradient echo axial image of the left shoulder. The low signal anterior labrum (*arrowhead*) and posterior labrum (*arrow*) are well shown, but the lack of joint distention limits labral/capsular evaluation overall.

MUSCLE

Normal Appearance

The normal appearance of muscle is intermediate signal intensity on all sequences.

Useful Sequences (Fig. 1-25)

1. *T1:* Good depiction of overall muscle architecture and of fatty atrophy of the muscle
2. *STIR:* Extremely sensitive for detecting most types of muscle pathology other than atrophy

SYNOVIUM

Normal Appearance

The synovium is not usually evident unless it is pathologically thickened.

Useful Sequences (Fig. 1-26)

1. T1W fat-saturated images after the administration of IV Gd-DTPA
2. T1W images without Gd-DTPA enhancement show synovial pannus as intermediate signal intensity tissue that is slightly higher in signal intensity than adjacent joint fluid or muscle. This slightly higher signal intensity can be detected with careful scrutiny of the images but is much less conspicuous than after Gd-DTPA enhancement.

Pitfalls

It usually is impossible to distinguish hypertrophied synovium from joint fluid on T2W and STIR images.

Applications

Because each anatomic site contains multiple different structures within the volume being imaged (eg, tendons, carti-

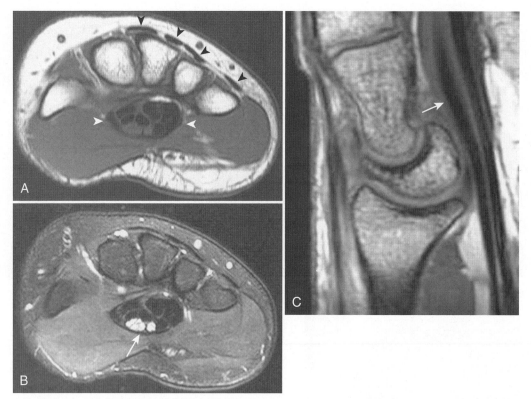

Figure 1-23 **Normal tendons. A,** T1 axial image of the wrist. The low signal flexor tendons are well shown within the carpal tunnel (*white arrowheads*), as are the extensor tendons along the dorsum of the wrist (*black arrowheads*). **B,** FSE-T2 axial image of the wrist. The flexor and extensor tendons remain low signal intensity. Note the high signal bifid median nerve within the carpal tunnel, a normal variant (*arrow*). **C,** Gradient echo T2* sagittal image of the wrist. The low signal intensity flexor tendons are well displayed in the carpal tunnel (*arrow*).

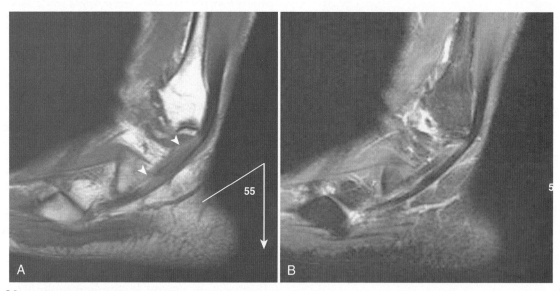

Figure 1-24 **Magic angle artifact. A,** Spin echo–T1 sagittal image of the ankle. There is intermediate signal intensity within the peroneus tendons (*arrowheads*) where they course near 55 degrees to the main magnetic field (*arrow* aligned with main magnetic field, B⁰). **B,** STIR sagittal image of the ankle. The intermediate signal intensity disappears, and the tendons display normal size and low signal intensity.

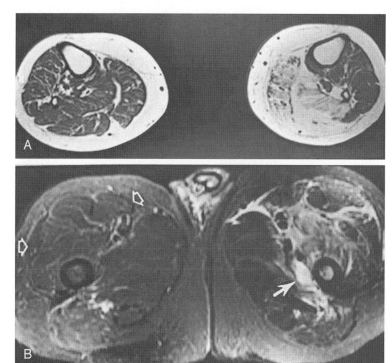

Figure 1-25 Muscle. **A,** T1 axial image of the proximal lower legs. There is extensive muscular atrophy in the left calf, as evidenced by high signal intensity fatty infiltration of the gastrocnemius and soleus muscles. Note the normal fatty septa distributed within the muscles of the right calf. **B,** STIR axial image of the proximal thighs. Note the normal low signal muscles in the anterior compartment of the right thigh (*short arrows*). There is extensive intramuscular and perifascial fluid within the proximal left thigh of this patient with necrotizing fasciitis. There also is a small abscess (*long arrow*) along the medial aspect of the femoral shaft.

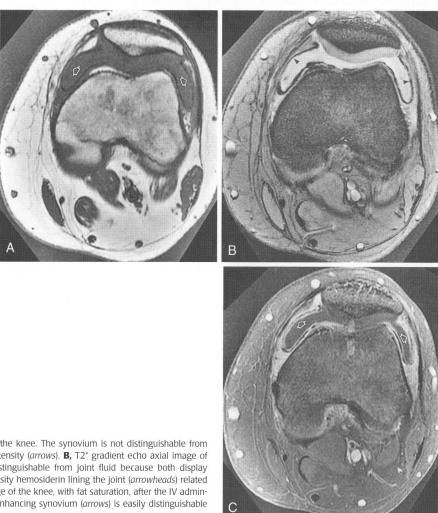

Figure 1-26 Synovium. **A,** T1 axial image of the knee. The synovium is not distinguishable from joint fluid because both are intermediate signal intensity (*arrows*). **B,** T2* gradient echo axial image of the knee (same patient). The synovium is not distinguishable from joint fluid because both display increased signal intensity. Note the low signal intensity hemosiderin lining the joint (*arrowheads*) related to the patient's known hemophilia. **C,** T1 axial image of the knee, with fat saturation, after the IV administration of Gd-DTPA (same patient). A thin rim of enhancing synovium (*arrows*) is easily distinguishable from the low signal intensity joint fluid.

lage, bone, muscle, spinal cord), it is necessary to use protocols that adequately show all of these varied structures. Pulse sequences and imaging planes must be selected carefully to show these structures optimally in a relatively short time. The clinical indications for obtaining an MRI examination further help to determine which pulse sequences and imaging planes should be selected. There is no added value in obtaining every pulse sequence or imaging plane known; it would not improve your ability to make a diagnosis compared with using tailored protocols. Clinicians also appreciate the use of standardized protocols because this consistency allows them to become familiar with the anatomy and pathology shown on the studies.

It is hoped that the basic information presented in this chapter regarding MRI as it relates to the musculoskeletal system will allow you to be street smart about MRI without being plagued by details of the physics (unless you want to be). It is our impression that name dropping various MRI terms in front of clinicians serves little to no useful purpose. Our orthopedists are not impressed if they hear us discussing flip angles, TRs, TEs, and signal intensity. They are much more pleased if we point to a white line traversing the black triangle of a meniscus and assure them that they will find a meniscal tear at arthroscopy.

The protocols presented in each subsequent chapter are based on our approach to musculoskeletal MRI. These work well for us, but we recognize that there is more than one way to perform any given MRI examination properly. Our protocols are meant to serve as a useful guide. Because of the different types of equipment available, we cannot specify all of the parameters, such as repetition times (TR) and echo times (TE). Instead, we have concentrated on the field of view, section thickness, imaging planes, and pulse sequences used for different indications. The precise TR, TE, number of signal averages, and matrix size would need to be optimized for the particular machine with which you work.

Remember, all scanners are *not* created equal. If you try to duplicate the results from an article written by investigators using one type of MRI scanner by using their protocol on a different brand of scanner, it probably will not work because each machine uses different methods to acquire and display the data. First, you need to work at understanding the fundamentals that go into producing a high-quality MR image, then work just as hard at understanding how this can be achieved with your particular machine.

REFERENCES

1. Weishaupt D, Koechli VD, Marincek B. *How does MRI work? An Introduction to the Physics and Function of Magnetic Resonance Imaging.* Berlin: Springer; 2006.
2. NessAvier M. *All You Really Need to Know About MRI Physics.* Baltimore: Simply Physics; 1997.
3. Elster AD. *Questions and Answers in Magnetic Resonance Imaging.* St. Louis: Mosby; 1994.
4. Jacobs MA, Ibrahim TS, Ouwerkerk R. MR imaging: brief overview and emerging applications. *RadioGraphics* 2007; 27:1213-1229.
5. Pooley RA. Fundamental physics of MR imaging. *RadioGraphics* 2005; 25:1087-1099.
6. Broome DR, Girquis MS, Baron PW, et al. Gadodiamide-associated nephrogenic systemic sclerosis: why radiologists should be concerned. *AJR Am J Roentgenol* 2007; 188:586-592.
7. Erickson SJ, Cox IH, Hyde JS, et al. Effect of tendon orientation on MR imaging signal intensity: a manifestation of the "magic angle" phenomenon. *Radiology* 1991; 183:389-392.

Glossary: Common Terms in Musculoskeletal MRI

Coil	Piece of hardware that can transmit or receive radiofrequency pulses during MRI. All scanners are equipped with a large body coil within the scanner itself. For most musculoskeletal applications, a surface coil is used. This is a smaller coil that can be placed on or around the body part of interest for improved imaging.
Cross talk	Phenomenon that occurs as a result of some "spillover" of radiofrequency excitation between adjacent tissue slices during MRI and results in increased image noise. This effect can be minimized by inserting small "gaps" of nonimaged tissue between adjacent slices.
Echo	Refers to the radiofrequency returning from tissues, which is used to create the final image. Various types of echoes (eg, spin echo, gradient echo) are produced, depending on which pulse sequence is used.
Echo train	Specialized rapid pulse sequences can produce a series of echoes, known as an *echo train,* in the same amount of time that conventional sequences produce a single echo. The reduction in imaging time is directly proportional to the length of the echo train (typically 2-16). See also *fast spin echo.*
Fast spin echo (FSE)	Family of pulse sequences that include RARE, fast spin echo (General Electric term), and turbo spin echo (Siemens/Phillips term). These pulse sequences produce images with contrast similar to conventional spin echo sequences, but in less time.
Fat saturation	Certain scanning techniques result in the suppression (reduction) of the signal intensity arising from fat. The two main techniques are inversion recovery imaging and frequency-selective fat suppression.
Field of view	Amount of tissue included on each cross-sectional image. Typically expressed in mm^2 or cm^2.
Gadolinium	Paramagnetic compound that forms the basis for most MR contrast agents. Its primary effect is to cause increased signal intensity on T1-weighted images within tissues (if administered intravenously) or within a joint (if administered intra-articularly after being diluted in saline).
Gap	Small slice of nonimaged tissue inserted between two adjacent imaging slices to reduce cross talk.
Gradient echo	Family of pulse sequences originally developed to produce T2-weighted images in less time than with the spin echo technique. Because of differences between these two types of sequences, gradient echo-T2W images are designated T2*W and are especially useful for imaging ligaments, fibrocartilage, and hyaline articular cartilage. They also are useful for identifying areas of hemorrhage, metal, bone, or air owing to heightened susceptibility effects.
Inversion recovery	Commonly known as STIR (short tau inversion recovery). This technique results in excellent fat suppression and high signal intensity from areas of fluid or edema; it is extremely sensitive for detecting many types of acute pathology.
Matrix	Grid of voxels that compose each MR image. Typical matrix values range from 128 × 128 to 512 × 512 (width × height).
Noise	The quality of an MR image is determined largely by two competing factors—signal and noise. Image noise refers to the background graininess that results from several factors, including the background electrical noise of the imaging system, the presence of the patient in the magnet, the imaging coil used, and other factors. For a given patient, the noise is constant, and maneuvers employed to improve the signal of the image result in an improved signal-to-noise ratio (SNR) and a better image.
Proton density sequence	Pulse sequence that is relatively balanced in terms of T1 and T2 weighting (TR <1000, TE >30). Tissue contrast on these images is based on the number of protons within each tissue, rather than their T1 or T2 relaxation properties. (Fat is relatively bright, whereas fluid is gray because of the higher number of protons per unit volume in the fat.)
Pulse sequence	Combination of imaging parameters that are selected at the MRI console to produce images of predictable tissue contrast. The most common families of pulse sequences include spin echo, FSE, gradient echo, and inversion recovery (STIR).
Resolution	Ability to distinguish between two objects. The better the resolution of an image, the easier it is to distinguish objects of increasingly smaller size. Generally, the smaller the voxels in an image, the better the resolution, but this also results in decreased image signal.
Signal average	Number of times each portion of tissue (voxel) is sampled to generate an MR image. Increasing the number of signal averages improves the signal-to-noise ratio of an image, but also prolongs imaging time proportionately.
Slice thickness	Thickness of the MR image. Although each image is projected two-dimensionally on a monitor or film, it represents a three-dimensional slice of tissue, typically ranging from 1 to 10 mm in depth. The smaller the slice thickness, the better the resolution.
Spin echo sequence	Family of pulse sequences that includes T1-weighted, proton density–weighted, and T2-weighted sequences.
STIR (short tau inversion recovery)	See *inversion recovery.*
Susceptibility	Degree to which a tissue distorts the magnetic field around it. Certain materials, such as surgical hardware, metal fragments, or the iron-containing hemoglobin found within areas of hemorrhage, have large susceptibilities and tend to create artifactual signal loss on MR images. Gradient echo pulse sequences accentuate these artifacts. FSE sequences tend to minimize them.
T1, T2	Inherent properties of tissue that define how a proton would react during MRI. Each tissue has unique T1 and T2 values. As a result, contrast between tissues on an MR image is based primarily on differences in T1 or T2 properties, depending on the imaging parameters selected (ie, T1 or T2 "weighting").
TE	Also known as *echo time,* a parameter selected at the imaging console that controls the T2 weighting of an image. A short TE minimizes T2 differences, whereas a long TE maximizes T2 weighting.
TR	Also known as *repetition time,* an imaging parameter selected at the console that controls the amount of T1 weighting in an image. A short TR maximizes T1 differences, whereas a long TR minimizes T1 weighting.
Turbo spin echo	See *fast spin echo.*
Voxel	Basic unit of the MR image, this represents a small portion of tissue within the patient that is sampled during the MR examination. The size of each voxel is determined by the field of view, imaging matrix, and slice thickness. Also known as *volume elements.*
Weighting	Refers to the contrast properties of a particular imaging sequence. This is determined by selecting specific scanning parameters at the console that emphasize contrast differences between tissues based on tissue-specific properties (eg, T1-weighted or T2-weighted images).

Marrow

2

How to Image Bone Marrow

Imaging of bone marrow has not changed much since the first edition of this book. Screening of marrow with T1 and fat-suppressed T2 images has helped to evaluate marrow processes. Where appropriate, references have been updated, and the text has been modified to include recent advances.

MRI of suspected bone marrow abnormalities should be directed to the site of clinical symptoms or to where abnormalities or confusing findings are present on bone scintigraphy or other imaging studies. The selection of coil, position of patient, planes of imaging, and field of view vary for each site. The parameters generally should be the same as those used for imaging the nearest joint.

When diffuse marrow disease is suspected, a marrow survey of the entire body or, more commonly, of the entire spine, pelvis, and proximal femora is performed. These areas are surveyed because they are where the bulk of hematopoietic marrow (and marrow pathology) exists. The following imaging parameters are for a marrow survey of the spine, pelvis, and proximal femora:

- *Coils and patient position:* For a marrow survey, the patient is supine in the magnet. Spine phased array coils are used for the spine, and the body coil is used for the pelvis and proximal femora.
- *Image orientation:* Sagittal images of the spine and coronal images of the pelvis and proximal femora are obtained.

- *Pulse sequences and regions of interest:* Large field-of-view sagittal T1W images of the cervical and upper thoracic spine and of the lower thoracic and entire lumbar spine are routine. We also use coronal T1W and STIR images of the pelvis and proximal femora. Section thickness in the spine is 4 mm and in the pelvis is 7 mm.
- *Contrast:* IV Gd-DTPA generally serves no useful purpose for routine diagnosis of marrow disorders. It may camouflage the lesions by giving them signal characteristics similar to fatty marrow on T1W images, unless fat suppression is used.

NORMAL MARROW ANATOMY AND FUNCTION (Box 2-1)

It is important to understand the function and distribution of normal marrow to be able to diagnose abnormalities and understand how best to image for marrow disease. In simplest terms, bone marrow consists of three components:

1. Trabecular bone
2. Red marrow
3. Yellow marrow

Red marrow is the hematopoietically active fraction of marrow that produces blood cells. Yellow marrow is hematopoietically inactive and composed mainly of fat cells, the purpose of which is uncertain. Red and yellow marrow elements are supported by a system composed of reticulum cells, nerves, and vascular sinusoids. The trabecular bone

Table 2-1 CHARACTERISTICS OF RED AND YELLOW MARROW

Red Marrow	Yellow Marrow
Rich vascular supply	Poor vascular supply
Reticulin stroma	Paucity of reticulin
Small fraction of fat cells	Small fraction of red marrow elements
Increases if demand for hematopoiesis increases (reconversion)	Increases with age

Table 2-2 PROGRESSION OF CONVERSION FROM RED TO YELLOW MARROW

Entire Skeleton (Extremities to Axial Skeleton)	Individual Long Bones (Peripheral to Central)
Hands/feet	Epiphyses/apophyses
↓	↓
Forearms/lower legs	Diaphysis
↓	↓
Humeri/femora	Distal metaphysis
↓	↓
Pelvis/spine	Proximal metaphysis

serves as a framework to support the red and yellow marrow elements.[1-3]

Trabecular Bone

Synonyms for trabecular bone include cancellous, spongy, and medullary bone. It is composed of primary and bridging secondary trabeculae that serve as architectural support and as a mineral depot. The number of trabeculae decreases with age.

Red Marrow (Table 2-1)

Synonyms for red marrow are cellular, active, myeloid, or hematopoietic marrow. Red marrow is composed of cellular elements that include erythrocytes (red blood cells), granulocytes (white blood cells), and thrombocytes (platelets), which are responsible for satisfying an individual's needs for oxygenation (erythrocytes), immunity (granulocytes), and coagulation (thrombocytes). Within islands of red marrow, there is a supporting stroma—the reticulin (or reticulum)—which includes two major groups of cells: phagocytes (or macrophages) and undifferentiated nonphagocytic cells. There is a rich sinusoidal vascular supply in red marrow.

Yellow Marrow

Synonyms for yellow marrow include fatty or inactive marrow. The theory for the purpose of fat cells in yellow

marrow is that they provide surface or nutritional support for red marrow elements. The vascular supply to yellow marrow is sparse.

For convenience, red and yellow marrow generally are discussed as if they are completely separate entities that exist in precise anatomic locations; however, this is not the case. Red marrow is not composed entirely of hematopoietic cells but always has a significant amount of fat cells scattered throughout the active cellular elements. Conversely, normal yellow marrow is never composed entirely of fat cells but always has some small amount of active cellular elements present. Red marrow is the portion of marrow where the largest concentrations of active cellular elements exist, and

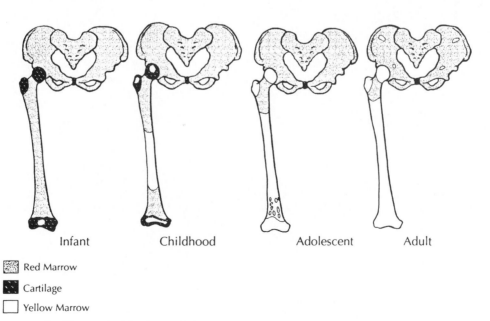

Infant   Childhood   Adolescent   Adult

▨ Red Marrow

▦ Cartilage

☐ Yellow Marrow

Figure 2-1 Marrow conversion. Diagram of axial and appendicular marrow distribution as a function of age, as red marrow progressively converts to yellow marrow.

Table 2-3   RATE OF CONVERSION FROM RED TO YELLOW MARROW

Age Group		Marrow Findings
Infants (<1 yr)	→	Diffuse red marrow except for ossified epiphyses and apophyses
Children (1-10 yr)	→	Yellow marrow below knees and elbows, and in diaphyses of femora and humeri
Adolescents (10-20 yr)	→	Progressive yellow marrow in distal and proximal metaphyses of proximal long bones
Adults (>25 yr)	→	Yellow marrow except in axial skeleton and proximal metaphyses of proximal long bones

BOX 2-2

Normal Variations in Red Marrow

- Amount and distribution vary from person to person but are symmetric in the same person
- Persistent curvilinear, subchondral red marrow in proximal epiphyses of humeri and femora
- Heterogeneous, focal islands of red marrow

yellow marrow is the portion of marrow where fat cells predominate. This composition of marrow elements accounts for the MRI appearance discussed later in this chapter. The fraction of yellow marrow increases with age as trabecular bone resorbs from osteoporosis, and fat fills in the spaces created.

Marrow Conversion (Table 2-2)

The amount and distribution of red and yellow marrow change with age.[4-10] This normal conversion from red to yellow marrow occurs in a predictable and progressive manner and is completed by an individual's middle 20s (Fig. 2-1). At birth, nearly the entire osseous skeleton is composed of red marrow. When epiphyses and apophyses ossify, they have red marrow within them only transiently, for a few weeks, before conversion to yellow marrow occurs. Conversion of the remainder of the skeleton occurs over the following 2 decades.

Conversion from red to yellow marrow proceeds from the extremities to the axial skeleton, occurring in the distal bones of the extremities (feet and hands) first, and progressing finally to the proximal bones (humeri and femora). This process occurs in a roughly symmetric manner on each side in an individual.

Progression of conversion from red to yellow marrow within an individual long bone occurs in the following sequence: epiphyses and apophyses first, then the diaphysis, followed by the distal metaphysis, and finally the proximal metaphysis. Conversion also occurs in a centripetal fashion within a bone, with fat predominating centrally, whereas red marrow predominates at the outer margins or periphery (subcortical region) of the medullary space of flat bones, long bones, and vertebral bodies.

The rate of conversion may vary from one individual to another, but generalities have been established that are important to know (Table 2-3). The reverse process of

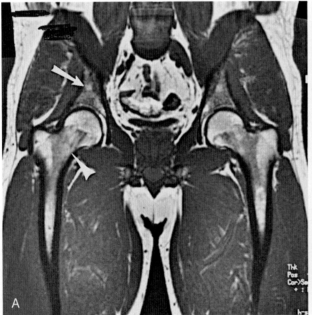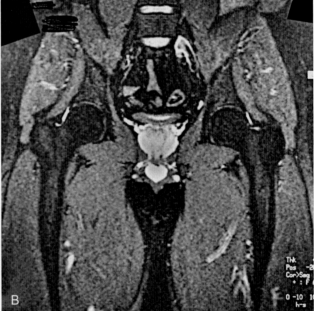

Figure 2-2   Normal red and yellow marrow. A, T1 coronal image of the pelvis and femora. Yellow marrow has signal identical to that of the high signal subcutaneous fat. It is present in apophyses, epiphyses, the femoral diaphyses, and focal regions in the pelvis (*arrow*). Red marrow is intermediate signal (higher signal than muscle) and located in the pelvis and proximal femoral metaphyses (*arrowhead*). Note the striking symmetry of the distribution of red and yellow marrow bilaterally. **B,** STIR coronal image of the pelvis and femora. Fatty marrow becomes black from fat suppression in this sequence. Red marrow is intermediate signal, similar in appearance to muscle; this is best seen in the pelvis.

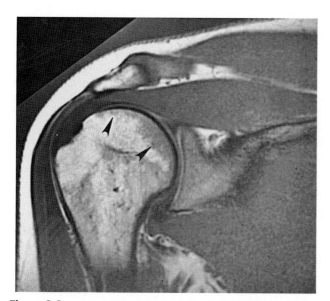

Figure 2-3 **Normal red marrow: variation in distribution.** T1 coronal oblique image of the shoulder. Intermediate signal normal red marrow is seen in the scapula and proximal humeral metaphysis, as expected. Curvilinear red marrow in the subchondral bone of the humeral head (*arrowheads*) is present. This can be seen as a normal variation in the humeral and femoral heads without disease being present.

conversion can occur, called *reconversion*. This is a process of yellow marrow being reconverted to red marrow when there is an increased demand for hematopoiesis. Reconversion affects marrow in the entire skeleton and in individual long bones in exactly the reverse sequence as conversion.

Variations in Normal Red Marrow (Box 2-2)

There are several normal variations in appearance of red marrow that are important to know so as not to misinterpret them as pathology. Variations in red marrow distribution may be confusing.

Some individuals have virtually no red marrow in the femora or humeri, whereas others have large amounts; most fall somewhere between these two extremes (Fig. 2-2). Small differences in the amount and distribution of red marrow from side to side are normal, but marked asymmetry is suspicious for a disease process.

An important and common exception to early and complete conversion in the epiphyses occurs in the proximal humeral and femoral epiphyses, where a small amount of red marrow may persist normally throughout life. This normal epiphyseal red marrow is curvilinear in configuration and located in the subchondral regions of these bones (Fig. 2-3).[11]

Variations in the red marrow pattern commonly are encountered and could be a source of error if not recognized as normal. Heterogeneous patterns of red and yellow marrow distribution occur with isolated islands of red marrow in predominately yellow marrow, or foci of yellow marrow in regions of predominately red marrow.[12] Foci of red marrow are often juxtacortical and located around the periphery of the marrow space (Fig. 2-4). Central foci of yellow marrow within islands of red marrow indicate a benign appearance. Focal islands of conversion to fatty marrow may be the result of chronic stress and biomechanical stimuli causing decreased vascularity at involved sites, which stimulates conversion.[13,14]

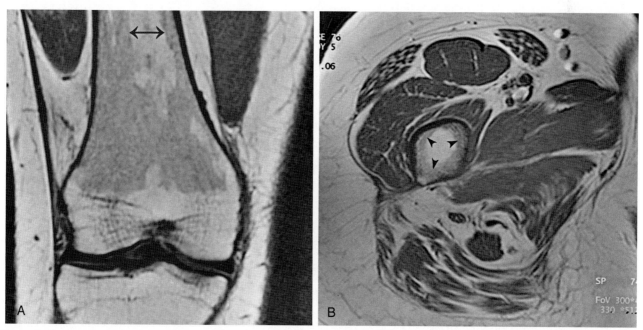

Figure 2-4 **Normal red marrow: variation in pattern. A,** T1 coronal image of the knee. Patchy foci of intermediate signal red marrow are located in the peripheral juxtacortical region of bone (*arrow*). **B,** T1 axial image of the thigh. *Arrowheads* point to the red marrow located around the periphery of the marrow space, just deep to the low signal cortical bone of the femur.

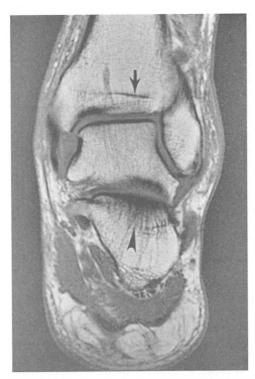

Figure 2-5 **Normal yellow marrow.** T1 coronal image of the ankle. In the distal extremities, high signal fatty marrow predominates. The yellow marrow is interrupted by low signal normal structures, including the physeal scar (*arrow*) where the growth plate closed, and stress trabeculae in the calcaneus (*arrowhead*). There also is a low signal bone island evident just above the distal tibial epiphyseal scar.

MRI OF NORMAL MARROW

The most important pulse sequence used to evaluate marrow is the T1W–spin echo sequence. T2W and STIR sequences commonly are used also.[1-3,15-17] Gd-DTPA has no apparent effect on normal adult yellow or red marrow; children's abundant red marrow may show mild enhancement. Red and yellow marrow should be distributed in predictable locations, based on age, as discussed earlier in the section on normal marrow anatomy.

Yellow Marrow

On T1W MR images, yellow marrow has signal characteristics similar to subcutaneous fat, with relatively high signal intensity. On T2W or STIR images, the signal intensity follows that of subcutaneous fat, being relatively intermediate signal intensity on T2W images and completely suppressed and showing low signal intensity on fat-suppressed images (see Fig. 2-2).

Fat signal in marrow is interrupted by groups of low signal intensity stress trabeculae. A thin, low signal intensity line where a physeal plate closed (the "physeal scar") often is evident (Fig. 2-5). Bone islands are oval, low signal intensity regions on all pulse sequences (Fig. 2-6).

Red Marrow

When red marrow exists in enough concentration, it is evident on T1W and T2W images as intermediate signal

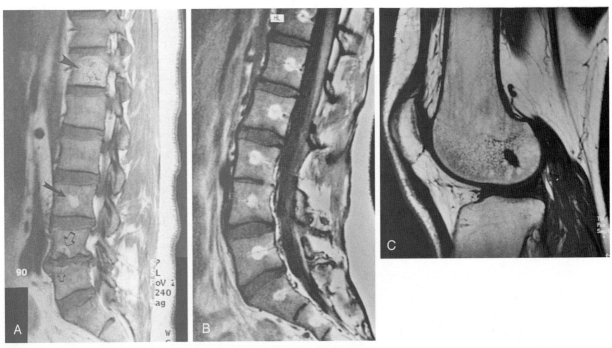

Figure 2-6 **Normal marrow heterogeneity: foci of fatty marrow. A,** T1 sagittal image of the lumbar spine. Overall, the marrow has intermediate signal (higher signal than intervertebral disks) from normal red marrow. In addition, several foci of high signal fat that are of no real clinical significance are evident. There is a large hemangioma in T12 (*arrowhead*) and a central focus of fat in L3 (*solid arrow*) from either focal marrow conversion or a small hemangioma; curvilinear fat surrounds a Schmorl's node in the inferior end plate of L4 (*large open arrow*), and linear fat along the superior end plate of L5 (*small open arrow*) is the result of adjacent degenerative disk disease. **B,** T1 sagittal image of the lumbar spine. Focal conversion to high signal fatty marrow in the center of each vertebral body at the level of the basivertebral vessels is present. **C,** T1 sagittal image of the knee. Numerous foci of high signal fatty marrow are scattered throughout the distal femoral metaphysis and epiphysis from disuse ("aggressive") osteoporosis. The oval, low signal structure in the epiphysis is a benign bone island (enostosis).

Focal Regions of Fatty Marrow of Minimal or No Significance

- Central venous channels, vertebral bodies
- Posterior elements, spine
- Vertebral bodies adjacent to degenerated disk
- Centrally in islands of red marrow ("bull's-eye")
- Healed lesion
- Hemangioma
- Disuse ("aggressive") osteoporosis

intensity (see Fig. 2-2). On T1W images, it would be lower in signal intensity than yellow marrow and easy to identify. Because yellow and red marrow show intermediate signal intensity on T2W images, they can be difficult to distinguish from each other on this sequence.

On STIR or fat-suppressed T2W images, red marrow shows intermediate signal intensity that is more hyperintense than yellow marrow and similar in appearance to muscle (see Fig. 2-2).

An important feature of normal red marrow is that it is always slightly higher in signal intensity than normal muscle or normal intervertebral disks on T1W images (see Figs. 2-2 and 2-6). It is never normal for marrow to have lower signal intensity than normal muscle or disk on the same T1W image. The reason red marrow is always slightly higher in signal intensity than muscle or disk on T1W images is because of the normal red marrow composition, where a significant number of fat cells are scattered throughout the red marrow elements, contributing to the higher signal intensity. When red marrow becomes equal or lower in signal intensity than normal disk or muscle on T1W images, pathology is almost certainly present.

Marrow Heterogeneity (Box 2-3)

Red and yellow marrow may be either homogeneous or focal in appearance. The focal marrow patterns sometimes are difficult to distinguish from pathology without careful analysis of the location and signal intensity involved. Focal islands of red marrow may have high signal intensity fat centers of a benign nature on T1W images from focal conversion, known as the *bull's-eye appearance.*[18] Focal islands of yellow marrow are common in the spine, especially in the posterior elements, around the central venous channels in the vertebral bodies, or adjacent to the end plates of vertebral bodies (see Fig. 2-6).[12]

Generally, identification of focal areas of fat within the marrow on MRI should never be a cause for concern. Focal regions of fat in marrow are common in normal marrow or may result from extremely common disease-related alterations, but they never result from anything of a serious nature (see Fig. 2-6). Chronic stresses and biomechanical stimuli cause a decrease in the vascularity to specific sites in marrow and stimulate conversion of red to yellow marrow, which probably accounts for many focal areas of conversion to fat. A classic example of this phenomenon occurs in the marrow adjacent to vertebral end plates that border on a

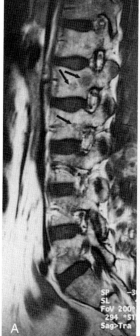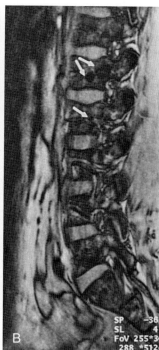

Figure 2-7 **Normal marrow heterogeneity: foci of red marrow. A,** T1 sagittal image of the lumbar spine. Foci of low signal in the vertebral bodies of L1 and L2 (*arrows*) were suspicious for metastases in this elderly woman with a history of breast and colon cancer. The suspicious areas are slightly higher signal than the disks; islands of red marrow should be strongly considered for the diagnosis. **B,** Out-of-phase gradient echo sagittal image of the lumbar spine. This special sequence determines if fat is present in the marrow lesions. Any lesion with fat cells remaining should be benign and low signal on this sequence (*arrows*). The larger lesion at L1 was biopsied and was normal red marrow.

degenerated disk. A bandlike focal alteration in marrow signal occurs as a result of the ischemia associated with the disk disease.

Focal areas of red marrow can be particularly difficult to distinguish from pathologic lesions, such as metastases. Articles have been published regarding the use of certain "designer" pulse sequences to try to determine if such lesions are red marrow or not (in-phase and out-of-phase gradient echo imaging and diffusion imaging).[19,20] The theory behind these sequences is that foci of red marrow have some fat intermixed, whereas neoplasm completely replaces normal marrow, including the fatty elements. On in-phase and out-of-phase gradient echo imaging, the signal contribution of fat and water cycle in and out of phase with respect to each other as the echo time increases. The signal generated from tissue that has fat in it differs from the signal generated from tissue without fat in it. Benign foci of red marrow (which has some fat cells in it) are low signal intensity on the out-of-phase images, whereas neoplasm should be high signal intensity compared with the in-phase images because of the lack of fat in the lesion (Fig. 2-7).[21]

MARROW PATHOLOGY

Abnormalities of bone marrow sometimes have a diagnostic appearance, but they often are nonspecific in their MRI fea-

Proliferative Marrow Disorders

Arise from existing marrow elements
Diffuse disease, usually; major exception: focal multiple myeloma

Benign

Myelofibrosis
Reconversion
Polycythemia vera
Mastocytosis
Myelodysplastic syndrome

Malignant

Leukemia
Multiple myeloma
Amyloidosis
Waldenström's macroglobulinemia

MRI

Normal signal and distribution (low tumor burden, higher signal than muscle or disk on T1)
Abnormal signal: Equal or lower than muscle on T1; variable on T2, usually some increased signal
Abnormal distribution: Replacement of yellow marrow
Abnormal signal and distribution

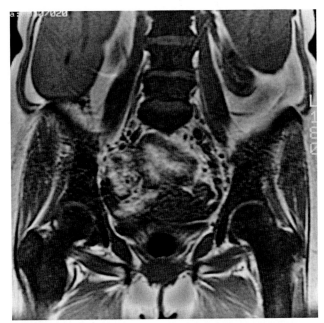

Figure 2-8   **Marrow proliferative disorders: mastocytosis.** T1 coronal image of the pelvis. The marrow, including the epiphyses and apophyses, is diffusely lower signal than disks and muscle. The spleen is enlarged. The marrow is abnormal in signal and distribution, which is typical of a marrow proliferative disorder. This patient has mastocytosis.

tures.[1-3,22] It is best to have an approach to the lesions and offer a reasonable differential diagnosis in the many instances where a specific diagnosis is impossible. Five broad categories of marrow disease can be used to facilitate an approach to evaluating the images and forming an appropriate differential diagnosis:

1. Marrow proliferative disorders
2. Marrow replacement disorders
3. Marrow depletion
4. Vascular abnormalities
5. Miscellaneous marrow diseases

Marrow Proliferative Disorders (Box 2-4)

Marrow proliferative disorders are considered as benign and malignant diseases that arise from proliferation of cells that normally exist in the marrow. These diseases should be distinguished from the closely related category of marrow replacement disorders, which consists of replacement of normal marrow by implantation of cells that do not arise from normally existing marrow elements.

Benign. Benign marrow proliferative abnormalities include myelodysplastic syndrome, polycythemia vera, myelofibrosis, mastocytosis, and reconversion from yellow to red marrow. Malignant conditions that arise from existing marrow elements are leukemias, multiple myeloma, primary amyloidosis, and Waldenström's macroglobulinemia. The general MRI appearance of these entities is discussed first, and specifics of some of the diseases are delineated later. Generally, marrow proliferative disorders involve the marrow in a diffuse manner rather than with focal lesions, except for the focal form of multiple myeloma.

MRI of marrow proliferative disorders can have several appearances. First, the normal appearance of marrow on MRI does not eliminate the possibility of a significant marrow disease being present. Proliferation of abnormal cells may be indistinguishable from normal red marrow early in the disease when the tumor burden is low because of the fact that not all fat cells have yet been replaced. This is the situation in about 10% to 20% of patients with multiple myeloma and leukemia, and it is important to understand this weakness of the imaging technique.

The major abnormalities we look for on MRI to indicate a marrow proliferative disease are listed:

1. Abnormal signal intensity
2. Abnormal distribution of what appears to be normal signal intensity red marrow
3. Both abnormal marrow distribution and signal intensity (Figs. 2-8 and 2-9)

Only if there is an abnormal distribution of what appears to be red marrow can the disease be diagnosed on MRI before the signal intensity becomes abnormal. Conversely, only if the signal intensity is abnormal compared with normal red marrow can the disease be diagnosed if there is a normal red marrow distribution. As abnormal numbers of cells continue to proliferate, fat cells in the marrow are replaced, and the signal intensity becomes equal to or lower than muscle or disk on T1W images. The cells appear in areas where red marrow should not exist for the age of the patient (distal femora or humeri, diaphyses of long bones, below the knee or elbow, in epiphyses or apophyses along the central venous channels in the vertebral body). Increased cellular elements generally lead to STIR or T2W images showing increased signal intensity relative to muscle.

A potential pitfall when imaging marrow abnormalities occurs when evaluating a FSE sequence without fat suppres-

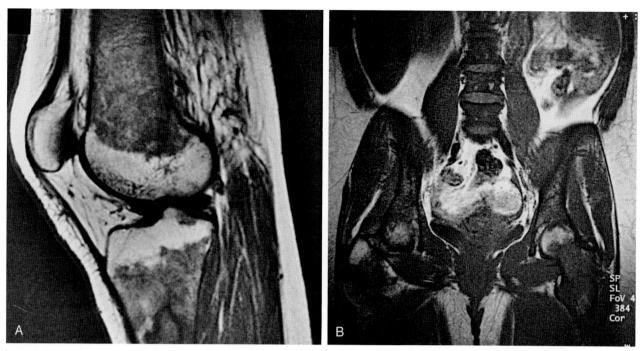

Figure 2-9 **Marrow proliferative disorders: reconversion due to sickle cell anemia. A,** T1 sagittal image of the knee. The red marrow in the distal femur and proximal tibia of this 27-year-old woman has normal signal that is higher than muscle, but the distribution is abnormal for her age. There also is a low signal serpiginous line in the tibial diametaphysis from osteonecrosis. **B,** T1 coronal image of the pelvis. The signal of the marrow in the spine is lower than disk, and in the femora and pelvis it is equal to or lower than muscle. These findings are from reconversion from yellow to red marrow in response to sickle cell anemia. The linear signal in the left femoral head is from osteonecrosis.

sion. The increased signal of the pathologic marrow-based process on fast spin echo sequence can blend into the background mixture hematopoietic marrow, allowing the process to be overlooked. This is due to the fact that on fast spin echo imaging, both fluid and fat can be of increased signal intensity. Careful evaluation of T1W images and fat-suppressed images should assist with this potential pitfall (Fig. 2-10).

Several of these diseases alter the appearance of the marrow for reasons other than proliferation of the abnormal cellular elements, and the MRI appearance may vary. When the cells proliferate, they replace normal marrow elements and cause induction of reconversion from yellow to red marrow to increase hematopoiesis; reconversion affects the appearance of marrow in ways indistinguishable from proliferation of cells from other benign or malignant causes. Also, some of

the marrow proliferative disorders, such as mastocytosis and myelofibrosis, stimulate fibrosis of the reticulin of the marrow, and sclerosis of adjacent trabecular bone occurs, which results in extremely low signal intensity on all pulse sequences. Finally, some patients have hemolysis (eg, sickle cell anemia and thalassemia) and develop hemosiderosis, which causes diffuse, very low signal intensity (black) in marrow from deposition of hemosiderin.

Reconversion of Yellow to Red Marrow (Box 2-5)**.** If existing red marrow cannot meet an individual's needs for hematopoiesis, hyperplasia of red marrow elements occurs in exactly the reverse sequence in which conversion from red to yellow marrow occurred during normal maturation (Fig. 2-11). Marrow reconversion starts in areas that are predominantly red marrow and progresses to areas that are predominantly

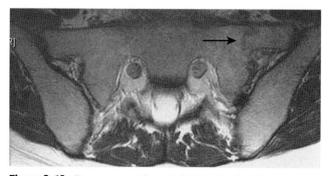

Figure 2-10 **Bone marrow edema.** Axial fast spin echo–T2W image. This image through the sacrum in a collegiate tennis player with back pain does not show obvious bone marrow edema. The fracture line is evident (*arrow*).

BOX 2-5

Reconversion of Yellow to Red Marrow

Increased Demand for Hematopoiesis
- Incidental finding, obese women
- Hemolytic anemias (sickle cell, thalassemia, sports)
- Increased oxygen requirements
  - High altitudes
  - High-level athletes
- Replacement/destruction of normal red marrow from marrow proliferative or replacement disorders
- Granulocyte colony-stimulating factor given as part of chemotherapy

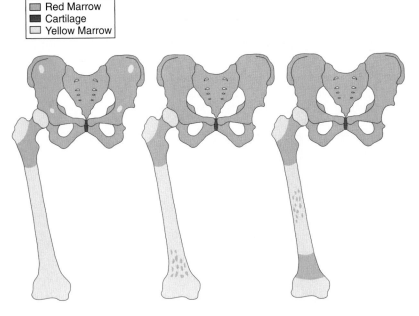

Red Marrow
Cartilage
Yellow Marrow

Figure 2-11 Marrow proliferative disorders: reconversion. Diagram of the response of the axial and appendicular skeleton to an increased demand for hematopoiesis, which leads to marrow reconversion from yellow to red marrow. This occurs in exactly the reverse order as normal conversion from red to yellow marrow. If severe enough, even the epiphyses undergo reconversion.

yellow marrow. Regarding the progression of changes in the entire skeleton, the axial skeleton undergoes red marrow hyperplasia earliest, followed by the peripheral (appendicular) skeleton. The humeri and femora are affected before the bones of the forearm and lower leg. In an individual long bone, marrow reconversion first affects the proximal metaphysis, followed by the distal metaphysis and then the diaphysis. If there is an extreme need to recruit red marrow in response to an increased demand for hematopoiesis, the epiphyses and apophyses of long bones convert to cellular red marrow.

MRI of marrow reconversion shows an abnormal distribution of marrow signal, with replacement of areas expected to be composed of yellow marrow by focal or diffuse areas of red marrow that have signal characteristics identical to normal red marrow (see Fig. 2-9). If red marrow hyperplasia is massive, the signal intensity is abnormal and isointense or even lower signal than muscle and disk on T1W images because of near-complete replacement of all fatty elements in the marrow.

An increased demand for hematopoiesis may exist in circumstances of replacement or destruction of normal red marrow by diffuse marrow proliferative disorders or marrow replacement disorders. It also may be seen in severe anemias, such as sickle cell anemia and thalassemia from hemolysis; in high-level athletes with increased oxygen requirements (marathon runners); in high altitudes; or as an incidental finding, usually in obese female smokers. Hematopoiesis also is stimulated by administration of human hematopoietic growth factors in patients being treated with high-dose chemotherapy.

Mild marrow reconversion as an incidental finding in women who are obese (and who are often smokers) is probably the most common cause of marrow reconversion seen on MRI. The proposed theory for this incidental marrow expansion is that these patients have a leukocytosis, possibly on the basis of chronic bronchitis, which may cause recruitment of myeloid elements in marrow. These women are of menstruating age, and this may contribute to the increased requirement for red marrow hyperplasia.

Sickle cell anemia results in an altered configuration of the red blood cells, preventing them from flowing through small vessels, which causes vascular obstruction and tissue infarction. The two MRI features of sickle cell anemia in the marrow are those of reconversion with red marrow hyperplasia and bone infarction (Box 2-6; see Fig. 2-9). Other severe anemias, such as thalassemia, cause identical changes as sickle cell anemia regarding marrow reconversion, but bone infarctions are not typical.

Monoclonal Gammopathies. Monoclonal gammopathies consist of a spectrum of diseases, categorized by severity. The *aggressive monoclonal gammopathies* are multiple myeloma, primary amyloidosis, Waldenström's macroglobulinemia, and lymphoproliferative disorder.

The *nonmyelomatous monoclonal gammopathies* (further divided into monoclonal gammopathy of undetermined significance and monoclonal gammopathy of borderline significance) are less aggressive marrow disorders. These two

---

BOX 2-6

Osteonecrosis Superimposed on Diffuse Marrow Abnormalities

- Sickle cell anemia
- Waldenström's macroglobulinemia
- Gaucher's disease
- Marrow proliferative or replacement disorders treated with steroids

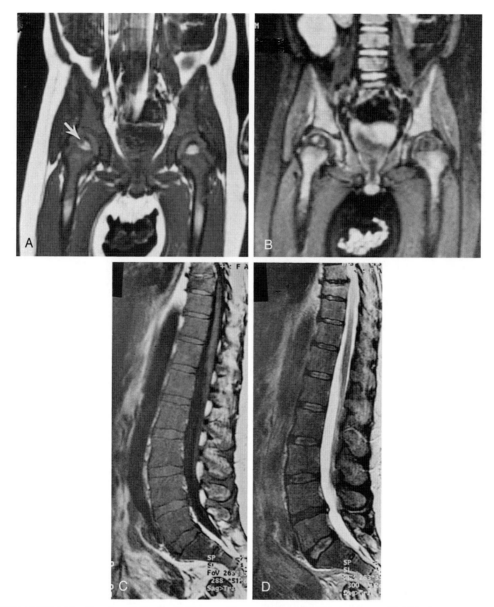

Figure 2-12 **Marrow proliferative disorders: leukemia. A,** T1 coronal image of the pelvis. This is a 2-year-old child who presented with a limp and had normal radiographs and an abnormal radionuclide bone scan at the right iliac wing above the acetabulum. MRI shows diffuse marrow signal that is equal to muscle, which is abnormal. In addition, there is an abnormal distribution with a focal round area of abnormal signal in the right femoral head (*arrow*), which should be entirely fat at this age. **B,** STIR coronal image of the pelvis. The marrow becomes significantly higher signal than muscle, which is abnormal. Abnormal signal in the soft tissues adjacent to the right iliac wing corresponds to the only abnormal focus on bone scan. The high signal between the legs is the dirty diaper (similar to almost everything else, a dirty diaper is low signal on T1 and high signal on T2). Biopsy of the iliac crest showed leukemia. **C,** T1 sagittal image of the lumbar spine (different patient). There is diffuse abnormal signal throughout the vertebral bodies that is slightly lower signal than adjacent intervertebral disks. There is a fracture at T9, which is why the patient presented with back pain. Marrow aspirate showed leukemia. **D,** Fast spin echo–T2 sagittal image of the lumbar spine (same patient as in **C**). There is no increased signal except in the fractured T9 vertebral body. This is the typical appearance of most leukemias on T2 types of sequence.

types of gammopathy constitute a large subgroup of asymptomatic patients who are discovered, usually incidentally, to have small amounts of monoclonal protein in their blood; they require no therapy. Within 10 years, 19% of these patients progress to an aggressive monoclonal gammopathy, however, which requires treatment. The current method to determine which patients progress to aggressive disease is by routine measurements of monoclonal protein in the urine and blood, and often by bone marrow aspirates as well. MRI has been shown to be a valuable adjunct in predicting which patients are likely to have disease progression, allowing for more appropriate management of patients. Patients who are likely to progress to an aggressive gammopathy have MRI abnormalities that consist of diffuse or focal marrow lesions in the spine or pelvis, similar to abnormalities seen in multiple myeloma.[23,24]

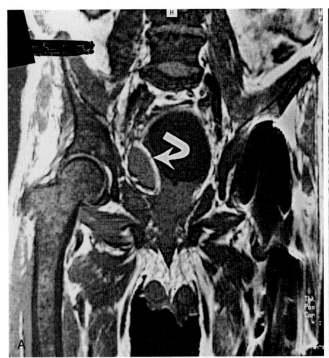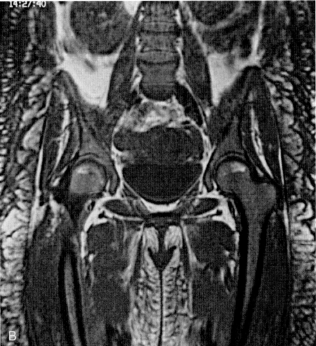

Figure 2-13 Marrow proliferative disorders: aggressive gammopathies. **A,** T1 coronal image of the pelvis. There is diffuse marrow signal and distribution abnormalities from Waldenström's macroglobulinemia. The marrow is equal to or lower in signal to muscle and disks, and involves the diaphysis of the femur and the epiphysis. There is a hematoma (*arrow*) adjacent to a fracture in the pubic ramus. **B,** T1 coronal image of the pelvis (different patient). This woman has primary amyloidosis. The marrow distribution is abnormal, with replacement of fatty marrow in the diaphyses of the femora and of the greater trochanters, and patchy replacement in the femoral heads. The signal of the marrow is normal, being slightly higher than muscle. There is diffuse subcutaneous edema.

Malignant

Leukemias. The proliferation of leukemic cells in bone marrow replaces normal red marrow elements, ultimately leading to anemia, neutropenia, and thrombocytopenia. Marrow aspiration or biopsy is required for definitive diagnosis.

MR images of marrow in patients with leukemia show focal or, much more commonly, diffuse abnormalities, usually in the metaphyses and diaphyses of bones. Infiltration of marrow by leukemic cells also may extend into the epiphyses and apophyses of patients with leukemia, which is an indication of a large tumor load. Abnormal signal intensity in epiphyses and apophyses also may represent red marrow hyperplasia occurring because of replacement of red marrow elsewhere by leukemic infiltrate. On T1W images, there is abnormal marrow signal intensity that is lower than muscle and disk; the signal intensity increases so that it is higher than fat on T2W images (or higher signal than muscle on STIR images) because of the high water content of leukemic cells (Fig. 2-12). The T2W findings vary; often, leukemic infiltrate has little increased signal intensity and may resemble an excessive amount of red marrow (see Fig. 2-12). Serial MRI has been shown to allow accurate monitoring of the disease for remission and relapse in children with acute lymphocytic leukemia.

Aggressive Gammopathies (Plasma Cell Dyscrasias). Multiple myeloma, amyloidosis, and Waldenström's macroglobulinemia are very closely related to one another and have essentially identical MRI appearances (Fig. 2-13). One difference that may be evident with Waldenström's macroglobulinemia is bone infarctions, which occur as a result of the hyperviscosity of the blood.

Multiple myeloma is a common disease of uncontrolled, malignant proliferation of plasma cells in the absence of an antigenic stimulus. Proliferation of plasma cells causes production of an osteoclastic stimulating factor and inhibition of osteoblastic activity, which leads to trabecular destruction and diffuse osteopenia. Radionuclide bone scans are often normal because of the lack of osteoblastic response in this disease. Laboratory findings are extremely important for making the diagnosis of myeloma, but they are not always present or conclusive, either initially or later in the disease. Bone biopsy or marrow aspiration is an important method of documenting the diagnosis. MRI is probably the most valuable imaging technique to establish the presence and precise location of abnormalities to guide a marrow biopsy because the process may be focal or diffuse, and blind marrow aspirates in the pelvis may not reflect the nature of the problem accurately. MRI may be useful in patients with a presumed solitary plasmacytoma[25]; more than one marrow lesion is seen on MRI in 25% of these patients, which may alter therapy.[23]

The marrow patterns of multiple myeloma on MRI, in increasing order of severity of disease, are listed:

1. Normal marrow pattern
2. Focal lesions (Fig. 2-14)
3. Variegated pattern (Fig. 2-15)
4. Diffuse homogeneous pattern (Fig. 2-16 and Box 2-7)[3,26]

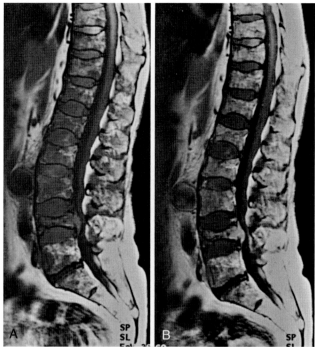

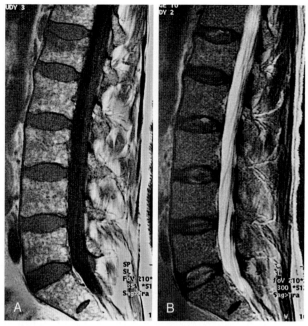

Figure 2-15 Marrow proliferative disorders: variegated pattern of myeloma. **A,** T1 sagittal image of the lumbar spine. There is a diffuse, stippled appearance to the marrow that looks like pepper has been sprinkled on fatty marrow. This is a more aggressive pattern of myeloma than focal lesions. There is a fracture of L1. **B,** Fast T2 sagittal image of the lumbar spine. The marrow appears normal on this sequence.

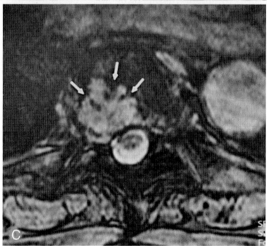

Figure 2-14 Marrow proliferative disorders: focal multiple myeloma. **A,** T1 sagittal image of the lumbar spine. There are multiple focal marrow lesions, indistinguishable from metastases. Many vertebral bodies are compressed as a result of the myeloma. There is an epidural mass posterior to the L4 vertebral body. **B,** T1 contrast-enhanced sagittal image of the lumbar spine. Many of the lesions show contrast enhancement, obscuring the lesions. If the patient has received therapy for the myeloma, this indicates a poor response. The epidural mass is easier to see because of the enhancement. **C,** T2* axial image of the spine (different patient). A focal lesion of multiple myeloma shows the "mini-brain" appearance that, when present, helps to distinguish myeloma from metastatic disease. Thick bone struts (*arrows*) are radiating into the lesion from its outer margin, creating the sulci and gyri pattern.

Focal lesions on MRI from myeloma may be equal to or lower in signal intensity than muscle or disk on T1W images; hemorrhage into a lesion occasionally results in high signal intensity in a focal lesion on T1W images. On T2W images, lesions may be either low or high signal intensity in approximately equal numbers in untreated patients. The findings are identical to the findings of metastatic disease, unless a pattern known as the *mini-brain* is present (see Fig. 2-14). The mini-brain appearance occurs in some focal myeloma lesions as thick bone struts radiating inward from the outer margins of a focal lesion, resembling the sulci and gyri pattern of the brain.[25]

The variegated pattern of myeloma has the appearance of many small, low signal intensity foci on T1W images, as if cracked black pepper were sprinkled on the marrow. There may be some mild, increased signal intensity on T2W images. This pattern is relatively specific for myeloma (see Fig. 2-15).

The diffuse pattern of myeloma is a homogeneous pattern of marrow replacement without features to distinguish it from many other marrow proliferative entities (see Fig. 2-16). There may be a mix of more than one of the four marrow patterns in a single patient with myeloma, as a result of the disease progressing or regressing.

A successful response to therapy can be inferred in patients with myeloma who initially have high signal intensity lesions on T2W images that become low signal intensity after treatment. Because 50% of myeloma lesions are low signal intensity on T2W images before treatment, this finding is of no significance, unless patients have had pretreatment and post-treatment scans. Because of this confusing picture, Gd-DTPA has been used after therapy to try to determine if there has been a successful response.

The preliminary work with Gd-DTPA after therapy for myeloma suggests it is useful for predicting therapeutic response and prognosis. Complete response to chemotherapy includes the following postcontrast enhancement patterns:

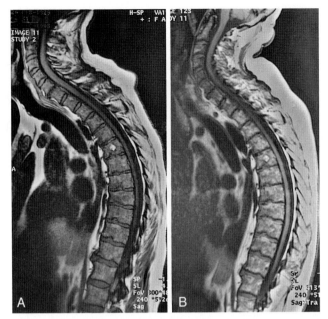

Figure 2-16 Marrow proliferative disorders: diffuse pattern of myeloma. A, T1 sagittal image of the cervical and upper thoracic spine. The marrow is diffusely and homogeneously intermediate signal, similar to the intervertebral disks. This is a 70-year-old man who should have much more fatty marrow present. **B,** T1 postcontrast sagittal image of the spine. There is heterogeneous marrow with many areas of contrast enhancement. Normal red marrow in adults does not show contrast enhancement. This patient has received therapy for myeloma, and the enhancement indicates a poor response.

1. Complete resolution of abnormality
2. Persistent abnormality with no enhancement
3. Peripheral rim enhancement only[26]

A partial response to chemotherapy showed conversion of a diffuse to a focal or variegated pattern with persistent contrast enhancement.

The Bottom Line. The benign and malignant proliferative disorders arising from existing marrow elements may have a variable appearance—focal or diffuse or both. All of the disorders have a similar appearance to one another, and cellular red marrow hyperplasia may look like benign or malignant cellular deposition. So, why do MRI?

MRI establishes that a disease is present, which is not always easy on a clinical or laboratory basis. Even if laboratory findings are abnormal, a marrow biopsy or aspirate often is required to establish the diagnosis. Blind marrow aspirates usually are performed for this purpose. Sampling error can be great, considering the variability in extent and location of disease as shown on MRI. A biopsy can be properly directed toward an abnormal site in the marrow based on MRI. Response of a disease to therapy can be monitored with serial MRI examinations.

Marrow Replacement Disorders (Box 2-8)

In contrast to marrow proliferative diseases, which usually are diffuse and arise from cells that originate in the bone marrow, the most common marrow replacement diseases usually are focal abnormalities that arise from cells other than those inherent in the bone marrow. Major marrow replacement disorders include metastatic disease, lymphoma, primary bone tumors, and osteomyelitis.

Skeletal Metastases. The typical MRI appearance of metastatic disease in the bone marrow is that of focal, often multiple lesions characterized by low signal intensity on T1W images that become higher signal intensity than surrounding marrow on T2W sequences (Fig. 2-17). Sclerotic metastases usually, but not always, show low signal intensity on all pulse sequences. Marrow and soft tissue edema surrounding a metastatic lesion may be extensive or nonexistent. Benign lesions, such as bone islands, Paget's disease, and hemangiomas, can have appearances similar to metastases, and evaluation of MRI studies should always be done by correlating with other imaging examinations to avoid errors. Although most metastatic lesions are focal, metastases also may show a diffuse pattern in the marrow that is either homogeneous or heterogeneous in appearance (Fig. 2-18).

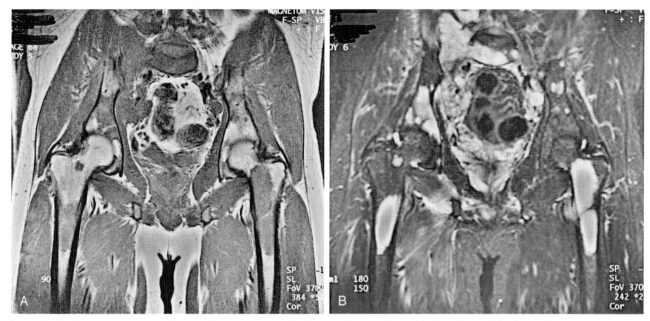

Figure 2-17 Marrow replacement disorders: focal metastases. **A,** T1 coronal image of the pelvis. This 32-year-old patient with adenocarcinoma of the urachus had pain in the posterior pelvis but a normal bone scan and radiographs. MRI shows multiple intermediate signal focal bone metastases involving the proximal femora and scattered throughout the pelvic bones and the sacrum. **B,** STIR coronal image of the pelvis. The metastatic lesions become very high signal on this sequence, which is typical of most metastases.

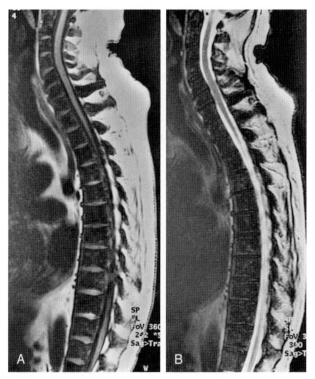

Figure 2-18 Marrow replacement disorders: diffuse metastases. **A,** T1 sagittal image of the cervical and upper thoracic spine. This is a patient with prostate cancer and diffuse skeletal metastases. The image gives an appearance identical to many marrow proliferative disorders. The metastases are sclerotic, which gives the very low signal on the MRI. **B,** Fast T2 sagittal image of the spine. The diffuse metastases remain low signal on the T2 sequence, which is typical of most sclerotic metastases.

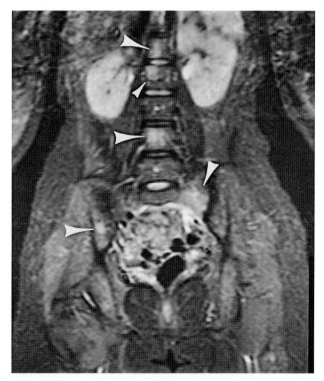

Figure 2-19 Marrow replacement disorders: screening for metastases. STIR coronal image of the spine and pelvis. This is part of an MRI marrow survey that covers the entire body from head to toe. Multiple high signal bone metastases (*arrowheads*) were discovered in this 41-year-old patient with breast cancer, whereas bone scintigraphy was negative.

MRI is exquisitely sensitive to detecting metastatic disease and surpasses all other imaging techniques in this regard. Screening MRI studies of the entire skeleton for metastases (see Fig. 2-18) may become the standard of practice in the future, but currently MRI generally is used as a problem-solving tool to clarify abnormalities of uncertain significance detected by other imaging.[25] Patients with bone pain or abnormal laboratory values may have metastases not evident on other studies, whereas MRI shows lesions (Fig. 2-19; see Fig. 2-17).[27-29]

MRI can show that lesions change in size with time. Monitoring the response of metastases to therapy may allow appropriate and early alteration of therapy (Box 2-9). A focal lesion surrounded by a halo of high signal intensity edema on T2W images (the T2 halo sign) indicates an active lesion (Fig. 2-20). A rim of high signal intensity yellow marrow surrounding a focal marrow lesion on T1W images (the T1 halo sign) is observed in treated lesions that have responded (see Fig. 2-20).[18] Complete fatty replacement of marrow where lesions previously existed can occur after treatment for metastases (Fig. 2-21).[30] MRI also is useful in showing the extent of a lesion in the bone and relative to other adjacent structures, such as the spinal cord (Fig. 2-22).

Areas of increased activity on a radionuclide bone scan in patients with a known primary carcinoma have been shown to be from benign causes in many instances.[31] The superior anatomic resolution of MRI compared with radionuclide

studies allows more specific diagnoses to be made. Many patients with cancer are older and osteoporotic. Chemotherapy (especially steroids) and radiation therapy contribute to osteoporosis. Insufficiency fractures, often multiple, are common in this group. Osteonecrosis from steroid therapy also is common. Bursitis, fasciitis, tendinopathy, and other soft tissue inflammatory changes can incite a hyperemic response in adjacent marrow that may be suspicious for metastases on a bone scan but is clearly from a benign process on MRI. The nonspecificity of bone scans has led us to require an MRI study before biopsy of bone lesions in patients who have normal conventional radiographs to establish that there is a lesion present that should be biopsied.

Osteoporotic Versus Pathologic Vertebral Compression Fracture (Table 2-4). Determining if an acute fracture of a vertebral body occurred on the basis of tumor from metastasis or from osteoporosis is a commonly encountered dilemma, especially in patients with a known primary tumor. Both entities would show a fractured vertebral body with replacement of normal marrow indicated by low signal intensity on T1W MRI. The low signal in the marrow represents either tumor or hemorrhage and edema from a nonpathologic fracture (Figs. 2-23 and 2-24). T2W features vary and are not helpful in making a distinction between benign and malignant. Features that suggest tumor are abnormal low signal intensity extending into the pedicles and other posterior spinal elements, involvement of the entire vertebral body by abnormal signal intensity, associated soft tissue mass, and multiple bone lesions. Features suggestive of an osteoporotic fracture are absence of the aforementioned features; abnormal signal does not involve the entire vertebral body but has a horizontal straight line or band separating the abnormal signal intensity from the normal fatty marrow signal (Fig. 2-25).[3,32,33] A linear horizontal fracture line from compressed trabeculae also has been proposed as a sign of benignancy because a vertebral body that collapses from tumor would not have a fracture line evident because the

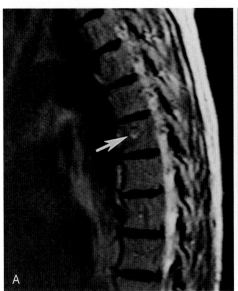
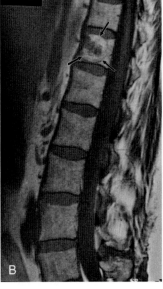

Figure 2-20 Marrow replacement disorders: the halo signs. A, Fast T2 sagittal image of the thoracic spine. There is a small lesion with surrounding edema (the T2 halo sign; *arrow*). This indicates active disease, and this proved to be metastatic lung cancer. **B,** T1 sagittal image of the lumbar spine (different patient). There is a low signal lesion in the T12 vertebral body surrounded by fat (*arrows*). This is the T1 halo sign, which indicates a positive response of a metastasis to therapy. The fatty rim is where tumor previously existed. This patient was undergoing treatment for metastatic carcinoid.

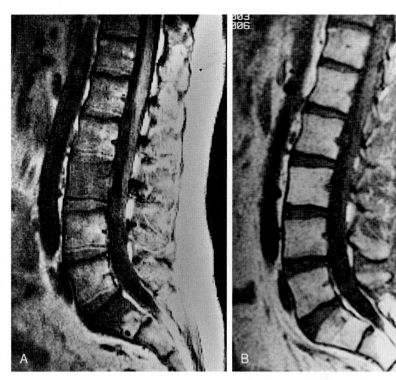

Figure 2-21 **Marrow replacement disorders: treated lesions replaced by fat. A,** T1 sagittal image of the lumbar spine. Several focal marrow replacement lesions are seen, most pronounced at L3 and S1, from Hodgkin's lymphoma. This MRI study was done before treatment. **B,** T1 sagittal image of the lumbar spine. Following therapy, all of the focal marrow lymphoma lesions have disappeared (as has the red marrow). Complete fatty replacement where the lesions previously existed indicates a positive response.

trabeculae are destroyed by tumor. The posterior vertebral body wall often has an angled, concave appearance from a benign fracture, whereas fractures related to metastases more often result in a bowed or convex posterior wall (see Fig. 2-25).

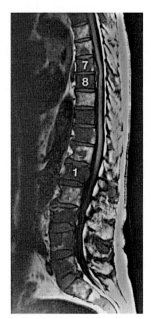

Figure 2-22 **Marrow replacement disorders.** T1 sagittal image of the thoracic and lumbar spine. MRI shows the presence of metastatic lesions in the spine of this woman with breast cancer. In addition, it shows the relationship of the lesions to adjacent structures. Epidural masses extend into the anterior epidural space posterior to T7 and T8 with compression of the spinal cord, and posterior to L1.

The signs that help differentiate tumor from osteoporotic compression fractures are interesting, and it is valuable to be aware of them. For an individual patient, however, the difference between having metastatic disease or not is of such importance that it is usually not adequate to depend on these signs to declare a patient tumor-free or not (see Figs. 2-23 and 2-24). In patients who are at risk for having metastatic disease, we recommend following the lesion with a limited MRI examination in about 8 weeks, or performing a biopsy to establish a definitive diagnosis. Osteoporotic fractures show partial or complete resolution of the marrow abnormalities on follow-up MRI, whereas tumors are unchanged or progress during the same interval.

Lymphoma. About 95% of lymphomas in bone are deposited in the marrow from circulating blood, which carried the cells from an extraskeletal primary site. MRI characteristics are indistinguishable from those of metastatic carcinoma. Generally, lymphoma affecting bone has low signal intensity

Table 2-4 OSTEOPOROTIC VERSUS PATHOLOGIC VERTEBRAL FRACTURES

Osteoporotic	Pathologic
Abnormal signal limited to vertebral body	Abnormal signal in pedicles, other posterior elements
Usually no soft tissue hematoma/mass	Associated soft tissue mass
Some fatty marrow persists in vertebral body	Entire vertebral body involved
Usually solitary	
Concave posterior wall	Convex posterior wall
Fracture line	No fracture line

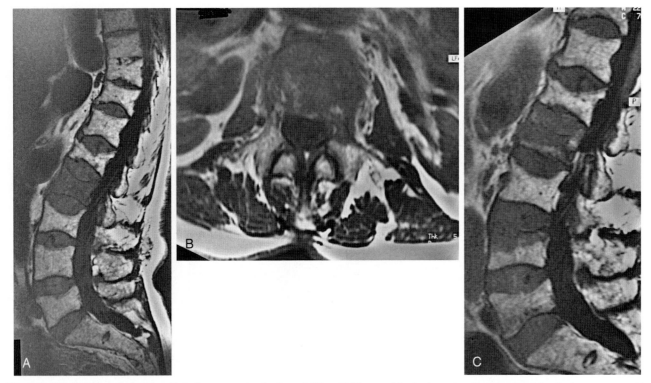

Figure 2-23 Osteoporotic versus pathologic compression fracture. **A,** T1 sagittal image of the lumbar spine. Several compression fractures are present in this woman with a history of primary malignancy. The L2 vertebral body is fractured and completely replaced by low signal, a feature suspicious for tumor. **B,** T1 axial image through L2. Abnormal signal extends from the vertebral body into the left pedicle, another sign suspicious for tumor as the basis for the fracture. **C,** T1 sagittal image of the lumbar spine. This follow-up MRI study was obtained 8 weeks after the study in **A** and **B**. The L2 vertebral body has collapsed a bit more in the interval, but there is partial regression of the low signal so that the inferior vertebral body shows linear high signal, paralleling the end plate. This could occur only with a benign fracture because untreated tumor would not regress spontaneously in this short interval. The L4 vertebral body has collapsed partially since the first study, and it has a straight line separation between fat marrow (below) and low signal marrow (above). This is a typical acute benign fracture.

on T1W and T2W images. Osseous dissemination of lymphoma is seen in 20% to 50% of patients with a primary extraskeletal lymphoma at postmortem examination. Blind marrow aspirates in patients with lymphoma show marrow involvement much less frequently. The focal nature of lymphoma accounts for this discrepancy, and biopsies directed to a specific lesion seen on MRI would allow more accurate staging and treatment of the disease to occur.

Benign and Malignant Primary Bone Tumors. Benign and malignant primary bone tumors are focal lesions of bone marrow. The precise nature of the lesions is best diagnosed by conventional radiographs. The extent of the tumor in the marrow and the relationship to adjacent structures can be determined best with MRI. Monitoring the response to therapy with MRI is valuable. This is a varied and large group of diseases, and this topic and osteomyelitis are marrow replacement diseases that are covered elsewhere.

Marrow Depletion (Box 2-10)

Diffuse or regional absence of normal red marrow may occur as a consequence of aplastic anemia, chemotherapy, and radiation therapy. We do not image to diagnose these entities. Rather, we often image patients who have had radiation therapy or chemotherapy to look for evidence of tumor. The typical reason to image patients with aplastic anemia is that they have pain from osteonecrosis secondary to the steroids they took as part of the treatment for their disease.

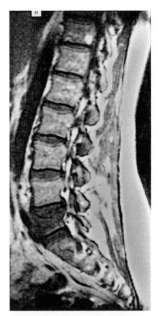

Figure 2-24 Osteoporotic versus pathologic compression fracture. T1 sagittal image of the lumbar spine. There is a straight line cutoff between low signal in the upper portion of the fractured L5 vertebral body and high signal fat in the lower portion, paralleling the end plate. This suggests a benign osteoporotic fracture. The angled posterior vertebral body wall fragments also suggest this fracture is benign. The vertebra was biopsied because of a history of breast cancer. This was metastatic disease. The point is to follow or biopsy these lesions in patients at risk because the rules for differentiating these lesions are not very good.

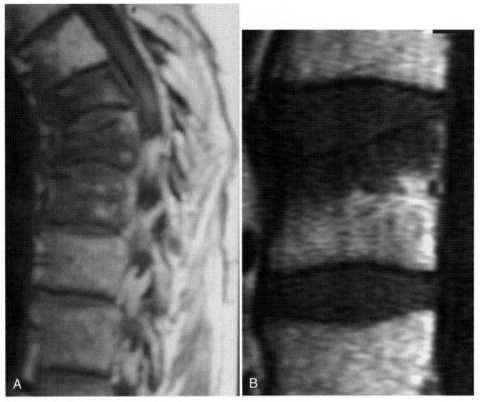

Figure 2-25   **Osteoporotic collapse. A,** Sagittal T1W image. This image through the thoracic spine shows areas of preservation of some normal marrow signal consistent with osteoporotic collapse. **B,** Sagittal T1W image. This image through the mid thoracic spine shows superior collapse as evidenced by a band of low signal intensity.

We must recognize the findings of marrow depletion and subsequent marrow regeneration so as not to misinterpret the findings.

Aplastic Anemia. Two marrow MRI patterns may be seen in patients with aplastic anemia.[34,35] One pattern is that of diffuse yellow marrow throughout the skeleton in areas where red marrow is expected to exist (Fig. 2-26A). This pattern may be difficult to recognize as abnormal in older individuals, who normally have large proportions of fatty marrow. The second pattern is seen in patients who have been treated for aplastic anemia and develop focal islands of red marrow regeneration scattered throughout the yellow marrow (see Fig. 2-26B). These islands of red marrow can be very focal in appearance and may simulate other diseases.

Chemotherapy. There may be no changes in the MRI study of some patients receiving chemotherapy. Other patients have diffuse ablation of the red marrow elements and an appearance identical to that of untreated aplastic anemia, with diffuse fatty marrow that has MRI signal characteristics that follow those of subcutaneous fat on all pulse sequences (Fig. 2-27).

An important caveat regarding chemotherapy is that some patients being treated for musculoskeletal malignancies (usually primary bone tumors) receive human hematopoietic growth factor (granulocyte or granulocyte-macrophage colony-stimulating factor) with their neoadjuvant chemotherapy regimen.[36] This growth factor is given to boost the patient's red marrow production and to prevent the negative sequelae of chemotherapy-induced myelosuppression, allowing earlier and more intense therapy to be administered. This iatrogenic red marrow stimulation appears as diffuse or patchy areas of low signal intensity on T1W images similar to muscle, and unchanged or slightly high signal intensity on T2W images, similar to normal red marrow in its signal intensity (Fig. 2-28). The changes in the marrow can be striking and rapid from this therapy (Box 2-11).

Radiation. Metastases and multiple myeloma often are treated with local radiation. Red marrow elements are pref-

---

BOX 2-10

Marrow Depletion

- Ablation of red marrow elements
- Diffuse or regional distribution
- Causes
  - Chemotherapy
  - Radiation therapy
  - Aplastic anemia
- MRI
  - T1: Diffuse or regional high signal, typical of fat
  - T2: Marrow signal follows fat (low signal on STIR or fat saturation, intermediate on T2, high on turbo T2 without fat saturation)

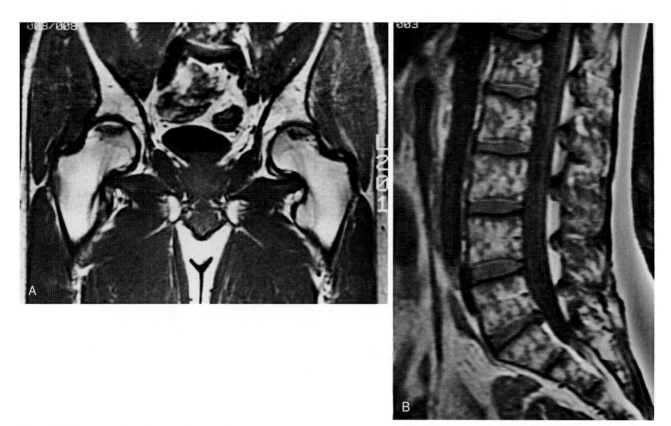

Figure 2-26 **Marrow depletion: aplastic anemia. A,** T1 coronal image of the pelvis. There is high signal fatty marrow throughout the pelvis and hips (with the exception of avascular necrosis in both femoral heads). The marrow normally should be more intermediate signal. This is from aplastic anemia. **B,** T1 sagittal image of the lumbar spine (same patient). There is diffuse heterogeneous marrow signal. The lumbar spine was biopsied and showed islands of regenerating red marrow in this patient, who was treated for aplastic anemia.

erentially destroyed compared with fatty marrow cells because of the greater sensitivity of the immature red marrow cells to radiation. The extent of ablation of red marrow and its ability to recover is dose-dependent. Changes in marrow signal intensity on MRI relate to the dose of radiation received and to the amount of time elapsed since treatment (Fig. 2-29).[37]

Patients who receive radiation to the spine usually show no marrow changes by MRI during the first 2 weeks after treatment. Most of the red marrow disappears 3 to 6 weeks post-treatment, and there is diffuse fatty marrow centrally in the vertebral body. A second pattern that may be seen is that of an increased heterogeneity of the marrow because of partial red marrow ablation. After 6 weeks, all patients have homogeneous high signal intensity fatty marrow on T1W images because of ablation of the red marrow elements. Within 1 year of cessation of radiation therapy that was less than 30 Gy (relatively low dose), red marrow regeneration occurs diffusely in the radiated marrow so that it looks normal, or there may be a peripheral distribution of red marrow in the margins of the vertebral body only (Fig. 2-30). This pattern must not be confused with tumor. Marrow that receives doses greater than 50 Gy never shows regeneration of red marrow. MRI shows diffuse fatty marrow in the region of the treatment portal with a straight line cutoff between normal cellular red marrow and abnormal fatty marrow at the margin of the radiation port (Fig. 2-31).

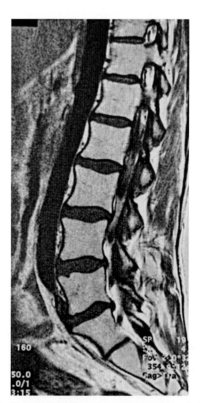

Figure 2-27 **Marrow depletion: chemotherapy.** T1 sagittal image of the lumbar spine. The marrow is diffusely high signal intensity from fat as a result of ablation of the red marrow elements from systemic chemotherapy.

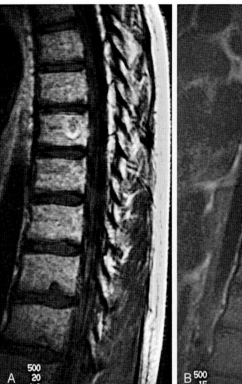
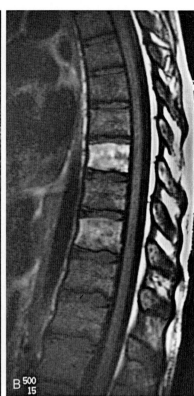

Figure 2-28 **Increased red marrow from hematopoietic growth factor chemotherapy. A,** T1 sagittal image of the thoracic spine. The marrow is generally a patchy intermediate signal intensity that is higher than in adjacent disks. There are no definite signs of metastases in this 16-year-old patient with a primitive neuroectodermal tumor. **B,** T1 sagittal image of the thoracic spine. The marrow has become diffusely intermediate signal and much lower signal than on the original MRI study done 9 months earlier (**A**). The diffuse intermediate signal is from red marrow stimulation that occurred from receiving granulocyte colony-stimulating factor. The high signal fatty marrow in the two vertebral bodies indicate there was tumor present at the time of the original MRI study that has been destroyed by the therapy.

Vascular Abnormalities (Hyperemia and Ischemia)

The underlying cause of extracellular bone marrow edema is probably hyperemia. Different clinical abnormalities may lead to localized bone marrow edema, including trauma (bone contusions, stress and insufficiency fractures), transient osteoporosis of the hip, regional migratory osteoporosis, reflex sympathetic dystrophy syndrome, osteonecrosis (early), infection, tumors, and joint abnormalities (cartilage abrasion in degenerative joint disease).

The MRI appearance of marrow edema is that of intermediate signal intensity on T1W images and very high signal intensity on T2W images. The signal characteristics are the result of fatty marrow cells intermixed with the edema fluid (Fig. 2-32). It has a heterogeneous appearance without a discrete pattern. Tumor and infection generally have edema at the periphery of the underlying lesion (Fig. 2-33). Marrow edema from the other causes is not associated with an underlying mass (Box 2-12).

Transient Osteoporosis of the Hip/Painful Bone Marrow Edema Syndrome. Mainly young and middle-aged men are affected in either hip by transient osteoporosis of the hip/painful bone marrow edema syndrome. Women with transient osteoporosis of the hip often are affected in the last trimester of pregnancy, with a predilection for the left hip. Osteoporosis may be so severe that fractures occur. The

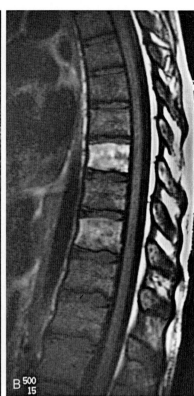

Figure 2-29 **Prostate metastatic disease.** Sequential imaging after radiation therapy showing nearly 100% yellow marrow at 28 days after radiation therapy.

BOX 2-11

Marrow Regeneration

- Occurs after
  - Chemotherapy
  - Treatment of aplastic anemia
  - Low-dose radiation
- MRI
  - T1: Intermediate/low signal (higher or equal to muscle, disk)
  - T2: Usually mildly increased signal
  - Patterns: Focal islands, periphery of bone only, diffusely in bone

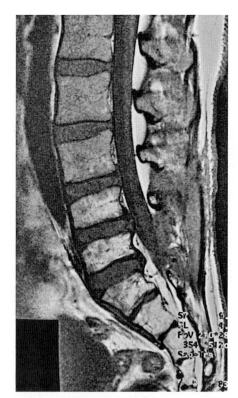

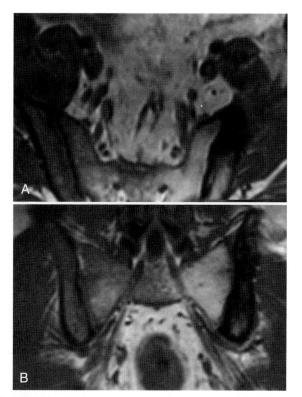

Figure 2-30 Marrow depletion: radiation. T1 sagittal image of the lumbar spine. This patient received pelvic radiation as a child for a sarcoma. The lower two lumbar vertebrae and the sacrum are hypoplastic as the result of radiation given during growth. The sacrum and lower lumbar spine also have more fatty marrow than the normal lumbar spine, seen from L1 through L3. A small amount of red marrow exists in the periphery of the radiated vertebral bodies, but most of the red marrow has been ablated and will never regenerate.

Figure 2-31 Radiation changes. A, Axial T1W image. This image shows yellow marrow in the left hemipelvis with associated cortical hyperostosis, which also can be seen with radiation changes. **B,** Coronal T1W image. This image in the same patient shows evidence of the radiation port. (Note the yellow marrow in the left hemipelvis compared with the yellow/red marrow mixture in the right hemipelvis.)

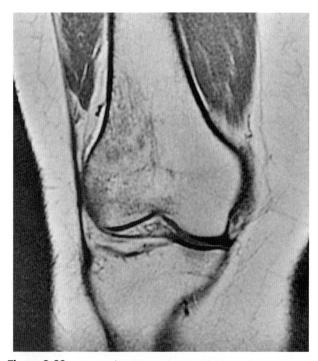

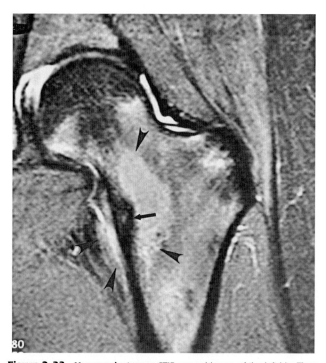

Figure 2-32 Hyperemia: trauma. T1 coronal image of the knee. This image shows intermediate signal with no discrete pattern in the marrow of the lateral and distal aspects of the femur. This is typical of marrow edema, in this case from a lateral patellar dislocation that traumatized the femur.

Figure 2-33 Hyperemia: tumor. STIR coronal image of the left hip. There is a large area of high signal marrow edema from hyperemia involving the medial aspect of the femoral neck and the soft tissues adjacent to the neck (*arrowheads*). This edema surrounds an underlying osteoid osteoma (*arrow*).

joint space remains normal, but joint effusions are common. Bone marrow edema usually affects the femoral head and neck down to the intertrochanteric region (Fig. 2-34). Follow-up studies show resolution of edema and osteoporosis as the clinical symptoms subside in 3 to 12 months.[38,39]

Regional Migratory Osteoporosis. Regional migratory osteoporosis has the same MRI and clinical features as transient osteoporosis of the hip. The major difference is that abnormalities are not confined to the hip and are migratory in nature. The subchondral regions of the knee, ankle, and hip each may be affected in turn, and both extremities may be involved over several years (Fig. 2-35). Spontaneous recovery also occurs in this entity.

The pathogenesis of transient osteoporosis of the hip and regional migratory osteoporosis is unknown, but clinical similarities to reflex sympathetic dystrophy syndrome are striking. The MRI findings for all of these entities are compatible with ischemic changes of the small vessels that supply proximal nerve roots, with loss of control of the normal vascular supply more distally, leading to localized hyperemia. If any abnormalities are seen in marrow from reflex sympathetic dystrophy, they are similar to the other two diseases, with patchy areas of intermediate signal intensity (isointense or higher than muscle or disk) on T1W images that become bright on T2W images.

The relationship between transient osteoporosis of the hip and regional migratory osteoporosis to osteonecrosis is unclear. Biopsy of these lesions shows areas of bone necrosis. There have been reports of typical changes of transient osteoporosis of the hip that, rather than undergoing spontaneous resolution, went on to develop typical MRI and biopsy changes of osteonecrosis in the femoral heads. Why this should occur in some patients, and in which patients, is unclear.[40]

Ischemia (Box 2-13). The causes of bone marrow infarction are numerous and include traumatic disruption of the blood supply, steroids, sickle cell anemia, Gaucher's disease, alcoholism, pancreatitis, dysbaric causes, systemic lupus erythematosus, idiopathic causes, and other causes. Many clinicians refer to ischemic changes in the epiphyses as avascular necrosis and to changes in the shafts of bone as bone infarction. The MRI findings are the same regardless of the location of the lesions, and here we use the term *osteonecrosis* to mean ischemic changes to bone and do not differentiate further by name as to the location of the lesions.

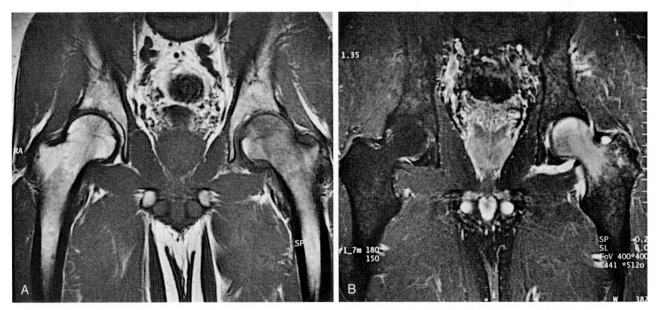

Figure 2-34 **Hyperemia: transient osteoporosis of the hip. A,** T1 coronal image of the pelvis. There is abnormal intermediate signal in the left femoral head and neck, down to the intertrochanteric region. **B,** STIR coronal image of the pelvis. The abnormality in the left hip becomes very high signal so that it looks like a light bulb, and there is a left hip joint effusion. The distribution of marrow edema is typical of transient osteoporosis of the hip/painful bone marrow edema syndrome.

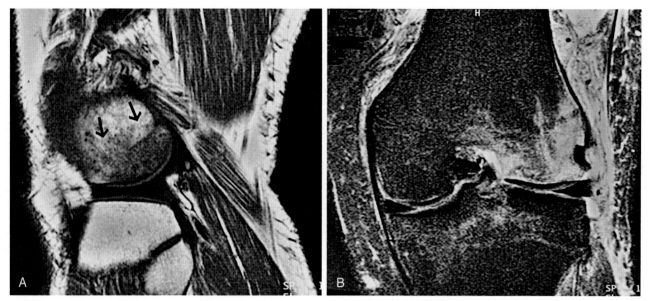

Figure 2-35 **Hyperemia: regional migratory osteoporosis. A,** T1 sagittal image of the knee. There is intermediate signal in the lateral femoral condyle with fat mixed in (*arrows*), an appearance typical of marrow edema. **B,** STIR coronal image of the knee. The marrow edema becomes very high signal, and there is edema in the adjacent soft tissues. This patient previously had transient osteoporosis of the hip and later had it in the ankle.

Osteonecrosis most commonly affects areas where yellow marrow (with its poor vascular supply) predominates: the epiphyses and diaphyses of long bones. Patients with osteonecrosis of the femoral head were shown by MRI to have more fatty than red marrow elements at an earlier age in the femoral neck and intertrochanteric region than a control group, and this indicates a decreased blood supply to the region, which may predispose to developing osteonecrosis.[41]

The sensitivity of MRI for osteonecrosis exceeds that of all other imaging techniques. In addition to a high sensitivity, MRI also usually allows a specific diagnosis to be made. Early diagnosis is difficult by other imaging techniques and can resemble subtle metastases or infection.[42] An accurate and early diagnosis by MRI can avoid inappropriate therapy and allow early core decompression or other treatment, which would give the patient the best chance for recovery without the debilitating sequelae of bone collapse and secondary degenerative joint disease.

The MRI appearance of osteonecrosis varies, based on the age and stage of the lesion. The earliest manifestation seen with MRI is a nonspecific focal area of what looks like marrow edema, intermediate signal intensity on T1W images and high signal intensity on T2W images, in the typical anatomic locations for infarction, that is, in the epiphyses and diametaphyses (Fig. 2-36).[43,44] This appearance rapidly progresses to a distinctive, well-defined pattern that allows a specific diagnosis to be made.

A characteristic, low signal intensity serpentine rim develops in greater than 90% of cases on T1W and T2W images (Fig. 2-37).[45-52] This rim forms what has been called a *geographic pattern* because the areas of osteonecrosis resemble the shapes of different countries and states on a map. This serpentine line represents the interface at the junction between living and dead bone. This is the site of active bone repair, where new bone and an advancing front of granulation tissue is seen histologically. In approximately 80% of cases of osteonecrosis, a high signal intensity line is present on T2W images just inside the low signal intensity serpentine line, producing the *double-line sign* (Fig. 2-38). This line probably occurs as a result of chemical shift misregistration or perhaps reflects the pathologic changes at the reactive bone interface.[53] A *double-line sign* is not required to make the diagnosis of osteonecrosis. The area of bone within the infarcted segment usually has signal intensity identical to fat. Occasionally, the infarcted bone has signal that is low intensity on T1W images and high signal on T2W images (edema), or low signal intensity on T1W and T2W images (fibrosis,

---

BOX 2-13

Vascular Abnormalities (Ischemia)

- Ischemia causes osteonecrosis in poorly vascularized fatty marrow
- Focal lesions in epiphyses or diaphyses
- Usual causes
  - Trauma
  - Steroids
  - Sickle cell anemia
  - Dysbaric causes
  - Systemic lupus erythematosus
  - Gaucher's disease
  - Alcoholism
  - Pancreatitis
  - Idiopathic

MRI

- Marrow edema early (intermediate signal, T1; high signal, T2)
- Serpiginous, geographic patterns later
  - T1: Low signal margin; center usually isointense to fat or may be low signal
  - T2: Low signal margin (± double-line sign); center isointense to fat or may be low or high signal

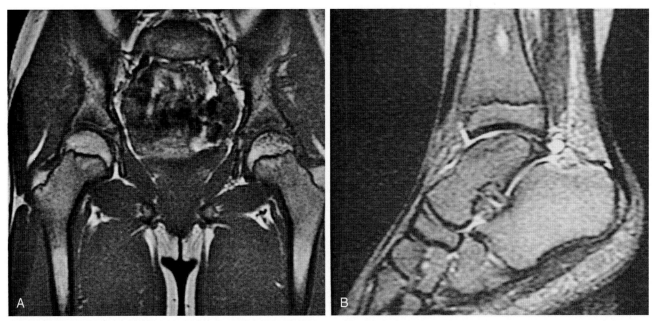

Figure 2-36 **Ischemia: early changes. A,** T1 coronal image of the pelvis. Vague, patchy abnormal signal is present in the left femoral head of this child, with early MRI evidence of osteonecrosis. **B,** Spin echo–T2 sagittal image of the ankle. There is an oblong high signal abnormality in the distal tibial diametaphysis from early changes of osteonecrosis in this 5-year-old patient, who had a bone marrow transplant and was on steroids.

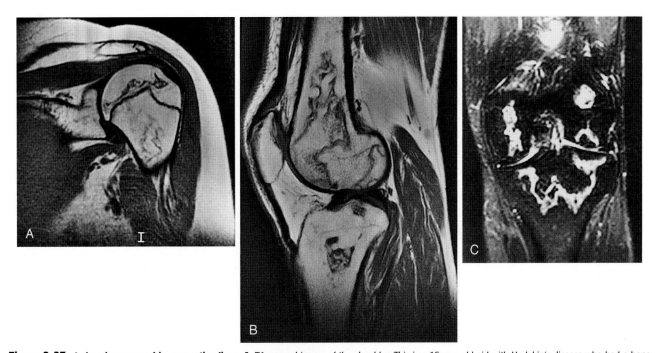

Figure 2-37 **Ischemia: geographic, serpentine lines. A,** T1 coronal image of the shoulder. This is a 16-year-old girl with Hodgkin's disease who had a bone marrow transplant. She had bone pain and a positive bone scan at multiple sites, with negative radiographs. MRI shows several areas of serpentine low signal lines involving the proximal humeral epiphysis and diametaphysis from osteonecrosis. The thickest of the low signal lines is the growth plate. There is high signal fatty marrow in the scapula and proximal humerus, which is abnormal at any age, as a result of the therapy that ablated the patient's red marrow. **B,** T1 sagittal image of the knee (different patient). Serpiginous lines from osteonecrosis secondary to steroid therapy are evident in the distal femur and proximal tibia. This forms the geographic pattern typical of osteonecrosis (look closely and you can see Canada in the distal femur, with Hudson Bay dipping down to the articular surface). **C,** STIR coronal image of the knee (same patient as in **B**). The serpiginous lines can become high signal on heavily T2W sequences, as seen here in both femoral condyles and the proximal tibia.

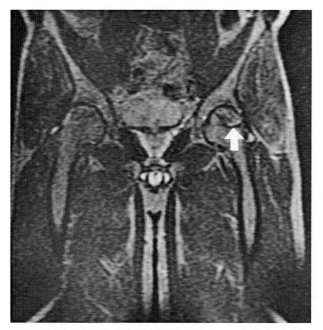

Figure 2-38   Ischemia: the double-line sign. Spin echo–T2 coronal image of the pelvis. There is osteonecrosis of the left femoral head (*arrow*), with a high signal line just proximal to a low signal line. This is the "double-line sign" of osteonecrosis. This sign is not necessary to make the diagnosis and is not always present. It is frequently discussed, however.

sclerosis, trabecular collapse). Symptoms tend to be least severe in lesions that are isointense with fat and most severe in lesions with low signal intensity on all pulse sequences. Joint effusions usually are present in cases of painful osteonecrosis that involve the epiphysis of a bone that makes up the joint.

MRI can be used to determine the volume and location of bone involved with osteonecrosis. MRI also can show if there is collapse of bone or if degenerative changes are present.

Miscellaneous Marrow Diseases

There is an important group of abnormalities that affects bone marrow, but these abnormalities do not fit neatly into the other categories of marrow disease. This group includes Gaucher's disease, Paget's disease, osteopetrosis, hemosiderosis, and serous atrophy (gelatinous transformation) of marrow.

Gaucher's Disease. Gaucher's disease is a rare disease of cerebroside metabolism, in which the enzyme glucocerebroside hydrolase is absent. Lipid material (glucocerebroside) accumulates in histiocytes throughout the reticuloendothelial system. Infiltration of marrow in the axial and proximal appendicular skeleton is common.

MRI findings of the marrow infiltration are nonspecific; however, there often are areas of osteonecrosis that significantly limit the differential diagnostic possibilities (Fig. 2-39). The marrow infiltration may be patchy or diffuse, and the signal intensity is low on T1W and T2W images. Erlenmeyer flask deformities of the distal femora are obvious on MRI. Occasionally, the Gaucher cells can be seen breaking out of the cortex and into the soft tissues surrounding the bone.

Treatment of Gaucher's disease may consist of administration of an enzyme to break down the glucocerebroside. MRI often is used for monitoring the changes in the liver, spleen, and marrow in these patients. Decreased amounts of marrow infiltration are evident on serial images in patients who respond to the therapy (Fig. 2-40).

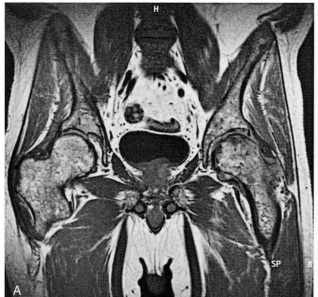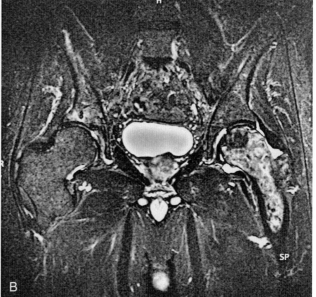

Figure 2-39   Miscellaneous: Gaucher's disease. A, T1 coronal image of the pelvis. There is diffuse, patchy abnormal intermediate signal throughout the visualized marrow, including the femoral epiphyses and apophyses. There also is osteonecrosis of the left femoral head and low signal serpiginous lines in the right supra-acetabular region from osteonecrosis. **B,** STIR coronal image of the pelvis. The Gaucher cells in the marrow remain low signal. There is high signal in the left femoral neck and the right supra-acetabular regions from the osteonecrosis.

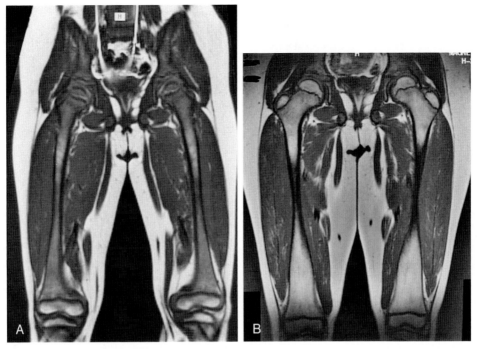

Figure 2-40   **Miscellaneous: Gaucher's disease. A,** T1 coronal image of the pelvis and femora. This is a 5-year-old child with Gaucher's disease before treatment with enzyme therapy. There is abnormal marrow distribution with intermediate signal in the proximal and distal femoral epiphyses, in the apophyses, and in the diaphyses. **B,** T1 coronal image of the femora. Slightly more than 1 year after initiating enzyme therapy for treatment of Gaucher's disease, the marrow distribution has returned to normal, with fatty epiphyses and apophyses in the proximal and distal femora, and the marrow is not as low signal as it was pretreatment. Erlenmeyer flask deformities of the femora remain.

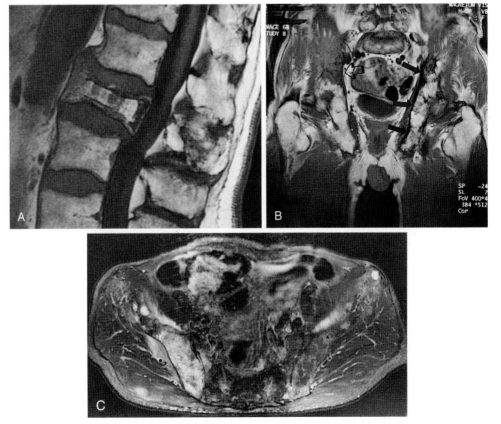

Figure 2-41   **Miscellaneous: Paget's disease. A,** T1 sagittal image of the spine. There is a fracture of L1, and mixed regions of intermediate signal and high signal, with a peripheral rim of intermediate signal (the "picture frame" seen on radiography). Taking the fracture into account, the vertebra is still enlarged. There are thickened trabeculae. **B,** T1 coronal image of the pelvis (different patient). The bones of the pelvis are enlarged with thickened cortex (*solid arrows*) and thickened trabeculae. The signal of the marrow is high on the left side from fat in the pagetic bone, but on the right side there are focal areas of intermediate signal (*open arrow*). **C,** STIR axial image of the pelvis (same patient as in **B**). The fatty marrow is suppressed on this sequence, but large focal areas of high signal on the right side are evident with surrounding soft tissue edema. Biopsy of the right iliac showed metastatic disease to pagetic bone.

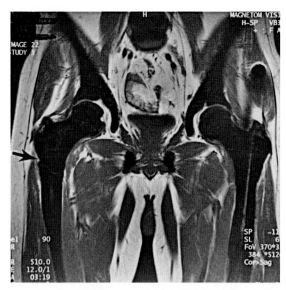

Figure 2-42 **Miscellaneous: osteopetrosis.** T1 coronal image of the pelvis. The bone is diffusely very low signal intensity. This is the result of osteopetrosis with lack of medullary bone and the presence of cortical bone diffusely. There is a pathologic fracture (*arrow*) in the right subtrochanteric region, which was much better seen on the STIR sequence. The left femur previously had an intramedullary rod placed for a pathologic fracture.

BOX 2-14

Diffuse Very Low Signal (Black) Marrow

Focal
- Bone islands
- Sclerotic metastases
- Vacuum phenomenon (intraosseous)

Diffuse
- Mastocytosis
- Hemosiderosis
- Myelofibrosis
- Osteopetrosis

Paget's Disease. The MRI appearance of Paget's disease varies, depending on the balance between osseous matrix and normal marrow. Common MRI findings in pagetic bone include areas of normal high signal intensity from fat and areas of intermediate or low signal intensity on T1W images (Fig. 2-41). The low signal intensity reflects fibrovascular connective tissue, dilated vascular channels, or uncalcified osteoid. Thick bone trabeculae and cortical bone can be seen but not as easily as on conventional radiographs or CT. This diagnosis often is overlooked or misinterpreted as a hemangioma in the spine because of the large areas of fatty marrow that result in a near-normal appearance. The diagnosis is so easy to make by correlating the MR images with conventional radiographs that there is no excuse to misdiagnose it, unless there are no existing radiographs. Sarcomatous degeneration of pagetic bone, giant cell tumors within it, or metastases to areas of Paget's disease can be easily shown on T1W images as low signal intensity marrow lesions or soft tissue masses replacing the bone; these lesions are high signal intensity on T2W images (see Fig. 2-41). There is a higher incidence of metastases to pagetic bone because of its hypervascularity.

Osteopetrosis. Osteopetrosis is a hereditary bone dysplasia with different manifestations, depending on the severity of disease. There is a decreased level of osteoclastic activity so that the normal differentiation between cortical and medullary bone is not present. Cortical bone predominates, with mild or near complete obliteration of the marrow space, depending on which type of disease is present (there are four types, of varying severity). The recessive or lethal form has been successfully treated with bone marrow transplants.

MRI of the most severe cases shows low signal cortical bone on all pulse sequences with little to no high signal intensity fatty bone marrow on T1W images (Fig. 2-42). After marrow transplant, the modeling abnormalities disappear, and a marrow space with normal-appearing marrow develops. Milder forms of osteopetrosis have greater amounts of marrow (although still decreased), and the characteristic bone-in-bone appearance seen on conventional radiographs can be seen on MRI as low signal intensity within higher signal intensity marrow on T1W images. Stress fractures are common in bones weakened by osteopetrosis, and these can be shown easily on MRI, if the diagnosis is unclear from radiographs.

Hemosiderin Deposition (Box 2-14). Hemosiderin (iron) deposition in macrophages located in bone marrow and other organs occurs from chronic breakdown of red blood cells (sickle cell anemia, thalassemia), chronic blood transfusions, or metabolic abnormalities in chronic inflammatory disorders and acquired immunodeficiency syndrome (AIDS). The marrow appears extremely low signal intensity (signal void, black marrow) on all pulse sequences, and there is the blooming effect on gradient echo imaging (Fig. 2-43). The liver and spleen have the same low signal intensity as bone marrow, which helps to distinguish this process from similar-appearing diseases on MRI.

Serous Atrophy (Gelatinous Transformation). Severely cachectic patients, patients with anorexia nervosa, and AIDS patients all may develop serous atrophy, which consists of bone marrow essentially turning to mush. The process occurs in exactly the same progression and sequence as does conversion of red to yellow marrow. The hands and feet, followed by the bones of the forearms and lower legs, are affected first. Ultimately, the proximal long bones and axial skeleton become abnormal. The MRI signal characteristics are identical to those of water, with low signal intensity (equal to or lower than muscle) on T1W images that becomes high signal on T2W images (Fig. 2-44). This process may start out as focal lesions, but it rapidly progresses to large, confluent regions of abnormality on MRI. Histologically, the marrow is necrotic and composed of serous fluid.[54]

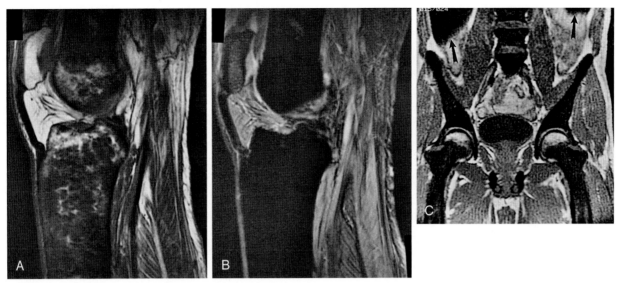

Figure 2-43 **Miscellaneous: hemosiderin deposition. A,** T1 sagittal image of the knee. There is diffuse abnormal low signal in the femur and tibia, involving the epiphyses and the shafts of the bones in this patient with sickle cell anemia. **B,** T2* sagittal image of the knee. The bones become diffusely very low signal from blooming that occurs from the hemosiderin deposited in the marrow. **C,** T1 coronal image of the pelvis (different patient). The bones are diffusely black except for the femoral heads. The liver and spleen also are black (*arrows*). This patient has hemosiderosis.

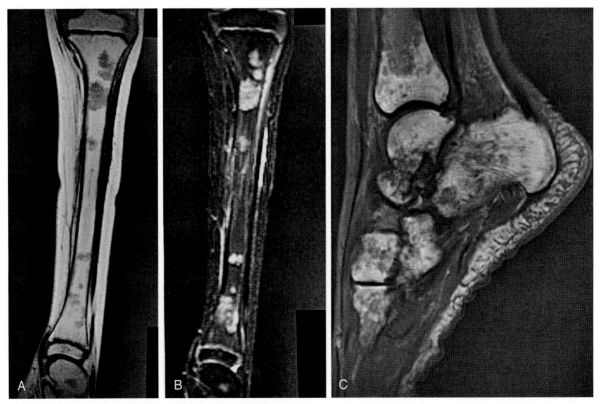

Figure 2-44 **Miscellaneous: serous atrophy (gelatinous transformation). A,** T1 coronal image of the lower leg. This patient was previously treated for Ewing's sarcoma and was cachectic (note the lack of muscle in the calf). The focal areas of intermediate signal intensity were of concern for metastatic disease. **B,** STIR coronal image of the lower leg. The focal marrow abnormalities are high signal. Biopsy of the proximal large lesion showed fluid in the marrow, and this was diagnosed as serous atrophy. **C,** T1 sagittal image of the foot. This patient (different patient than in **A** and **B**) had AIDS. There are multiple foci of intermediate signal in the marrow of the foot and tibia and in the subcutaneous fat, compatible with serous atrophy.

REFERENCES

1. Vogler JB, Murphy WA. Bone marrow imaging. *Radiology* 1988; 168:679-693.
2. Steiner RM, Mitchell DG, Rao VM, Schweitzer ME. Magnetic resonance imaging of diffuse bone marrow disease. *Radiol Clin North Am* 1992; 31:383-409.
3. Kaplan PA, Dussault RG. Magnetic resonance imaging of the bone marrow. In Higgins CB, Hricak H, Helms CA (eds). *Magnetic Resonance Imaging of the Body*, ed 3. New York: Lippincott-Raven; 1997:101-126.
4. Dooms GC, Fisher MR, Hricak H, et al. Bone marrow imaging: magnetic resonance studies related to age and sex. *Radiology* 1985; 155:429-432.
5. Jaramillo D, Laor T, Hoffer FA, et al. Epiphyseal marrow in infancy: MR imaging. *Radiology* 1991; 180:809-812.
6. Ricci C, Cova M, Kang YS, et al. Normal age-related patterns of cellular and fatty bone marrow distribution in the axial skeleton: MR imaging study. *Radiology* 1990; 177:83-88.
7. Dawson KL, Moore SG, Rowland JM. Age-related marrow changes in the pelvis: MR and anatomic findings. *Radiology* 1992; 183:47-51.
8. Kricun ME. Red-yellow marrow conversion: its effect on the location of some solitary bone lesions. *Skeletal Radiol* 1985; 14:10-19.
9. Moore SG, Dawson KL. Red and yellow marrow in the femur: age-related changes in appearance at MR imaging. *Radiology* 1990; 175:219-223.
10. Moore SG, Bisset GS, Siegel MJ, Donaldson JS. Pediatric musculoskeletal MR imaging. *Radiology* 1991; 179:345-360.
11. Mirowitz SA. Hematopoietic bone marrow within the proximal humeral epiphysis in normal adults: investigation with MR imaging. *Radiology* 1993; 188:689-693.
12. Hajek PC, Baker LL, Goobar JE, et al. Focal fat deposition in axial bone marrow: MR characteristics. *Radiology* 1987; 162:245-249.
13. Roos AD, Kressel H, Spritzer C, Dalinka M. MR imaging of marrow changes adjacent to end plates in degenerative lumbar disk disease. *AJR Am J Roentgenol* 1987; 149:531-534.
14. Modic MT, Steinberg PM, Ross JS, et al. Degenerative disk disease: assessment of changes in vertebral body marrow with MR imaging. *Radiology* 1988; 166:193-199.
15. Jones KM, Unger EC, Granstrom P, et al. Bone marrow imaging using STIR at 0.5 and 1.5 T. *Magn Reson Imaging* 1992; 10:169-176.
16. Sebag GH, Moore SG. Effect of trabecular bone on the appearance of marrow in gradient-echo imaging of the appendicular skeleton. *Radiology* 1990; 174:855-859.
17. Vande Berg BC, Malghem J, Lecouvet FE, Maldague B. Magnetic resonance imaging of the normal bone marrow. *Skeletal Radiol* 1998; 27:471-483.
18. Schweitzer ME, Levine C, Mitchell DG, et al. Bull's-eyes and halos: useful MR discriminators of osseous metastases. *Radiology* 1993; 188:249-252.
19. Disler DG, McCauley TR, Ratner LM, et al. In-phase and out-of-phase MR imaging of bone marrow: prediction of neoplasia based on the detection of coexistent fat and water. *AJR Am J Roentgenol* 1997;169:1439-1447.
20. Baur A, Stäbler A, Brüning R, et al. Diffusion-weighted MR imaging of bone marrow: differentiation of benign versus pathologic compression fractures. *Radiology* 1998; 207:349-356.
21. Erly WK, Oh ES, Outwater EK. The utility of in-phase/opposed-phase imaging in differentiating malignancy from acute benign compression fractures of the spine. *AJNR Am J Neuroradiol* 2006; 27:1183-1188.
22. Vande Berg BC, Mallghem J, Lecouvet FE, Maldague B. Classification and detection of bone marrow lesions with magnetic resonance imaging. *Skeletal Radiol* 1998; 27:529-545.
23. Vande Berg BC, Lecouvet FE, Michaux L, et al. Stage I multiple myeloma: value of MR imaging of the bone marrow in the determination of prognosis. *Radiology* 1996; 201:243-246.
24. Vande Berg BC, Michaux L, Lecouvet FE, et al. Nonmyelomatous monoclonal gammopathy: correlation of bone marrow MR images with laboratory findings and spontaneous clinical outcome. *Radiology* 1997; 202:247-251.
25. Major NM, Helms CA, Richardson WJ. The "mini brain": plasmacytoma in a vertebral body on MR imaging. *AJR Am J Roentgenol* 2000; 175:261-263.
26. Moulopoulos LA, Dimopoulos MA, Alexanian R, et al. Multiple myeloma: MR patterns of response to treatment. *Radiology* 1994; 192:441-446.
27. Eustace S, Tello R, DeCarvalho V, et al. A comparison of whole-body TurboSTIR MR imaging and planar ^{99m}Tc-methylene diphosphonate scintigraphy in the examination of patients with suspected skeletal metastases. *AJR Am J Roentgenol* 1997; 169:1655-1661.
28. Frank JA, Ling A, Patronas NJ, et al. Detection of malignant bone tumors: MR imaging vs scintigraphy. *AJR Am J Roentgenol* 1990; 155:1043-1048.
29. Algra PR, Bloem JL, Tissing H, et al. Detection of vertebral metastases: comparison between MR imaging and bone scintigraphy. *RadioGraphics* 1991; 11:219-232.
30. Lien HH, Holte H. Fat replacement of Hodgkin disease of bone marrow after chemotherapy: report of three cases. *Skeletal Radiol* 1996; 25:671-674.
31. Mink J. Percutaneous bone biopsy in the patient with known or suspected osseous metastases. *Radiology* 1986; 161:191-194.
32. Yuh WTC, Zachar CK, Barloon TJ, et al. Vertebral compression fractures: distinction between benign and malignant causes with MR imaging. *Radiology* 1989; 172:215-218.
33. Baker LL, Goodman SB, Inder P, et al. Benign versus pathologic compression fractures of vertebral bodies: assessment with conventional spin-echo, chemical shift, and STIR MR imaging. *Radiology* 1990; 174:495-502.
34. Kaplan PA, Asleson RJ, Klassen LW, Duggan MJ. Bone marrow patterns in aplastic anemia: observations with 1.5-T MR imaging. *Radiology* 1987; 164:441-444.
35. McKinstry CS, Steiner RE, Young AT, et al. Bone marrow in leukemia and aplastic anemia: MR imaging before, during, and after treatment. *Radiology* 1987; 162:701-707.
36. Fletcher BD, Wall JE, Hanna SL. Effect of hematopoietic growth factors on MR images of bone marrow in children undergoing chemotherapy. *Radiology* 1993; 189:745-751.
37. Stevens SK, Moore SG, Kaplan ID. Early and late bone-marrow changes after irradiation: MR evaluation. *AJR Am J Roentgenol* 1990; 154:745-750.
38. Wilson AJ, Murphy WA, Hardy DC, Totty WG. Transient osteoporosis: transient bone marrow edema? *Radiology* 1988; 167:757-760.
39. Bloem J. Transient osteoporosis of the hip: MR imaging. *Radiology* 1988; 167:753-755.
40. Vande Berg BC, Malghem JJ, Lecouvet FE, et al. Idiopathic bone marrow edema lesions of the femoral head: predictive value of MR imaging findings. *Radiology* 1999; 212:527-535.
41. Mitchell DG, Rao VM, Dalinka M, et al. Hematopoietic and fatty bone marrow distribution in the normal and ischemic hip: new observations with 1.5-T MR imaging. *Radiology* 1986; 161:199-202.
42. Munk PL, Helms CA, Holt RG. Immature bone infarcts: findings on plain radiographs and MR scans. *AJR Am J Roentgenol* 1989; 152:547-549.
43. Turner DA, Templeton AC, Selzer PM, et al. Femoral capital osteonecrosis: MR finding of diffuse marrow abnormalities without focal lesions. *Radiology* 1989; 171:135-140.
44. Guerra JJ, Steinberg ME. Distinguishing transient osteoporosis from avascular necrosis of the hip. *J Bone Joint Surg [Am]* 1995; 77:616-624.
45. Totty WG, Murphy WA, Ganz WI, et al. Magnetic resonance imaging of the normal and ischemic femoral head. *AJR Am J Roentgenol* 1984; 143:1273-1280.
46. Mitchell MD, Kundel HL, Steinberg ME, et al. Avascular necrosis of the hip: comparison of MR, CT, and scintigraphy. *AJR Am J Roentgenol* 1986; 147:67-71.
47. Mitchell DG, Rao VM, Dalinka MK, et al. Femoral head avascular necrosis: correlation of MR imaging, radiographic staging, radionuclide imaging, and clinical findings. *Radiology* 1987; 162:709-715.
48. Bettran J, Herman LJ, Burk JM, et al. Femoral head avascular necrosis: MR imaging with clinical-pathologic and radionuclide correlation. *Radiology* 1988; 166:215-220.
49. Genez BM, Wilson MR, Houk RW, et al. Early osteonecrosis of the femoral head: detection in high risk patients with MR imaging. *Radiology* 1988; 168:521-524.

50. Coleman BG, Kressel HY, Dalinka MK, et al. Radiographically negative avascular necrosis: detection with MR imaging. *Radiology* 1988; 168:525-528.

51. Tervonen O, Mueller DM, Matteson EL, et al. Clinically occult avascular necrosis of the hip: prevalence in an asymptomatic population at risk. *Radiology* 1992; 182:845-847.

52. Glickstein MF, Burk DL, Schiebler ML, et al. Avascular necrosis versus other diseases of the hip: sensitivity of MR imaging. *Radiology* 1988; 169:213-215.

53. Sugimoto H, Okubo RS, Ohsawa T. Chemical shift and the double-line sign in MRI of early femoral avascular necrosis. *J Comput Assist Tomogr* 1992; 16:727-730.

54. Van de Berg BC, Malghem J, Devuyst O, et al. Anorexia nervosa: correlation between MR appearance of bone marrow and severity of disease. *Radiology* 1994; 193:859-864.

Tendons and Muscles

How to Image Tendons

- *Coils and patient position:* Whether or not a coil should be used is based entirely on the anatomy to be imaged. Generally, surface coils improve images and should be used. For large areas, such as the thighs or pelvis, this approach is not practical, and surface coils are not used. Patients should be positioned as if the nearest joint were being imaged. Ankle tendons are imaged by positioning the patient and using a coil for an ankle examination.
- *Image orientation:* Generally, tendons are best imaged transversely (perpendicular to their long axis). Occasionally, other planes are helpful to image tendons in their entire length. The triceps, quadriceps, and Achilles tendons are depicted well on axial and sagittal images. The hamstring tendons in the pelvis and the supraspinatus tendon in the shoulder are shown well on coronal and axial images. Given only one option for an imaging plane through a tendon, axial images generally are the most useful.
- *Pulse sequences and regions of interest:* T1W and some type of T2W images are required for complete evaluation of tendons. T2W sequences are useful for showing abnormal fluid surrounding the tendon (tenosynovitis) and tears and most other kinds of tendon pathology. We prefer fast spin echo with fat saturation or STIR sequences for T2W images of tendons. Slice thickness and fields of view are determined by the size of the body

part being imaged. A good rule of thumb is that the same field of view and slice thickness that are used to image the adjacent joint would suffice to image a tendon in that same region.
- *Contrast:* There is no need to do contrast-enhanced studies for tendon evaluation except to evaluate possible active tendon disease in inflammatory conditions (eg, rheumatoid arthritis).[1]

NORMAL TENDONS

Anatomy

Tendons are avascular structures that attach muscles to bones. They are made of dense fascicles of collagen fibers. The fascicles of collagen are composed of smaller units, called *microfibrils.* Microfibrils interdigitate with one another in a regular and structured fashion to form extremely tight bonds, giving tendons their strength. The microfibrils are made of a protein called *tropocollagen,* which consists of three polypeptide chains arranged in a triple-helix configuration. The helical configuration of the protein tightly binds molecules of water so that tendons have low signal intensity because the hydrogen ions in water are not mobile.

Most tendons are invested with a tendon sheath, which either partially or completely covers the tendon. Tendon sheaths are present where tendons pass through fascial slings, beneath ligamentous bands, or through fibro-osseous

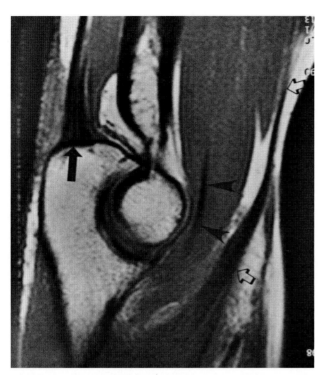

Figure 3-1   Normal tendons. T1 sagittal image of the elbow. The anteriorly located biceps tendon (*open arrows*) is low signal and has a long segment that is not surrounded by muscle. The brachialis tendon (*arrowheads*) is also a typical low signal tendon, but it is surrounded by muscle with little exposed tendon. The triceps (*solid arrow*), in contrast to most tendons, normally has vertical striations of low and intermediate signal.

tunnels. They exist where closely apposed structures move relative to one another, to decrease friction. The microscopic structure of a tendon sheath is similar to the synovial membrane that lines joints. During fetal development, the tendon invaginates the tendon sheath so that there are inner (visceral) and outer (parietal) layers of the sheath that are closely

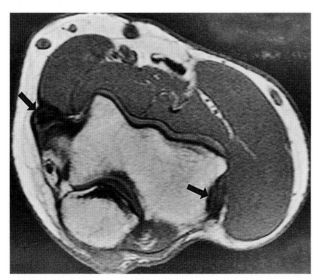

Figure 3-2   Normal tendon intermediate signal. T1 axial image of the elbow. The attachment sites of some tendons to bone (*arrows*) result in areas of intermediate signal within the tendon, which is normal and is caused by diverging collagen fascicles, rather than partial tendon tears.

BOX 3-1

High Signal Within Tendons

Normal Causes

- Coarse fascicles or several tendon layers fusing
  - Quadriceps and distal triceps tendons
- Osseous insertions
  - Tendons spread, change orientation
- Magic angle phenomenon
  - Tendon orientation at 55 degrees to bore of magnet

Abnormalities

- Myxoid degeneration
- Partial or complete tears
- Xanthoma, tumor, gout deposits

apposed to each other. A mesotendon is formed where the tendon invaginated the sheath. The mesotendon carries blood vessels and is located on the nonfrictional surface of the tendon. A thin layer of synovial fluid exists between the visceral and parietal layers of the tendon sheath and allows for smooth gliding of the tendon.

Some tendons are located mainly outside of the muscle, such as the distal biceps tendon at the elbow. Other tendons have long segments that are surrounded by muscle and have very little exposed tendon, such as the brachialis at the elbow (Fig. 3-1).

MRI of Normal Tendons

Normal tendons have so few mobile protons that they are usually low signal intensity on all pulse sequences. The major exceptions to this rule include the quadriceps tendon at the knee and distal triceps tendon at the elbow, which have a striated appearance with alternating areas of linear low and intermediate signal intensity (similar to the distal anterior cruciate ligament in the knee) (see Fig. 3-1). This striated appearance is caused by the longitudinal arrangement of coarse fasciculi and by the fact that several tendons are fusing to form a single, conjoined tendon.[2] The longitudinal striations in the triceps and quadriceps tendons must not be mistaken for pathology. Similarly, there is a solitary vertical line of high signal intensity in the midsubstance of many normal Achilles tendons, which probably represents the site where the soleus and gastrocnemius tendons (which make up the Achilles tendon) are apposed to one another, or else a vascular channel in the tendon.

There are certain other exceptions to the rule that normal tendons are low signal intensity on all pulse sequences (Box

BOX 3-2

Tendon Abnormalities

- Degeneration*
- Tenosynovitis*
- Partial or complete tears*
- Subluxation or dislocation
- Xanthoma formation
- Gout, hydroxyapatite, or other crystals
- Giant cell tumor of tendon sheath
- Clear cell sarcoma

*Most common.

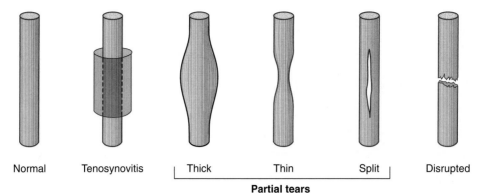

| Normal | Tenosynovitis | Thick | Thin | Split | Disrupted |

Partial tears

Figure 3-3 **Tendon inflammation/tears.** Diagram showing the changes that occur in tendons from inflammatory tenosynovitis through different types of partial tears and complete tendon disruption.

3-1). Many tendons may show slightly increased signal intensity near their osseous insertions. This increased signal intensity occurs because tendons may fan out as they come to attach to a bone, and nontendinous fatty material is interposed between tendon fibers (Fig. 3-2).

A second major reason for a normal tendon having increased signal intensity is the result of the magic angle phenomenon.[3] The magic angle phenomenon results from the fact that tendons are anisotropic structures. When tendons are oriented at an angle of about 55 degrees to the bore of the magnet, there is high signal intensity within the tendon on short TE sequences (eg, T1W, proton density, and gradient echo sequences). Whether high signal on short TE sequences is from the magic angle phenomenon or from pathology generally can be determined in various ways:

1. Use a pulse sequence with a long TE, in which case the high signal intensity disappears and the tendon appears normal.
2. Observe that the tendon is of normal caliber.
3. Reposition the body part being imaged so that the tendon is imaged at a different angle relative to the bore of the magnet.

Most tendons are round, oval, or flat when imaged transversely. Tendon sheaths are not normally seen on MRI, unless fluid is present in the sheath. Small amounts of fluid may be seen in certain tendon sheaths, particularly in the ankle and wrist. Our general rule is that the fluid should not be considered abnormal unless it completely surrounds the circumference of the tendon.

TENDON ABNORMALITIES (Box 3-2)

The major abnormalities that may affect tendons include tendon degeneration, tenosynovitis, partial tears, complete tears, subluxation or dislocation, xanthoma formation, deposits of calcium hydroxyapatite or calcium pyrophosphate crystals, gouty tophi, and clear cell sarcoma. Giant cell tumor of the tendon sheath is a common mass that arises from the tendon sheath. The most common tendon abnormalities seen on MRI are degeneration, tenosynovitis, and tears (Fig. 3-3).

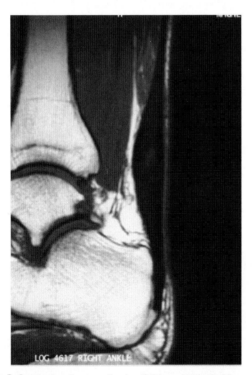

Figure 3-4 **Tendon degeneration/partial tears.** T1 sagittal image of the ankle. The Achilles tendon is markedly thickened in this middle-aged patient and shows intermediate signal within its fibers representing myxoid degeneration and partial tears.

BOX 3-3

Tenosynovitis

Causes
- Overuse, increased stresses
- Inflammatory arthritis
- Infection

Stenosing Tenosynovitis
- Focal, loculated fluid collections in tendon sheath, often with septations in fluid

MRI
- Underlying tendon may be normal or abnormal
- Fluid (low signal, T1; high signal, T2) must surround the entire circumference of a tendon—meaningless if tendon sheath communicates with adjacent joint
- Septations in loculated fluid of stenosing tenosynovitis are thin, linear, low signal structures; do not confuse with mesotendon
- Pannus may be present in tendon sheaths in rheumatoid arthritis

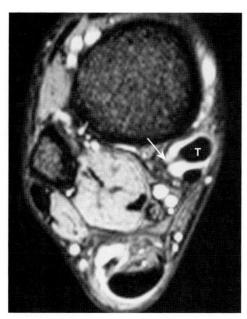

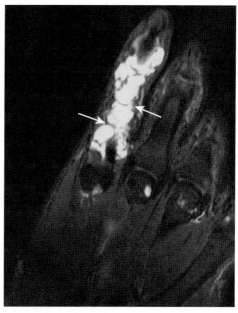

Figure 3-5 **Tenosynovitis.** T2* axial image of the ankle. The posterior tibial tendon (T) is mildly enlarged, but of normal signal intensity. It is surrounded by high signal fluid, representing tenosynovitis. The thin line within the fluid (*arrow*) is the mesotendon, where the tendon invaginated the tendon sheath during fetal development.

Figure 3-6 **Stenosing tenosynovitis.** Fat-saturated T2 coronal image of the finger. High signal fluid from tenosynovitis surrounds the flexor tendons of the index finger. There are lobulated margins of the tendon sheath and small, linear septations within it (*arrows*) indicating this is stenosing tenosynovitis with scarring and inflammatory changes of the sheath.

Degeneration

Myxoid degeneration of tendons occurs with aging or from chronic overuse (Fig. 3-4). This is a painless process, but it weakens the tendon so that it is predisposed to partial or complete tears with minimal trauma. The quadriceps, patellar, and Achilles tendons are good examples of tendons that may rupture with no or minimal trauma because of preexisting underlying tendon degeneration.

On MRI examination, a degenerated tendon has high signal intensity within the substance of the tendon on T1W and any type of T2W sequences. The tendon is generally normal or enlarged in caliber; this cannot be distinguished from partial tears of a tendon. Many clinicians use terms such as *tendinitis, tendinopathy,* or *tendinosis* to indicate that such abnormal signal intensity of a tendon exists, but that it is impossible to give the precise cause for the findings. The term *tendinitis* probably should not be used because an inflammatory response in the tendon does not occur. Another way to describe the nonspecific findings of intrasubstance high signal in a tendon is simply to state that it is compatible with degeneration or partial tears because they generally coexist anyway.

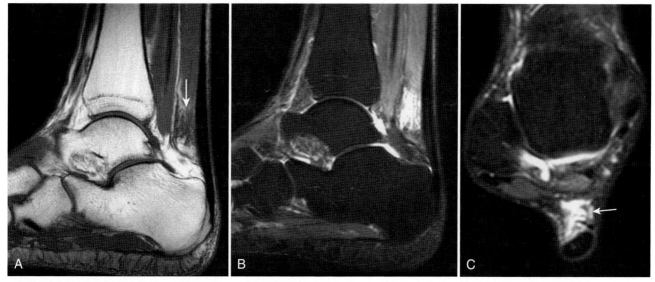

Figure 3-7 **Paratendinitis. A,** T1 sagittal image of the ankle. The Achilles tendon does not have a tendon sheath, so inflammatory changes appear as edema in the fat adjacent to the tendon (*arrow*). **B** and **C,** STIR sagittal and axial images of the ankle. Edema anterior to the Achilles tendon manifests as high signal in Kager's fat (*arrow* in **C**), indicating paratendinitis.

- Tendon degeneration—occurs with age and from chronic stresses
- Chronic, repetitive stresses (overuse)
- Acute major trauma
- Diabetes
- Systemic steroids and other medications
- Rheumatoid arthritis and other inflammatory arthritides
- Chronic renal failure/hyperparathyroidism
- Infection of tendon sheath
- Gout

Tenosynovitis (Box 3-3)

Fluid that completely surrounds the circumference of a tendon indicates an inflammatory process of the tendon sheath, called *tenosynovitis*. The underlying tendon may be normal or abnormal. The abnormal presence and amount of fluid is required to make this diagnosis regardless of the status of the tendon fibers. Tenosynovitis may occur from chronic repetitive motion or stress on the tendon from overuse, from an inflammatory arthritis, or from a purulent infection.

Stenosing tenosynovitis can occur when there are focal, loculated collections of fluid in the tendon sheath. This is a common finding in the flexor hallucis longus tendon around the ankle in patients with the os trigonum syndrome and in the wrist from de Quervain's stenosing tenosynovitis.

MRI of tenosynovitis shows a rounded collection of fluid that is low signal intensity on T1W and high signal intensity on T2W images, completely surrounding a tendon on images obtained transversely through it. The mesotendon may be identified as a thin, low signal intensity line extending from the tendon to the outer layer of the tendon sheath (Fig. 3-5). The underlying tendon may be normal or abnormal in signal intensity and caliber. Stenosing tenosynovitis can be diagnosed on MRI by the presence of focal distention of a tendon sheath with fluid and thin, linear low signal intensity septations that course through the fluid in the sheath (Fig. 3-6).

Tendon sheaths that communicate directly with an adjacent joint (eg, the long head of the biceps tendon in the shoulder and the flexor hallucis longus tendon at the ankle) should not be considered to have tenosynovitis simply because of the finding of fluid surrounding the circumference of the tendon. If there is an effusion of the joint, fluid can surround the tendon without the tendon or its sheath being abnormal. We consider fluid around these specific tendons to have possible clinical significance only if there is no adjacent joint effusion.

Tendons that do not have a sheath may have inflammatory changes surrounding the tendon, which is called *paratendinitis* (Fig. 3-7). MRI shows abnormal signal intensity typical of edema (low signal intensity on T1W and hyperintense on T2W images) in the soft tissues surrounding the tendon. The Achilles tendon is a classic location for these findings because it has no tendon sheath.

Tendon Tears (Box 3-4)

Several conditions cause weakened tendons and predispose to tears, including chronic repetitive stresses, tendon degen-

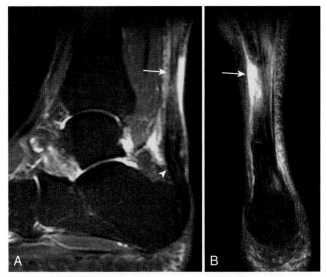

Figure 3-8   Partial tendon tear. A, STIR sagittal image of the ankle. There is marked thickening of the distal Achilles tendon related to chronic tendinopathy and hypertrophic partial tendon tears (*arrowhead*). The tendon is markedly thinned proximally at the site of a high-grade partial tear (*arrow*). **B,** STIR coronal image of the ankle. The degree of tendon disruption is better shown (*arrow*).

eration, inflammatory processes of tendons (eg, from rheumatoid arthritis, seronegative spondyloarthropathies, systemic lupus erythematosus, or infection of the tendon sheath), chronic renal disease, use of long-term systemic steroids and certain other medications, diabetes, and gout.[4] Partial tendon tears represent incomplete disruption of the fibers. Complete tendon tears indicate total disruption of the fibers of the tendon so that there are two separate fragments. Partial tears often are difficult to diagnose on clinical grounds, whereas complete tears are more obvious.

Partial tendon tears can have a variable appearance on MRI (Fig. 3-8). The tendon may be thickened (hypertrophic partial tear) or thinned (atrophic partial tear), or remain of normal caliber with abnormal signal being the only evidence of the partial tear. An attenuated tendon is closer to complete rupture than a thickened tendon. A classification system has been proposed to describe tears based on the caliber of the tendon; we prefer simply to describe the findings (partial tear with a normal-caliber, thickened, or attenuated tendon), rather than assign a number from a classification system, because we cannot remember the system ourselves and especially because referring physicians are unaware of the classification system. Tendons sometimes become partially torn in a longitudinal or vertical manner, rather than transversely (Fig. 3-9). A split tendon may be functionally incompetent and act as if it is completely torn, even though it is still in continuity with the muscle and the bone. Another type of partial tear involves delamination of the tendon fibers.[5] This diagnosis is made when fluid is seen to extend through a partial-thickness tear and track within the substance of a tendon, with partial retraction of the fibers along one of its surfaces (Fig. 3-10).

Usually there is high signal intensity in the tendon on all pulse sequences with partial tendon tears, but with chronic partial tears, there may be low signal intensity because of

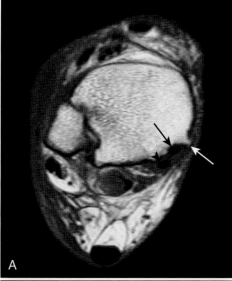

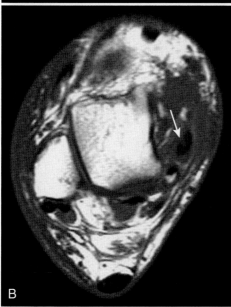

Figure 3-9 **Partial tendon tear: longitudinal split. A,** T1 axial image of the ankle. The posterior tibial tendon (*black arrow*) is the same size as the adjacent flexor digitorum longus tendon (*arrowhead*), indicating atrophic partial tendon tearing (it should be approximately twice the size of the flexor digitorum tendon at this level). Note also the prominent spur arising from the medial malleolus (*white arrow*), a finding often present in cases of posterior tibial tendon dysfunction. **B,** T1 axial image of the ankle. The posterior tibial tendon has a splitlike tear (*arrow*), which extended along the length of the tendon, representing a longitudinal split tear.

scarring and fibrosis. An abnormal tendon size and tenosynovitis are the only ways to recognize the tendon as abnormal in this situation. Tenosynovitis often coexists with partial tendon tears.

Complete tendon rupture on MRI appears as a focal disruption with absence of the tendon fibers for variable distances (Fig. 3-11). MRI is valuable in documenting the presence of a complete tear, showing the quality of the remnants of tendon, and showing how far retracted the remnants are; all of these features may contribute to determining how to manage the patient. Careful search for

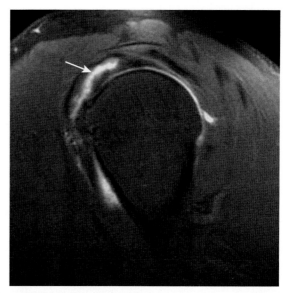

Figure 3-10 **Partial tendon tear: delamination.** Fat-saturated T1 oblique sagittal image of the shoulder (MR arthrogram). There is a large partial-thickness tear of the supraspinatus tendon with horizontal splitting of the tendon (*arrow*) indicating delamination.

tendons on every image is essential not to overlook tears because abnormalities may be present on only one image.

Tendon Subluxation/Dislocation (Box 3-5)

Most tendons maintain a normal relationship to adjacent osseous structures by way of retinacula that hold them in place. If the retinacula become disrupted, the tendons may sublux or dislocate from their normal positions (Fig. 3-12). The tendons may have no intrinsic, underlying abnormalities, but partial tears, complete tears, and tenosynovitis are common from irritation with chronic subluxation and wear and tear on adjacent bones. The tendons that may sublux or dislocate include the extensor carpi ulnaris in the wrist, the long head of the biceps in the shoulder, the peroneal tendons over the lateral malleolus at the ankle, and the posterior tibial tendon on the medial side of the ankle.[6,7]

Miscellaneous Tendon Lesions

Abnormalities other than tears, tenosynovitis, and dislocations are uncommon. Xanthomas occur in patients with familial hyperlipidemia syndrome and most commonly affect the Achilles tendon and the extensor tendons of the hand (Fig. 3-13).

Deposits of gout crystals also may affect tendons (Fig. 3-14). It is usually impossible to distinguish gouty tophi or xanthomas from partial tendon tears by MRI, and they should simply be kept in mind in the appropriate setting. Calcific tendinitis from deposition of calcium hydroxyapatite crystals is common and easy to diagnose on radiographs, which is a good thing because MRI does not usually show the abnormality well. The hydroxyapatite crystals have low signal intensity on all pulse sequences that are usually difficult or impossible to distinguish from the low signal intensity tendon.[8] If the crystal deposit is large enough, it may show lower signal than the tendon on all pulse sequences, making it visible on MRI (Fig. 3-15).

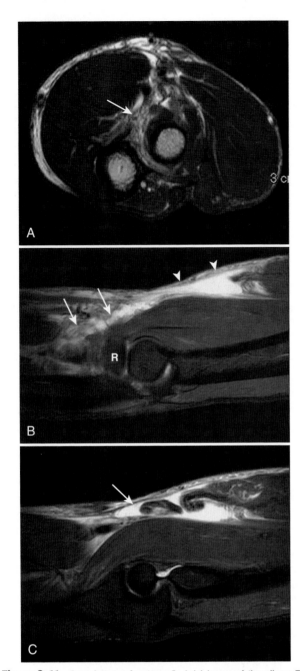

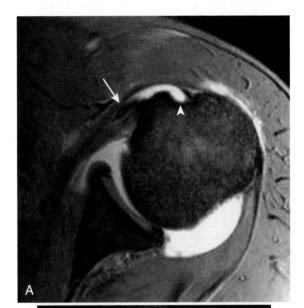

Tendons That Sublux or Dislocate

- Wrist
  - Extensor carpi ulnaris (medial)
- Shoulder
  - Long head of biceps (medial)
- Ankle
  - Peroneal tendons (lateral or medial)
  - Posterior tibial (medial and anterior)

Figure 3-11   Complete tendon tear. A, Axial image of the elbow. The distal end of the distal biceps tendon is not present in its expected location (*arrow*). **B,** STIR sagittal image of the elbow. Fluid is evident in the expected location of the tendon (*arrows*), with high signal fluid and/or hemorrhage proximally (*arrowheads*). R, radial head. **C,** STIR sagittal image (adjacent to image in **B**). The thickened, torn biceps tendon is retracted several centimeters above its insertion site (*arrow*).

Tumors of tendons are exceedingly rare, but clear cell sarcoma (malignant melanoma of soft parts) should be considered if one is considering a tumor at all. Tumors arising from the tendon sheath are much more common than a tumor of the tendon itself. Giant cell tumor of the tendon sheath is a common cause of a mass in the hands and feet. It is a localized and extra-articular form of pigmented villonodular synovitis. It manifests as a nonpainful, soft tissue mass. On MRI, it usually is lobulated with intermediate signal on T1W and T2W images, closely apposed to a low signal tendon (Fig. 3-16).

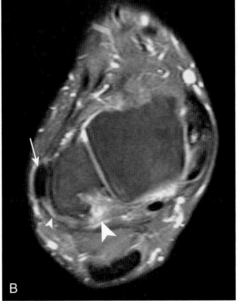

Figure 3-12   Dislocated tendons. A, T2* axial image of the shoulder. The long head of the biceps tendon (*arrow*) has dislocated medially from the bicipital groove (*arrowhead*) and lies within a partially torn subscapularis tendon. **B,** Fat-saturated T1 axial image (postgadolinium administration) of the ankle. The peroneus tendons (*arrow*) have dislocated laterally from the retrofibular groove (*large arrowhead*) where they normally lie. The superior peroneal retinaculum has stripped away from its attachment on the fibula (*small arrowhead*).

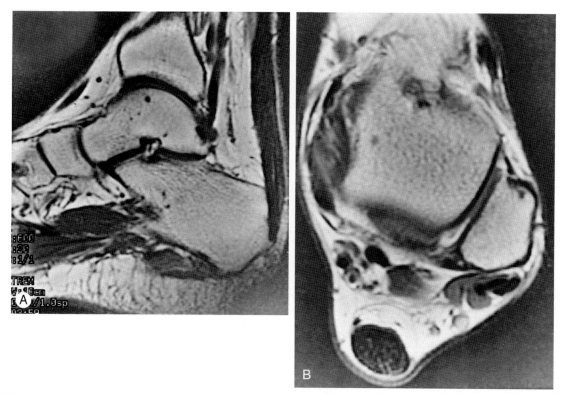

Figure 3-13 Xanthoma of the tendon. **A,** T1 sagittal image of the ankle. The Achilles tendon is thickened and has abnormal high signal striations within it. **B,** T1 axial image of the ankle. The Achilles tendon has a stippled appearance of low and high signal and is thickened with a convex anterior margin. These findings are from familial hyperlipidemia with xanthoma formation, but cannot be distinguished from partial tendon tears by MRI.

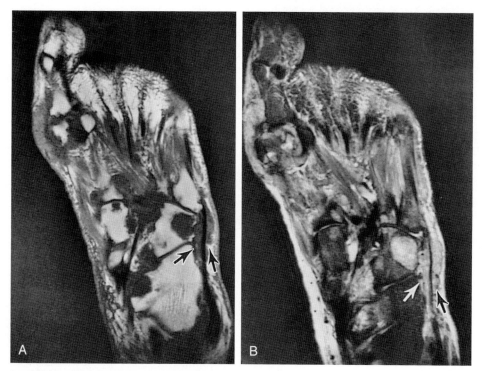

Figure 3-14 Gout that affects tendons. **A,** T1 coronal image of the foot. An intermediate signal lobulated mass (*arrows*) representing a gouty tophus surrounds a tendon. Intraosseous gout deposits can be seen in several bones as well. **B,** STIR coronal image of the foot. Findings are the same as in **A,** but the gouty tophi change signal slightly. They are intermediate signal on this STIR image, but may be even lower signal on other types of T2W sequences.

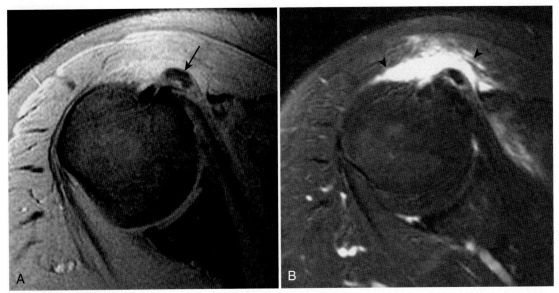

Figure 3-15   **Calcium hydroxyapatite in tendons. A,** T2* axial image of the shoulder. A low signal intensity focus is present within the distal subscapularis tendon (*arrow*) from calcium hydroxyapatite crystal deposition (calcific tendinitis). **B,** Fat-saturated T2 axial image of the shoulder. The low signal calcific focus is seen again, and the adjacent inflammatory fluid and edema are better shown (*arrowheads*).

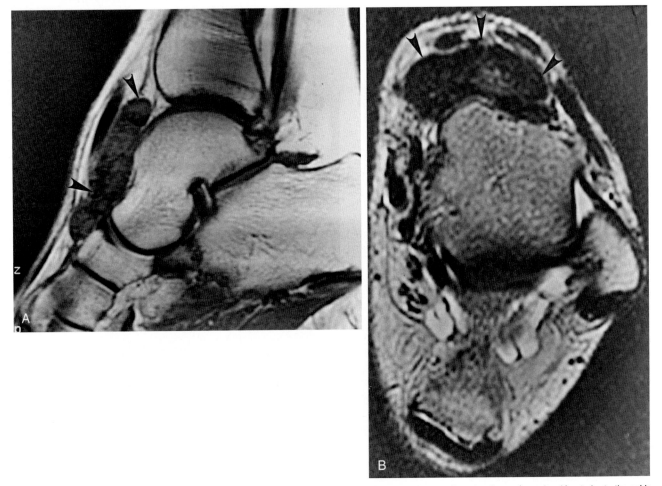

Figure 3-16   **Giant cell tumor of the tendon sheath. A,** T1 sagittal image of the ankle. There is an intermediate signal mass (*arrowheads*) anterior to the ankle. **B,** Spin echo–T2 axial image of the ankle. The mass remains intermediate to low signal intensity on this sequence (*arrowheads*) and is seen just deep to the extensor tendons.

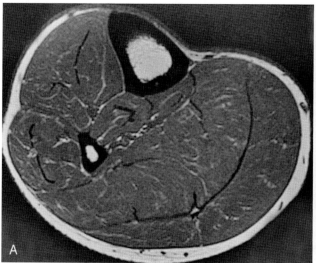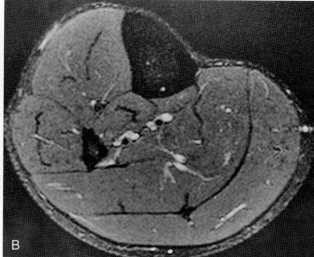

Figure 3-17   Normal skeletal muscle. A, T1 axial image of the calf. Muscle has intermediate signal intensity with a feathery appearance created by small amounts of interspersed fat. Little to no intermuscular fat is present in this individual, making identification of specific muscles difficult. **B,** STIR axial image of the calf. Muscle remains intermediate signal on this sequence, but the feathery pattern disappears because of suppression of the fat.

How to Image Muscles

- *Coils and patient position:* Injury or other types of pathology often affect large muscles in large body parts where surface coils are not used. The use of coils depends on the size of the region being imaged. Generally, the patient should be imaged in the same position as if the adjacent joint were being imaged.
- *Image orientation:* Generally, most muscles and muscle groups are best evaluated in the axial plane. Longitudinal (coronal or sagittal) planes are used for orientation of abnormalities relative to osseous landmarks and to show the extent of the disease.
- *Pulse sequences and regions of interest:* T1W and some type of T2W imaging is required. For the T2 sequence, we prefer using STIR because this sequence is exquisitely sensitive to most muscle pathology. T1 sequences also are necessary to show anatomic detail and configuration of the muscle, subacute hemorrhage, and fatty atrophy of muscle. Fields of view and slice thickness depend entirely on the body part being imaged and the extent of the suspected abnormality. We often do a large field-of-view coronal, fast STIR sequence as a scout view. The edema that is present indicates the region that needs to be covered with a smaller field of view and other pulse sequences, and whether or not a surface coil can be used.
- *Contrast:* Contrast-enhanced sequences are unnecessary, unless one is attempting to identify abscesses or areas of muscle necrosis.

NORMAL MUSCLE

MRI Appearance

Normal skeletal muscle has intermediate signal intensity on all pulse sequences (Fig. 3-17). T1W images show a feathery

---

BOX 3-6

Indirect Muscle Injuries

Delayed-Onset Muscle Soreness (Muscle Stiffness)
- Pain peaks 2 days after unaccustomed activity
- No acute injury or painful event
- Damage is at ultrastructural level and reversible

Muscle Strains (Partial or Complete Tears)
- Sudden onset of pain occurs during activity
- Occurs during eccentric muscle contraction (ie, muscle lengthens as it contracts, such as the biceps while lowering a weight)
- Often affects muscles crossing two joints (rectus femoris, biceps femoris, gastrocnemius) and affects myotendinous junction
- Three grades
  - Grade I—few muscle fibers torn, no functional loss, interstitial blood
  - Grade II—more fibers torn, some loss of strength, focal defect and interstitial blood in muscle, blood surrounding tendon from myotendinous junction injury
  - Grade III—muscle completely torn, loss of strength, focal and interstitial blood

MRI of Muscle Strains
- DOMS and grade I (T2)
  - Feathery, interstitial signal in muscle
  - ± ↑ signal between muscles
- Grade II (T2)
  - Feathery, interstitial ↑ signal in muscle
  - ↑ signal between muscles
  - ± focal muscle defect
  - Tendon thinned, irregular, lax
  - ↑ signal surrounding tendon
- Grade III (T2)
  - Feathery, interstitial ↑ signal in muscle
  - Complete muscle disruption with ↑ signal in gap between retracted segments
  - ↑ signal between muscle fragments—discontinuity of tendon within muscle

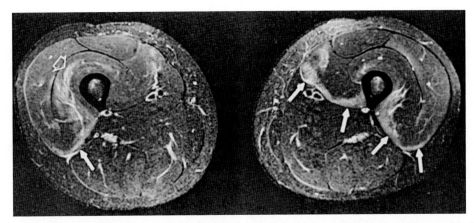

Figure 3-18 **Delayed-onset muscle soreness.** STIR axial image of the thighs. One of our fellows ran a marathon, and these are her thighs less than 2 days later (she said they felt as bad as they look). High signal edema is seen in the periphery of some of the vastus musculature (*solid arrows*). More diffuse interstitial muscle edema is seen in the right vastus intermedius (*open arrow*). Intermuscular (perifascial) edema was not present at the time of this MRI.

or marbled appearance because of fat that is interposed between adjacent muscles and between muscle fibers within a muscle. In some locations, individual muscle groups can be distinguished because of interposed fat. Where intermuscular fat is sparse, such as in the calf, individual muscle groups blend together and are difficult to identify. Low signal intensity tendons may course through a muscle for long distances, or may arise near the periphery of a muscle; this myotendinous junction is usually the weakest link in the chain from a perspective of strength of the entire unit. On T2W sequences, normal muscle remains intermediate signal intensity, and no high signal is evident between muscles, with the exception of normal vascular structures.

MUSCLE ABNORMALITIES

Several abnormalities of muscle occur that can be evaluated well by MRI, including abnormalities from trauma, inflammatory disorders, tumors, denervation, muscular dystrophies, neuromuscular disorders, and ischemia. Despite the wide variety of pathology that may affect it, muscle responds in only a few ways, and this is reflected in the MRI appear-

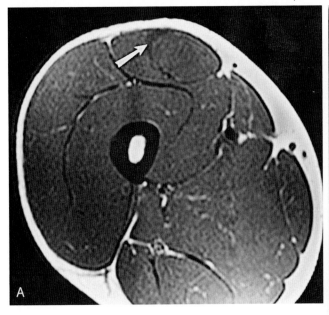

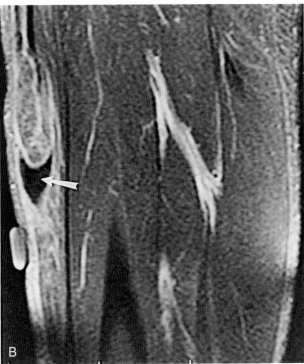

Figure 3-19 **Muscle tear masquerading as a tumor. A,** T1 axial image of the thigh. This patient was referred for work-up of a tumor (painless mass) in the anterior thigh. The rectus femoris muscle is enlarged focally, and there is a defect within it (*arrow*), indicating a grade II muscle strain (tear), rather than a tumor mass. **B,** T1 sagittal image of the thigh, with fat suppression after gadolinium enhancement. The gap in the muscle (*arrow*) from the tear is seen again. Hyperemia surrounds the torn muscle. No mass is evident. This patient was a runner, which is typically the inciting event for (often painless) tears of this muscle.

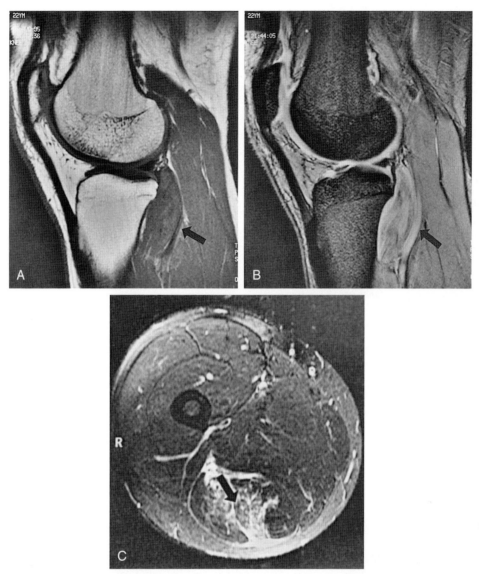

Figure 3-20 **Grade I muscle strains. A,** T1 sagittal image of the knee. The popliteus muscle (*arrow*) is enlarged, and the feathery fat pattern is absent compared with adjacent muscles. **B,** T2* sagittal image of the knee. High signal within the enlarged popliteus muscle (*arrow*) has a feathery pattern from interstitial edema or hemorrhage, and there is perifascial edema anterior and posterior to the muscle. **C,** STIR axial image of the thigh (different patient than in **A** and **B**). The interstitial feathery pattern from edema or hemorrhage is seen well in this grade I strain of the hamstrings (*arrow*). There is also intermuscular (perifascial) edema.

ances of most of these entities. Generally, *acute* muscle pathology manifests as high signal intensity on *STIR* or fat-saturated *T2W* images (edema, hemorrhage), whereas *chronic* muscle pathology typically results in fatty atrophy that is evident as high signal intensity on *T1W* images. As a result, MRI is exquisitely sensitive to muscle abnormalities, but is usually nonspecific. Because of this, it is important to have a list of differential diagnoses available when a muscle abnormality is encountered on MRI (eg, the abnormalities listed in the outline for this chapter). Clinical findings and biopsy of abnormal tissue play important roles in making a specific diagnosis when abnormalities are proved by MRI, and MRI is useful in directing where a biopsy specimen should be obtained.

Abnormal muscle may have a normal, increased, or decreased size. As mentioned previously, there may be fatty replacement, manifested as high signal intensity in the

muscle on T1W images, or there may be areas of high signal intensity on T2W images. A focal mass within muscle is another manifestation of disease.

MUSCLE TRAUMA

Traumatic muscle injuries are extremely common and can be divided into indirect muscle injuries, direct muscle injuries, and miscellaneous muscle injuries. Usually, traumatic injuries are imaged to assess the exact cause of pain and the extent of the injured area.

Indirect Muscle Injuries (Box 3-6)

Indirect muscle injuries include (1) delayed-onset muscle soreness (DOMS) and (2) strains (muscle tears). When the force of a contracting muscle exceeds the load placed on it, the muscle shortens, and this is called *concentric action* (eg,

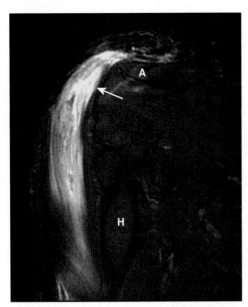

Figure 3-21 **Grade II muscle strain.** STIR oblique coronal image of the shoulder. There is diffuse high signal compatible with edema or hemorrhage or both within the deltoid muscle after an injury. There also is an area of focal disruption of the muscle fibers (*arrow*) compatible with a grade II strain. A, acromion; H, humeral shaft.

the action of the biceps when lifting a weight). Conversely, *eccentric action* is when a muscle lengthens or stretches as it contracts (eg, the action of the biceps when lowering a weight). Concentric contractions produce fatigue, whereas eccentric contractions are responsible for indirect muscle injuries with muscle strains (partial or complete muscle tears).

Injuries often occur along the myotendinous junction and are generally sports related.[9-11] Muscles at highest risk for indirect injuries are muscles that span two joints and are eccentrically activated, such as the biceps femoris, gastrocnemius, and rectus femoris muscles in the lower extremity.

Delayed-Onset Muscle Soreness. DOMS refers to stiff muscles. We all have experienced this problem, which begins hours or days after participating in an unaccustomed exertional activity. Symptoms peak 2 to 3 days after the activity. Serum creatine kinase levels are elevated because of the myonecrosis that is present, and although there is ultrastructural damage to the contractile elements of muscle, no irreversible damage is done. Training prevents or reduces DOMS.

MRI is never done to diagnose DOMS because we all are familiar with what it is, and it poses no diagnostic dilemma. We might inadvertently image a patient, however, who happens to have DOMS for unrelated reasons. DOMS is in the differential diagnosis for a certain constellation of MRI findings, and that is the main reason to be aware of it.

T1W images show no abnormality with DOMS. On T2W images, increased signal intensity may be seen around the periphery of muscles or in the perifascial and intermuscular spaces in close proximity to the injured muscle (Fig. 3-18). This abnormal rim develops 3 to 5 days after the inciting event. A feathery interstitial pattern of increased signal intensity also may be evident throughout the entire muscle from the extracellular fluid that causes increased intramuscular pressure.

MRI abnormalities persist long after clinical symptoms abate and after creatine kinase levels return to normal; however, the abnormalities on MRI persist for the same

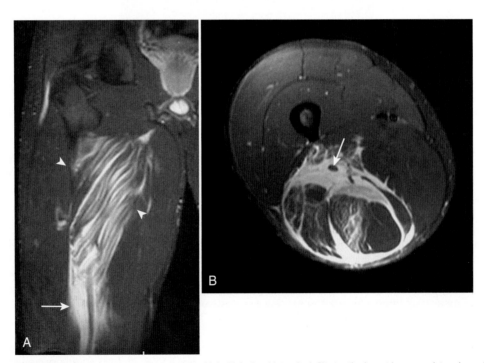

Figure 3-22 **Grade II muscle strain. A,** STIR coronal image of the thigh. High signal intensity infiltrates the hamstring musculature (*arrowheads*) in this college football player who felt a "pop" while running. Note the focal disruption of muscle fibers along the myotendinous junction (*arrow*). **B,** STIR axial image of the thigh. Intramuscular high signal intensity is seen as extensive fascial fluid, which surrounds the sciatic nerve (*arrow*).

period that biopsy-proved ultrastructural damage is identified.[12] Findings may take weeks to resolve on MRI.

Muscle Strains. Strains are muscle tears, either partial or complete, that result from a sudden event during eccentric muscle contraction. DOMS and certain types of muscle strains can have identical appearances on MRI, but the history serves to distinguish the two entities. Muscle strains occur with an acute onset during activity versus delayed onset of symptoms for DOMS. Muscles can absorb more energy and be protected from muscle strains by warming up and stretching; these activities have no protective effect for DOMS.

Muscle strains are the most frequent injuries in sports. Powerful, eccentric muscle contraction while a muscle is being stretched tears the muscle fibers at and just proximal to the myotendinous junction. With healing, the muscle can regain most of its strength. Until full recovery, the muscle is at increased risk for a second injury because of the decreased strength and stiffness of the injured muscle. The myotendinous junction is the weakest point because it has less ability to absorb energy than either the muscle or the tendon. At the myotendinous junction, the muscle cells have multiple projections that form intervening recesses, into which collagen fibrils from the tendon insert. This ultrastructural arrangement allows for increased contact area between the muscle and tendon that helps to dissipate forces and lessen the risk of injury; however, the myotendinous junction remains the area most susceptible to injury.

One exception to muscle strains manifesting as an acute painful event relates to the rectus femoris muscle in the anterior thigh. Chronic repetitive stresses, usually in runners, may result in a nonpainful muscle strain that manifests as a palpable mass. Many of these patients come to medical attention for work-up of a tumor mass (Fig. 3-19).

Strains are divided into three grades. Grade I and grade II strains can be difficult to distinguish from each other, or from DOMS or a direct blow to muscle, on MRI. A grade I strain consists of tearing of only a few muscle fibers, with no loss of function or permanent defect in the muscle (essentially, the muscle was stretched). There is edema, which causes enlargement of the muscle; a feathery, interstitial pattern of increased signal intensity on T2W images; and

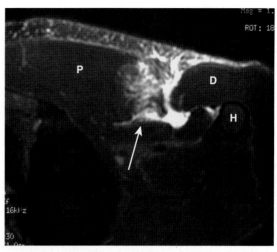

Figure 3-23 **Grade III muscle strain.** STIR axial image of the anterior chest wall. There is complete disruption of the pectoralis major muscle at the point indicated by the *arrow*. High signal hematoma fills the gap. D, deltoid muscle; H, humeral shaft; P, pectoralis major muscle.

perifascial edema (Fig. 3-20). We rarely seem to do MRI for grade I strains, probably because the symptoms are not severe enough to warrant the imaging examination. A grade II strain is a larger partial tear of the muscle with some loss of muscle strength. On MRI, there is the same feathery increased signal intensity from edema and hemorrhage in muscle as in grade I strains; additionally, a focal, masslike lesion or stellate defect in the muscle may be found as the result of a focal disruption of muscle fibers, and perifascial edema or hemorrhage is evident between muscles (Fig. 3-21). A grade II strain has a myotendinous junction that is partially torn so that mild thinning, irregularity, or laxity of the tendon may be evident (Fig. 3-22). Hematoma involving the myotendinous junction is diagnostic of a grade II partial tear, indicating a true defect in the muscle tissue.

A grade III strain is a complete rupture of the muscle with near-complete loss of function (strength). MRI shows discontinuity of muscle and of the tendon traversing the muscle, retraction of fragments with wavy margins, and a hematoma that forms between the fragments (Fig. 3-23).[13,14]

BOX 3-7

Direct Muscle Injuries

Muscle Contusions
- Interstitial hemorrhage
- Intraparenchymal bleeding
- High signal on T2 with muscle fibers coursing through the abnormal area
- No focal defect; muscle may be enlarged

Hematoma
- Confined, masslike collection of blood
- No muscle fibers coursing through mass
- Focal, heterogeneous mass with muscle enlargement
- Signal of blood on T1 and T2 is age dependent

Myositis Ossificans
- Intramuscular granulation tissue that may ossify or calcify
- Acute (<8 wk)
  - Heterogeneous mass
  - T1: isointense to muscle
  - T2: mixed high and low signal lesion; surrounding high signal edema
- Chronic (>8 wk)
  - Variable appearance
  - Fatty marrow—T1 and T2: low signal rim, center isointense with fat
  - T1: diffuse, intermediate signal center
  - T2: slight increased signal in center
  - Low signal rim, all sequences

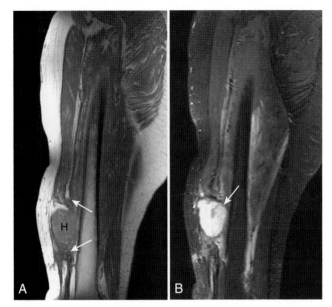

Figure 3-24 Muscle laceration with hematoma. **A,** T1 sagittal image of the thigh. The quadriceps muscles are divided at the site of a prior chainsaw injury (*arrows*). The intermediate signal mass at the site of the laceration represents a post-traumatic hematoma (H). **B,** STIR sagittal image of the thigh. The hematoma displays heterogeneous signal, especially in its dependent portion (*arrow*).

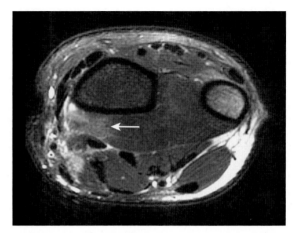

Figure 3-25 Intramuscular (interstitial) muscle hemorrhage (direct blow). Axial T2 image with fat saturation. Faint high signal intensity is present in the lateral aspect of the pronator quadratus muscle (*arrow*) compatible with interstitial hemorrhage (contusion) at the site of a direct blow from a lacrosse stick.

MRI is useful for defining the extent and location of the injury within the muscle, two features that have been correlated with prognosis for recovery.[15,16] Generally, muscle strains take a long time to heal because it is so difficult to put a muscle at rest for purposes of healing. Persistent contractions of the injured muscle can result in repeated microtears and hemorrhage months after the initial injury. For this reason, it is not unusual to see fatty infiltration from muscle atrophy secondary to disuse or injury, with superimposed blood products of varying age at the site of the muscle strain.

Direct Muscle Injuries (Box 3-7)

Direct trauma to muscles can be blunt or penetrating. Blunt trauma results in muscle contusions with intraparenchymal (interstitial) bleeds, hematoma formation, or myositis ossificans as a late sequela. Direct muscle lacerations can occur from penetrating injuries. Blunt trauma and lacerations produce hemorrhage within the muscle belly at the point of insult (Fig. 3-24). Lacerations also may cause denervation with muscle abnormalities distal to the injury.

Acutely, T2W images show increased signal intensity within the muscle as a result of the blood, edema, and inflammation that accompany bleeding from a contusion. This signal intensity may have a feathery pattern within the muscle. Hematomas less than 48 hours old are usually isointense to muscle on T1W images, whereas subacute hemorrhage characteristically has high signal intensity on T1W images.

Intramuscular (Intraparenchymal or Interstitial) Hemorrhage. When blood dissects freely between muscle fibers, it is referred to as *intraparenchymal, interstitial,* or *intramuscular hemorrhage.* The integrity of the muscle is not violated. Interstitial hemorrhage is caused by direct injury to the muscle with a contusion, usually by a blunt object, rather than from exertional physical activity (indirect muscle injury).

MRI shows focal muscle enlargement, which may be subtle, and separation of fibers by blood, creating a feathery pattern on T2W images (Fig. 3-25). T1W images may appear normal or may show the enlarged muscle. No focal collections of blood or edema are evident. Muscle fibers are always evident coursing through the abnormal area in the muscle. This hemorrhage can have an appearance similar to grade I muscle strains, and the history is necessary for reliable differentiation of the two entities.

Hematoma (Table 3-1). Injury to soft tissues can cause subcutaneous or intramuscular hematomas. Hematomas are confined collections of blood that are well defined with a masslike character and no interspersed muscle parenchyma or stroma.

The appearance of hematomas on MRI is highly variable, is age dependent, and follows the same changes as blood in the brain and spinal cord, but the time course tends to be longer and less predictable because of the lower oxygen tension outside of the brain (Figs. 3-26 and 3-27). What is considered isointense signal relative to the brain or cord can be considered as intermediate signal intensity in the extremities, similar to muscle. Hyperacute blood is rarely imaged, but is intermediate signal intensity on T1W (similar to muscle) and high signal intensity on T2W images. Acute blood has intermediate signal intensity on T1W and T2W images. Subacute hematomas show hyperintensity on T1W images, similar to that of fat. Early subacute hematomas have low signal intensity on T2W images, whereas older subacute hematomas and chronic hematomas have high signal intensity on T2W images. Chronic hematomas may have low signal intensity, especially around their rims, because of hemosiderin deposition and fibrosis (see Fig. 3-27).

Table 3-1   PROGRESSION OF HEMATOMA SIGNAL ON MRI

	Blood Products	T1 Signal	T2 Signal	Mnemonic	
Hyperacute	Oxyhemoglobin/serum	Intermediate	Bright	It Be	(IB)
Acute	Deoxyhemoglobin	Intermediate	Dark	IdDy	(ID)
Subacute, early	Intracellular methemoglobin	Bright	Dark	BiDdy	(BD)
Subacute, late	Extracellular methemoglobin	Bright	Bright	BaBy	(BB)
Chronic	Hemosiderin	Dark	Dark	Doo Doo	(DD)

The easiest way we know to remember the progression of signal intensity changes in hematomas that occurs over time is by using a sophisticated mnemonic imported by one of our fellows from Canada (who clearly had nothing better to do on those long, cold northern nights): "**It Be IdDy BiDdy BaBy DooDoo**." This phrase helps to organize the sequence of events: I, intermediate signal; B, bright signal; and D, dark (low) signal; and the bold letters in the phrase refer to the signal intensity on T1W and T2W images in each of the five stages of hematoma progression (hyperacute, acute, early subacute, late subacute, and chronic) (see Table 3-1).

There often is heterogeneity of the hematoma, probably from repeated bleeding from recurrent injury, because placing muscles at rest is difficult (Fig. 3-28; see Figs. 3-26 and 3-27). Fat and subacute blood can cause high signal intensity on T1W images in the musculoskeletal system and could have a similar appearance; fat-suppressed images allow differentiation of fat (which suppresses) from blood (which does not).

With healing, scarring with fibrosis is produced along with muscle regeneration. The amount of fibrosis produced can be monitored with MRI examinations and predicts whether full tensile strength and functional recovery would occur. Chronic scar tissue and fibrosis have low signal intensity on all MRI pulse sequences. A defect in muscle from a tear may eventually fill in with fat, rather than fibrosis (Fig. 3-29).

Hemorrhage Into Tumor. The presence of a hematoma in or between muscle may be the manifestation of bleeding into a necrotic soft tissue tumor, rather than simply being a benign post-traumatic hematoma (Fig. 3-30). It can be difficult sometimes to determine if a hematoma exists within or between muscles because intermuscular masses may sig-

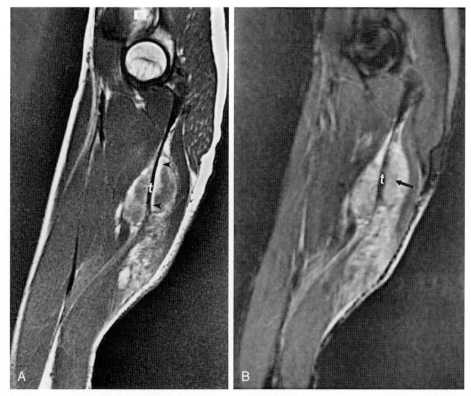

Figure 3-26 **Hematoma with blood at different stages. A,** T1 sagittal image of the thigh. There is a hematoma surrounding the biceps femoris tendon (t) from a large grade II muscle strain. The outer rim of the hematoma (*arrowheads*) has high signal from late subacute blood products. The inner portion of the hematoma is intermediate signal. **B,** STIR sagittal image of the thigh. The hematoma around the biceps femoris tendon (t) has a heterogeneous pattern. The areas that were high signal on T1 remain high signal on STIR (late subacute blood). Some of the area that was intermediate signal on T1 became high signal on STIR (hyperacute blood), and other areas were intermediate on T1 and remained low signal on STIR (*arrow*) (acute blood).

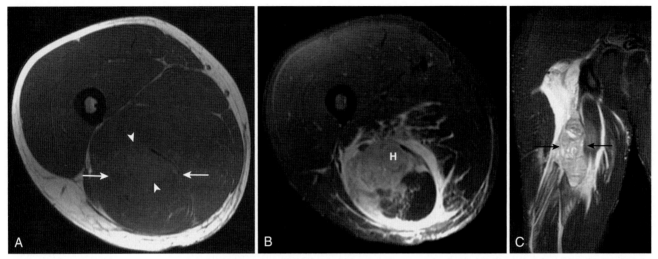

Figure 3-27 Hematoma with blood at various stages (same patient as Fig. 3-22). **A,** T1 axial image of the thigh. The biceps femoris muscle is enlarged (*arrows*) and contains faintly increased signal intensity adjacent to its tendon (*arrowheads*). **B,** STIR axial image of the thigh. Masslike tissue replaces the normal muscle architecture at the site of intramuscular hematoma formation (H). **C,** STIR coronal image of the thigh. Note the heterogeneous signal within the hematoma (*arrows*) indicating blood products of various ages. The extent of the hematoma is better defined in this imaging plane.

nificantly displace and thin overlying muscle so that the appearance in both circumstances is very similar. If the history is inconsistent so that the patient reports minimal trauma, but a large hematoma is present, or if there is any solid-appearing component in the hematoma, one must suspect a soft tissue sarcoma and evaluate it by other means, such as angiography or biopsy. Other helpful signs to differentiate a hematoma from a hemorrhagic neoplasm are that neoplasms do not have complete or partial tears of the tendon, and the mass effect of the neoplasm causes displacement of the tendon, rather than abnormal signal surrounding it, the latter finding being more typical of a traumatic hematoma at the myotendinous junction.

Myositis Ossificans. Blunt trauma to muscle can cause myositis ossificans, which is a circumscribed mass of granulation tissue that may calcify or ossify with time. If the trauma is not recalled, and no calcification is seen on radiographs, this entity is generally not thought of, and patients undergo a work-up for a soft tissue mass.

The MRI appearance depends on the histology and the stage of evolution of the lesion (Fig. 3-31).[17] Generally, the appearance varies and is nonspecific, and it can be confused with a soft tissue tumor, especially early on. Acute lesions less than 2 months old are isointense to muscle on T1W images and mixed signal (mainly high signal) intensity on T2W images, especially centrally, because of proliferating

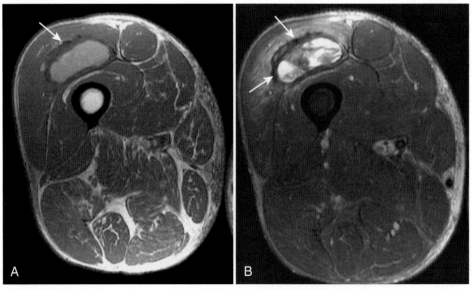

Figure 3-28 Chronic hematoma. **A,** T1 axial image of the thigh. Diffusely increased signal is seen within this quadriceps hematoma surrounded by a thick rim containing foci of low signal intensity (*arrow*). **B,** STIR axial image of the thigh. The internal blood products show more pronounced heterogeneous signal intensity, and the marginal low signal intensity is more apparent (*arrows*), typical of a chronic hematoma with fibrosis and hemosiderin deposition.

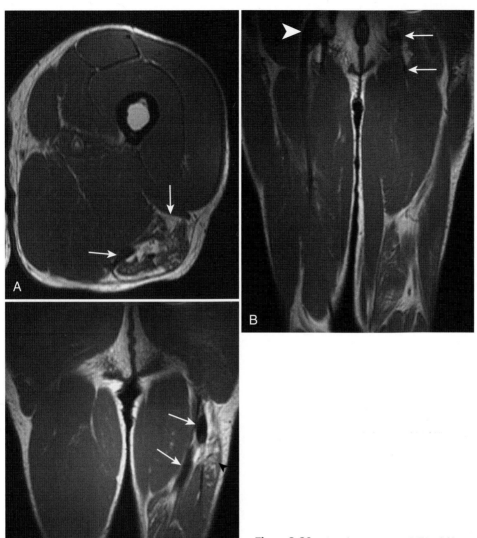

Figure 3-29 **Chronic muscle tear. A,** T1 axial image of the thigh. Focal fatty atrophy of the biceps femoris muscle is evident (*arrows*). **B,** T1 coronal image of the thighs. The proximal hamstring tendon is absent (*arrows*), compatible with a prior tear. Compare the normal tendon on the right (*arrowhead*). **C,** T1 coronal image of the thighs. The thickened, retracted tendon is evident (*arrows*) adjacent to the area of muscle atrophy (*arrowhead*).

cellular fibroblasts and myofibroblasts. There may be a large area of surrounding edema.

Lesions of myositis ossificans more than 8 weeks old may have two different patterns on MRI: (1) central signal intensity that is isointense with fat on T1W and T2W images, representing bone marrow surrounded by a low signal intensity rim of lamellar bone, or (2) diffuse intermediate signal intensity on T1W images from fibrosis that is slightly high signal intensity on T2W images. Edema generally is not present surrounding the mass after the first few weeks postinjury. Radiographs and computed tomography can be helpful in making the specific diagnosis of myositis ossificans if it is unclear on MRI.

Miscellaneous Traumatic Injuries

Compartment syndromes and fascial herniation of muscle are considered here. Denervation of muscle and

rhabdomyolysis may occur from trauma, but are discussed elsewhere.

Compartment Syndromes (Box 3-8)**.** Acute traumatic compartment syndrome can affect the calf after trauma with a fracture. Compartment syndrome occurs when hemorrhage or edema within closed fascial boundaries leads to increased pressure with compromise of the circulation. MRI can show the extent of edema and rhabdomyolysis because necrotic muscle is much higher signal intensity than normal muscle on T2W images. This is a surgical emergency, and MRI generally does not play a role in the work-up of this entity.

In chronic compartment syndrome, muscles are atrophied and may be densely fibrotic. Calcification of the involved muscle compartment may exist, and this is especially common in the peroneal compartment. A chronic

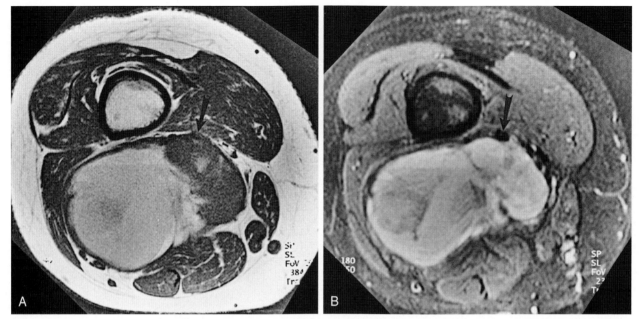

Figure 3-30 Hemorrhage into a tumor. **A,** T1 axial image of the distal thigh. There is a large mass posteriorly with high signal throughout most of it, indicating blood. There is a tendon displaced by the hemorrhagic mass (*arrow*). **B,** STIR axial image of the distal thigh. The posterior mass is heterogeneous, but mainly high signal, and consistent with blood. The displaced tendon is seen (*arrow*). This initially was diagnosed elsewhere as a hematoma and left alone for 1 year. The patient came to see our orthopedists because the mass did not decrease in size. The fact that the blood does not surround the tendon is a good clue that this is not a traumatic hematoma. The medial portion of this mass (on the side where the tendon is displaced) is actually solid, and a synovial sarcoma was shown at biopsy.

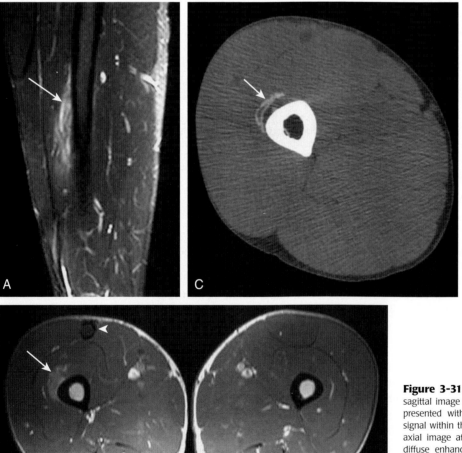

Figure 3-31 Myositis ossificans. **A,** T2 fat-saturated sagittal image of the thigh. This college basketball player presented with thigh pain. There is diffusely increased signal within the vastus intermedius muscle (*arrow*). **B,** T1 axial image after IV gadolinium administration. There is diffuse enhancement within that portion of the muscle (*arrow*). **C,** Axial computed tomography scan of the thigh (obtained subsequently). Mature shell-like ossification is present at the site of the MRI abnormality (*arrow*) compatible with a diagnosis of myositis ossificans.

Exertional Compartment Syndrome. During intense activity, extracellular free water increases in the affected muscles, particularly in concentrically exercised muscles. This increased intramuscular fluid leads to increased pressure in the anatomic compartment that contains the muscles. MRI can show this normal, exercise-induced phenomenon, which causes no changes on T1W images, but shows increased signal intensity on T2W images immediately after exercise. The signal intensity returns to baseline by 10 minutes after cessation of exercise. The increased signal intensity is seen diffusely throughout the affected muscles.[18]

Intramuscular pressure increases more than normal in some patients after exercise and does not quickly return to baseline. Such changes may lead to an acute or chronic exertional compartment syndrome, requiring fasciotomy for cure. Chronic exertional compartment syndromes are difficult to diagnose because symptoms abate between episodes of exertion. Intramuscular wick pressure measurements before and after exercise may be useful for diagnostic purposes, but it is an invasive test, and pressure criteria for the diagnosis are not universally accepted.

On MR images, exertional compartment syndromes are characterized by swelling within a compartment, which manifests as intramuscular diffuse high signal intensity on T2W images (Fig. 3-33). Performing the MRI examination immediately after a provocative exercise may be necessary. Failure of the edematous muscles to return to a baseline normal appearance by 15 to 25 minutes after the completion of exercise is diagnostic.

compartment syndrome may rarely lead to calcific myonecrosis. There is typically a remote history of trauma, usually several decades before the development of calcific myonecrosis. Patients have a painless mass, usually in the calf. The mass consists of liquefied necrotic muscle surrounded by a thin shell of calcification (Fig. 3-32). Peripheral peroneal nerve damage commonly is associated with this condition. MRI is useful for showing the anatomic extent of the abnormalities and the extent of muscle loss that exists.

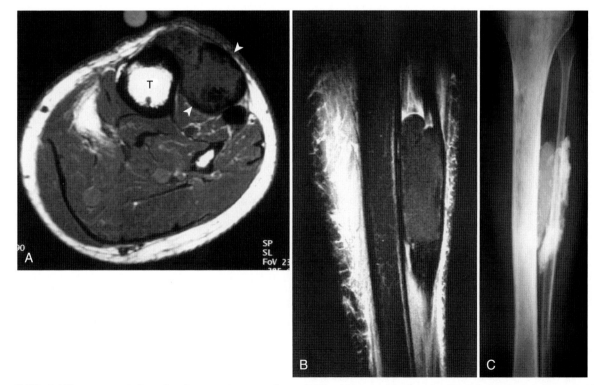

Figure 3-32 **Calcific myonecrosis from chronic compartment syndrome. A,** T1 axial image of the lower leg. The patient presented with a palpable mass. There is enlargement of the anterior compartment muscles with a masslike area of intermediate signal intensity bordered by a thick, low signal intensity rim (*arrowheads*). T, tibia. **B,** STIR coronal image of the lower leg. The mass shows similar signal characteristic along with diffuse edema within the soft tissues of the calf. **C,** Anteroposterior radiograph of the lower leg. The mass is shown to contain extensive, mature calcification, compatible with calcific myonecrosis.

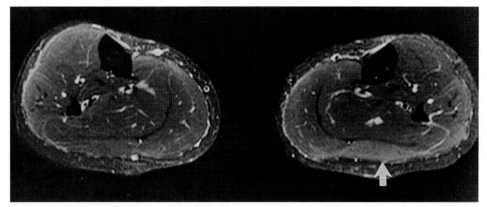

Figure 3-33   Exertional compartment syndrome. STIR axial image of the calves. There is diffuse intramuscular high signal in the lateral head of the left gastrocnemius muscle 30 minutes after provocative exercise (*arrow*). The T1 images were normal, as were the STIR images obtained before exercise (not shown). Postexercise muscle edema normally disappears within about 10 minutes of the activity.

Fascial Herniation of Muscle. Muscle can herniate through a traumatic fascial defect and manifest clinically as a soft tissue mass (Fig. 3-34). The lesions are usually asymptomatic, although pain or cramping may occur with activity. It sometimes is difficult to show the mass during the MRI examination without contracting the muscle by placing the foot in dorsal and plantar flexion, but this may lead to motion and degraded images. Very short pulse sequences during muscle contraction may show muscle tissue protruding in the region of the patient's palpable mass. The mass may disappear on images obtained without muscle contraction. MRI can confirm the diagnosis by showing normal muscles with no mass, even though the herniated muscle is not shown on the study. In other cases, the muscle remains herniated at all times and is not significantly affected by muscle contraction; the diagnosis is easier to make in this circumstance.

Occasionally, a defect in the low signal intensity fascia through which the muscle herniates can be seen by MRI. This is a traumatic injury and most commonly is seen in the anterior lower leg or thigh in athletes, may be multiple, and usually is asymptomatic.

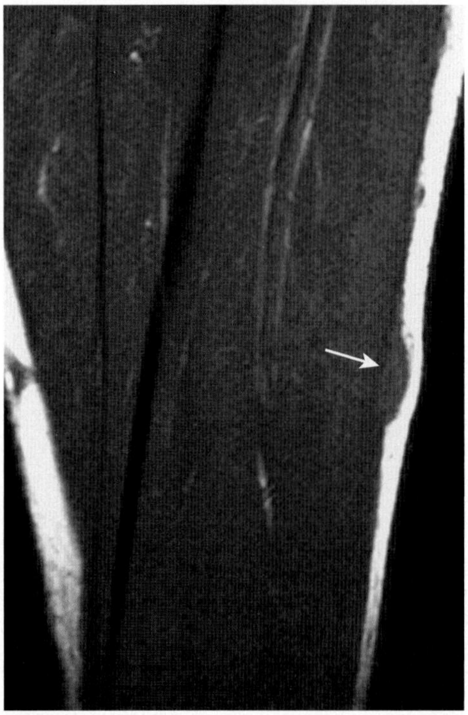

INFLAMMATORY MYOPATHIES

Bacterial or viral pyomyositis, necrotizing fasciitis, sarcoidosis, and the autoimmune idiopathic inflammatory polymyopathies all are unusual diseases that may affect muscle. MRI has proved to be useful for evaluating these conditions.[19]

Pyomyositis (Box 3-9)

Infection of muscle may be introduced either during a penetrating injury or by hematogenous spread and must be

Figure 3-34   Muscle herniation. T1 coronal image of the calf. There is a soft tissue mass (*arrow*) protruding into the subcutaneous fat at the site of a painless, palpable abnormality. The signal intensity followed that of muscle on all pulse sequences, and this represents herniation of the peroneus longus muscle through fascia.

BOX 3-9

Infection

Pyomyositis
- Penetrating injury or hematogenous
- Rare; usually in immunocompromised host
- Nonspecific MRI with high signal on T2 images in and around muscle

Necrotizing Fasciitis
- Infection of intermuscular fascia, pyomyositis rarely associated
- Severe systemic toxicity, high mortality
- Difficult clinical distinction from cellulitis, which affects only subcutaneous fat
- MRI
- T2: increased signal between muscles; possible increased signal in muscles (from hyperemia)
- Easy distinction from cellulitis that shows strandlike abnormal signal (low on T1, high on T2) limited to subcutaneous fat

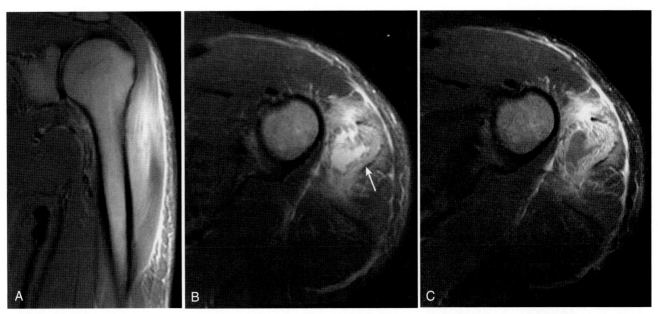

Figure 3-35 **Pyomyositis. A,** STIR coronal image of the shoulder. There is diffuse edema within the deltoid muscle of this immunocompromised patient. **B,** STIR axial image of the shoulder. A thick-walled focal fluid collection is present within the muscle, compatible with an intramuscular abscess (*arrow*). **C,** T1 axial image with fat saturation after IV gadolinium administration. There is a lack of central enhancement within the abscess with prominent enhancement of its irregular wall and adjacent soft tissues.

considered as a cause for abnormal size and signal intensity in musculature by MRI.

Bacterial myositis is unusual except in immunocompromised hosts, such as transplant patients and patients with acquired immunodeficiency syndrome.

Pyomyositis generally occurs where there was blunt trauma, with a coexisting source in the body for bacteremia, usually in someone who is immunocompromised.[20] There is diffuse muscle involvement, sometimes with a focal abscess (Fig. 3-35). Nothing specific is seen on MRI in pyomyositis. There is increased signal intensity throughout the affected muscle on T2W images. The muscle often is enlarged, and there may be high signal intensity fluid in fascial planes surrounding the abnormal muscle.

Muscle abscesses are fluid-filled cavities that are bright on T2W images, with a thick rim (Box 3-10). The center does not enhance with intravenous (IV) contrast material, whereas the rim typically does. Such a pattern is typical of an abscess, but it may be seen in other entities, including ischemic foci in muscle and necrotic soft tissue tumors.

BOX 3-10

Rim Enhancement of Focal Muscle Lesion

MRI
- Low signal on T1
- High signal on T2
- Rim enhancement postcontrast

Differential Diagnosis
- Abscess
- Necrotic tumor
- Ischemic foci (diabetics)

Necrotizing Fasciitis

Necrotizing fasciitis is a rare, rapidly progressive infection characterized by extensive necrosis of subcutaneous tissue and the fascia between muscles, and usually accompanied by severe systemic toxicity (see Box 3-9). The mortality rate is greater than 70% if not recognized and appropriately treated.

Early clinical recognition of necrotizing fasciitis may be difficult, and the differentiation between this entity and cellulitis may be impossible on clinical grounds. Cellulitis involves infection of only subcutaneous fatty tissue and can be treated adequately with antibiotics in most cases. Necrotizing fasciitis requires early surgical intervention in addition to antibiotics. Early fasciotomy and débridement in necrotizing fasciitis have been associated with improved survival compared with delayed surgical exploration.

Before MRI, the only way to diagnose necrotizing fasciitis was at the time of surgery, when no resistance to probing was discovered in the fascial planes between muscles. MRI is able to make the differentiation between cellulitis and necrotizing fasciitis in a noninvasive manner and constitutes a legitimate reason for an emergency MRI examination (Figs. 3-36 and 3-37).[21,22]

The MRI appearance in necrotizing fasciitis is that of high signal intensity and thickening between muscles along deep fascial sheaths on T2W images. The adjacent muscles also may have high signal intensity secondary to hyperemia and edema from the adjacent inflammatory process. Contrast-enhanced images show high signal intensity on T1W images in fascial planes because of the hyperemia associated with the infection; occasionally, muscle abscesses or focal necrotic tissue with ring enhancement also can be seen. Generally, there is no need to do contrast-enhanced imaging for this

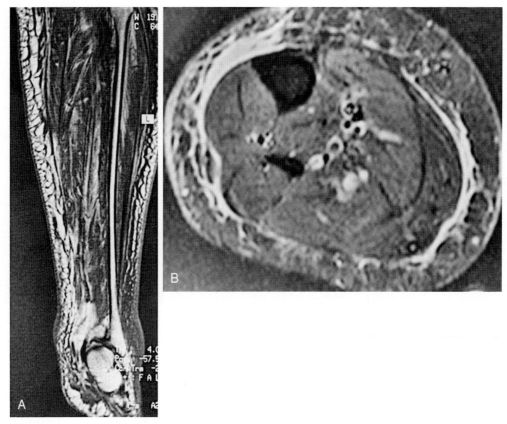

Figure 3-36   Cellulitis. **A,** T1 coronal image of the calf. There is a low signal reticular pattern throughout the subcutaneous fat from edema as the result of cellulitis. **B,** STIR axial image of the calf. The reticular edema pattern in the subcutaneous fat becomes high signal on this sequence. Of key importance is that there is no high signal in or between muscles.

diagnosis, especially because muscle pyomyositis is rarely associated with this disease.

MRI has a high sensitivity for detecting necrotizing fasciitis and showing its extent, but the findings are nonspecific. This lack of specificity is not a real problem, however, because the clinical setting in conjunction with the typical MRI appearance allows the diagnosis to be made, even though the MRI findings are seen in other entities.

Idiopathic Inflammatory Polymyopathies

The common diseases among the idiopathic inflammatory polymyopathies are polymyositis and dermatomyositis. Active myositis shows increased signal intensity on T2W images, which is more conspicuous with fat-suppression techniques (Fig. 3-38). Burned-out disease shows fatty replacement of muscles that is high signal intensity on T1W images.

Muscle involvement is typically nonuniform in these diseases, and MRI is useful to direct a biopsy to an abnormal muscle early in the disease process to make a diagnosis. Non–image-guided biopsies can have a 25% false-negative rate because the needle is in abnormal muscle only by chance.[23-25]

When disease is established, increased weakness in these patients can be from several sources, such as an inflamma-

tory flare involving the muscles (which responds to steroid therapy), a steroid-induced myopathy, or progressive muscle atrophy. MRI is useful to distinguish among these possibilities.

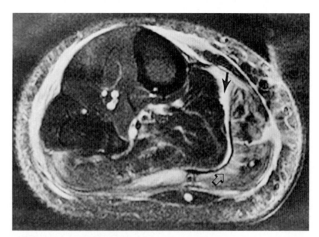

Figure 3-37   Necrotizing fasciitis. STIR axial image of the calf. There is edema in the subcutaneous fat. There is also high signal between muscles (*solid arrow*) in deep fascial planes, and diffuse interstitial edema in the gastrocnemius muscle (*open arrow*) from hyperemia and edema as a result of the adjacent fascial infection.

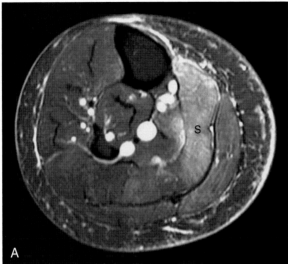

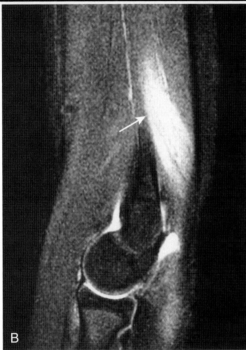

Figure 3-38 Idiopathic inflammatory polymyopathies. A, STIR axial image of the lower leg. There is patchy high signal within multiple muscles, most prominent in the medial portion of the soleus muscle (S) in this patient with known polymyositis. **B,** STIR sagittal image of the elbow. A focal area of diffusely increased signal intensity is evident within the triceps musculature (*arrow*). This child presented with elbow pain and a skin rash. Subsequent biopsy of the rash revealed dermatomyositis.

PRIMARY MUSCLE DISEASES

Dystrophies and Myopathies

Muscular dystrophies and congenital myopathies can sometimes be differentiated on the pattern of muscle involvement. Duchenne's muscular dystrophy tends to have symmetrical involvement progressing from proximal to distal, whereas myotonic dystrophy tends to progress from distal to proximal.[26,27]

MRI can show the pattern of muscle involvement, which may help to confirm a diagnosis; MRI also can be valuable

---

> **BOX 3-11**
> **Fatty Atrophy of Muscle**
>
> - High signal intensity on T1 images
> - Differential diagnoses
>   - Denervation
>   - Burned-out dermatomyositis or polymyositis
>   - Disuse
>   - Muscular dystrophies
>   - Congenital myopathies

in guiding a biopsy to an involved muscle. Similarly, MRI can identify muscles that are selectively spared by the disease process and can be used for muscle transfer operations. MRI more accurately depicts progression of disease than serum enzyme levels.

Early in the disease, MRI generally shows increased signal intensity on T2W images as a result of edema and inflammation in the abnormal muscle. Atrophy of the muscle is the predominant finding late in the disease, and high signal intensity from fatty infiltration of the atrophied muscle is seen on T1W images.

DENERVATION (Boxes 3-11 and 3-12)

Muscles and the nerves that supply them can be considered as a single motor or neuromuscular unit. Damage to a nerve causes changes in the muscle supplied by that nerve. Several traumatic, vascular, congenital, metabolic, and infiltrative processes can disrupt the nerve supply to muscle.

The MRI changes after denervation follow a predictable course. Acutely, MRI may be normal. After about 2 weeks, extracellular water increases within muscle, resulting in increased signal intensity on T2W images, especially fat-suppressed images such as STIR (Fig. 3-39). This appearance tends to persist for about 1 year after the insult. If the nerve heals, the signal intensity returns to normal.[28] If reinnervation does not occur, fatty atrophy develops in the muscle, which is easily detected on T1W images as high signal intensity replacing muscle fibers (Fig. 3-40). These early and late changes in muscle are not specific, unless the pattern of muscle involvement correlates with a known nerve distribution, which would suggest the diagnosis.[29,30]

MRI can predict that a muscle would not be salvageable from reinnervation or nerve grafting by showing that the muscle has undergone fatty atrophy, which is irreversible at that point. MRI can be useful to map out muscles that are

---

> **BOX 3-12**
> **MRI Appearance of Denervation**
>
> - Acute (<2 wk)
>   - Normal signal in muscle
> - 1-12 mo
>   - High signal in affected muscles on T2 from extracellular, intramuscular edema
> - >12 mo
>   - High signal on T1 from fatty infiltration of atrophied muscle

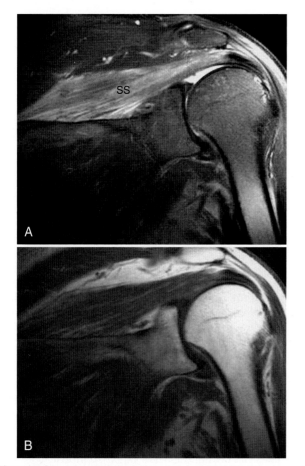

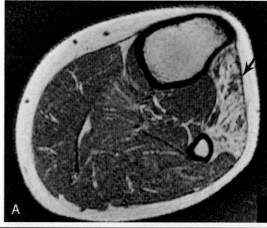

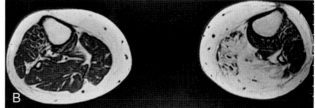

Figure 3-40 **Late denervation. A,** T1 axial image of the calf. The tibialis anterior muscle shows fatty atrophy (*arrow*) compared with the normal adjacent muscles. **B,** T1 axial image of the calves (different patient than in **A**). Profound fatty replacement of the posterior calf musculature on the left is evident from long-standing denervation in this diabetic patient.

Figure 3-39 **Subacute denervation. A,** Fat-saturated T2 oblique coronal image of the shoulder. Diffuse edema is present within the supraspinatus muscle (SS) in this patient who sustained a traumatic injury to the suprascapular nerve. **B,** T1 oblique coronal image of the shoulder. Mild, streaky increased signal is noted within the muscle indicating minimal fatty atrophy.

spared and could be used in muscle-tendon transfer operations. Occasionally, the cause of the neuropathy can be shown with MRI. MRI has several advantages over electromyographic evaluation: It is noninvasive, has excellent resolution, and can show pathology in muscles with aberrant or dual nerve supplies.

TUMORS (Table 3-2)

MRI frequently is used in the work-up of soft tissue masses, many of which arise in muscle. The MRI appearance of some masses, such as intramuscular lipomas, hematomas, and hemangiomas, is sufficiently specific so that no further tests are necessary. Most disorders have a nonspecific appearance, however, with increased signal on T2W images and variable enhancement. Although biopsy is often necessary, MRI is still useful to localize the most viable and diagnostic tissues for biopsy.

Common intramuscular tumors include hemangioma, lipoma, myxoma, neurofibroma, sarcoma, metastases, and lymphoma. Hemangiomas usually have serpiginous channels surrounded by fat that are diagnostic by MRI (Fig. 3-41). Lipomas also are easily diagnosed as masses with fat

signal intensity on all pulse sequences (Fig. 3-42). Lymphoma often infiltrates an entire muscle, but also may appear as a rounded mass (Fig. 3-43); metastases to muscle are rounded masses that often have large areas of edema surrounding them (Fig. 3-44).[31] Metastases from malignant melanoma may have a classic MRI appearance, consisting of focal lesions in muscle that are high signal intensity on T1W images and very low signal on STIR or T2W images, as a consequence of melanin (see Fig. 3-44). Soft tissue sarcomas are rounded masses, but they generally do not have edema surrounding them; they may become necrotic, and hemorrhage into the necrotic tumor could be mistaken for a traumatic hematoma. Myxomas have signal characteristics that resemble fluid (very low signal on T1W, and very bright signal on T2W images) with heterogeneous or only peripheral enhancement when contrast material is administered (Fig. 3-45). Intramuscular neurofibromas generally have a nonspecific appearance—a mass that is low signal on T1W images that is difficult to distinguish from normal surround-

Table 3-2 INTRAMUSCULAR TUMORS

Lesion	Discriminators
Hemangioma	Contains fat
Lipoma	Is fat
Myxoma	Many cyst characteristics
Sarcoma	No surrounding edema
Metastases	Often surrounding edema
Lymphoma	Infiltrates entire muscle
Neurofibroma	Target sign possible; resembles myxoma, but diffuse enhancement

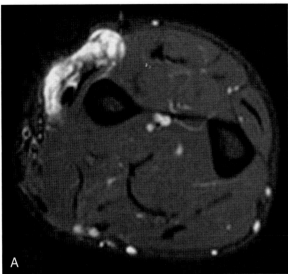

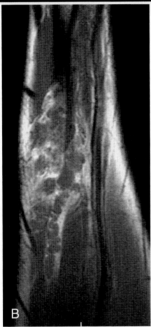

Figure 3-41 **Intramuscular tumor: hemangioma. A,** STIR axial image of the forearm. A mass showing lobular areas of high signal is present within the extensor carpi radialis brevis muscle. **B,** T1 coronal image of the forearm. The lobular components are separated by fat, an appearance compatible with a soft tissue hemangioma.

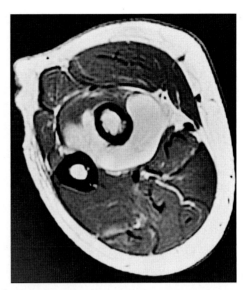

Figure 3-42 **Intramuscular tumor: lipoma.** T1 axial image of the forearm. There is a high signal fatty mass replacing most of the supinator muscle and extending between the radius and the ulna.

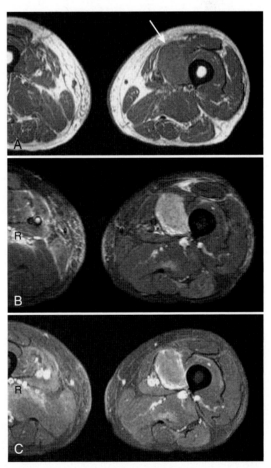

Figure 3-43 **Intramuscular tumor: lymphoma. A,** T1 axial image of the thigh. A masslike area of intermediate signal intensity is evident within the medial aspect of the vastus intermedius (*arrow*). **B,** STIR axial image of the thigh. The mass shows diffusely increased signal intensity. **C,** T1 axial image with fat saturation after IV gadolinium administration. There is prominent enhancement along the margins of the mass with less enhancement centrally. Note the nonspecific signal characteristics and well-defined margins of this intramuscular lymphoma.

ing muscle, and diffuse increased signal on T2W images. It has an MRI appearance similar to a myxoma, but there should be diffuse enhancement of a neurofibroma after IV gadolinium is given. A target sign may be evident on T2W or contrast-enhanced images (low signal in the center of the mass).

MISCELLANEOUS MUSCLE ABNORMALITIES

Rhabdomyolysis

Many entities may cause massive destruction of muscle with increased serum levels of creatine kinase enzyme, including

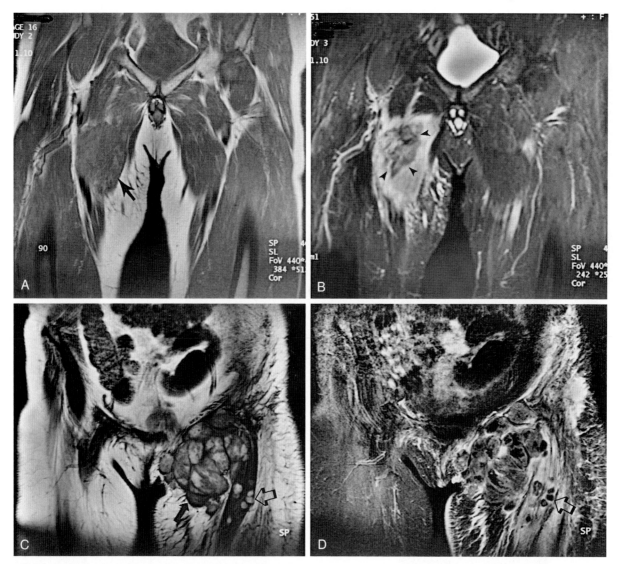

Figure 3-44 **Intramuscular tumor: metastases. A,** T1 coronal image of the pelvis. A mass is in the right adductor muscles (*arrow*). **B,** STIR coronal image of the pelvis (same patient as in **A**). The mass is heterogeneous and intermediate to high signal (*arrowheads*). The mass is surrounded by a large amount of high signal edema. This was metastatic transitional cell cancer from the bladder. **C,** T1 coronal image of the pelvis (different patient than in **A** and **B**). A mass of enlarged lymph nodes is present in the left groin. Several rounded high signal masses are evident in the left sartorius muscle (*open arrow*). **D,** STIR coronal image of the pelvis (same patient as in **C**). The intramuscular masses in the sartorius (*open arrow*) and several focal areas in the enlarged lymph nodes demonstrate profoundly low signal intensity. In addition, there is edema in the sartorius muscle surrounding the focal lesions. These masses are from metastatic malignant melanoma, and the signal intensity changes are typical for that tumor.

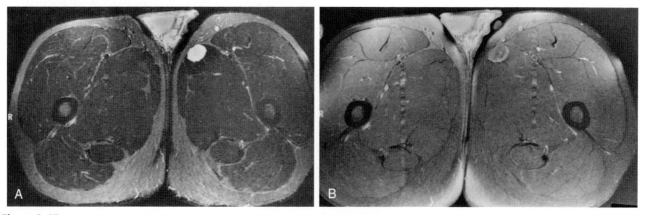

Figure 3-45 **Intramuscular tumor: myxoma. A,** STIR axial image of the thighs. There is a very high signal mass in the left adductor musculature. **B,** T1 contrast-enhanced axial image of the thighs with fat suppression. This myxoma shows peripheral enhancement.

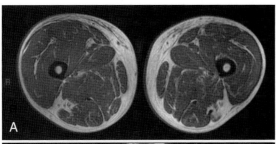

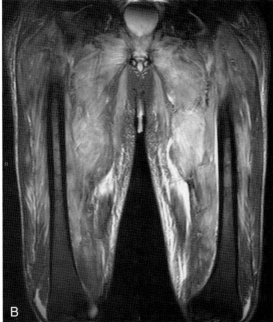

Figure 3-46   **Rhabdomyolysis. A,** T1 axial image of the thighs. No abnormality is evident in this patient with a history of lipid therapy with statin and fibrate drugs. **B,** STIR coronal image of the thighs. Diffuse, high signal intensity is seen throughout the thigh musculature compatible with extensive rhabdomyolysis.

- Common in diabetes and sickle cell anemia
- Diabetic muscle infarction
  - Severe pain with or without swelling/mass
  - Normal white blood cell count
  - Thigh involved in 80%; calf involved in 20%
  - Bilateral in one third of patients
- MRI appearance
  - T1: muscle swelling, obliteration of fat planes
  - T2: diffuse intramuscular and intermuscular increased signal
  - Contrast: diffuse enhancement of affected area or ring enhancement of necrotic foci

massive trauma, prolonged immobilization, vascular ischemia, excessive exercise, drug or alcohol overdose, and metabolic disorders such as hypokalemia, among others. The involved muscles show diffuse increased signal intensity on T2W images resulting from edema, necrosis, and hemorrhage (Fig. 3-46). T1W images are not helpful, and the muscles usually are not enlarged.[32]

Muscle Infarction (Box 3-13)

Muscle ischemia is particularly common in diabetics and patients with sickle cell anemia. Ischemic changes are very painful and result in edema with focal and diffuse areas of increased signal intensity in and surrounding muscle on T2W images.[33,34]

Diabetic muscle infarction occurs from thrombosis of medium and small arterioles in patients with atherosclerosis and poorly controlled diabetes. Clinical symptoms consist of severe pain with or without swelling or a mass. The white blood cell count is normal. More than half of patients have coexistent diabetic nephropathy, neuropathy, and retinopathy.

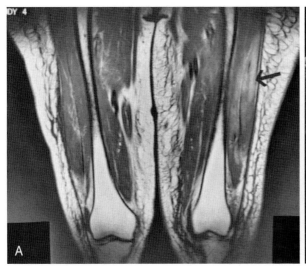

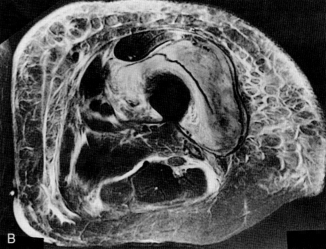

Figure 3-47   **Muscle infarction. A,** T1 coronal image of the thighs. Both thighs are abnormal, but the findings are much more pronounced on the left. There is subcutaneous edema with a reticular pattern. The muscles are enlarged, and high signal in a left thigh muscle (*arrow*) indicates hemorrhage from the muscle infarction in this diabetic patient. **B,** STIR axial image of the left thigh. Subcutaneous edema with reticular high signal is present diffusely. There is increased signal within the vastus musculature, and intermuscular septa show high signal as well.

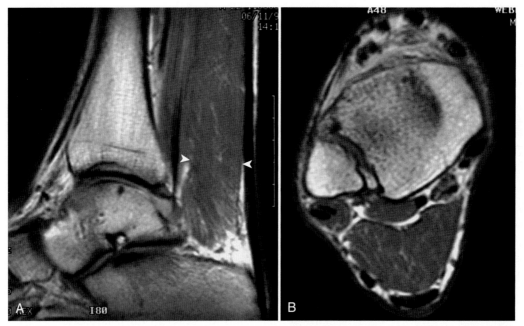

Figure 3-48   Anomalous muscle. A, T1 sagittal image of the ankle. This is a basketball player who presented with a pre-Achilles mass. Intermediate signal intensity tissue with fatty striations is present within the pre-Achilles fat (*arrowheads*), an appearance compatible with skeletal muscle, in this case, an accessory soleus muscle. **B,** T1 axial image of the ankle. The accessory muscle fills the pre-Achilles space.

The thigh, especially the vastus musculature, is involved most commonly (~80%); the calf is next most frequently affected (~20%). The ischemia may start in the calf and progress to the thigh. There is bilateral involvement in more than one third of cases.

MRI shows diffuse enlargement of several muscles, and more than one compartment often is involved (Fig. 3-47). The intermuscular fatty septa may be obliterated, and subfascial edema often is evident. On T2W images, there is increased signal intensity diffusely in and between muscles. There may be foci of hemorrhage. Gadolinium administration shows diffuse enhancement, but there also may be focal areas of rim enhancement, probably from hyperemia around an area of infarcted or necrotic muscle.

The diagnosis is not specific based on MRI alone, but in conjunction with the clinical history, a specific diagnosis often can be made. If there is any question about the diagnosis, percutaneous biopsy for culture and histology can be performed.

Accessory Muscles

Accessory muscles may be an incidental finding on MRI examinations; they also may manifest clinically as a mass or cause compression of an adjacent nerve. Accessory muscles occur in many locations throughout the body. The diagnosis of an accessory muscle is easy with MRI because the signal intensity and feathery texture are identical to other adjacent muscles (Fig. 3-48).

Radiation, Surgery, and Chemotherapy

Lesions in the extremities that are treated with surgery, local radiation therapy, or chemotherapy often develop diffuse high signal intensity in the muscle and subcutaneous fat with the typical feathery appearance in muscle on T2W images (Fig. 3-49). These findings are nonspecific, but they should not be confused with persistent or recurrent tumor because it is a common "normal" finding after treatment. Only the presence of a rounded mass should be of concern for persistent or recurrent tumor in the site of previous surgery or radiation. Often, a mass at a surgical site is a hematoma or seroma, rather than tumor; this can be determined by administering IV contrast material to determine if the mass is cystic or solid.

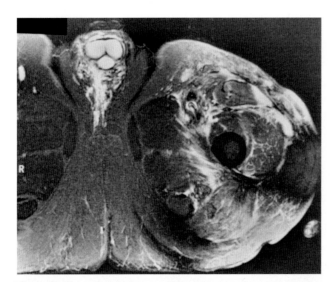

Figure 3-49   Radiation changes. STIR axial image of the proximal thigh. There is diffuse intramuscular and subcutaneous high signal. This man received radiation and surgery for a tumor in this region. These findings are expected after therapy. The lack of a round, high signal mass essentially excludes recurrent tumor.

REFERENCES

1. Tehranzadeh J, Ashikyan O, Anavim A, Tramma S. Enhanced MR imaging of tenosynovitis of hand and wrist in inflammatory arthritis. *Skeletal Radiol* 2006; 35:814-822.

2. Zeiss J, Saddemi SR, Ebraheim NA. MR imaging of the quadriceps tendon: normal layered configuration and its importance in cases of tendon rupture. *AJR Am J Roentgenol* 1992; 159:1031-1034.

3. Erickson SJ, Cox IH, Hyde JS, et al. Effect of tendon orientation on MR imaging signal intensity: a manifestation of the "magic angle" phenomenon. *Radiology* 1991; 181:389-392.

4. Kannus P, Joaazsa L. Histopathological changes preceding spontaneous rupture of a tendon. *J Bone Joint Surg [Am]* 1991; 73:1507-1524.

5. Walz DM, Miller TT, Chen S, Hofman J. MR imaging of delamination tears of the rotator cuff tendons. *Skeletal Radiol* 2007; 36:411-416.

6. Chan TW, Dalinka MK, Kneeland JB, Chervrot A. Biceps tendon dislocation: evaluation with MR imaging. *Radiology* 1991; 179:649-652.

7. Ferran NA, Oliva F, Maffuli N. Recurrent subluxation of the peroneal tendons. *Sports Med* 2006; 36:839-846.

8. Zubler C, Mengiardi B, Schmid MR, et al. MR arthrography in calcific tendonitis of the shoulder: diagnostic performance and pitfalls. *Eur Radiol* 2007; 17:1603-1610.

9. Fleckenstein JL, Weatherall PT, Parkey RW, et al. Sports-related muscle injuries: evaluation with MR imaging. *Radiology* 1989; 172:793-798.

10. Shellock FG, Fukunaga T, Mink JH, Edgerton VR. Acute effects of exercise on MR imaging of skeletal muscle: concentric vs eccentric actions. *AJR Am J Roentgenol* 1991; 156:765-768.

11. Shellock FG, Fukunaga T, Mink JH, Edgerton VR. Exertional muscle injury: evaluation of concentric versus eccentric actions with serial MR imaging. *Radiology* 1991; 179:659-664.

12. Nurenberg P, Giddings CJ, Stray-Gundersen J, et al. MR imaging–guided muscle biopsy for correlation of increased signal intensity with ultrastructural change and delayed-onset muscle soreness after exercise. *Radiology* 1992; 184:865-869.

13. De Smet AA. Magnetic resonance findings in skeletal tears. *Skeletal Radiol* 1993; 22:479-484.

14. El-Khoury GY, Brandser EA, Kathol MH, et al. Imaging of muscle injuries. *Skeletal Radiol* 1996; 25:3-11.

15. Askling CM, Tengvar M, Saartok T, Thorstensson A. Acute first-time hamstring strains during high-speed running: a longitudinal study including clinical and magnetic resonance imaging findings. *Am J Sports Med* 2007; 35:197-206.

16. Cross TM, Givvs N, Jouang MT, Cameron M. Acute quadriceps muscle strains: magnetic resonance imaging features and prognosis. *Am J Sports Med* 2004; 32:710-719.

17. Kransdorf MJ, Meis JM, Jelinek JS. Myositis ossificans: MR appearance with radiologic-pathologic correlation. *AJR Am J Roentgenol* 1991; 157:1243-1248.

18. Amendola A, Rorabeck CH, Vellette D, et al. The use of magnetic resonance imaging in exertional compartment syndromes. *Am J Sports Med* 1990; 18:29-34.

19. Kuo GP, Carrino JA. Skeletal muscle imaging and inflammatory myopathies. *Curr Opin Rheumatol* 2007; 19:530-535.

20. Gordon BA, Martinez S, Collins AJ. Pyomyositis: characteristics at CT and MR imaging. *Radiology* 1995; 197:279-286.

21. Schmid MR, Kossmann T, Duewell S. Differentiation of necrotizing fasciitis and cellulitis using MR imaging. *AJR Am J Roentgenol* 1998; 170:615-620.

22. Rahmouni A, Chosidow O, Mathieu D, et al. MR imaging in acute infectious cellulitis. *Radiology* 1994; 192:493-496.

23. Conner A, Stebbings S, Hung NA, et al. STIR MRI to direct muscle biopsy in suspected idiopathic inflammatory myopathy. *J Clin Rheumatol* 2007; 13:341-345.

24. Hernandez RJ, Sullivan DB, Chenevert TL, Keim DR. MR imaging in children with dermatomyositis: musculoskeletal findings and correlation with clinical and laboratory findings. *AJR Am J Roentgenol* 1993; 161:359-366.

25. Schweitzer ME, Fort J. Cost-effectiveness of MR imaging in evaluating polymyositis. *AJR Am J Roentgenol* 1995; 165:1469-1471.

26. Murphy WA, Totty WG, Carroll JE. MRI of normal and pathologic skeletal muscle. *AJR Am J Roentgenol* 1986; 146:565-574.

27. Lie G-C, Jong Y-J, Chiang C-H, Jaw T-S. Duchenne muscular dystrophy: MR grading system with functional correlation. *Radiology* 1993; 186:475-480.

28. Wessig C, Koltzenburg M, Reiners K, et al. Muscle magnetic resonance imaging of denervation and reinnervation: correlation with electrophysiology and histology. *Exp Neurol* 2004; 185:254-261.

29. Fleckenstein JL, Watumull D, Conner KE, et al. Denervated human skeletal muscle: MR imaging evaluation. *Radiology* 1993; 187:213-218.

30. Uetani M, Hayashi K, Matsunaga N, et al. Denervated skeletal muscle: MR imaging—work in progress. *Radiology* 1993; 189:511-515.

31. Williams JB, Youngberg RA, Bui-Mansfield LT, Pitcher JD. MR imaging of skeletal muscle metastases. *AJR Am J Roentgenol* 1997; 168:555-557.

32. Moratalla MB, Braun P, Fornas GM. Importance of MRI in the diagnosis and treatment of rhabdomyolysis. *Eur J Radiol* 2008; 65:311-315.

33. Chason DP, Fleckenstein JL, Burns DK, Rojas G. Diabetic muscle infarction: radiologic evaluation. *Skeletal Radiol* 1996; 25:127-132.

34. Jelinek JS, Murphey MD, Aboulafia AJ, et al. Muscle infarction in patients with diabetes mellitus: MR imaging findings. *Radiology* 1999; 211:241-247.

Peripheral Nerves

How to Image Nerves

- *Coils and patient position:* High-resolution images of the small peripheral nerves require the use of phased array surface coils. The large sciatic nerve can be evaluated without a surface coil, but better resolution is possible if surface coils are used. Positioning of the patient is determined by which nerve is being evaluated. Generally, the nerve can be imaged with the same surface coils, in the same position, and with the same field of view and section thickness as would be used for the nearby joint.

- *Image orientation:* If possible, images of nerves should be obtained in two orthogonal planes. Images that run parallel to the long axis of the nerve (in-plane or longitudinal images) are good for an overview of the course of the nerve and to detect displacement or enlargement. Partial volume artifacts may complicate interpretation of these images, however. Images obtained with the nerve in cross section (perpendicular to the long axis of the nerve) avoid partial volume averaging artifacts and allow for assessment of the size, configuration, signal intensity, and fascicular pattern of the nerve.

- *Pulse sequences:* T1W and some types of T2W fat-suppressed (turbo T2 with fat suppression or STIR) images are best to evaluate the peripheral nerves. T1W images show the anatomy adjacent to the nerve, and T2W sequences are good for showing pathology of the nerve and the fascicular pattern. MR neurography is a specialized technique for depicting the anatomy and course of a nerve similar to how a vessel is displayed on an MR angiogram. The technique requires attention to certain technical details and sophisticated postprocessing of the imaging data. Although the images obtained can be impressive, we do not currently use this technique because of its cumbersome requirements. A few references have been provided, however, for the interested reader.[1-3]

- *Contrast:* Contrast enhancement is generally of no added value in the evaluation of nerves with the exception of determining whether a mass is cystic or solid.

Normal and Abnormal

BACKGROUND

Electrophysiologic studies are a widely used invasive technique for detecting a conduction abnormality in peripheral nerves. These tests are sensitive, but they lack specificity and cannot show anatomic detail that would delineate the precise location of an abnormality, which often affects treatment planning. Microsurgery for repair of damaged nerves has gained acceptance, and a means of documenting the presence and extent of a nerve abnormality by direct visualization in a noninvasive way before surgery has value.

MRI is the best imaging technique available at this time to evaluate peripheral nerves. Given its ability to display directly the anatomy and course of a nerve and any compressive lesion or other adjacent pathology, MRI has proved to be a useful, complementary adjunct to electromyography.[4] Additionally, if a nerve is difficult to assess directly on a given scan, abnormal signal intensity within the muscles it supplies is important, indirect evidence of nerve pathology.[5]

Nerves are present on every MRI examination of an extremity, and it is important to be aware of the normal and abnormal appearances of peripheral nerves to be able to offer differential diagnoses for the findings.

NORMAL ANATOMY AND MRI APPEARANCE

The fundamental unit of a peripheral nerve is the axon, which may be either myelinated or unmyelinated, and which carries efferent (motor) or afferent (sensory) electrical impulses. Peripheral nerves have a mixture of myelinated and unmyelinated axons. A myelinated fiber exists when a

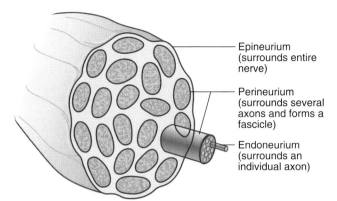

- Epineurium (surrounds entire nerve)
- Perineurium (surrounds several axons and forms a fascicle)
- Endoneurium (surrounds an individual axon)

Figure 4-1   **Anatomy of a peripheral nerve.** Fascicles are the smallest unit of a nerve visible on MRI. Fascicles are composed of several axons wrapped in a layer of perineurium. Several fascicles form a nerve, which is surrounded by a layer of epineurium. Individual axons are covered by endoneurium, but are not visible on MRI.

single axon is encased by a single Schwann cell; unmyelinated fibers result if a single Schwann cell encases multiple axons. Layers of Schwann cells form the myelin sheaths.[6,7]

Large peripheral nerves have three connective tissue sheaths that support and protect the axons and myelin sheaths (Fig. 4-1). The innermost sheath is the endoneurium, which invests each individual myelinated axon. Several axons, along with their Schwann cells and endoneurial sheaths, are bundled together into fascicles that are each wrapped in a dense sheath of perineurium, which serves as

a protective barrier to infectious agents or toxins. The third layer is the epineurium, which surrounds the entire peripheral nerve and protects the axons during stretching forces on the nerve. The connective tissue sheaths cannot be detected with MRI; nerve fascicles are the smallest units of nerves that currently can be identified.

Variable amounts of fat are present between fascicles, with more being present in nerves of the lower extremities than in nerves of the upper extremities. Large peripheral nerves contain about 10 fascicles. Each fascicle is composed of motor, sensory, and sympathetic fibers.

MRI shows normal nerves as round or oval in cross section (Fig. 4-2). The rodlike fascicles in the nerves are seen end on in transverse images as a stippled or honeycomb-like appearance, called a *fascicular pattern*. The fascicles are uniform in size and similar to, or slightly hyperintense to, muscle on T2W images. On T1W images, the fascicles are similar in signal intensity to muscle with intervening areas of relatively high signal similar to fat (see Fig. 4-2). The fascicular pattern is much easier to detect on T2W than on T1W images, especially in small nerves (Fig. 4-3).

Large nerves, such as the sciatic nerve, may have a striated appearance when imaged longitudinally (resembling strands of hair or spaghetti), with signal intensity typical of fat separating the fascicles (see Fig. 4-2). Nerves are easy to identify if they are surrounded by fat; however, if they lie adjacent to muscle, without intervening fat, they can be difficult to detect. T2W images in the axial plane give the best chance of identifying and following the nerve in the latter situation.

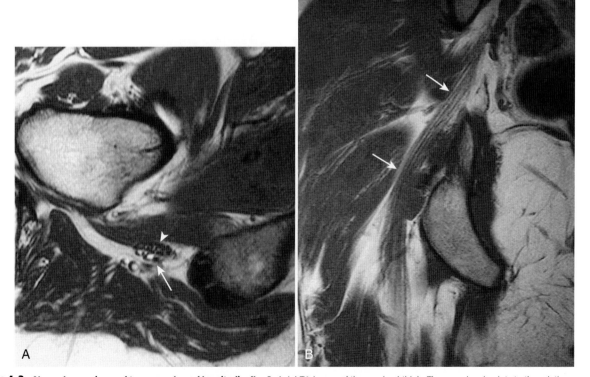

Figure 4-2   **Normal nerve imaged transversely and longitudinally. A,** Axial T1 image of the proximal thigh. The *arrowhead* points to the sciatic nerve, which is oval in cross section. The uniform stippled appearance is the result of intermediate signal fascicles separated by high signal fat. Note the small vessels along its posterior margin (*arrow*). **B,** Coronal T1 image of the pelvis. The sciatic nerve imaged longitudinally appears striated (looks like spaghetti or strands of hair) (*arrows*).

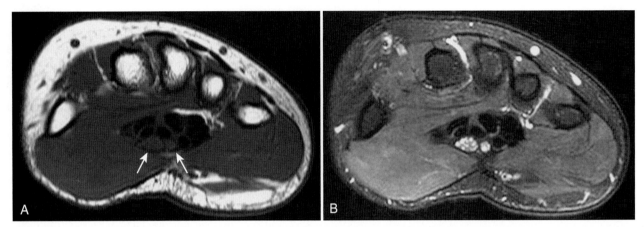

Figure 4-3 **Normal nerve with fascicles more evident on T2 than T1. A,** Axial T1 image of the hand. The individual fascicles of the two components (*arrows*) of this bifid median nerve, a normal variant, are difficult to see. **B,** Axial fat-saturated T2 image of the hand. The fascicles are much easier to identify with this sequence.

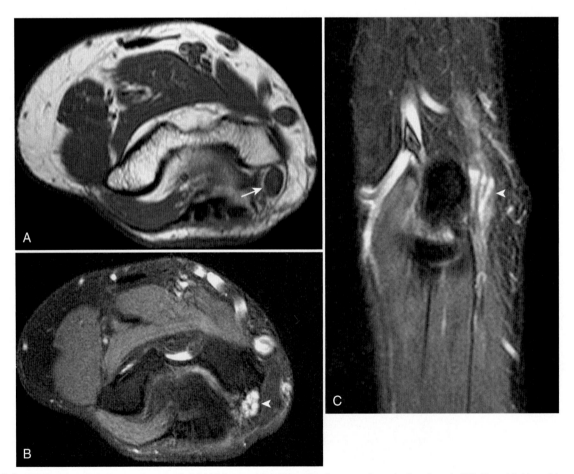

Figure 4-4 **MR features of an abnormal nerve. A,** Axial T1 image of the elbow. The ulnar nerve is markedly enlarged within the cubital tunnel (*arrow*) in this patient with symptoms of an ulnar neuropathy. **B,** Axial STIR image of the elbow. Abnormal, enlarged fascicles (*arrowhead*) are better shown within the nerve, compatible with an ulnar neuritis. **C,** Sagittal STIR image of the elbow. The prominent fascicles and focal enlargement of the nerve (*arrowhead*) are well shown in this plane as well.

ABNORMALITIES OF NERVES

Peripheral nerves can be affected by trauma, compression or encasement by an adjacent mass or infiltrative process, nerve entrapment syndromes, nerve sheath tumors, inflammatory neuritis, radiation, hereditary hypertrophic neuropathies, and inflammatory pseudotumors. Nerve problems are evaluated on MRI by directly imaging the nerve and looking for abnormalities in position, size, or signal intensity, and by looking for abnormalities that would indicate denervation in the muscles supplied by the nerve (Fig. 4-4).

Nerves are abnormal if they have diffuse or focal enlargement or diffuse or focal high signal intensity on T2W images. Determining if the signal intensity is too high is a subjective

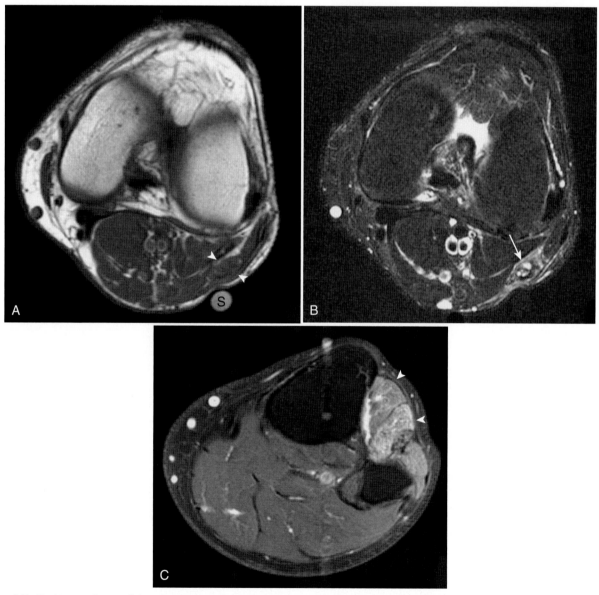

Figure 4-5 Post-traumatic nerve injury. **A,** Axial T1 image of the knee. The patient sustained a dog bite along the lateral knee at the level of the skin marker (S). Note the enlarged, amorphous-appearing common peroneal nerve at that level (*arrowheads*). **B,** Axial STIR image of the knee. Foci of increased signal are evident within the nerve (*arrow*) with an absence of normal fascicular architecture, compatible with injury. **C,** STIR axial image of the proximal calf. Associated edema is present within the anterior compartment muscles (*arrowheads*) compatible with denervation injury.

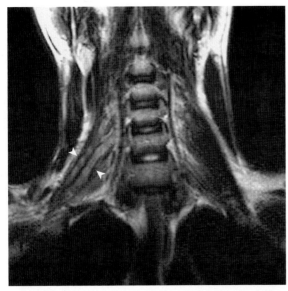

Figure 4-6 **Post-traumatic nerve injury: brachial plexus.** Coronal T2 image of the neck. The right C5 and C6 nerves in the proximal brachial plexus (*arrowheads*) are markedly enlarged in this patient with neurologic symptoms in the right upper extremity after trauma. At surgery, the nerves were found to be edematous and scarred together in this region.

exercise. Alteration in the fascicular pattern also may occur in an abnormal nerve (see Fig. 4-4). Fascicles in an abnormal nerve may be difficult to identify, even if enlarged or hyperintense. A nonuniform pattern of fascicles results, which is also virtually always accompanied by increased signal intensity in the nerve on T2W images. Nerves have limited ways to appear abnormal on MRI, and the findings are usually nonspecific, requiring a differential diagnosis, but MRI still adds significant information that can help in the management of patients (Box 4-1).

Traumatic Nerve Injury

Neurologic symptoms may be present after a nerve injury from disruption of axonal conduction, but the nerve remains intact (neurapraxia). MRI generally is not performed in this setting.

More severe trauma to nerves can result in partial or complete transection of the nerve. With an acute injury, MRI can show the precise location of the nerve abnormality because of the presence of high signal intensity edema on T2W images, and it can show the site of nerve disruption. The nerve may respond by forming a neuroma within the first year after the injury, which is sometimes painful.

Trauma to a nerve may result in a focal neuritis with nerve swelling and surrounding soft tissue edema in the acute setting; this appears as focal nerve enlargement with intraneural and perineural high signal intensity on T2W MR images (Fig. 4-5). Enlargement of the nerve can be recognized by comparing the caliber from proximal to distal because it should gradually decrease in size as images progress distally. Similarly, if both sides of the body are imaged (eg, in the spine or pelvis), a side-to-side comparison can be helpful for recognizing pathologic enlargement (Fig. 4-6).

Additionally, when a peripheral nerve is severely injured, the muscles it serves undergoes denervation changes, which

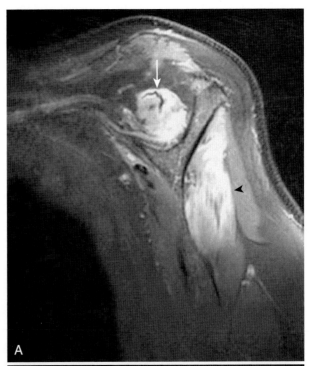

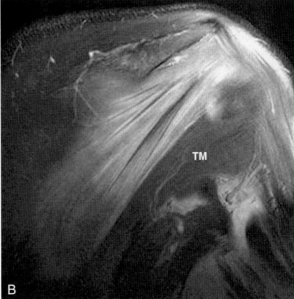

Figure 4-7 **Post-traumatic nerve injury: denervation changes in muscle. A,** Oblique sagittal STIR image of the shoulder. This patient sustained trauma to the shoulder. Diffusely increased signal within the supraspinatus (*arrow*) and infraspinatus (*arrowhead*) muscles is compatible with denervation changes related to suprascapular nerve injury. **B,** The high signal edema is well shown throughout the infraspinatus muscle. Note the absence of edema within the teres minor muscle (TM), which is innervated by the axillary nerve. The sharp demarcation between muscles supplied by different nerves is a useful imaging finding for identifying denervation injuries.

manifest on MR images as high signal intensity ("edema") on fat-saturated T2W images in the acute to subacute phases, and fatty atrophy (high signal on T1W images) later if the nerve does not regenerate. The detection of these signal abnormalities within muscles served by one nerve is a useful secondary sign of probable nerve injury, and the specific nerve can be evaluated more closely (Fig. 4-7).

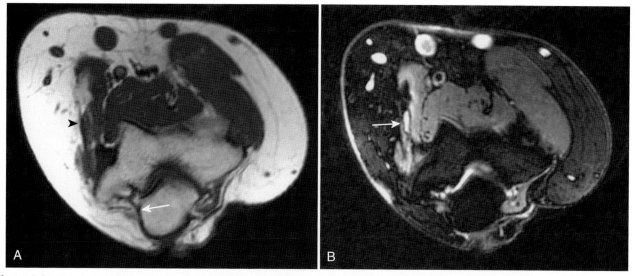

Figure 4-8 **Abnormal position of a nerve from surgical transposition. A,** Axial T1 image of the elbow. The ulnar nerve is not present in its usual position within the cubital tunnel (*arrow*). Instead, it is located far anterior to its normal position (*arrowhead*) where it is difficult to separate from adjacent muscle. This is not from an injury or subluxation, but from surgical transfer of the nerve to prevent chronic irritation. **B,** Axial fat-saturated T2 image of the elbow. The nerve is more easily identified on this T2W image (*arrow*) because of its high signal intensity.

Nerves can sublux over an adjacent bone; the ulnar nerve subluxing around the medial epicondyle of the humerus is a classic example. This subluxation may lead to stretching of the nerve, irritation from friction, and swelling of the nerve (neuritis) with increased nerve size and increased signal intensity seen on T2W images. A nerve in an abnormal location from subluxation or traumatic transection of a nerve must not be confused with surgical transposition of a nerve to a new anatomic location to avoid chronic irritation. Transfer of the ulnar nerve at the elbow is a standard surgical procedure that results in the nerve being positioned anterior to its usual location (Fig. 4-8).

Nerve Tumors

Neuromas. Neuromas frequently occur as a consequence of an injury with traumatic (or iatrogenic) transection of a nerve. These tumors may be painful and occur within 1 year of the injury. This phenomenon is well known in the setting of an amputation of an extremity, where a neuroma develops at the distal end of a severed nerve. There is no malignant potential for a traumatic neuroma, which simply represents the attempt of the nerve to repair by disorganized proliferation of cells in multiple directions.

A neuroma appears as a fusiform or bulbous mass of the nerve end with heterogeneous signal intensity, and there may or may not be strandlike regions (disorganized fascicular appearance) of low signal intensity interspersed in the mass. The normal nerve proximal to the mass can be detected entering the mass; if the nerve has not been completely transected, an exiting nerve may be seen distal to the mass. Chronic friction or irritation of an intact nerve also can result in a neuroma with fusiform swelling in a nerve that is not disrupted. A neuroma has intermediate signal intensity on T1W images and intermediate to high signal on T2W images. Diffuse enhancement of the mass can be expected after intravenous contrast administration (Figs. 4-9 and 4-10).

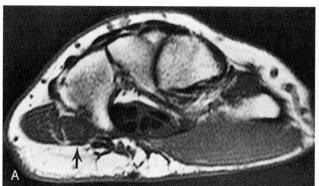
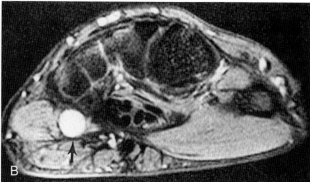

Figure 4-9 **Neuroma from chronic irritation. A,** Axial T1 image of the wrist. There is an intermediate signal mass (*arrow*) adjacent to the hook of the hamate that blends with the adjacent muscle. **B,** Axial T2* image of the wrist (same level as in **A**). A high signal round mass (*arrow*) is obvious on this sequence. This was a neuroma of the deep branch of the ulnar nerve, likely caused by chronic irritation against the hook of the hamate.

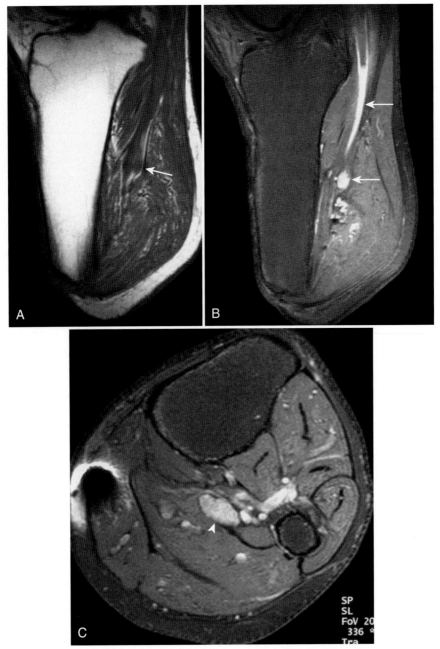

Figure 4-10 **Amputation neuroma. A,** T1 sagittal image of the proximal calf. The *arrow* points to an intermediate signal bulbous mass at the cut end of the posterior tibial nerve in this patient, who had a below-the-knee amputation 18 months previously and now has pain symptoms. **B,** Sagittal T1 fat saturation with contrast image, same location as in **A**. The nerve and distal bulbous neuroma enhance (*arrows*). **C,** Axial STIR image through neuroma of posterior tibial nerve. The nerve (*arrowhead*) is markedly enlarged, has high signal intensity, and is devoid of the normal fascicular pattern.

Neurofibroma and Neurilemoma (Box 4-2). Aside from post-traumatic neuromas, the tumors of significance that involve peripheral nerves are neurilemomas (also called *schwannomas*) and neurofibromas. These are benign lesions that are usually difficult or impossible to distinguish from each other; they often are lumped together by referring to them as *nerve sheath tumors*. The major difference between the two is that neurilemomas arise from the surface of a nerve, whereas neurofibromas arise centrally, with the nerve coursing through the tumor. Both entities have an association with neurofibromatosis, but most lesions are solitary

---

BOX 4-2

Nerve Sheath Tumors: Suggestive MRI Features

String Sign
- Fusiform mass with vertical, soft tissue "string" extending from either or both ends of the mass; the string represents normal entering or exiting nerve

Split Fat Sign
- Peripheral rim of fat surrounding mass, from displacement of fat in neurovascular bundle

Target Pattern
- T2 and postcontrast T1 MRI with low signal centrally and high signal in the periphery of the mass

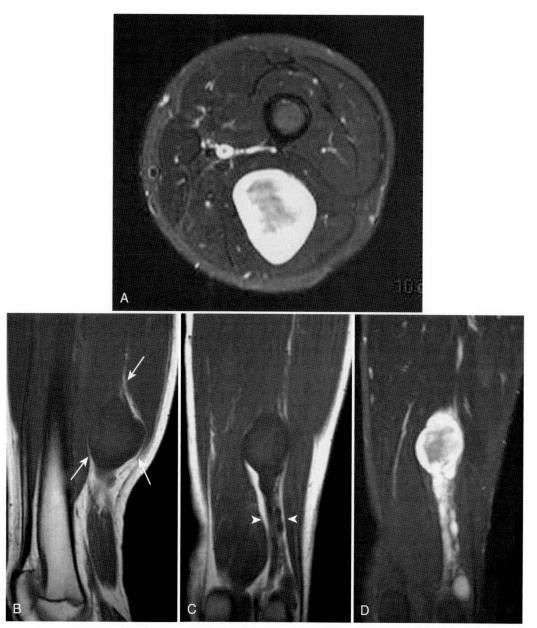

Figure 4-11 Neurofibroma: target sign, split fat sign, and string sign. **A,** STIR axial image of the mid thigh. There is a large high signal mass in the posterior thigh in this patient with a history of neurofibromatosis. Note the high signal margin surrounding the lower signal centrally ("target sign"). **B,** Sagittal T1 image of the thigh. Note the fat diverging around the margins of the mass (*arrows*) indicating its intermuscular location ("split fat sign"). **C,** Coronal T1 image of the thigh (same patient as in **A** and **B**). There is vertically oriented soft tissue (*arrowheads*) extending from the distal end of the mass related to additional, smaller neurofibromas, creating a "string sign." **D,** Coronal STIR image of the thigh. The individual tumors are more easily discerned on this image. Note the "target sign" in the large proximal mass.

and unrelated to that disease. Patients with neurofibromatosis tend to have multiple nerve sheath tumors or diffuse plexiform neurofibromas. Malignant degeneration rarely may occur; differentiation of benign from malignant nerve sheath tumors generally is impossible with MRI.

On MRI, both of these nerve sheath tumors appear as well-defined, smooth, fusiform-shaped masses. The mass is intermediate to low signal intensity on T1W images and generally shows a diffuse, increased signal intensity on T2W images. Nerve sheath tumors may become necrotic, with a cystic or hemorrhagic appearance; this occurs much more commonly with schwannomas than with neurofibromas.

Contrast enhancement is diffuse in the tumor, unless it has a necrotic or cystic center, or if the target sign is present (see later) (Fig. 4-11).

Three additional signs on MRI may be present and help to limit the differential diagnosis of a mass to a nerve sheath tumor, if identified (see Fig. 4-11)[7-9]:

1. String sign
2. Split fat sign
3. Target sign

The string sign consists of the appearance of a fusiform mass with a "string" of vertically oriented soft tissue extending from one or both ends of the mass. The string represents

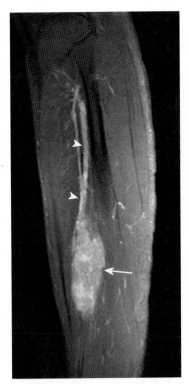

Figure 4-12 Pseudostring sign. Vertically oriented tissue appears to extend proximally from an enhancing fusiform mass (*arrow* and *arrowheads*) simulating a "string sign" of a nerve sheath tumor. The mass was a Ewing's sarcoma, and the vertically oriented tissue was the anterior tibial neurovascular structures.

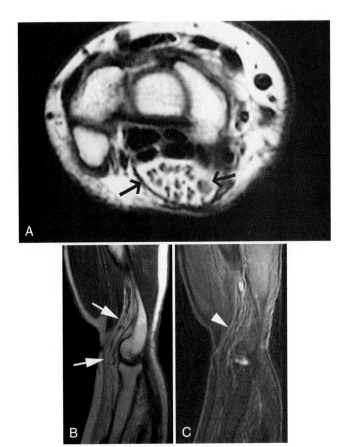

Figure 4-13 Fibrolipomatous hamartoma. A, T1 axial image of the wrist. The median nerve (*arrows*) is gigantic in the carpal tunnel. The fascicles are larger than normal, but otherwise normal in appearance and surrounded by normal high signal fat. This is typical of the appearance and location of a fibrolipomatous hamartoma. **B,** T1 sagittal image of the elbow. A similar lesion is present in a different patient involving the radial nerve (*arrows*). At surgery, an enlarged nerve with extensive fatty infiltration was found. **C,** T2 fat-saturated sagittal image of the elbow. The fascicles of the enlarged nerve show increased signal (*arrowhead*), whereas signal from the infiltrating fat is suppressed.

the normal entering or exiting nerve that is in continuity with the nerve sheath tumor. Masses that are not of neural origin may have features that mimic a nerve sheath tumor and must be carefully evaluated to avoid a mistake. Vessels adjacent to a mass may create an appearance similar to the string sign and lead to a misdiagnosis (Fig. 4-12).

The split fat sign describes the peripheral rim of fat that often is seen surrounding the margins of a nerve sheath tumor. The appearance of this rim of fat is thought to relate to the displacement of the fat that normally surrounds the neurovascular bundle, the site of origin of these lesions (see Fig. 4-11).

The target sign consists of low signal intensity centrally and high signal intensity peripherally on T2W and post–contrast-enhanced T1W images (see Fig. 4-11). The target pattern probably reflects the histology of these lesions, with peripheral myxomatous tissue and central fibrous tissue creating the signal characteristics. This sign has been described in neurofibromas, but it probably can occur in other nerve tumors.

Fibrolipomatous Hamartoma. Fibrolipomatous hamartoma is a rare lesion of major nerves and their branches. There is gradual infiltration of the nerve by fibrofatty tissue. These lesions occur in children or young adults. They can cause an enlarging mass, macrodactyly, and compression neuropathy. The hand is the site most commonly involved, especially the median nerve. MRI shows an enlarged nerve composed of tubular, serpentine-like,

longitudinal low signal intensity structures, representing the fascicles with perineural fibrosis, coursing through a nerve that has signal characteristics typical of fat (Fig. 4-13).[10]

Pseudotumors of Nerves. Ganglion cysts can develop in a nerve sheath and cause compression of the underlying nerve. The ganglion cyst has the same appearance as elsewhere, with low signal intensity on T1W images and high signal intensity on T2W images, frequently with lobulated margins and thin septations within the mass. If the ganglion follows a nerve, the diagnosis should be suggested. The peroneal nerve at the knee joint is most commonly affected (Fig. 4-14).

Morton's neuromas are not true neuromas or neoplasms of the nerve. Morton's neuromas cause severe pain between the toes, most commonly in the second and third web spaces, and they occur as a reaction to the plantar digital nerves in the foot being compressed and irritated between metatarsal heads, resulting in perineural fibrosis, neural degeneration, and inflammatory changes surrounding the nerve. Morton's neuroma manifests as a teardrop-shaped mass that projects

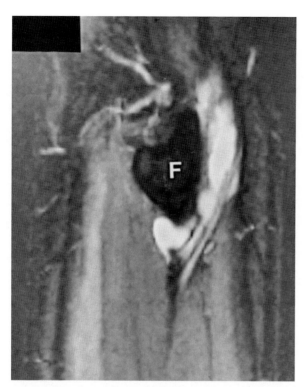

Figure 4-14   **Ganglion cyst of the peroneal nerve.** STIR sagittal image at the knee shows a high signal, lobulated, elongated mass wrapping around the neck of the fibula (F), following the distribution of the peroneal nerve. This is a ganglion cyst that caused compression of the nerve.

between and plantar to the metatarsal heads. The MRI appearance is delineated in detail in Chapter 16.

Compressive Neuropathy and Entrapment Syndromes

Compression or entrapment of a short segment of nerve at specific and predictable anatomic sites, as the nerves pass through openings in muscular or fibrous tissue or fibro-osseous tunnels, can cause symptoms that vary with the site

involved. MRI can be used to detect objective findings of nerve compression by demonstrating alterations in the size, signal intensity, or position of a peripheral nerve.[11-14] Osseous or soft tissue lesions that cause the compression neuropathy can be depicted, if present (Fig. 4-15). Findings of muscle denervation may be evident; when compression is acute, these findings consist of increased signal intensity on T2W images of the muscles innervated by the affected nerve (Fig. 4-16).[5] Denervation progresses to muscle atrophy with fatty infiltration on a more chronic basis, manifested by high signal intensity typical of fat infiltrating muscle on T1W images.[15]

Common sites of compression and entrapment neuropathies are as follows:

- Brachial plexus at insertion of anterior scalene muscle on first rib (scalenus anticus syndrome), or at the crossing of a cervical rib (cervical rib syndrome)
- Suprascapular nerve in the suprascapular or spinoglenoid notch of the scapula (suprascapular notch syndrome)
- Axillary nerve in the quadrilateral space of the axilla (quadrilateral space syndrome)
- Radial nerve in the axilla (sleep palsy), spiral groove of the distal humerus (from a fracture), or deep to the supinator muscle at the elbow (posterior interosseous nerve syndrome)
- Median nerve in the distal humerus deep to the ligament of Struthers, deep to the pronator teres muscle at the elbow (pronator syndrome), or in the carpal tunnel at the wrist (carpal tunnel syndrome)
- Ulnar nerve in the cubital tunnel of the elbow (cubital tunnel syndrome), or Guyon's canal in the wrist (ulnar tunnel syndrome)
- Sciatic nerve at the greater sciatic foramen in the pelvis (piriformis syndrome)
- Lateral femoral cutaneous nerve at the attachment of the inguinal ligament to the anterior superior iliac spine (meralgia paresthetica)
- Posterior tibial nerve in the tarsal tunnel of the hindfoot and ankle (tarsal tunnel syndrome)

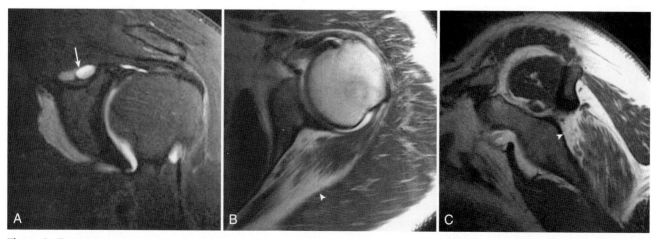

Figure 4-15   **Compressive neuropathy from a mass. A,** T2 fat-saturated oblique coronal image of the shoulder. A bilobed high signal paralabral cyst (*arrow*) extends into the suprascapular notch. **B,** T1 axial image of the shoulder. There is marked fatty atrophy of the infraspinatus muscle (*arrowhead*) indicating chronic compressive neuropathy of the suprascapular nerve. **C,** T1 oblique sagittal image of the shoulder again demonstrates profound atrophy of the infraspinatus muscle (*arrowhead*).

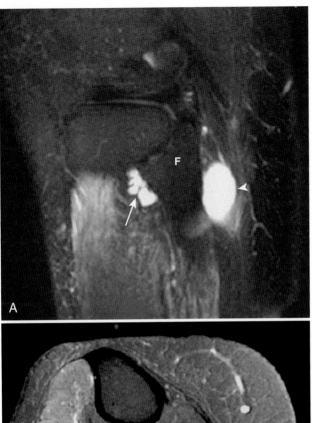

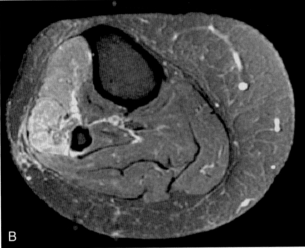

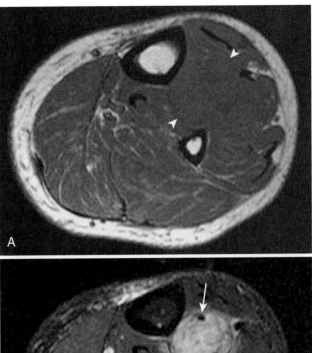

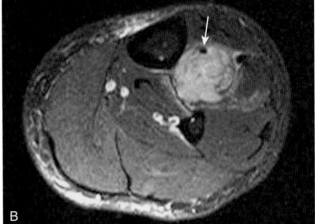

Figure 4-17 **Tumor encasing the neurovascular bundle. A,** T1 axial image of the calf. An intermediate signal intensity mass is present (*arrowheads*), but is difficult to distinguish from adjacent muscles. **B,** STIR axial image of the calf. The mass is more easily identified because of its increased signal, as is the anterior tibial neurovascular bundle (*arrow* points to the anterior tibial artery) that has been engulfed by this soft tissue sarcoma.

Figure 4-16 **Compressive neuropathy from a mass. A,** T2 fat-saturated sagittal image of the knee. A high signal mass shown to represent a ganglion cyst (*arrowhead*) lies posterior to the fibular head (F). Note the additional smaller ganglia along the anterior margin of the proximal tibiofibular joint (*arrow*). **B,** STIR axial image of the proximal calf. Diffuse edema within the anterior and peroneus muscles indicates an associated compressive neuropathy of the common peroneal nerve.

Miscellaneous Nerve Abnormalities

Tumor Encasement/Radiation Changes. Nerves may be encased or displaced by adjacent tumor, such as a primary carcinoma, lymphoma, or desmoid tumors, which can cause neurologic symptoms and pain. MRI can show the tumor and its relationship to nerves (Fig. 4-17). Patients who receive radiation therapy for a tumor may develop radiation-induced neuritis as an inflammatory reaction of the nerve to the radiation. The symptoms are not distinguishable from encasement by tumor. MRI shows if there is tumor present or not and can show increased signal intensity and enlargement of the nerves in the radiation portal on T2W images from radiation neuritis unrelated to tumor.

Inflammatory Neuritis. Nerves may become inflamed and symptomatic for unknown reasons. It is believed that this inflammation often is the result of a viral infection, and it is referred to as *idiopathic inflammatory neuritis.* There is often a history of a recent flulike syndrome that preceded the onset of neural symptoms. These acute neuromuscular disorders have not shown abnormalities of the nerves on MRI, but have shown abnormalities in the affected muscles.

Acute brachial neuritis, also called *Parsonage-Turner syndrome,* is a painful neuromuscular disorder that affects the shoulder with marked weakness and pain, and which probably is the result of a viral neuritis. The clinical symptoms may be similar to the many other causes of shoulder pain, and MRI may help to make the diagnosis. The findings are those of muscle edema with high signal intensity on T2W images, or of muscle atrophy with high signal intensity on T1W images in the supraspinatus, infraspinatus, or deltoid muscles (Fig. 4-18).[16]

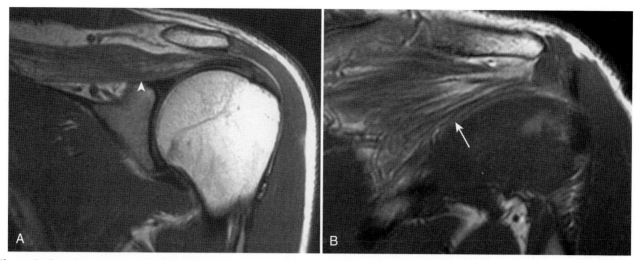

Figure 4-18   Inflammatory neuritis. **A,** T1 oblique coronal image of the shoulder. There is fatty infiltration of the supraspinatus muscle (*arrowhead*) without a tear of the rotator cuff, indicating a nerve abnormality. This patient had profound weakness and pain, and this was believed to be from a viral neuritis (Parsonage-Turner syndrome). **B,** T1 oblique coronal image of the shoulder. This image at a more posterior level shows similar, extensive fatty atrophy of the infraspinatus muscle as well (*arrow*), related to the brachial neuritis.

Unexplained Neuropathy. Focal or diffuse nerve abnormalities may be seen from an inflammatory pseudotumor of the nerve or from hereditary hypertrophic neuropathies (Charcot-Marie-Tooth disease, Dejerine-Sottas syndrome). The findings are nonspecific on MRI, consisting of nerve enlargement, heterogeneity in size of the fascicles, and hyperintense signal on T2W images.

REFERENCES

1. Filler AG, Maravilla KR, Tsuruda JS. MR neurography and muscle MR imaging for image diagnosis of disorders affecting the peripheral nerves and musculature. *Neurol Clin* 2004; 22:643-682.
2. Moore KR, Tsuruda JS, Dailey AT. The value of MR neurography for evaluating extraspinal neuropathic leg pain: a pictorial essay. *AJNR Am J Neuroradiol* 2001; 22:786-794.
3. Freund W, Brinkmann A, Wagner F, et al. MR neurography with multiplanar reconstruction of 3D MRI datasets: an anatomical study and clinical applications. *Neuroradiology* 2007; 49:335-341.
4. Bendszus M, Wessig C, Reiners K, et al. MR imaging in the differential diagnosis of neurogenic foot drop. *AJNR Am J Neuroradiol* 2003; 24:1283-1289.
5. Lisle DA, Johnstone SA. Usefulness of muscle denervation as an MRI sign of peripheral nerve pathology. *Australas Radiol* 2007; 51:516-526.
6. Maravilla KR, Bowen BC. Imaging of the peripheral nervous system: evaluation of peripheral neuropathy and plexopathy. *AJNR Am J Neuroradiol* 1998; 19:1011-1023.
7. Murphey MD, Smith WS, Smith SE, et al. Imaging of musculoskeletal neurogenic tumors: radiologic-pathologic correlation. *RadioGraphics* 1999; 19:1253-1280.
8. Kransdorf MJ, Murphey MD. *Imaging of Soft Tissue Tumors.* Philadelphia: Saunders; 1997.
9. Suh JS, Abenoza P, Galloway HR, et al. Peripheral (extracranial) nerve tumors: correlation of MR imaging and histologic findings. *Radiology* 1992; 183:341-346.
10. Cavallaro MC, Taylor JAM, Gorman JD, et al. Imaging findings in a patient with fibrolipomatous hamartoma of the median nerve. *AJR Am J Roentgenol* 1993; 161:837-838.
11. Kim S, Choi J-Y, Huh Y-M, et al. Role of magnetic resonance imaging in entrapment and compressive neuropathy—what, where, and how to see the peripheral nerves on the musculoskeletal magnetic resonance image, part 1: overview and lower extremity. *Eur Radiol* 2007; 17:139-149.
12. Kim S, Choi J-Y, Huh Y-M, et al. Role of magnetic resonance imaging in entrapment and compressive neuropathy—what, where, and how to see the peripheral nerves on the musculoskeletal magnetic resonance image, part 2: upper extremity. *Eur Radiol* 2007; 17:509-522.
13 Dunn AJ, Salonen DC, Anastakis DJ. MR imaging findings of anterior interosseous nerve lesions. *Skeletal Radiol* 2007; 36:1155-1162.
14. Ferdinand BD, Rosenberg ZS, Schweitzer ME, et al. MR imaging features of radial tunnel syndrome: initial experience. *Radiology* 2006; 240:161-168.
15. Sallomi D, Janzen DL, Munk PL, et al. Muscle denervation patterns in upper limb nerve injuries: MR imaging findings and anatomic basis. *AJR Am J Roentgenol* 1998; 171:779-784.
16. Helms CA, Martinez, S, Speer KP. Acute brachial neuritis (Parsonage-Turner syndrome): MR imaging appearance—report of three cases. *Radiology* 1998; 207:255-259.

Musculoskeletal Infections

How to Image Infection (Box 5-1)

Musculoskeletal infections affect bones, soft tissues, and joints. Infection often is considered a therapeutic emergency, and MRI is used to determine the presence or absence of disease and its extent. The MRI study should be directed to the site of involvement based on clinical grounds or where abnormalities on other imaging studies have been found. The coil used, the patient's position, the planes of imaging, and the field of view vary for each site.

- *Coils and patient position:* The patient is usually supine in the magnet, unless the region affected involves mainly the posterior soft tissues, such as the buttocks or posterior thoracic cage. Spine phased array coils are used for any portion of the spine; the body coil or, preferably, a large field-of-view phased array coil is used for the thorax, pelvis, and femora; and smaller surface coils are used for the other extremities and joints.
- *Image orientation:* The best imaging planes for the spine are sagittal and axial; for the pelvis, coronal and axial images are preferred; generally, axial and coronal images are used for lesions near the hip, foot, shoulder, and wrist; and lesions near the knee, ankle, and elbow are evaluated best with axial and sagittal images.
- *Pulse sequences and regions of interest:* In the spine, sagittal and stacked axial T1W, fast T2W, and post-gadolinium T1W images of the region of interest are obtained. In the pelvis and extremities, our routine protocols include T1, STIR, and postgadolinium T1W images.[1-4] Section thickness in the spine is 4 mm; in the pelvis, 7 mm; and in the extremities, 4 mm (or larger, depending on the volume to be covered).
- *Contrast:* Intravenous (IV) gadolinium routinely is used for diagnosing musculoskeletal infections. It allows differentiation of an abscess from cellulitis or phlegmon in the soft tissues, or an abscess from bone marrow edema

in the marrow space.[4] Gadolinium also increases the conspicuity of sinus tracts and sequestra.

Osteomyelitis

MRI allows for early detection of osteomyelitis, the extent of involvement, and the activity of the disease in cases of chronic osteomyelitis.[5,6]

DEFINITION OF TERMS (Box 5-2)

Sequestrum: A fragment of necrotic (dead) bone separated from living bone by surrounding granulation tissue is a sequestrum. This is seen on a radiograph as a dense bone fragment (sequestrum) surrounded by a radiolucency (granulation tissue); on MRIs, the sequestrum is a low signal intensity structure on T1W and STIR sequences, whereas the surrounding granulation tissue is intermediate to low signal intensity on T1W images and high signal intensity with STIR or T2W sequences (Fig. 5-1). With gadolinium, the granulation tissue is enhanced, whereas the sequestrum remains low signal intensity.

Involucrum: An envelope of thick, wavy periosteal reaction formed around the cortex of an infected tubular bone is known as the involucrum. It commonly is found in bones of infants and children with osteomyelitis. As the infection is controlled, the dead cortical bone is incorporated with the involucrum, forming a thickened cortex (see Fig. 5-1). On MRI, the ossified periosteal shell and the dead tubular cortical bone are low signal intensity on all pulse sequences; periosteal reaction and cortical bone are separated by linear intermediate to high signal intensity on T2W or STIR images (Fig. 5-2), until the periosteal reaction and cortical bone are incorporated.

BOX 5-1

MRI for Musculoskeletal Infections

Sequences
- T1
- STIR or fast T2
- T1 postcontrast with fat saturation

Imaging Planes
- Spine: axial and sagittal
- Pelvis, hip, shoulder, wrist: axial and coronal
- Knee, ankle, elbow: axial and sagittal
- Foot: axial, sagittal, and coronal

BOX 5-2

Definition of Terms

Cloaca: Defect in the periosteum created by infection
Involucrum: Thick sleeve of periosteal new bone surrounding dead cortical bone
Sequestrum: Fragment of dead bone surrounded by granulation tissue
Sinus tract: Channel extending from bone to skin surface, lined with granulation tissue
Fistula: Channel between two internal organs

Cloaca: An opening through the periosteum that permits pus from the infected bone to enter the soft tissues is called a *cloaca*. On MRI, the linear low signal intensity periosteum that is elevated from the cortical bone or the thickened cortex is interrupted by a high signal intensity gap (cloaca) on T2W images (see Fig. 5-1). On T2W images, the high signal intensity pus can be seen extending into the soft tissues from the cloaca and may form a sinus tract or abscess.[7]

Sinus Tract/Fistula: A sinus tract is a channel between an infected bone and the skin surface, whereas a fistula is a tract or channel between two internal organs. Sinus tracts and fistulae are lined by vascular granulation tissue, and they function as conduits for pus to flow away from the infected bone. On MRI, a sinus tract or fistula is linear low signal intensity on T1W images, best seen if the subcutaneous fatty tissues are not infiltrated with edema. On T2W images, the channel shows linear high signal intensity as a result of the granulation tissue

and pus (Fig. 5-3). The granulation tissue is enhanced after IV injection of gadolinium, and the channel is most conspicuous with a fat-suppressed T1W sequence after contrast enhancement.

Abscess/Phlegmon: A cavity filled with pus that is surrounded by a capsule and lined with granulation tissue is an abscess, whereas a phlegmon is a solid mass of inflammatory tissue. An abscess may be limited to the medullary bone, the cortex, the soft tissues, or more than one of these compartments (Fig. 5-4). On MRI, the abscess and the phlegmon are intermediate to low signal intensity on T1W and high signal intensity on T2W images. After IV injection of gadolinium, the rim of an abscess is enhanced, whereas the center of the mass that contains the pus remains low signal intensity. A phlegmon enhances diffusely.

Penumbra Sign: One imaging finding reported to be helpful in differentiating a subacute or chronic abscess from tumor has been called the *penumbra sign*.[8] This sign was originally described in cases of subacute osteomyelitis, but it has been found to be useful in identifying soft tissue abscesses as well. It consists of a thin,

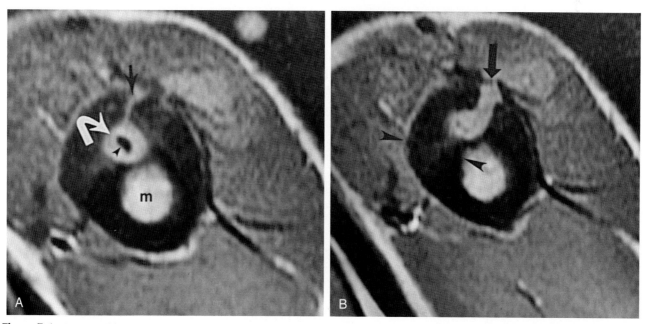

Figure 5-1 **Osteomyelitis: sequestrum, abscess, cloaca, periosteal new bone. A,** Spin echo–T2 axial image of the upper arm. There is high signal in the medullary cavity of the humerus (m) from osteomyelitis. A low signal sequestrum (*arrowhead*) is surrounded by high signal granulation tissue and pus (*curved arrow*). A high signal cloaca extends through the thickened cortex (*straight arrow*). **B,** Spin echo–T2 axial image of the upper arm. A cut adjacent to that in **A** shows the markedly thickened cortex (between *arrowheads*) formed by periosteal reaction/involucrum formation incorporated with the underlying cortex. A high signal linear cloaca extends through the cortex as well (*arrow*).

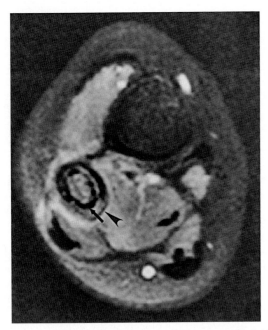

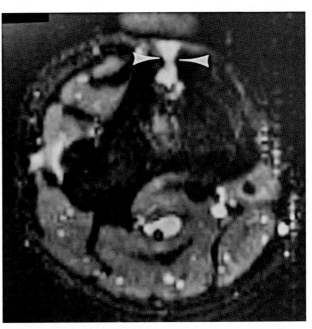

Figure 5-2   **Osteomyelitis: involucrum.** Fast T2 fat-suppressed axial image of the calf. The low signal linear periosteal reaction (involucrum) (*arrowhead*) and low signal cortical bone (*arrow*) are separated by high signal pus in this infected fibula in a child.

Figure 5-3   **Osteomyelitis: sinus tract.** STIR axial image of the calf. There is a linear high signal channel (between *arrowheads*) extending through the cortex of the tibia to the skin surface.

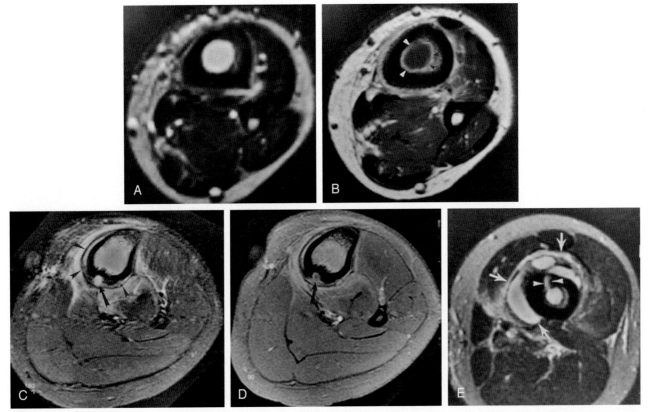

Figure 5-4   **Osteomyelitis: abscess. A** and **B,** Medullary abscess. **A,** Spin echo–T2 axial image of the calf. The medullary canal of the tibia is diffusely high signal. **B,** T1 contrast-enhanced axial image of the calf. There is a thin line of enhancing tissue (*arrowheads*) surrounding a low signal collection of pus in this abscess of the medullary cavity. **C** and **D,** Cortical abscess. **C,** STIR axial image of the calf. A round focus of high signal is present in the posterior cortex of the tibia (*arrow*), representing a cortical abscess. The medullary canal also demonstrates diffusely high signal from inflammation. The periosteum is elevated (*arrowheads*) from the cortical bone. **D,** T1 contrast-enhanced fat-suppressed axial image of the calf. The cortical abscess displays high signal peripherally with a low signal center that contains pus. The medullary canal and soft tissues surrounding bone all show enhancement, indicating there is no abscess in these locations, only inflammatory hyperemia. **E,** Soft tissue abscess. Spin echo–T2 axial image of the thigh. There is a focal area of high signal in the medullary canal of the femur from an abscess with a cloaca in the lateral femoral cortex (between *arrowheads*). A fluid collection surrounding a large portion of the femur (*arrows*) caused by a soft tissue abscess also is present.

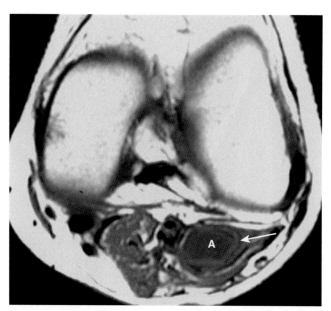

Figure 5-5 **Abscess: penumbra sign.** T1 axial image of the knee. A small abscess (A) is visible within the lateral head of the gastrocnemius muscle in this patient with pyomyositis. Note the intermediate signal intensity rim (*arrow*) ("penumbra sign") around the central low signal intensity fluid.

BOX 5-3
Routes of Bone Infection

Hematogenous
- Infants (<1 yr)
  - Metaphysis/epiphysis
- Children (1 yr to growth plate closure)
  - Metaphysis
- Adults
  - Epiphysis

Direct Implantation
- Puncture wounds
- Human/animal bites
- Open fractures
- Surgery

Contiguous Spread
- Infection starts in soft tissues
  ↓
  - Periostitis (periosteal involvement)
    ↓
  - Osteitis (cortical involvement)
    ↓
  - Osteomyelitis (marrow involvement)
- Reverse sequence from hematogenous spread

intermediate signal intensity rim along the periphery of a bone or soft tissue abscess on unenhanced T1W images (Fig. 5-5). Although this appearance is not specific for an abscess, it is highly suggestive, and is thought to be related to a layer of granulation tissue along its wall.

ROUTES OF CONTAMINATION
(Box 5-3)

Osteomyelitis can develop via three routes:
1. Hematogenous seeding
2. Contiguous spread from an adjacent infection
3. Direct implantation of microorganisms

Hematogenous Seeding

The location of lesions from hematogenous seeding is related to the vascular supply of tissues; in some patients, involvement may be multifocal. In hematogenous osteomyelitis, the contamination begins in the bone marrow and extends secondarily through the cortex and then to the adjacent soft tissues. In the spine, the common initial site of involvement is the subchondral bone of the vertebral body, which is supplied by nutrient arterioles. This process eventually extends to the disk (spondylodiscitis). In children, vascular channels perforate the vertebral end plates, allowing direct access of microorganisms to the intervertebral disk (diskitis) without initial contamination of the vertebral bodies. In tubular bones, the vascular anatomy changes with age and is different for infants, children, and adults.[7,9] This particular vascular distribution explains the location of lesions for the different age groups.

The infantile pattern (0-1 year) is related to the fetal vascular arrangement that persists up to age 1 year. The metaphyseal and diaphyseal vessels penetrate the growth plate and extend into the epiphysis. In infants, infection affects primarily the epiphysis and the growth plate because of this

vascular anatomy. Profuse involucrum formation is characteristic, reflecting the ease with which the periosteum is lifted from the underlying bone in infants and the presence of a rich vascularity. Development of soft tissue abscesses and

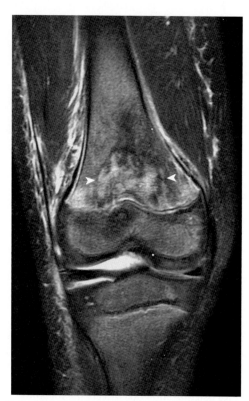

Figure 5-6 **Osteomyelitis: hematogenous spread.** STIR coronal image of the knee. An irregular focus of heterogeneous signal intensity within the distal femoral metaphysis (*arrowheads*) is from hematogenous spread of infection to the region of terminal arterial ramifications in this child with open growth plates. This patient also was found to have a septic knee joint that resulted from contiguous spread of infection through the bone.

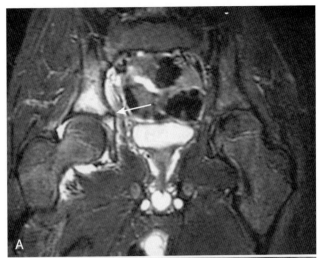

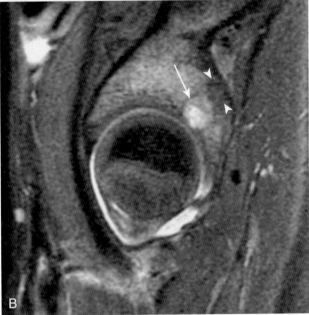

Figure 5-7 **Osteomyelitis: pelvis. A,** STIR coronal image of the pelvis. There is a right hip effusion in this 12-year-old boy who presented with hip pain on that side. Extensive bone marrow edema also is present in the adjacent acetabulum bordering the triradiate cartilage (*arrow*). **B,** STIR sagittal image of the right acetabulum. A small subarticular abscess is present along the posterior acetabular roof (*arrow*). A portion of the triradiate cartilage (*arrowheads*) abuts the posterior margin of the abscess.

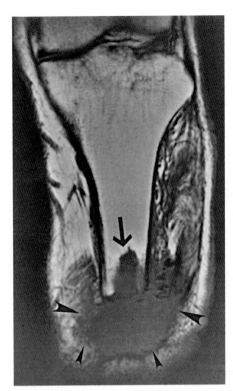

Figure 5-8 **Osteomyelitis: contiguous spread.** T1 coronal image of the knee. This patient had a below-the-knee amputation in the remote past. An ulcer developed in the distal soft tissues over the tibia. Infection spread from the soft tissue abscess (*arrowheads*) through the periosteum and cortex into the medullary canal, where there is now osteomyelitis (*arrow*).

extension into the joint also are common. Group A streptococcus is the most common organism affecting infants with osteomyelitis.

The childhood pattern is from 1 year of age to closure of the growth plates (Fig. 5-6). The metaphyseal vessels become terminal ramifications of nutrient arteries, with the capillaries forming large sinusoidal lakes in the metaphysis. The slow blood flow in this area contributes to the increased incidence of osteomyelitis that affects the metaphysis in the child. Later, extension into the epiphysis may occur from contiguous spread. Involucrum, sequestrum, and abscess formation are common. Articular extension (septic arthritis) occurs at sites where the growth plate is intra-articular, such

as in the hip, elbow, and shoulder. In flat bones, such as the pelvis, childhood osteomyelitis shows a predilection for metaphyseal-equivalent locations adjacent to apophyses (eg, the iliac crests), and for epiphyseal-equivalent locations adjacent to articular cartilage (eg, around the triradiate cartilage) (Fig. 5-7). *Staphylococcus aureus* (80%) and group A streptococcus are the most frequent organisms that affect children.

The adult pattern of hematogenous seeding of osteomyelitis is seen when growth plate closure has occurred. The diaphyseal and metaphyseal vessels penetrate the fused growth plate, which allows infection to localize in the subchondral bone regions (epiphyses). Septic arthritis may complicate this epiphyseal location. The spine, the pelvis, and the small bones of the hands and feet are the most common sites of infection.

Contiguous Spread

When soft tissues initially are infected, and the noncontained infection extends to adjacent osseous structures, it is considered contamination by contiguous spread (Fig. 5-8). Contamination of bone by contiguous spread most commonly is seen in debilitated patients, in diabetics, and in patients treated with corticosteroids. The soft tissue infection invades bone marrow by progressing in sequence from cellulitis in the soft tissues to periostitis to osteitis to osteomyelitis. Osteitis indicates involvement of cortical bone; extension of the cortical infection into the marrow cavity produces osteomy-

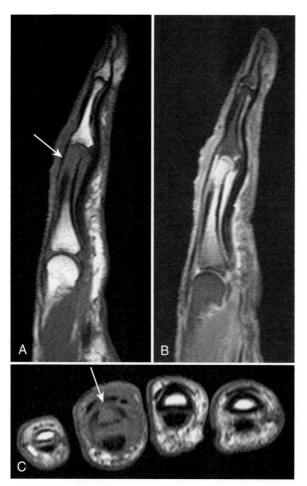

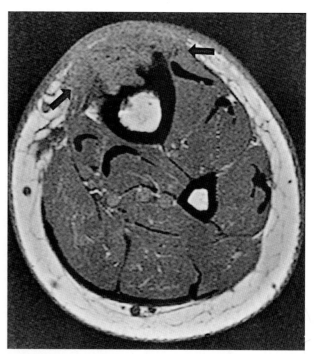

Figure 5-10   Osteomyelitis: direct implantation. T1 axial image of the calf. There is a soft tissue and cortical abscess in the anterior and medial aspect of the tibia with cortical destruction and a soft tissue mass (*arrows*). This occurred from direct implantation of bacteria when a shovel went through the skin and into the bone.

Figure 5-9   Osteomyelitis: direct implantation. **A,** T1 sagittal image of the finger. This patient had been bitten by a dog 6 months before this scan. Abnormal intermediate signal is present in the marrow of the distal portion of the proximal phalanx. There also is dorsal cortical destruction at that site (*arrow*), and these findings are compatible with osteomyelitis. **B,** Fat-saturated T1 sagittal image of the finger after IV gadolinium administration. There is diffuse, intense enhancement within the medullary cavity and adjacent soft tissues. **C,** T1 axial image of the finger. Diffuse swelling of the digit is evident at that level as is the focal breakthrough of the dorsal cortex (*arrow*).

elitis. The direction of contamination in contiguous spread of infection is the reverse of that which occurs with hematogenous osteomyelitis. With hematogenous osteomyelitis, marrow is affected initially, followed by cortical destruction, then periosteal contamination, and finally soft tissue cellulitis, phlegmon, or abscess.

Direct Implantation

Contamination of tissues by direct implantation of infectious agents is usually the result of puncture wounds, foreign bodies, open fractures, and surgery. Human bites (*S. aureus, Bacillus fusiformis*) and animal bites (*Pasteurella multocida, S. aureus,* and *Staphylococcus epidermidis*) also are common causes of infection from direct implantation (Fig. 5-9).[10] The infection starts at the site of implantation, which may be in the soft tissues, the periosteum, or the cortical or medullary bone; soft tissue involvement almost always is present (Fig. 5-10).

BOX 5-4
Osteomyelitis: MRI Findings

Bone Marrow Inflammation
- T1: Low signal intensity
- T2: High signal intensity
- T1 with contrast: High signal intensity

Intraosseous Abscess
- T1: Low signal intensity
- T2: High signal intensity
- T1 with contrast: High signal intensity only in periphery

Sequestrum
- T1: Low signal intensity
- T2: Low signal intensity
- T1 with contrast: High signal intensity surrounding sequestrum, which remains low signal

Cortical Destruction
- T1: Intermediate signal intensity
- T2: Intermediate or high signal intensity
- T1 with contrast: Intermediate signal intensity

Cloaca
- T1: Hard to see
- T2: High signal intensity defect in low signal periosteum
- T1 with contrast: Not seen

Sinus Tract
- T1: Not seen, or linear low signal intensity
- T2: High signal intensity
- T1 with contrast: High signal intensity in peripheral lining of low signal intensity tract

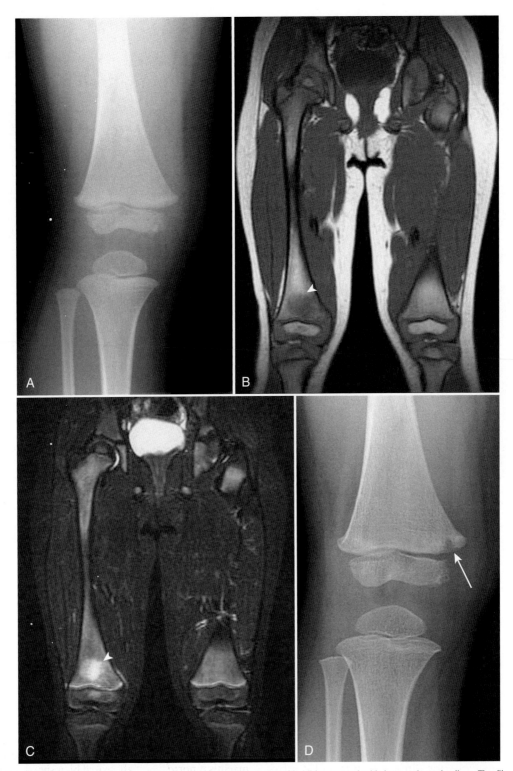

Figure 5-11   Osteomyelitis: acute. A, Frontal radiograph of the knee. This 3-year-old child presented with knee pain and a limp. The film is normal. **B,** T1 coronal image of the thighs. There is a rounded focus of abnormal, low signal intensity in the distal right femoral metaphysis (*arrowhead*). **C,** Coronal STIR image of the thighs. The lesion shows strikingly increased signal at this site of acute osteomyelitis. **D,** Frontal radiograph of the knee. This film, obtained 3 weeks after the first radiograph, now shows a small metaphyseal lucency abutting the medial aspect of the physis at the site of infection (*arrow*).

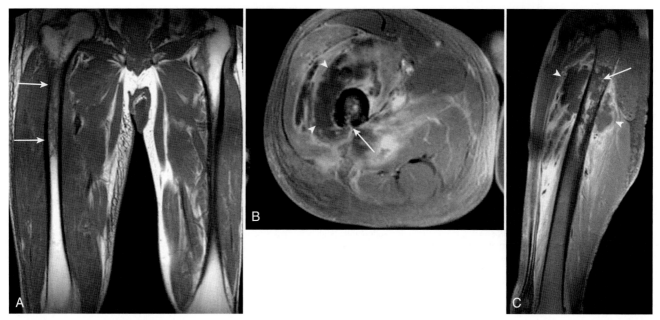

Figure 5-12   **Osteomyelitis: progression with cloaca and abscess formation. A,** T1 coronal image of the thighs. An elongated focus of decreased signal is evident in the proximal right femoral shaft (*arrows*). **B,** Fat-saturated T1 axial image of the thigh after IV administration of gadolinium. A defect in the posterior cortex represents a cloaca (*arrow*), and nonenhancing fluid is seen within the adjacent multilocular abscess (*arrowheads*). **C,** Fat-saturated T1 sagittal image of the thigh after the IV administration of gadolinium. The extent of the intraosseous (*arrow*) and extraosseous (*arrowheads*) abscesses are better shown in this plane. Note also the extensive, phlegmonous enhancement within the adjacent thigh muscles.

MRI OF OSTEOMYELITIS (Box 5-4)

Osteomyelitis classically is divided into three stages: acute, subacute, and chronic. These stages are based on the patient's clinical picture, on the duration of the disease, and on imaging findings.[11-19]

Acute Osteomyelitis

Acute osteomyelitis of hematogenous origin has normal radiographs in the first week, followed in the next 7 to 14 days by osteoporosis, fine linear periosteal reaction, and eventually permeative or moth-eaten bone destruction.[20] Before radiographic manifestations of infection, MRI shows obliteration of the medullary fat by bone marrow edema, which is high signal intensity on STIR images and low to intermediate signal intensity on T1W images (Fig. 5-11). These MRI features are not specific. MRI is highly sensitive, but not specific for diagnosing infection, with reported specificities for osteomyelitis ranging from 53% to 94%; however, MRI has a negative predictive value for osteomyelitis of close to 100%. As the disease progresses, MRI shows elevation of the periosteum, which is a low signal intensity line on all pulse sequences. The space between the periosteum and cortical bone has intermediate signal intensity on T1W and high signal intensity on STIR images; this usually is accompanied by adjacent soft tissue edema. Cortical destruction is a later finding and is depicted initially by blurring and eventually focal interruption of the cortical line, which is normally completely devoid of signal (low signal intensity) on all pulse sequences.

The infection may transgress the periosteum with formation of a cloaca. This is seen best on STIR images as a high signal intensity defect traversing the black periosteal line (Fig. 5-12). This defect may evolve into an abscess cavity or a sinus tract.[21-24] An abscess cavity is usually oval in shape, low signal intensity on T1W images, and high signal intensity on T2W images. It may blend in with, and be obscured by, diffuse surrounding edema. The use of gadolinium helps to distinguish an abscess from surrounding edema. The abscess shows high signal intensity enhancement of its capsule, whereas the cavity remains low signal intensity. Cellulitis shows diffuse contrast enhancement.

Osteomyelitis from contiguous spread manifests with the reverse sequence of events as hematogenous osteomyelitis. The soft tissues are affected initially with diffuse edema. There may be associated soft tissue ulcers and abscesses. Ulcers are identified as low signal intensity cutaneous defects. With soft tissue infection, there may be adjacent periosteal reaction and bone marrow edema, but these findings do not indicate osteomyelitis. Joints and bone marrow may develop sympathetic effusions or marrow edema from an adjacent inflammatory process. Distinguishing this sympathetic inflammatory reaction from true infection of these tissues is not always possible by MRI.

STIR and fat-saturated T2W images are usually assessed first in these cases. These images essentially exclude osteomyelitis if normal, but abnormal high signal intensity within the marrow may be related to osteomyelitis or the "reactive" marrow edema described earlier. In that case, the T1W images should be analyzed closely for further characterization because normal signal intensity or hazy decreased signal intensity within the marrow correlates strongly with reactive edema as an etiology for the T2 signal abnormality. Conversely, an area of geographic low signal intensity within the medullary cavity on a T1W image at the site of T2 abnormality is highly predictive for osteomyelitis.[25]

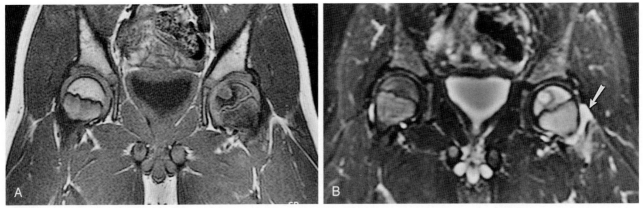

Figure 5-13 Osteomyelitis: subacute. **A,** T1 coronal image of the pelvis. There is a focal intermediate signal lesion (abscess) in the left femoral head surrounded by a rim of low signal (fibrosis or reactive new bone). The surrounding marrow is intermediate signal secondary to reactive marrow edema that surrounds the subacute osteomyelitis. **B,** STIR coronal image of the pelvis. The focal abscess becomes high signal, the thin line of surrounding reactive bone remains low signal, and the diffuse surrounding reactive marrow edema is high signal. In addition, there is a high signal joint effusion (*arrow*), which represents either a reaction to the adjacent inflammatory process or a septic joint.

Certain other characteristic MRI features of osteomyelitis also are helpful in this setting. The diagnosis of osteomyelitis can be made with even more confidence when the previously described findings are associated with one of the following[3]:

1. Sinus tract
2. Cortical destruction
3. An adjacent soft tissue abscess

Subacute Osteomyelitis

Subacute osteomyelitis is characterized on a radiograph by a geographic osteolytic lesion with or without sclerosis, often manifesting as a lucent serpiginous channel within the medullary cavity. There may be an associated periosteal reaction. Brodie's abscess is a form of subacute osteomyelitis that is especially common in children. Radiographic features of

Brodie's abscess are those of a well-circumscribed lytic lesion with sclerotic borders in the metaphysis of a long bone. Periosteal reaction and a sequestrum may sometimes be present. The most frequent sites of involvement are the tibia and femur.

MR images show a well-circumscribed, serpiginous or oval lesion of low to intermediate signal intensity on T1W images and high signal intensity on T2W images (Fig. 5-13). A focus of subacute osteomyelitis is surrounded by a low signal intensity rim of variable thickness, representing fibrous tissue and reactive bone. There is usually associated bone marrow edema surrounding the lesion. These MRI findings may be seen before any characteristic radiographic changes are shown. Periosteal reaction and adjacent soft tissue edema also may be present. Joint effusion may be seen, which may be sympathetic in origin or represent a true septic arthritis. When epiphyses or apophyses are involved with Brodie's abscess, the findings may resemble a chondroblastoma on radiographs and MR images. The use of IV gadolinium may help distinguish these two entities. Only the periphery of Brodie's abscess enhances, whereas a chondroblastoma shows heterogeneous enhancement of the entire lesion.

Chronic Osteomyelitis

Chronic osteomyelitis consists of an infection of more than 6 weeks' duration. In its florid state, it shows abundant sclerosis as manifested by periosteal and endosteal thickening, thickened and disorganized trabeculae, and cystic changes, with or without a sequestrum on radiographs. Chronic osteomyelitis of long duration with draining sinus tracts may

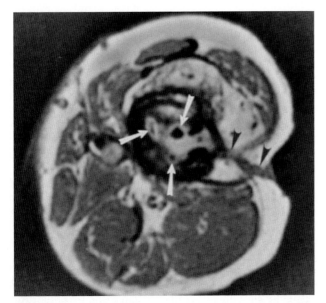

Figure 5-14 Osteomyelitis: chronic. Proton density axial image of the thigh. Several features of chronic infection are evident: sequestra (*arrows*), cloaca, sinus tract (*arrowheads*), and an abscess in the medullary canal (high signal diffusely except for the sequestra).

BOX 5-5
Cellulitis
• Abnormal signal limited to subcutaneous fat
• Reticulated pattern:
• Low signal on T1
• High signal on T2
• Enhancement with contrast
• No abnormality of deep fascial planes

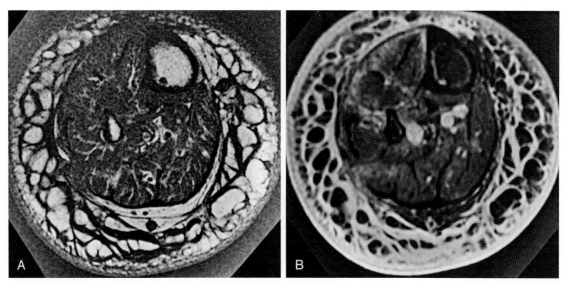

Figure 5-15 **Cellulitis. A,** T1 axial image of the lower leg. There is diffuse skin thickening and a reticular pattern of low signal edema in the subcutaneous fat. **B,** STIR axial image of the lower leg. The reticular pattern of edema and skin thickening become high signal on this sequence. There is no abnormal high signal in the intermuscular fascial planes, allowing distinction of cellulitis from necrotizing fasciitis.

develop into squamous cell carcinoma.[26,27] The most specific sign of active chronic osteomyelitis is the presence of a sequestrum, best shown with computed tomography. Other radiographic signs include the presence of poorly defined areas of osteolysis; osteolysis in areas of previous sclerosis; and development of a new, thin, linear periosteal reaction.

The MRI findings that indicate an active chronic osteomyelitis are listed[22,28]:

1. Identification of a sequestrum (Fig. 5-14) that is low signal intensity on all pulse sequences (injection of IV gadolinium increases its conspicuity because granulation tissue surrounding the sequestrum enhances, but the sequestrum remains low signal intensity)

2. Intramedullary abscess cavity, which is an oblong, well-delineated mass of low signal intensity on T1W and high signal intensity on T2W images (after IV injection of gadolinium, the rim of the intraosseous abscess enhances with high signal intensity, whereas the pus-filled cavity remains low signal intensity on T1W images)

3. Cloaca, which is seen on T2W images as a high signal intensity gap through the cortex and periosteum

4. Subperiosteal fluid collection (representing either pus or edema), seen on T2W images as a high signal intensity linear fluid collection elevating the periosteum and paralleling the cortex

5. Sinus tract, identified on T2W images as a high signal intensity channel extending from bone into the soft tissues or on contrast-enhanced T1W images as enhancement along its borders

Increased signal intensity of the bone marrow on T2W images may represent postsurgical or postinfectious granulation tissue and not persistent infection. Serial MRI studies showing progression of this process in the marrow indicates the presence of active osteomyelitis, however. The MRI diagnosis of healed osteomyelitis is based on the absence of the aforementioned signs and on the return of normal fatty marrow in the medullary cavity, seen as high signal intensity marrow on T1W and low signal intensity on fat-saturated T2W images.

Soft Tissue Infection

Soft tissue infections include cellulitis, septic tenosynovitis, septic bursitis, infectious myositis, and necrotizing fasciitis. Despite the fact that MRI findings are not specific, MRI is the best imaging modality to detect any soft tissue abnormality. It is used to evaluate the presence or absence of disease, evaluate its extent, and identify possible sites for biopsy.

CELLULITIS (Box 5-5)

Cellulitis represents diffuse inflammation of subcutaneous fat and skin. On MRI, cellulitis is seen as diffuse areas of low signal intensity on T1W and high signal intensity on T2W images, with a reticular (lacelike) pattern in the subcutaneous fat and skin thickening (Fig. 5-15). After injection of IV gadolinium, diffuse increased signal intensity is present in the same areas that are abnormal on unenhanced T1W and T2W sequences.[29]

SEPTIC TENOSYNOVITIS AND SEPTIC BURSITIS

Septic tenosynovitis and septic bursitis usually result from penetrating trauma, or may be a manifestation of tuberculosis.[30] Septic and aseptic causes of bursitis and tenosynovitis cannot be distinguished by imaging features. Fluid surrounding a tendon or within a bursa (Fig. 5-16) is low signal intensity on T1W and high signal intensity on any type of T2W images, and it shows enhancement of the synovial lining of these structures after injection of IV contrast material. These abnormalities usually are accompanied by adjacent cellulitis.

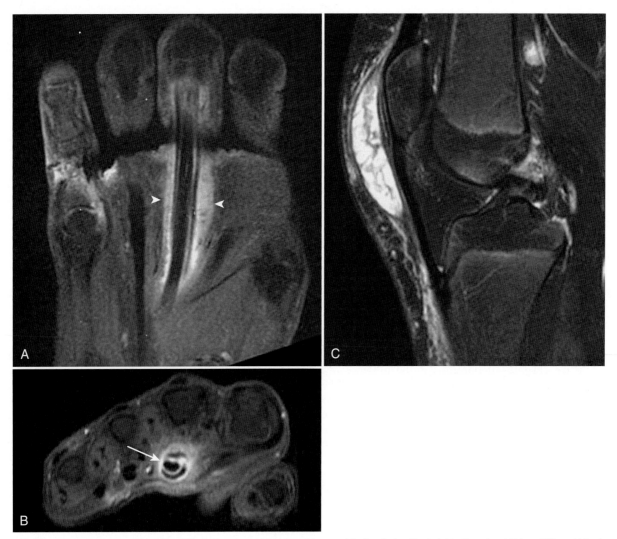

Figure 5-16 **Infected tenosynovitis and bursitis. A,** Fat-saturated T1 coronal image of the hand after IV administration of gadolinium. Diffuse thickening and enhancement of the flexor tendon sheath (*arrowheads*) were found to represent septic tenosynovitis in this patient. **B,** Fat-saturated T1 axial image of the hand after IV administration of gadolinium. The dark flexor tendons (*arrow*) are surrounded by low signal fluid (pus) and markedly enhancing tenosynovium. **C,** STIR sagittal image of the knee (different patient than in **A** and **B**). The prepatellar bursa is distended with material displaying heterogeneous signal intensity. This was subsequently found to be infected.

PYOMYOSITIS (INFECTIOUS MYOSITIS)

Pyomyositis is very rare, but it can result from penetrating trauma or from hematogenous seeding. In adults, pyomyositis most commonly affects IV drug abusers or immunocompromised patients.[31] In affected children, an underlying medical condition is less commonly present.[32] *S. aureus* is the most common causative agent. Lesions are multifocal in about half of patients.

The disease typically produces three clinical stages:

1. Invasive stage, in which the bacteria invade the muscle
2. Purulent stage, in which intramuscular abscesses form
3. Late stage, in which more severe systemic findings, such as septic shock, are common

In the invasive stage, MRI shows muscle enlargement with intermediate signal intensity on T1W images and increased signal intensity on T2W images. Associated changes of cellulitis occasionally may be present. In the purulent phase, solitary or multiple abscesses are seen (Fig. 5-17).[33-38] Abscesses may be surrounded by a high signal intensity rim on T1W images with contrast administration. A high signal intensity rim also has been described on T1W images without contrast in muscle abscesses (the penumbra sign described previously[8]); however, these findings are not specific, and the precise diagnosis usually is obtained by aspiration or biopsy and culture of the abnormal muscle. MRI is useful for directing therapy because antibiotics alone are often sufficient to treat the early stage of the disease, whereas percutaneous or surgical intervention is often required in the later stages.

NECROTIZING FASCIITIS (Box 5-6)

Necrotizing fasciitis is associated with a high mortality rate and represents a surgical emergency. Early diagnosis and

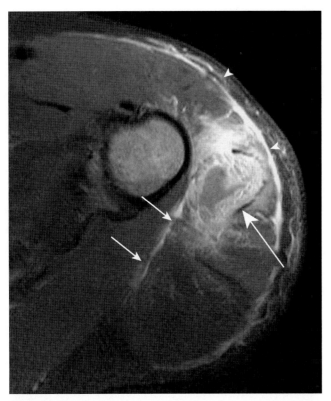

Figure 5-17 Pyomyositis. Fat-saturated T1 axial image of the shoulder after IV administration of gadolinium. There is patchy enhancement throughout the mid to posterior deltoid muscle with a focal intramuscular abscess in this 27-year-old immunocompromised man shown to have pyomyositis. Note the thick enhancing wall of the abscess (*large arrow*) surrounding the nonenhancing fluid centrally. There also is prominent enhancement along the superficial (*arrowheads*) and deep (*small arrows*) fascial layers.

BOX 5-6

Necrotizing Fasciitis

Deep Fasciae

- T2: High signal intensity
- T1 with contrast: High signal intensity

Subcutaneous Fat

- Diffuse reticulations
- T2 and T1 with contrast: Increased signal intensity

Muscle

- T2 and T1 with contrast: Increased signal intensity

Abscess in Muscle

- T2: Increased signal intensity
- T1 postcontrast: Rim enhancement with decreased signal intensity center

extensive débridement are associated with improved prognosis.[39] MRI is used to distinguish cellulitis from necrotizing fasciitis. In cellulitis, abnormal signal intensity is seen only in the subcutaneous fat.[29] With necrotizing fasciitis, the abnormal signal intensity extends into the deep fasciae between muscles, and occasionally into muscles. The abnormal signal intensity is best shown on STIR images. Linear high signal intensity is seen within the superficial and the deep fasciae from fascial necrosis. The associated muscle involvement, when present, is identified as poorly defined areas of high signal intensity on T2W or STIR images within the muscles, with or without hyperintense fluid collections representing abscesses (Fig. 5-18).

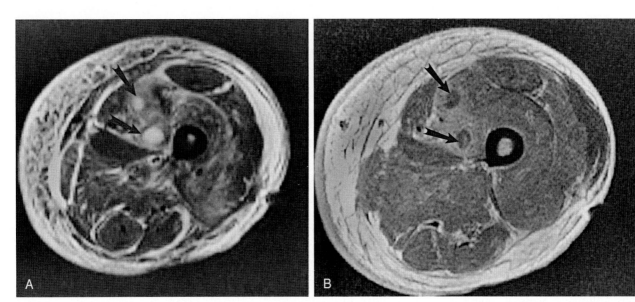

Figure 5-18 Necrotizing fasciitis. A, STIR axial image of the thigh. There is intermuscular fascial edema, subcutaneous edema, and intramuscular diffuse edema, all manifested as high signal intensity. In addition, there are two focal areas of high signal within muscle (*arrows*) from abscesses. Only intermuscular and subcutaneous high signal are required to make the diagnosis. **B,** T1 contrast-enhanced axial image of the thigh. There is mild diffuse enhancement of the muscle surrounding the two low signal abscesses (*arrows*). The other manifestations of this inflammatory process are masked with this sequence.

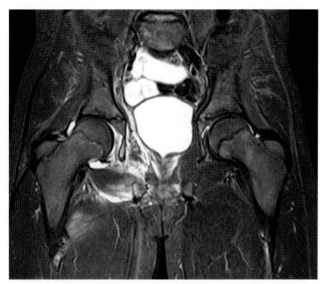

Figure 5-19   **Septic arthritis: hip.** STIR coronal image of the pelvis. There is a right hip effusion in this skeletally immature patient. Although this finding is nonspecific, the extensive fluid and edema involving the adjacent soft tissues is highly suggestive of a septic hip, which was confirmed clinically.

Muscle involvement is not required to make the diagnosis, but fascial involvement is.[40] Postcontrast T1W images show enhancement in the fascial planes, focal enhancement of the affected muscles, and peripheral enhancement of the abscess cavities, corresponding to the findings seen on STIR images. Contrast administration is not necessary to make the diagnosis in suspected cases of necrotizing fasciitis, and may underestimate the extent of disease owing to poor perfusion of devitalized and necrotic tissue. It is often helpful, however, for identifying associated abscesses.[41]

A word of caution: The MRI findings in necrotizing fasciitis are nonspecific and can be seen in other, less aggressive processes. Correlation with clinical findings is extremely important to determine the significance of the imaging findings. Given the high morbidity and mortality of this disease, if the clinical appearance is worrisome, early surgical intervention directed to the abnormal areas on MRI is usually indicated.[42]

Septic Arthritis

In the presence of a monarticular inflammatory process, the diagnosis of a septic joint should always be considered as a possibility (Fig. 5-19). Predisposing factors include diabetes, corticosteroid therapy, debilitating diseases, and IV drug abuse.[43-45] In IV drug abusers, the sites of predilection are the acromioclavicular, sternoclavicular, and sacroiliac joints, and the spine (Fig. 5-20). Whenever the diagnosis of septic arthritis is considered clinically, the joint should be aspirated for culture and sensitivity. In some instances, such as tuberculous arthritis, a synovial biopsy may be necessary to establish the diagnosis.

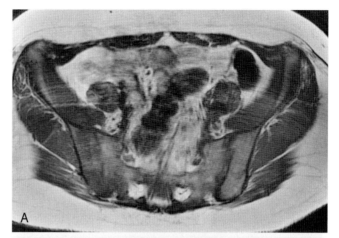

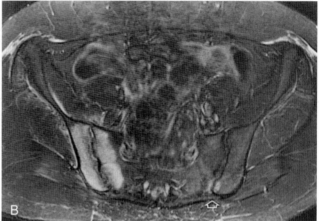

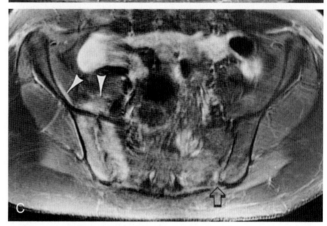

Figure 5-20   **Septic arthritis: sacroiliac joint. A,** T1 axial image of the pelvis. The black cortical lines in the right sacroiliac joint are obliterated (compare with the joint on the left). **B,** STIR axial image of the pelvis. Large bands of marrow edema are present on either side of the right sacroiliac joint. There is high signal within the joint and cortical destruction. Also, high signal is present in the soft tissues anterior to the joint and right iliac wing. Small areas of marrow edema are present on the posterior aspect of the left sacroiliac joint (*open arrow*) in this drug abuser with septic joints. **C,** T1 contrast-enhanced with fat suppression axial image of the pelvis. Almost identical features to the STIR image are seen, indicating hyperemia from infection, but no abscess formation. The high signal seen in the anterior soft tissues (*arrowheads*) is from either cellulitis or reactive hyperemia. There is bone marrow edema, granulation tissue, or synovitis in the joint, and cortical erosions and early changes of infection in the left sacroiliac joint (*open arrow*).

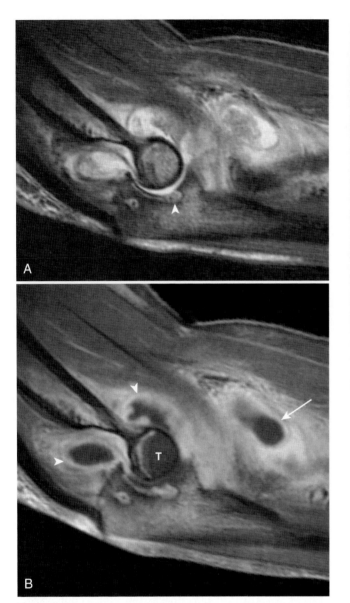

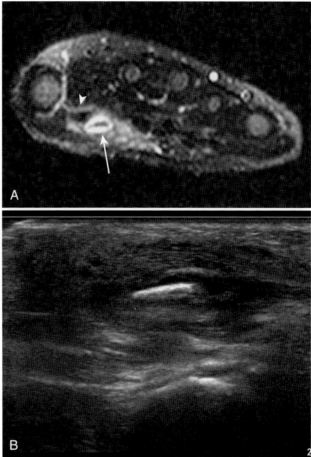

Figure 5-22 Foreign body: soft tissues. A, Fat-saturated T2 axial image of the hand. There is a focal region of high signal intensity (*arrow*) adjacent to the flexor pollicis longus tendon (*arrowhead*) in the palmar soft tissues of the hand. This 3-year-old child had fallen in the woods, and although a foreign body was suspected, it was not palpable on examination at the site of clinical pain and swelling. A small, linear low signal structure representing a foreign body (wood) is present in the center of the lesion (*arrow*). The high signal may be from focal cellulitis, abscess, or granulation tissue. **B,** Ultrasound of the hand. The location of the splinter was confirmed on a targeted ultrasound scan of this region.

Figure 5-21 Septic arthritis: elbow. A, Fat-saturated T2 sagittal image of the elbow. The joint is markedly distended with irregular, heterogeneous tissue. Note also the small erosion along the olecranon (*arrowhead*), and the faint marrow edema throughout the distal humerus and proximal ulna. **B,** Fat-saturated T1 sagittal image of the elbow after IV administration of gadolinium. Thick, enhancing synovium extends throughout the joint surrounding nonenhancing pockets of purulent material in this infected elbow (*arrowheads*). A loculated collection also is present within the extra-articular soft tissues anteriorly (*arrow*). The lack of enhancement in the trochlea (T) is compatible with an abscess or devitalized bone.

MRI findings of septic arthritis are not specific and are the same as for any inflammatory arthritis. Initially, there is a joint effusion and synovitis; later on, joint space narrowing and erosions may appear (Fig. 5-21). The joint effusion and synovitis are low signal intensity on T1W images and high signal intensity on T2W images, although synovitis is slightly higher signal intensity than joint fluid on T1W images. After IV contrast administration, the joint effusion remains low signal intensity, whereas synovitis becomes high signal intensity. Erosions are seen as marginal subchondral defects, low signal intensity on T1W and high signal intensity on T2W images. Adjacent soft tissue and bone marrow edema may be seen with a septic joint; these findings generally indicate a sympathetic hyperemia with edema, but occasionally the bone or soft tissues adjacent to the infected joint also may be infected.

Clinical evaluation of a child presenting with hip pain can be particularly challenging because transient synovitis may mimic a septic hip. Ultrasound or MRI usually shows an effusion in both conditions. The presence of associated abnormal marrow signal intensity and the finding of decreased perfusion of the femoral head on contrast-enhanced, fat-suppressed T1W images have been reported to be more suggestive of a septic joint, however.[46] In the case

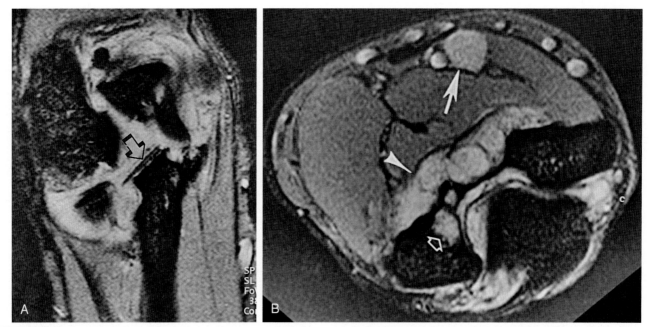

Figure 5-23   Foreign body: articular. **A,** T2* coronal image of the elbow. A linear foreign body (*open arrow*) is seen adjacent to the posterior ulna within the elbow joint. This was a thorn from a rosebush. High signal synovitis and joint effusion, and bone erosion in the ulna from the inflammatory process are present. **B,** T2* axial image of the elbow. The tremendous synovitis and joint effusion are evident (*arrowhead*). An enlarged lymph node is noted (*arrow*) as are bone erosions in the humerus (*open arrow*).

of other infectious entities that may mimic a septic hip, such as pyomyositis or osteomyelitis, MRI can help to differentiate these conditions and direct appropriate therapy.[47,48] Despite the usefulness of MRI in this scenario, if the clinical suspicion of a septic hip is high enough, image-guided aspiration is indicated.

Miscellaneous Conditions

Conditions that warrant special consideration include infection associated with foreign bodies, chronic recurrent multifocal osteomyelitis, acquired immunodeficiency syndrome (AIDS), and the diabetic foot.

FOREIGN BODIES

Soft tissue or intra-articular foreign bodies may cause an infection. These foreign bodies are most often wood, thorns, or glass, and are usually not radiopaque. Their sites of predilection are the feet and hands. Foreign bodies in the soft tissues create an inflammatory reaction (cellulitis), and eventually may lead to the formation of an abscess cavity or a sinus tract to permit the extrusion of the foreign body. The foreign body ultimately may cause osteomyelitis.

On MR images, foreign bodies are low signal intensity on all sequences and can be very subtle in appearance. Generally, they are linear in shape, which is a helpful criterion for identification. On T2W images, foreign bodies are surrounded by high signal intensity, representing granulation tissue, cellulitis, or abscess (Fig. 5-22). IV contrast material may increase the conspicuity of foreign bodies, which remain low signal intensity, surrounded by diffuse increased signal intensity in the case of granulation tissue or cellulitis, or abscess cavity, which remains low signal intensity except in its periphery.

Intra-articular foreign bodies are not as common as soft tissue foreign bodies, but they usually generate a marked reactive synovitis. On T1W images, the foreign bodies, synovitis, and joint effusion are low signal intensity, although the foreign bodies may be even lower signal intensity than the surrounding fluid. On T2W images, foreign bodies remain low signal intensity, whereas the joint effusion and the synovitis become high signal intensity. A high index of suspicion is necessary to identify foreign bodies, and their linear shape is a helpful clue for their identification (Fig. 5-23; see Fig. 5-22).

CHRONIC RECURRENT MULTIFOCAL OSTEOMYELITIS

Chronic recurrent multifocal osteomyelitis is a chronic osteomyelitis, usually affecting children and young adults. Any skeletal site can be involved, but there is a predilection for symmetrical involvement of the metaphyses of the lower extremity and/or the medial ends of the clavicles. Patients complain of pain and swelling in the affected areas, and 40%

BOX 5-7

Features of Osteomyelitis in Diabetic Feet

Virtual Requirements
- Abnormal marrow signal on T1 and T2
- Soft tissue ulcer or sinus tract overlying the abnormal bone and usually located at predictable pressure points (first and fifth metatarsal heads, calcaneal tuberosity, distal phalanges of toes, malleoli of ankles)

Other Possible Findings
- Cortical destruction (loss of the black cortical line)
- Intraosseous fluid collection (abscess)
- Sequestrum
- Soft tissue cellulitis, abscesses
- Adjacent joint effusion

Table 5-1 MARROW SIGNAL ABNORMALITIES IN DIABETIC FEET

T1 Marrow Signal	T2 (STIR) Marrow Signal	Diagnosis
↑ (fat)	↓	Definitely no osteomyelitis
↑ (fat)	↑	Mild reactive marrow edema, no osteomyelitis
↓	↑	Differential diagnosis Osteomyelitis Reactive marrow edema (marked) Acute neuropathic changes (use location of lesions to help distinguish, and sharpen your biopsy needles to prove)

of patients may have palmoplantar pustulosis.[49-52] This entity is included in the group of disorders designated as SAPHO (synovitis, acne, pustulosis, hyperostosis, and osteitis) syndrome. Laboratory findings are not specific, and blood and bone cultures are usually negative. Histologically, the osteolytic portion of the lesion contains a predominance of plasma cells, and the term *plasma cell osteomyelitis* has been used for this condition. The dominant radiographic feature is sclerosis, in combination with a variable amount of osteolysis and periostitis. No characteristic MRI findings have been described. The entity should be considered in the presence of multifocal involvement, or when the medial end of the clavicle is affected.

ACQUIRED IMMUNODEFICIENCY SYNDROME

Patients with human immunodeficiency virus infection are immunocompromised and have a susceptibility for bacterial and fungal infections. These patients are predisposed to osteomyelitis, septic arthritis, and pyomyositis with MRI changes as described previously.[53-55] A rare form of osteomyelitis that has a higher incidence in AIDS patients is bacillary angiomatosis,[56] caused by a gram-negative microorganism. Patients usually present with skin lesions characterized by multiple angiomatous papules. The bone lesions consist of multiple osteolytic foci involving cortex and medullary cavity, associated with soft tissue masses. The tubular bones of the extremities, in particular, the tibia, are the sites of predilection.

Radiographic findings of bacillary angiomatosis consist of poorly defined and well-defined cortical osteolytic defects associated with a variable amount of medullary osteolysis, sclerosis, and periosteal reaction. On MR images, lobulated soft tissue masses adjacent to cortical defects can be identified. These masses are intermediate signal intensity (higher than muscle) on T1W images and high signal intensity on T2W images. In addition to the cortical destruction and soft tissue masses, changes consistent with osteomyelitis in the adjacent marrow are evident.

DIABETIC FOOT INFECTION (Box 5-7 and Tables 5-1 and 5-2)

Foot disease in diabetics is common and usually is related to one or more of the following: vascular disease, infection, neuroarthropathy, and tendon rupture. MRI has proved to be extremely valuable for assessing these conditions.

Infection in diabetics is usually the result of a soft tissue injury, typically followed by cellulitis; the infection may remain limited to the soft tissues, extend to adjacent bone, or spread proximally within anatomic compartments or via tendon sheaths (Fig. 5-24). Soft tissue ulcerations usually are found under pressure areas of the foot, such as the plantar soft tissues beneath or adjacent to the first and fifth metatarsal heads, the calcaneal tuberosity, the distal phalanges,

Table 5-2 DIABETIC DILEMMA

	Osteomyelitis	Neuroarthropathy
Location	Adjacent to ulcers at pressure points	Always involves joints
	Metatarsal heads (first and fifth)	Tarsometatarsal (Lisfranc) joints and adjacent bones
	Calcaneal tuberosity	Talonavicular and calcaneocuboid (Chopart) joints and adjacent bones
	Distal phalanges of toes	Ankle and subtalar joints and adjacent bones
	Malleoli of ankle May or may not involve joints	
Other features	Cortical destruction Sequestrum Intraosseous fluid collection (abscess)	Bone fragmentation Malalignment
Nondiscriminatory features	Joint effusion Soft tissue edema Bone marrow edema Periosteal reaction	Joint effusion Soft tissue edema Bone marrow edema Periosteal reaction

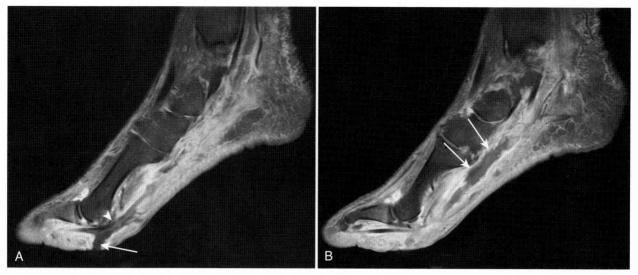

Figure 5-24 **Diabetic foot infection: proximal spread via tendon sheath. A,** Fat-saturated T1 sagittal image of the foot after IV injection of gadolinium. A nonenhancing sinus tract (*arrow*) extends from a cutaneous ulcer to the underlying flexor hallucis longus tendon sheath, which is mildly distended (*arrowhead*). **B,** Fat-saturated T1 sagittal image of the foot after IV injection of gadolinium. Distention of the tendon sheath is identified in the midfoot (*arrows*), compatible with proximal spread of infection.

and the malleoli. These ulcers are seen in most diabetic patients with foot infections, and osteomyelitis rarely is present without associated soft tissue ulcers.[3]

Ulcers can be identified on MRI as soft tissue defects of low signal intensity on T1W and T2W images. Cellulitis

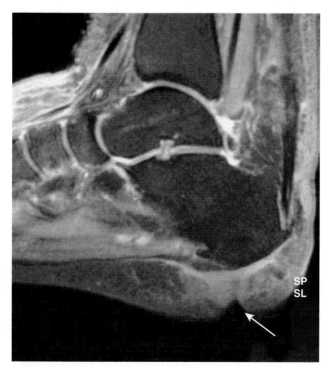

Figure 5-25 **Diabetic foot: ulcer, no osteomyelitis.** STIR sagittal image of the hindfoot. There is a large soft tissue defect (ulcer) within the plantar heel pad (*arrow*). The lack of signal abnormality in the underlying calcaneus excludes any associated osteomyelitis.

usually is associated with the soft tissue ulcers and is identified on MRI as diffuse areas of low signal intensity on T1W and high signal intensity on T2W images, with enhancement after gadolinium administration. Osteitis can be identified on MR images as blurring or destruction of the black cortical line on all pulse sequences, and osteomyelitis can be identified as abnormal low signal intensity marrow on T1W and high signal intensity on STIR images, with enhancement after gadolinium administration. Abnormal signal intensity in the bone marrow is not specific for infection, however, and can be seen with neuroarthropathy or from aseptic marrow edema (sympathetic reaction) secondary to hyperemia from the adjacent soft tissue inflammatory process.

MRI is useful for differentiating between these entities.[57] Absence of bone marrow changes on STIR images excludes the diagnosis of osteomyelitis (Fig. 5-25). If abnormal bone marrow signal intensity is identified, one or more of the following changes significantly increases the diagnostic confidence of osteomyelitis in a diabetic foot (Fig. 5-26)[58-65]:

1. Cutaneous ulcer overlying the bone abnormality
2. Sinus tract extending to bone
3. Cortical destruction
4. Intramedullary abscess
5. Sequestrum formation

Certain features help distinguish acute neuropathic changes from diabetic foot infections. Neuroarthropathy always affects joints. It often is associated with bone fragmentation and subluxation. The most common sites of involvement are the tarsometatarsal joints (Lisfranc joint), the talonavicular and calcaneocuboid joints (Chopart joint), and the subtalar joints. A biopsy is indicated whenever imaging features are inconclusive for either osteomyelitis or neuroarthropathy.

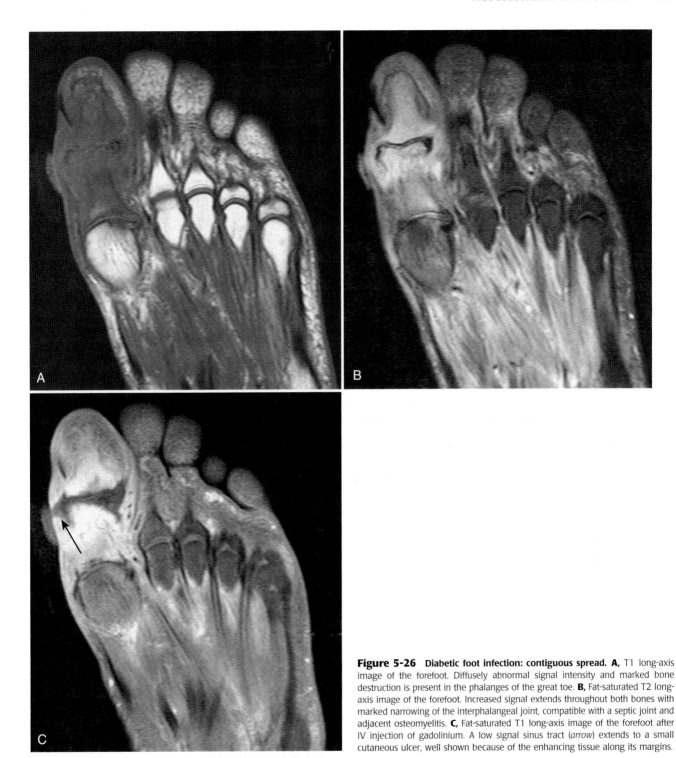

Figure 5-26 **Diabetic foot infection: contiguous spread. A,** T1 long-axis image of the forefoot. Diffusely abnormal signal intensity and marked bone destruction is present in the phalanges of the great toe. **B,** Fat-saturated T2 long-axis image of the forefoot. Increased signal extends throughout both bones with marked narrowing of the interphalangeal joint, compatible with a septic joint and adjacent osteomyelitis. **C,** Fat-saturated T1 long-axis image of the forefoot after IV injection of gadolinium. A low signal sinus tract (*arrow*) extends to a small cutaneous ulcer, well shown because of the enhancing tissue along its margins.

REFERENCES

1. Jones KM, Unger EC, Granstrom P, et al. Bone marrow imaging using STIR at 0.5 and 1.5T. *Magn Reson Imaging* 1992; 10:169-176.
2. Morrison WB, Schweitzer ME, Bock H, et al. Diagnosis of osteomyelitis: utility of fat-suppressed contrast-enhanced MR imaging. *Radiology* 1993; 189:251-257.
3. Morrison WB, Schweitzer ME, Batte WG, et al. Osteomyelitis of the foot: relative importance of primary and secondary MR imaging signs. *Radiology* 1998; 207:625-632.
4. Hopkins KL, Li KCP, Bergman G. Gadolinium-DTPA-enhanced magnetic resonance imaging of musculoskeletal infectious processes. *Skeletal Radiol* 1995; 24:325-330.
5. Lalam RK, Cassar-Pullicino VN, Tins BJ. Magnetic resonance imaging of appendicular musculoskeletal infection. *Top Magn Reson Imaging* 2007; 18:177-191.
6. Pineda C, Vargas A, Rodriguez AV. Imaging of osteomyelitis: current concepts. *Infect Dis Clin N Am* 2006; 20:789-825.
7. Resnick D, Niwayama G. Osteomyelitis, septic arthritis, and soft tissue infection: mechanisms and situations. In Resnick D (ed): *Diagnosis of Bone and Joint Disorders*, ed 3. Philadelphia: Saunders; 1995.

8. McGuinness B, Wilson N, Doyle AJ. The "penumbra sign" on T1-weighted MRI for differentiating musculoskeletal infection from tumor. *Skeletal Radiol* 2007; 36:417-421.

9. Trueta J. The three types of acute hematogenous osteomyelitis: a clinical and vascular study. *J Bone Joint Surg [Br]* 1959; 41:671-680.

10. Marcy SM. Infections due to dog and cat bites. *Pediatr Infect Dis* 1982; 1:351-356.

11. Beltran J, Noto AM, McGhee RB, et al. Infections of the musculoskeletal system: high-field strength MR imaging. *Radiology* 1987; 164:449-454.

12. Tumeh SS, Aliabadi P, Weissman BN, et al. Disease activity in osteomyelitis: role of radiography. *Radiology* 1987; 165:781-784.

13. Tang JS, Gold RH, Bassett LW, et al. Musculoskeletal infection of the extremities: evaluation with MR imaging. *Radiology* 1988; 166:205-209.

14. Unger E, Moldofsky P, Gatenby R, et al. Diagnosis of osteomyelitis by MR imaging. *AJR Am J Roentgenol* 1988; 150:605-610.

15. Wegener WA, Alavi A. Diagnostic imaging of musculoskeletal infection: roentgenography; gallium, indium-labeled white blood cell, gamma globulin bone scintigraphy; and MRI. *Orthop Clin North Am* 1991; 22:401-418.

16. Gold RH, Hawkins RA, Katz RD. Bacterial osteomyelitis: findings on plain radiography, CT, MR, and scintigraphy. *AJR Am J Roentgenol* 1991; 12:292-297.

17. Tehranzadeh J, Wang F, Mesqarzadeh M. Magnetic resonance imaging of osteomyelitis. *Crit Rev Diagn Imaging* 1992; 33:495-534.

18. Crim JR, Seeger LL. Imaging evaluation of osteomyelitis. *Crit Rev Diagn Imaging* 1994; 35:201-256.

19. Chew FS, Schulze ES, Mattia AR. Osteomyelitis. *AJR Am J Roentgenol* 1994; 162:942.

20. Capitanio MA, Kirkpatrick JA. Early roentgen observations in acute osteomyelitis. *AJR Am J Roentgenol* 1970; 108:488-496.

21. Chandnani VP, Beltran J, Morris DS, et al. Acute experimental osteomyelitis and abscesses: detection with MR imaging versus CT. *Radiology* 1990; 174:233-236.

22. Cohen MD, Cory DA, Kleiman M, et al. Magnetic resonance differentiation of acute and chronic osteomyelitis in children. *Clin Radiol* 1990; 41:53-56.

23. Dangman BC, Hoffer FA, Rand FF, et al. Osteomyelitis in children: gadolinium-enhanced MR imaging. *Radiology* 1992; 182:743-747.

24. Mazur JM, Ross G, Cummings RJ, et al. Usefulness of magnetic resonance imaging for the diagnosis of acute musculoskeletal infections in children. *J Pediatr Orthop* 1995; 15:144-147.

25. Collins MS, Schaar MM, Wenger DE, Mandrekar JN. T1-weighted MRI characteristics of pedal osteomyelitis. *AJR Am J Roentgenol* 2005; 185:386-393.

26. Fitzgerald RH, Brewer NS, Dahlin DC. Squamous-cell carcinoma complicating chronic osteomyelitis. *J Bone Joint Surg [Am]* 1976; 58:1146-1148.

27. Mason MD, Zlatkin MB, Esterhai JL, et al. Chronic complicated osteomyelitis of the lower extremity: evaluation with MR imaging. *Radiology* 1989; 173:355-359.

28. Quinn SF, Murray W, Clark RA, Cockran C. MR imaging of chronic osteomyelitis. *J Comput Assist Tomogr* 1988; 12:113-177.

29. Rahmouni A, Chosidow O, Mathieu D, et al. MR imaging in acute infectious cellulitis. *Radiology* 1994; 192:493-496.

30. Jaovisidha S, Chen C, Ryu KN, et al. Tuberculous tenosynovitis and bursitis: imaging findings in 21 cases. *Radiology* 1996; 201:507-513.

31. Crum NF. Bacterial pyomyositis in the United States. *Am J Med* 2004; 117:420-428.

32. Karmazyn B, Kleiman MB, Buckwalter K, et al. Acute pyomyositis of the pelvis: the spectrum of clinical presentations and MR findings. *Pediatr Radiol* 2006; 36:338-343.

33. Theodorou SJ, Theodorou DJ, Resnick D. MR imaging findings of pyogenic bacterial myositis (pyomyositis) in patients with local muscle trauma: illustrative cases. *Emerg Radiol* 2007; 14:89-96.

34. Yu C-W, Jsiao J-K, Hsu C-Y, Shih TT-F. Bacterial pyomyositis: MRI and clinical correlation. *Magn Reson Imaging* 2004; 22:1233-1241.

35. Yuh WTC, Schreiber AE, Montgomery WJ, et al. Magnetic resonance imaging of pyomyositis. *Skeletal Radiol* 1988; 17:190-193.

36. Fleckenstein JL, Burns DK, Murphy FK, et al. Differential diagnosis of bacterial myositis in AIDS: evaluation with MR imaging. *Radiology* 1991; 179:653-658.

37. Applegate GR, Cohen AJ. Pyomyositis: Early detection utilizing multiple imaging modalities. *Magn Reson Imaging* 1991; 9:187-193.

38. Gordon BA, Martinez S, Collins AJ. Pyomyositis: characteristics at CT and MR imaging. *Radiology* 1995; 197:279-286.

39. Freischlag JA, Ajalat G, Bussutil RW. Treatment of necrotizing soft tissue infections. *Am J Surg* 1985; 149:751-755.

40. Schmid MR, Kossmann T, Duewell S. Differentiation of necrotizing fasciitis and cellulitis using MR imaging. *AJR Am J Roentgenol* 1998; 170:615-620.

41. Fugitt JB, Puckett ML, Quigley MM, Kerr SM. Necrotizing fasciitis. *RadioGraphics* 2004; 24:1472-1476.

42. Arslan A, Pierre-Jerome C, Borthne A. Necrotizing fasciitis: unreliable MRI findings in the preoperative diagnosis. *Eur J Radiol* 2000; 36:139-143.

43. Roca RP, Yoshikawa TT. Primary skeletal infections in heroin users. *Clin Orthop Relat Res* 1979; 144:238-248.

44. Firooznia H, Golimbu C, Rafii M, et al. Radiology of musculoskeletal complications of drug addiction. *Semin Roentgenol* 1983; 18:198-206.

45. Zimmerman B III, Erickson AD, Mikolich DJ. Septic acromioclavicular arthritis and osteomyelitis in a patient with acquired immunodeficiency syndrome. *Arthritis Rheum* 1989; 32:1175-1178.

46. Kwack K-S, Cho JH, Lee JH, et al. Septic arthritis versus transient synovitis of the hip: gadolinium-enhanced MRI finding of decreased perfusion at the femoral epiphysis. *AJR Am J Roentgenol* 2007; 189:437-445.

47. Karmazyn B, Loder RT, Kleiman MB, et al. The role of pelvic magnetic resonance in evaluating nonhip sources of infection in children with acute nontraumatic hip pain. *J Pediatr Orthop* 2007; 27:158-164.

48. Connolly SA, Connolly LP, Drubach LA, et al. MRI for detection of abscess in acute osteomyelitis of the pelvis in children. *AJR Am J Roentgenol* 2007; 189:867-872.

49. Kahn M-F, Chamot A-M. SAPHO syndrome. *Rheum Dis Clin N Am* 1992; 18:225-246.

50. Carr AJ, Cole WG, Robertson DM, et al. Chronic multifocal osteomyelitis. *J Bone Joint Surg [Br]* 1993; 75:582-591.

51. Kasperczyk A, Freyschmidt J. Pustulotic arthrosteitis: spectrum of bone lesions with palmoplantar pustulosis. *Radiology* 1994; 191:207-211.

52. Sundaram M, McDonald D, Engel E, et al. Chronic recurrent multifocal osteomyelitis: an evolving clinical and radiological spectrum. *Skeletal Radiol* 1996; 25:333-336.

53. Steinbach LS, Tehranzadeh J, Fleckenstein JL, et al. Human immunodeficiency virus infection: musculoskeletal manifestations. *Radiology* 1993; 186:833-838.

54. Lee DJ, Sartoris DJ. Musculoskeletal manifestations of human immunodeficiency virus infection: review of imaging characteristics. *Radiol Clin North Am* 1994; 32:399-411.

55. Wyatt SH, Fishman EK. CT/MRI of musculoskeletal complications of AIDS. *Skeletal Radiol* 1995; 24:481-488.

56. Baron AL, Steinbach LS, LeBoit PE, et al. Osteolytic lesions and bacillary angiomatosis in HIV infection: radiologic differentiation from AIDS-related Kaposi sarcoma. *Radiology* 1990; 177:77-81.

57. Kapoor A, Page S, LaValley M, et al. Magnetic resonance imaging for diagnosing foot osteomyelitis. *Arch Intern Med* 2007; 167:125-132.

58. Yuh WTC, Corson JD, Baraniewski HM, et al. Osteomyelitis of the foot in diabetic patients: evaluation with plain film, 99mTc-MDP bone scintigraphy, and MR imaging. *AJR Am J Roentgenol* 1989; 152:795-800.

59. Wang A, Weinstein D, Greenfield L, et al. MRI and diabetic foot infections. *Magn Reson Imaging* 1990; 8:805-809.

60. Beltran J, Campanini DS, Knight C, et al. The diabetic foot: magnetic resonance imaging evaluation. *Skeletal Radiol* 1990; 19:37-41.

61. Durham JR, Lukens ML, Campanini DS, et al. Impact of magnetic resonance imaging on the management of diabetic foot infections. *Am J Surg* 1991; 162:150-153.

62. Eckman MH, Greenfield S, Mackey WC, et al. Foot infections in diabetic patients: decision and cost-effectiveness analyses. *JAMA* 1995; 273:712-720.

63. Gold RH, Tong DJ, Crim JR, et al. Imaging the diabetic foot. *Skeletal Radiol* 1995; 24:563-571.

64. Craig JG, Amin MB, Wu K, et al. Osteomyelitis of the diabetic foot: MR imaging-pathologic correlation. *Radiology* 1997; 203:849-855.

65. Tan PL, Teh J. MRI of the diabetic foot: differentiation of infection from neuropathic change. *Br J Radiol* 2007; 80:939-948.

Arthritis and Cartilage

How to Image Arthritis and Cartilage

- *Coils and patient position:* Which joint is being imaged determines which coil and which position are used. In the knee, the standard extremity coil is used in the same manner as imaging for a torn meniscus. The same would hold for the wrist, elbow, and so forth.
- *Image orientation:* Joints imaged for arthritis and for cartilage are best seen with the standard planes of imaging discussed in the other chapters. In the knee, three planes (axial, coronal, and sagittal) should be used to evaluate the cartilage adequately.
- *Pulse sequences and regions of interest:* For most entities involving the joints as in arthritis, it is recommended that T1W and some type of T2W sequence be used in each plane of imaging. Cartilage-sensitive sequences are discussed in greater detail later in this chapter.
- *Contrast:* There is no need to use contrast material for evaluating arthritis or cartilage, although it markedly increases the conspicuity of pannus.

Most joint abnormalities are discussed in the chapters under the specific joints (eg, avascular necrosis in the marrow or hip chapters). This short chapter discusses a few additional abnormalities that can affect any joint, such as pigmented villonodular synovitis (PVNS), synovial chondromatosis, and a few common arthritides; it also provides an overview of cartilage imaging.

MRI has little role in most cases of arthritis. Plain films seem to suffice for initial diagnosis and in follow-up to determine progression. Although MRI can depict erosive changes and cartilage loss in small joints in various arthritides, it currently does not seem to offer additional information over plain films in terms of initial diagnosis. Current trends in rheumatology suggest that MRI is a valuable tool in following synovitis to institute aggressive and earlier treatments. It is important to recognize, however, the changes encountered in the more common arthritides because these changes occasionally are seen in patients undergoing imaging for other reasons.

Rheumatoid Arthritis

The erosive changes in rheumatoid arthritis (RA) seen on MRI virtually mirror the changes seen on conventional radiographs (Fig. 6-1). MRI seems to show them to better advantage, and can be a useful clinical tool for showing the extent of disease. In the past, it was thought unnecessary to perform MRI in the setting of RA. Pannus cannot be reliably differentiated from synovium and joint fluid; however, with gadolinium administration, some investigators have reported that pannus can be easily identified because of the intense enhancement that occurs in the highly vascular pannus. More recent literature suggests contrast-enhanced T1W images identify more periarticular bone abnormalities than fat-suppressed T2W images.[1] If one looks at unenhanced images of joints very closely, pannus has a slightly higher signal than joint fluid on T1W images, allowing it to be identified without the expense and hassle of contrast administration. Previously, treatment of RA was not predicated on the amount of pannus present. Rheumatologists have become more aggressive, however, and MRI is often done to evaluate pannus to help determine a treatment plan.

Occasionally, a swollen joint in a patient with RA shows multiple small loose bodies, called *rice bodies* (Fig. 6-2). They are called this because of their resemblance at surgery to white rice. On MRI, rice bodies of RA can mimic another cause of multiple loose bodies, such as synovial chondromatosis, but typically rice bodies are much smaller than the loose bodies of synovial chondromatosis and remain low signal on T2W images. Most, but not all, patients already carry a diagnosis of RA, so the entity is easily recognized as rice bodies if the radiologist is familiar with this process. Rice bodies can be removed easily by a surgeon if they cause

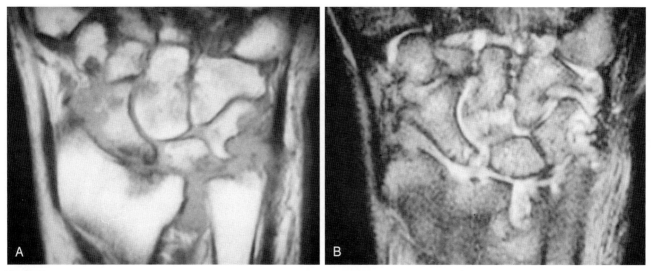

Figure 6-1 **Rheumatoid arthritis. A** and **B,** Coronal T1W (**A**) and gradient echo (**B**) images in a patient with advanced rheumatoid arthritis show the distended joints and multiple erosions throughout the wrist.

mechanical symptoms, but otherwise the treatment is the same as for any joint inflamed by RA.

Ankylosing Spondylitis

Generally, the changes of ankylosing spondylitis can be appreciated with conventional x-ray as has been discussed with other arthritides. The early changes, such as enthesopathy as evidenced by bone marrow edema at the tendinous insertion sites can be appreciated much earlier on MRI than conventional x-ray (Fig. 6-3).

Contrast enhancement may show the more subtle early changes around the sacroiliac joints before erosions are evident on plain films. Similarly, the MRI equivalent of "shiny corners" is reflected as bone marrow edema at the end plates of the ligament attachment. The presence of these

findings can help direct treatment for patients with this arthropathy.

Gout

As with RA, the radiographic findings in gout are sufficient for diagnosis, and MRI has little to offer in this disease. It is important to appreciate, however, that gouty tophi occasionally are seen in patients not known to have gout, in which case they can cause diagnostic confusion. Gouty tophi can occur in almost any soft tissue location, including intra-articularly. They can erode bones or can begin within bones (intraosseous tophi). In cases in which the tophus is large, and the diagnosis of gout is unknown, the tophus can be misdiagnosed as a tumor with resultant biopsy. Tophi are typically low in signal on T1W and T2W images (Fig. 6-4),

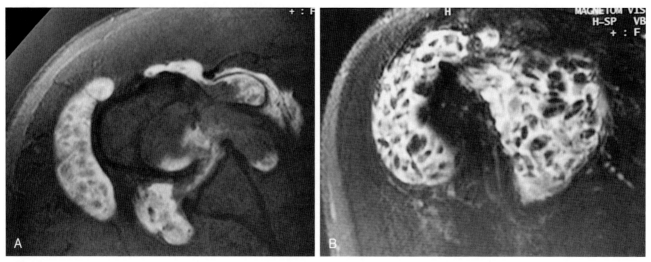

Figure 6-2 **Rheumatoid arthritis. A** and **B,** T1W images with fat suppression after a gadolinium arthrogram in the axial (**A**) and oblique (**B**) coronal planes through the shoulder show multiple small filling defects or loose bodies. At surgery, these were found to be rice bodies.

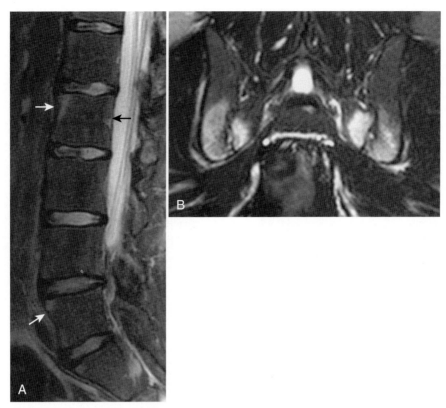

Figure 6-3   **Ankylosing spondylitis. A,** Sagittal fat-suppressed T2W image shows increased signal at anterior superior aspects of L2 and L5 (*white arrows*). Note the loss of the normal concave posterior margin of the vertebral body (*black arrow*). **B,** Coronal fat-suppressed T2W image shows bone marrow edema on both sides of the sacroiliac joint in this patient with ankylosing spondylitis.

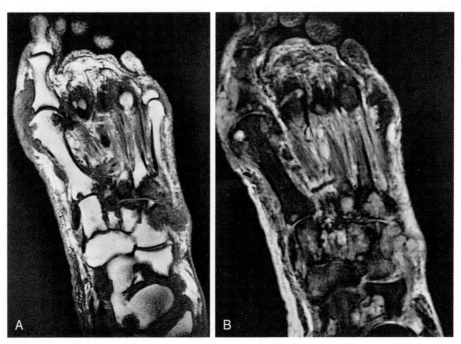

Figure 6-4   **Gout. A** and **B,** Coronal T1W (**A**) and STIR (**B**) images in the foot of a patient with advanced gout reveal multiple erosions and tophi, most of which are low in signal on both sequences.

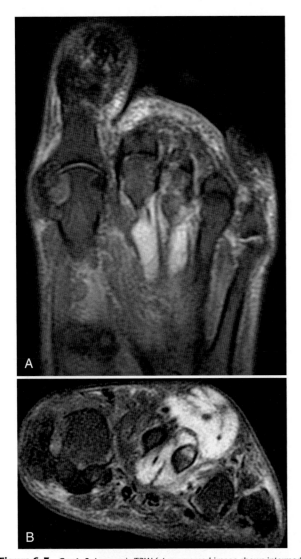

Figure 6-5 **Gout. A,** Long-axis T2W fat-suppressed image shows intermediate signal at the metatarsophalangeal joint consistent with the appearance of gout. Surrounding the third metatarsal head is a focus of increased signal, which is seen to better advantage in **B. B,** Short-axis T2W fat-suppressed image shows fluid signal around the third metatarsal with some increased signal within the metatarsal. Biopsy determined this to be gout.

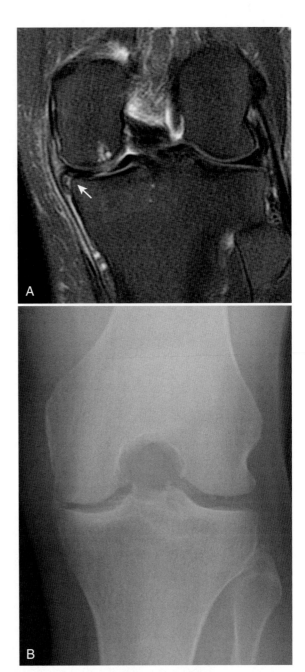

Figure 6-6 Calcium pyrophosphate dihydrate deposition. **A,** Coronal T2W image with fat suppression showing increased signal within the extruded medial meniscus (*arrow*). **B,** This is identified as calcification on the conventional x-ray.

which distinguishes them from most other joint problems and from most tumors (with the exception of fibrous tumors, PVNS, and amyloid). Images of tophi occasionally are increased signal intensity, however (Fig. 6-5).

Calcium Pyrophosphate Dihydrate Deposition

As with the aforementioned arthritides, MRI has little to offer in the diagnosis of calcium pyrophosphate dihydrate deposition, or pseudogout. The appearance of chondrocalcinosis in the menisci of the knee has been reported to have linear high signal that can mimic a meniscal tear (Fig. 6-6),

but this has not been a significant pitfall in our experience. One might intuitively think that calcification would produce low signal on MR images; however, in many cases, such as in the lumbar spine, calcification paradoxically causes intermediate to high signal on T1W images. The reason for this has not been explained, but several theories have been discussed in the literature.[2,3] Chondrocalcinosis also can appear as linear or punctate areas of low signal in hyaline cartilage, which are particularly noticeable on T2* sequences because of the blooming artifact.

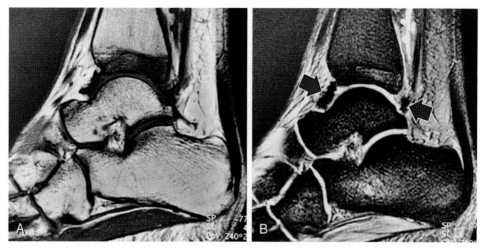

Figure 6-7 Hemophilia. **A** and **B,** Sagittal T1W (**A**) and gradient echo (**B**) images in the ankle of a patient with hemophilia show a large joint effusion that is low in signal on the T2* sequence (*arrows*), consistent with hemosiderin deposition.

Hemophilia

Although patients with hemophilia are not imaged with MRI often, some of the findings seen in hemophilia are worth mentioning. The joint destruction and cartilage loss seen on MRI are pretty much what one would expect from the conventional radiographs. Chronic joint hemorrhages leave deposits of hemosiderin, however, which is seen on MR images as clumps of low signal lining the synovium on T1W and T2W images (Fig. 6-7). This has been termed *hemosiderotic arthropathy.* The amount of hemosiderin seen varies from none to moderate; it is almost never as prominent as that seen in PVNS. In joints with a lot of hemosiderin, there typically is advanced joint destruction, which is uncommon in PVNS. It is virtually never a diagnostic dilemma to differentiate hemophilia from PVNS because patients with hemophilia are well aware of their diagnosis long before a joint is imaged. The main indications for imaging a hemophiliac joint are to determine the extent of cartilage destruction and the thickness of the synovium; these features help determine how to manage the joint abnormality.

Amyloid

Amyloid deposits tend to occur in and around large joints, and can cause significant joint swelling and pain (Figs. 6-8 and 6-9). Bony erosion can be prominent.[4] Amyloid also can

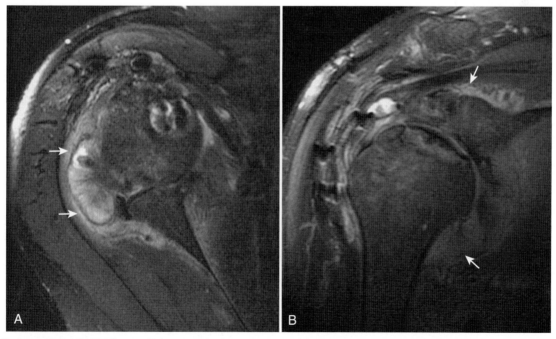

Figure 6-8 Amyloid. **A,** Axial T2W image with fat suppression in a patient with renal failure and prior rotator cuff surgery. Note the low and intermediate signal within the joint space (*arrows*). **B,** Coronal T2W image with fat suppression in the same patient as in **A** also shows the low and intermediate signal of amyloid within the joint space (*arrows*).

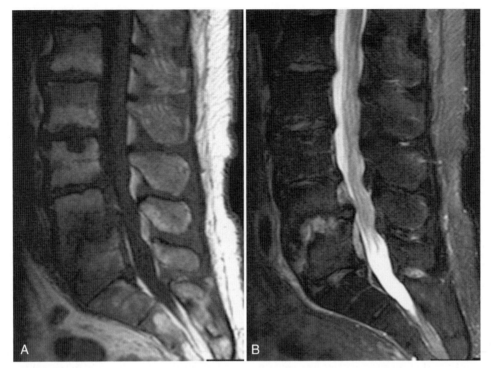

Figure 6-9   **Amyloid. A,** Sagittal T1W image in a patient with back pain and renal failure. End plate irregularity is noted with abnormal disk space. **B,** T2W image with fat suppression shows abnormal signal within the disk space. This process occasionally can be confused with diskitis because of the increased signal in the disk space.

occur in the spine (where it is much more common), where it may resemble a disk infection (Fig. 6-10). In the spine, the deposits can be either amyloid or an amyloid-like entity called *β₂-microglobulin.*[5] In a patient with suspected disk infection, it is imperative to inquire whether the patient has renal failure or is on dialysis because amyloid or β₂-

microglobulin deposits from renal disease can perfectly mimic infection on radiographs and MR images, resulting in an unnecessary biopsy. It is the only entity described that mimics a disk infection. Amyloid deposits have been reported to be low in signal on T1W and T2W images, which is distinctly unusual for most pathologic processes. Most examples

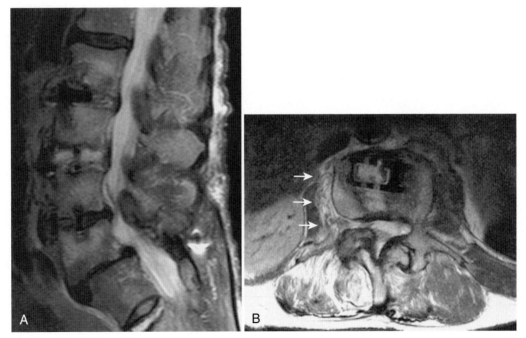

Figure 6-10   **Diskitis. A,** Sagittal T2W image shows fluid signal along the disk space in a patient who had a spacer device placed recently. **B,** Axial T2W image shows increased signal at the disk space level with extension of inflammatory process in a paraspinous location (*arrows*). The spacer device is noted as low signal at the disk space.

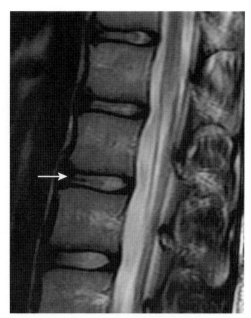

Figure 6-11   Intranuclear cleft. Sagittal T2W image in a normal lumbar spine shows the intermediate signal within the midsubstance of the disk (*arrow*). The intranuclear cleft is present within disks not affected by infection.

we have seen in the spine have shown high signal on T2W images. One helpful way of determining infection versus amyloid in the spine is noting the preservation of an intranuclear cleft within the disks. The cleft disappears in the setting of diskitis (Fig. 6-11).

Tumors

There are no tumors that originate in joints, but there are a few entities that are tumor-like and manifest as joint swelling. The most common of these are synovial chondromatosis and PVNS. Uncommon entities that can manifest similarly are synovial hemangioma and lipoma arborescens; these are rare enough that they are not mentioned further in this book.

Synovial Chondromatosis

There are two forms of synovial chondromatosis: primary and secondary. Primary synovial chondromatosis is an uncommon entity that is caused by metaplasia of the synovium, which produces multiple loose bodies within a joint. Initially, these are cartilaginous bodies that are not calcified; they generally progress to calcified loose bodies, all of which are the same size. They may cause mechanical symptoms, as with any loose body in a joint, or they may merely cause a feeling of swelling or fullness in the joint. Eventually, they become embedded in the synovium and do not float freely in the joint. Cartilage erosion from these loose bodies is a late finding if it occurs at all. Treatment is removal of the loose bodies and a synovectomy. MRI plays a role in the diagnosis because similar to on conventional x-rays, primary synovial chondromatosis resembles PVNS. MRI shows low signal of hemosiderin in PVNS and inter-

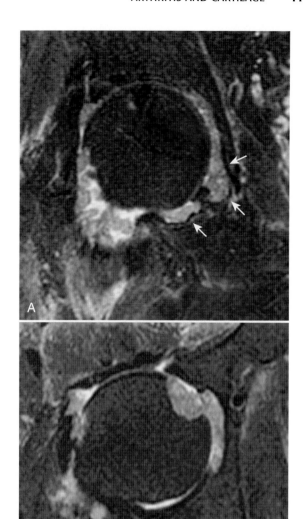

Figure 6-12   Primary synovial chondromatosis. A, Coronal T2W fat-suppressed image shows intermediate signal intensity in the joint space (*arrows*). **B,** Axial T2W fat-suppressed image of the same patient shows the erosions that also can be seen with this abnormality.

mediate signal bodies (same signal as cartilage) in synovial chondromatosis.

Secondary synovial chondromatosis is a much more common disorder. It is believed to be secondary to trauma, which causes shedding of bits of articular cartilage resulting in loose bodies in the joint. These bodies may or may not calcify. These loose bodies, in contrast to primary synovial chondromatosis, are of all different sizes and generally are fewer in number. Osteoarthritis typically is present because of the cartilage damage. Treatment is removal of the loose bodies (osteoarthrosis) and smoothing of the articular cartilage defects. A synovectomy is unnecessary because this condition is not caused by metaplasia of the synovium.

Synovial chondromatosis typically is an easy radiographic diagnosis, with the presence of multiple calcified loose bodies being virtually pathognomonic. It is not always that straight-

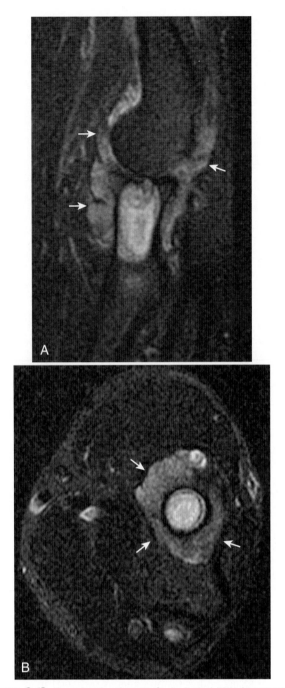

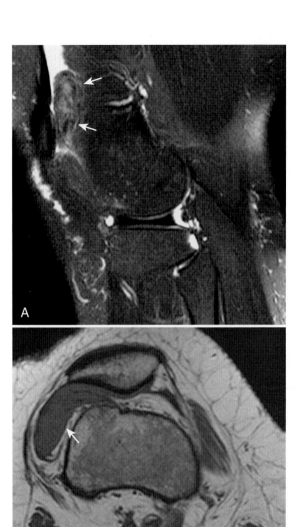

Figure 6-13 **Synovial chondromatosis. A,** Sagittal T2W fat-suppressed image shows intermediate signal within the joint space (*arrows*). Note the erosions within the radius. **B,** Axial T2W fat-suppressed image in the same patient shows the intermediate signal of the synovial chondromatosis (*arrows*). The increased signal in the radius consistent with the erosion seen in **A** is again identified.

Figure 6-14 **Pigmented villonodular synovitis. A,** Sagittal T2W fat-suppressed image shows intermediate signal focus within the suprapatellar pouch with low signal foci within this region (*arrows*). The low signal foci represent hemosiderin. **B,** Axial T1W image shows the intermediate signal of the focus of pigmented villonodular synovitis. The low signal of the hemosiderin can be seen on this sequence as well (*arrow*).

forward, however; 20% of cases may not have the loose bodies calcified, in which case the radiograph shows only joint swelling, if anything. MRI can show multiple loose bodies (see Fig. 6-16), but occasionally it has a second appearance that is not as easily recognized as synovial chondromatosis. In these cases, the MRI examination shows a confluent mass of tissue that can be high in signal on T2W images and looks more like a tumor than multiple loose bodies (Figs. 6-12 and 6-13). Biopsies performed in these

cases have incorrectly led to a diagnosis of chondrosarcoma, with extensive, radical surgery performed before the benign nature of the process was recognized. It is crucial that the radiologist recognize this benign disorder, rather than allow the pathologist to sort it out. There are no malignant tumors that begin in a joint, so a mass in a joint should raise concern for synovial chondromatosis and PVNS.

Pigmented Villonodular Synovitis

PVNS is a disorder of unknown cause that can affect any joint, bursa, or tendon sheath (when it affects a tendon

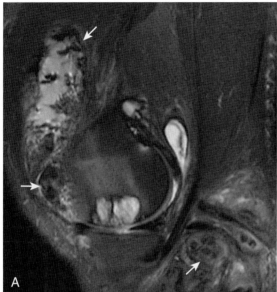

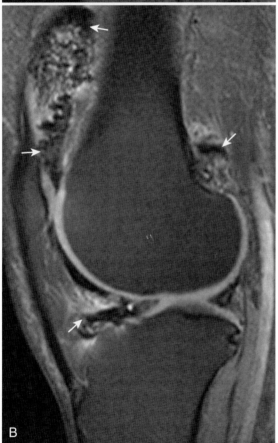

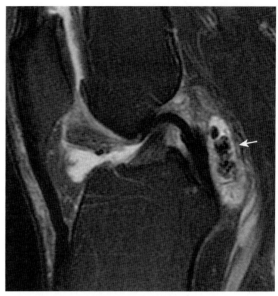

Figure 6-16 Synovial osteochondromatosis. Multiple ossified loose bodies of varying size (*arrow*) consistent with the diagnosis of secondary synovial chondromatosis.

Figure 6-15 Pigmented villonodular synovitis. A, Sagittal T2W fat-suppressed image through the medial aspect of the knee shows multiple low signal foci within the joint capsule and posterior portion of the knee (*arrows*). The blooming around the low signal foci is consistent with the appearance of hemosiderin. Note the erosion of the medial femoral condyle that can be seen in pigmented villonodular synovitis. **B,** Same patient as in **A**. Sagittal image through the lateral compartment, showing the involvement of the suprapatellar pouch with pigmented villonodular synovitis (*arrows*).

sheath, it is called *giant cell tumor of tendon sheath*). PVNS results in synovial hypertrophy with diffuse hemosiderin deposits within the joint. It virtually never calcifies and causes joint space narrowing only late in its course; radiographs simply show a swollen joint, if anything at all. When a large joint is affected, the hemosiderin can produce a dense effusion that can be seen radiographically.

MRI is virtually pathognomonic. A joint effusion with diffuse low signal lining hypertrophied synovium on T2W images is characteristic (Fig. 6-14). The process can erode into bone, making large cystic cavities, but typically is confined to the soft tissues within a joint.

PVNS has two presentations in joints: diffuse and focal. When PVNS is diffuse, it requires a total synovectomy for treatment, which is difficult to perform. Recurrence is common after attempted resection for diffuse PVNS. In focal PVNS (also called *focal nodular PVNS*), resection is considerably easier and more effective. When PVNS is identified within the joint, the remainder of the joint should be carefully inspected to identify other deposits. Occasionally, this inspection may necessitate increasing the field of view, particularly in the knee, to evaluate the suprapatellar location. Additional foci can change the management of the patient (Fig. 6-15).

Loose Bodies

Loose bodies in joints can be difficult to find with any imaging modality, but MRI seems to be better than almost any other technique.[6] MR arthrography is superior to plain MRI, unless a large joint effusion is present. Loose bodies can be composed of cartilage, cortical bone (Fig. 6-16), or cancellous bone (usually with some cortical bone attached). We try to include a gradient echo sequence in at least one plane when looking for loose bodies in the hope that, if they

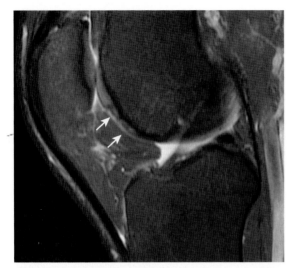

Figure 6-17 **Partial-width cartilage loss.** Sagittal T2W fat-suppressed image showing a partial-width cartilage abnormality within the trochlea (*arrows*).

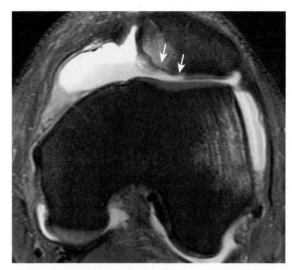

Figure 6-18 **Full-thickness cartilage loss.** Axial T2W fat-suppressed image in a patient who had a patella dislocation. Marked full-thickness cartilage loss at the apex of the patella (*arrows*). Recognizing cartilage loss in a patient with a patella dislocation has treatment implications and is an important observation.

have cortical bone attached to them, they will "bloom" and be more easily seen. Requests to image a patient for a loose body in the elbow and ankle occur, and we occasionally see loose bodies in the shoulder and in the hip. Loose bodies are most often encountered in the knee.

Cartilage

Perhaps the biggest impact in recent years in musculoskeletal research has been in the area of cartilage. Many articles have been published on MRI of cartilage with multiple comparisons of various imaging sequences for their utility in diagnosing cartilage abnormalities.[7-10] For the most part, the literature advocates several sequences, all of which seem superior to standard spin echo sequences. Which sequence is really the best is debatable, but so far no single sequence

is indisputably better than all the others, so it seems for now one can pick one of several available sequences that perform well at showing hyaline articular cartilage. It is imperative that every knee MRI examination have a cartilage-sensitive sequence. Some of the cartilage sequences promulgated in the literature are not readily available on commercial magnets, and others require inordinate imaging times, which renders them useless for routine use. Some authors recommend their use only when cartilage abnormalities are suspected. You had better suspect a cartilage abnormality in

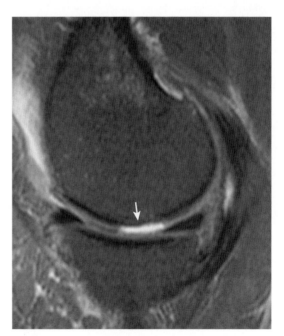

Figure 6-20 **Full-thickness cartilage loss.** Sagittal T2W fat-suppressed image shows a full-thickness cartilage defect as evidenced by the fluid signal replacing the intermediate signal of the hyaline articular cartilage along the weight-bearing portion of the medial femoral condyle.

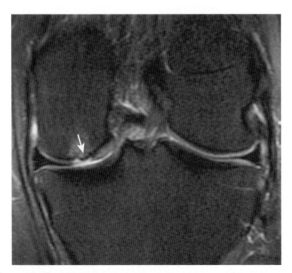

Figure 6-19 **Full-thickness cartilage loss.** Coronal T2W fat-suppressed image shows full-thickness cartilage loss (*arrow*) with adjacent bone marrow edema along the medial femoral condyle.

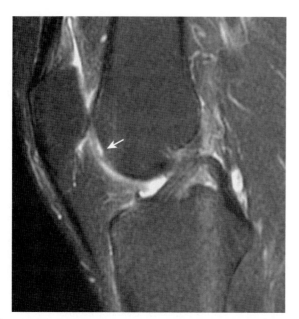

Figure 6-21 **Delamination.** Sagittal T2W fat-suppressed image shows fluid signal at the cartilage-bone interface (tidemark) (*arrow*).

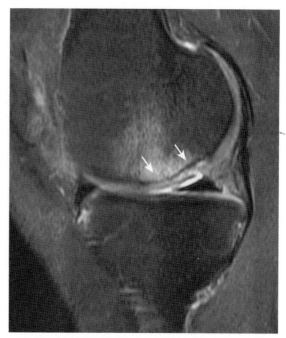

Figure 6-22 **Delamination.** Sagittal T2W fat-suppressed image shows delamination of the cartilage along the weight-bearing portion of the medial femoral condyle that resulted in a "flap" of cartilage (*arrows*).

every knee and have a sequence that shows the cartilage to good advantage, or your orthopedic surgeon will look elsewhere for an imaging diagnosis.

Cartilage treatment has become important in orthopedic surgery, and MRI is known to be useful in showing abnormal cartilage in the knee, ankle, and elbow. The use of color has become a good marketing tool for delineating cartilage defects.[11] Some of these postprocessing techniques are achievable through magnet upgrades. The use of color has not proved to be any more accurate than gray scale, and color is not widely available for general use. It seems that color is appealing to referring clinicians and is less exciting to the radiologist.

Multiple grading systems for cartilage abnormalities have been described in the radiology and the orthopedic surgery literature. One radiologist's grade 2 lesion is another's grade 3. Simply saying there is a grade 2 or 3 cartilage abnormality leaves one wondering which grading scale is being employed. It can get very confusing and often is misleading. No single grading system seems to have a majority of proponents; we do not recommend a description of the cartilage using a grading system except for research papers, unless everyone involved with that patient's care is using the same grading system—something that would be unlikely because one cannot predict where a patient might go next for treatment. A simple description of the MRI appearance would give the surgeon all he or she needs to treat the abnormality. Also, a description of the abnormality allows anyone who desires to place the lesion in his or her particular grading scale.

Descriptions of the cartilage should state if there is focal abnormal signal, surface fibrillation or irregularity (Fig. 6-17), a partial-thickness defect, or a full-thickness defect (Fig. 6-18), and if the underlying bone has abnormal signal (Figs. 6-19 and 6-20). We refrain from commenting on generalized thinning of the cartilage because it is virtually impossible to document at arthroscopy. Cartilage thickness seems to depend on patient age and activity, is not relevant

to any symptoms or therapy that has been described, and probably has a better than even chance of being an inaccurate assessment. One particular cartilage abnormality that is important to recognize, however, is that of delamination.[11] A delamination cartilage defect has a specific appearance and location. Fluid signal is identified along the tidemark (cartilage-bone interface) (Figs. 6-21 and 6-22).

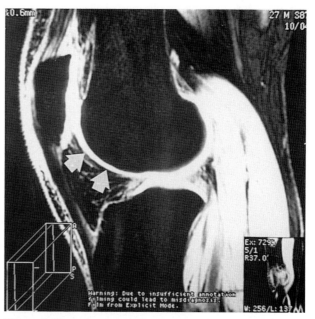

Figure 6-23 **Articular cartilage.** A sagittal 3D volume-spoiled GRASS image with fat suppression shows the articular cartilage to be very high in signal (*arrows*). Although the cartilage is elegantly depicted, this image takes more than 10 minutes to acquire.

The easiest part of diagnosing cartilage abnormalities is choosing an appropriate MRI sequence. Almost any sequence other than conventional spin echo T1W, proton density, and T2W images would suffice; this includes fast spin echo–T2 (TE > 40) with or without fat suppression, STIR, and gradient echo (either 2D or 3D). One sequence that is being strongly advocated in the radiology literature is a 3D volume-spoiled GRASS (gradient-recalled acquisition in the steady state) with fat suppression.[7] Although this sequence does provide elegant images of cartilage (Fig. 6-23), it has two drawbacks. First, it takes more than 10 minutes to acquire, which is too long for routine use. Second, it produces 60 images that need to be inspected. For most radiologists, that is information overload. One cannot examine all of the images with the diligence needed to have a high accuracy. We added this sequence to our standard knee protocol for about 6 months, and in hundreds of cases never found a single example in which a cartilage abnormality was seen on the GRASS images that we did not see on the fast spin echo–T2 images.

The hard part about diagnosing cartilage abnormalities is simply looking at all the cartilage surfaces. We have found that it is preferable to have a cartilage-sensitive sequence in all three planes because the conspicuity of the abnormality often is prominent in one of the planes and very subtle in the other two. It is dependent on the location of the abnormality. We probably spend as much time inspecting the knee for cartilage abnormalities as we do looking at the remainder of the entire knee.

Imaging with 3T was thought to have some of its greatest application for musculoskeletal imaging in the evaluation of cartilage. To date, 3T seems to allow slightly better resolution, and perhaps increased confidence, but even with 3T, it is imperative to have a proper sequence for evaluation. Perhaps the greatest utility of 3T would be the better resolution using 3D acquisition, which would allow timely evaluation of patients allowing visualization of all structures in all planes of imaging. The choice of coil can have an impact on resolution and signal-to-noise ratio, and should be a major consideration when placing patients (especially extremely large patients) on the magnet.

MRI has some utility in imaging for arthritis. Radiologists need to be familiar with the more common appearances of the arthritides. Cartilage imaging is considered an essential part of the imaging of the knee, ankle, and elbow. An appropriate sequence affords a good look at the cartilage, and a full description of the abnormality should be made, rather than placing it in a grading system.

REFERENCES

1. Yao L, Magalnick M, Wilson M, et al. Periarticular bone findings in rheumatoid arthritis: T2-weighted versus contrast-enhanced T1-weighted MRI. *AJR Am J Roentgenol* 2006; 187:358-363.
2. Major N, Helms C, Genant H. Calcification demonstrated as high signal intensity on T1-weighted MR images of the disks of the lumbar spine. *Radiology* 1993; 189:494-496.
3. Bangert B, Modic M, Ross J, et al. Hyperintense disks on T1-weighted MR images: correlation with calcification. *Radiology* 1995; 195:437-444.
4. Kurer M, Baillod R, Madgwick J. Musculoskeletal manifestations of amyloidosis. *J Bone Joint Surg [Br]* 1991; 73:271-276.
5. Naidich JB, Mossey RT, McHeffey AB, et al. Spondyloarthropathy from long-term hemodialysis. *Radiology* 1988; 167:761-764.
6. Brossmann J, Preidler KW, Daenen B, et al. Imaging of osseous and cartilaginous intraarticular bodies in the knee—comparison of MR imaging and MR arthrography with CT and CT arthrography in cadavers. *Radiology* 1996; 200:509-517.
7. Disler DG, McCauley TR, Kelman CG, et al. Fat-suppressed three-dimensional spoiled gradient-echo MR imaging of hyaline cartilage defects in the knee—comparison with standard MR imaging and arthroscopy. *AJR Am J Roentgenol* 1996; 167:127-132.
8. Gagliardi JA, Chung EM, Chandnani VP, et al. Detection and staging of chondromalacia patellae: relative efficacies of conventional MR imaging, MR arthrography, and CT arthrography. *AJR Am J Roentgenol* 1994; 163:629-636.
9. Hodler J, Resnick D. Current status of imaging of articular cartilage [review]. *Skeletal Radiol* 1996; 25:703-709.
10. Recht MP, Piraino DW, Paletta GA, et al. Accuracy of fat-suppressed three-dimensional spoiled gradient-echo flash MR imaging in the detection of patellofemoral articular cartilage abnormalities. *Radiology* 1996; 198:209-212.
11. Kendell SD, Helms CA, Rampton JW, et al. MRI appearance of chondral delamination injuries of the knee. *AJR Am J Roentgenol* 2005; 184:1486-1489.

Tumors

7

MRI plays a central role in the work-up of a patient presenting with a suspected musculoskeletal tumor.[1] MRI can confirm the presence of a lesion, allow for a specific diagnosis in some cases, define the extent of tumor spread, provide biopsy guidance, and assist in the evaluation of recurrent disease after therapy.

Therapeutic planning at the time of presentation is based primarily on the stage of the lesion. Local staging of a tumor depends on which anatomic structures and spaces (compartments) are involved, and this is best shown with MRI.[2,3] Because an understanding of tumor staging is an important precursor to designing an optimal MRI protocol for evaluating these lesions, this chapter begins with a section briefly describing the principles of tumor staging. Despite your understandable natural instinct to skip over this material, we strongly urge you to read it to understand better how to set up and interpret MRI studies for this important indication.

Staging of Musculoskeletal Tumors

PRINCIPLES OF STAGING

The primary goal of the oncologic surgeon is to provide local control of disease by obtaining adequate tumor margins at the time of resection. If possible, this goal is achieved through a limb-sparing procedure; but if the lesion is too advanced, an amputation or disarticulation is required. The decision to amputate or perform a limb-sparing procedure depends on many factors, including tumor size; relationship of the tumor to adjacent structures, such as nerves, vessels, and joints; and the overall stage of the tumor at the time of presentation.[4]

Although there are different staging systems, they all are based on three components[4,5]:
1. Grade of the tumor
2. Local extent of the tumor
3. Presence or absence of metastases

The Enneking staging system,[4] which has been adopted by the Musculoskeletal Tumor Society, is outlined in Table 7-1.

Grade

The grade of the tumor is a measure of its potential to metastasize.[5] It is based primarily on histologic features and requires a preoperative biopsy. A sarcoma is classified as either low grade or high grade. Generally, a low-grade lesion is less biologically active and requires a relatively conservative surgical procedure. Conversely, a high-grade lesion usually necessitates a more radical procedure because of its more aggressive nature.

Local Extent

Factors related to the local extent of the tumor include its size and degree of involvement of adjacent tissues. Sarcomas tend to grow centrifugally along pathways of least resistance and are contained in part by a pseudocapsule as they extend into adjacent tissues.[6] A malignant lesion may remain confined within the pseudocapsule (intracapsular); generally, however, malignant cells often extend beyond these capsular boundaries. If a lesion extends through its capsule, but is still confined within a single anatomic compartment, it is considered extracapsular and intracompartmental. If the tumor extends into an adjacent compartment, it is classified as extracompartmental. Extracompartmental spread may occur

Table 7-1 SARCOMA STAGING

Stage	Grade (G)	Site (T)	Metastases (M)
IA	Low (G1)	Intracompartmental (T1)	No (M0)
IB	Low (G1)	Extracompartmental (T2)	No (M0)
IIA	High (G2)	Intracompartmental (T1)	No (M0)
IIB	High (G2)	Extracompartmental (T2)	No (M0)
III	Any (G)	Any (T)	Yes (M1) Regional or distant

BOX 7-1

Checklist for Staging Musculoskeletal Tumor on MRI

- Intraosseous extent
- Extraosseous extent
- Neurovascular involvement
- Joint invasion
- Skip metastases in same bone
- Local adenopathy

via direct tumor invasion of an adjacent compartment or by contamination resulting from fracture, hemorrhage, or an operative procedure such as an unplanned resection or poorly planned biopsy.[5] Generally, lesions with more advanced local extension, including involvement of neurovascular structures or joints, require excision of more adjacent tissue than smaller tumors.

Metastases

The third component of the staging system is the presence or absence of nodal or distant metastases. Determination of metastases is usually accomplished with computed tomography (CT) and radionuclide bone scanning, but more recently, CT with positron emission tomography and whole-body MRI have been advocated as possible alternatives.[7-9] Regional lymph node involvement is much less common with musculoskeletal sarcomas than are pulmonary metastases, but both are equally poor prognostic factors.

PRINCIPLES OF IMAGING

Bone Tumors

MRI is the most sensitive imaging modality for detecting and delineating bone tumors, especially tumors involving the marrow cavity. The MRI appearance of most osseous lesions is very nonspecific, however, and conventional radiographs are essential for evaluating a primary bone tumor. Radiographs should be obtained early in the work-up of a symptomatic patient because they are inexpensive and provide the most specific information of any modality regarding the true nature of a lesion. The radiographic findings and degree of clinical suspicion dictate further work-up. If an aggressive osseous lesion is identified on conventional radiographs, MRI is useful in the preoperative assessment of these patients because it is the best modality for local staging.[10] If a bone lesion is clearly benign radiographically, MRI generally is unnecessary.

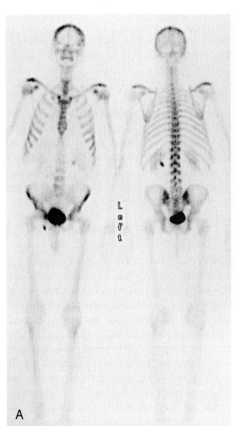

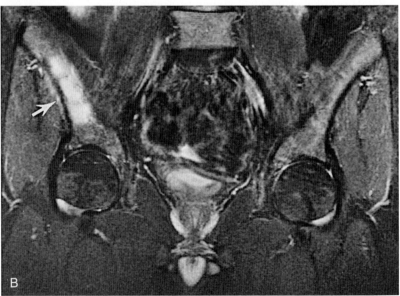

Figure 7-1 **Right iliac metastasis not detected on bone scan. A,** Whole-body bone scan image. There is no scintigraphic evidence of metastasis in this 54-year-old man with a history of colon cancer and recent right hip pain. **B,** STIR coronal image of the pelvis. There is abnormal signal intensity within the right iliac bone (*arrow*) at the site of an osseous metastasis.

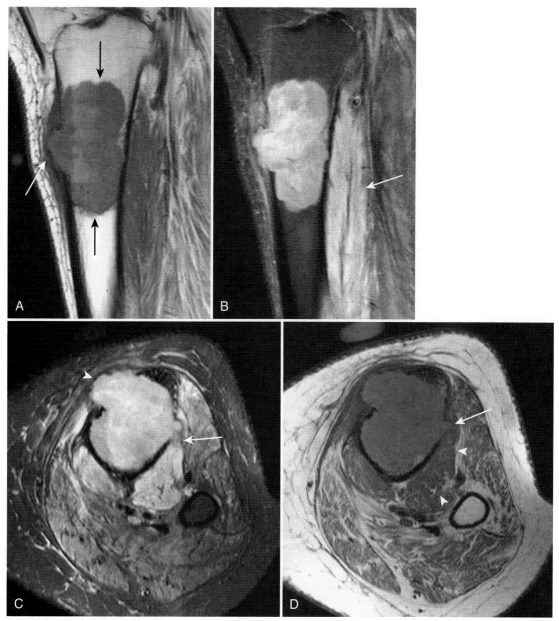

Figure 7-2 **MRI evaluation of local extent of tumor. A,** T1 sagittal image of the proximal tibia. A large tumor (plasmacytoma) is seen in the proximal tibia with intraosseous (*black arrows*) and extraosseous (*white arrow*) components. **B,** STIR sagittal image of the proximal tibia. The intraosseous and extraosseous components of the tumor are well shown. Note the associated edema within the adjacent musculature (*arrow*). **C,** STIR axial image of the proximal calf. The medial extraosseous tumor is well shown (*arrowhead*); however, the tumor is difficult to separate from adjacent muscle laterally (*arrow*). **D,** T1 axial image of the proximal calf. The lateral extraosseous component (*arrow*) is easier to delineate from adjacent edema and muscles. Note the normal fatty striations within the uninvolved skeletal muscle (*arrowheads*).

For a patient with normal radiographs, a radionuclide bone scan often is the next study obtained; if a focal abnormality is detected, MRI is useful for further characterization.[11] Even with a negative bone scan, MRI can detect radiographically occult intramedullary lesions and should be obtained in a patient with a known primary tumor and focal symptoms or laboratory abnormalities that suggest osseous metastases (Fig. 7-1).

Soft Tissue Tumors

In a patient with a suspected soft tissue mass, conventional radiographs still should be obtained because they may reveal bone involvement or soft tissue calcifications that might be missed with MRI. In many cases, the MRI appearance of a soft tissue mass is so characteristic that a confident, specific diagnosis can be provided, obviating further work-up. Even if the MRI features do not allow a specific diagnosis to be made, MRI is still useful for staging these lesions.

Important MRI Features (Box 7-1)

For osseous and soft tissue lesions, the crucial factors influencing resectability that should be addressed in the MRI report include intraosseous and extraosseous tumor extent, neurovascular or joint involvement, and nodes.

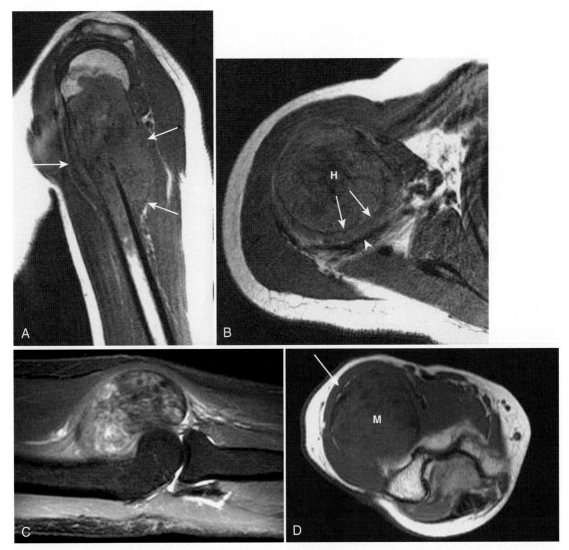

Figure 7-3 **Neurovascular involvement. A,** T1 sagittal image of the upper arm. A large tumor (osteosarcoma) involving the proximal humerus shows prominent extraosseous extension (*arrows*) and has resulted in a pathologic fracture. **B,** T1 axial image of the axilla. The tumor (*arrows*) is inseparable from and partially surrounds the circumflex humeral artery (H) and axillary nerve coursing through the quadrangular space (*arrowhead*). **C,** STIR sagittal image of the elbow (different patient than in **A** and **B**). A heterogeneous soft tissue mass (low-grade myxoid sarcoma) lies along the ventral surface of the distal humerus. **D,** T1 axial image of the elbow. The mass (M) displaces and compresses the radial neurovascular structures laterally. Although there appears to be preserved fat adjacent to the distorted radial nerve (*arrow*), tumor involvement is difficult to evaluate owing to the degree of compression.

Intraosseous Tumor Extent. Intraosseous tumor extent is best determined with T1W or STIR imaging (Fig. 7-2). The intraosseous extent of tumor may be overestimated with STIR because it can be difficult to separate intraosseous tumor from peritumoral edema on these images.[12] MRI also is able to detect skip lesions (foci of tumor that are not contiguous with the primary lesion) missed with scintigraphy.[13]

Extraosseous Tumor Extent. Extraosseous tumor extent is best evaluated with T2W or STIR imaging (see Fig. 7-2). Most tumors become hyperintense to fat on these sequences, and it may be difficult to separate tumor from adjacent soft tissue edema. MRI features of edema that help to differentiate it from neoplasm include feathery margins, an absence of mass effect, and no distortion of muscle planes (see Fig. 7-2).[14] Because a 5-cm "cuff" of normal tissue beyond the

tumor margins usually is desired at surgery, exact measurements of the intraosseous and extraosseous components should be provided with reference to an osseous landmark (eg, distance from the articular surface of the medial femoral condyle for a lesion involving the femoral shaft).

Neurovascular or Joint Involvement. Identification of neurovascular involvement is crucial (Fig. 7-3). Such involvement may preclude the possibility of a limb-sparing procedure because the functional status of a patient with a denervated limb after surgery may be worse than that achieved with an amputation. MRI is highly accurate in showing a lack of neurovascular involvement when a clear plane of normal tissue is shown between nerves or vessels and tumor. Gross tumor invasion usually is easily diagnosed, but if there is equivocal tumor involvement, this should be reported as such. The structures can be reassessed at the time

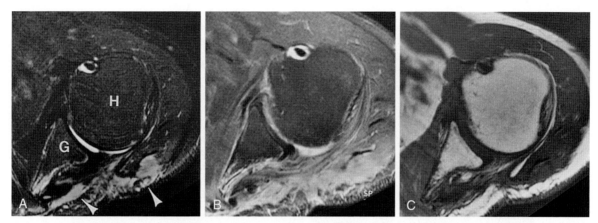

Figure 7-4 **Postsurgical changes. A,** STIR axial image of the left shoulder. There is high signal intensity infiltrating the posterior soft tissues (*arrowheads*) in this patient, who had undergone prior sarcoma resection in this region. G, glenoid; H, humeral head. **B,** T1 axial image with fat saturation of the left shoulder after IV gadolinium administration. There is diffuse enhancement within the posterior soft tissues. **C,** T1 axial image of the left shoulder. There is no evidence of focal mass effect or distortion of muscle architecture in the areas of abnormal signal and enhancement, indicating that these findings do not represent tumor recurrence.

of surgery.[15] On a practical note, an anatomic atlas should be consulted in most cases to determine the expected position of pertinent nerves and vessels. Otherwise, neurovascular involvement might be overlooked if these structures are completely obliterated by a tumor.

Because each joint is a distinct compartment, articular invasion changes the stage of a tumor and should be critically evaluated on every scan. MRI is very accurate for excluding joint involvement when the joint margins appear free of tumor, but is less accurate when the tumor is in close proximity to the joint. Close proximity results in a tendency to overcall joint invasion, which could result in an unnecessarily radical surgical procedure.[16]

Nodes. Local and, when possible, regional lymph nodes should be assessed because nodal involvement carries the same poor prognosis as distant metastases in a patient with a musculoskeletal sarcoma.

EVALUATION OF TUMOR AFTER THERAPY

Postchemotherapy

Survival of patients with musculoskeletal sarcomas has improved with the development of better adjuvant chemotherapeutic regimens. Assessing the degree of tumor response to chemotherapy is important for establishing the patient's prognosis and for planning further therapy.[17] If viable tumor cells constitute less than 10% of a lesion after therapy, this indicates a good response (a "responder"), whereas more than 10% represents a poor response (a "nonresponder"). Currently, this response is determined after resection of the tumor, but several series have evaluated the use of MRI in this setting with conflicting results.

Changes in tumor size, signal intensity, or adjacent edema on conventional sequences are not sufficiently predictive to separate responders from nonresponders.[17] Similarly, because tumor and non-neoplastic reactive tissue enhances on standard, postgadolinium T1W images, this technique

also is unreliable for this purpose.[17] Dynamic enhancement patterns on gadolinium-enhanced, rapid gradient echo–T1W sequences have shown a high degree of correlation with response or nonresponse because residual tumor enhances earlier than reactive tissue.[17,18] We do not use these methods, however, because they are time-consuming, technically challenging, and still not reliable enough to replace biopsy and histology.[19]

Postsurgery and Postradiation

MRI is valuable for detecting tumor recurrence after surgical or radiation therapy, primarily because of its superb soft tissue contrast. MRI is sometimes too sensitive in this regard because postsurgical and postradiation changes in tissues can produce signal intensity that may be mistaken for neoplasm. Careful analysis of T1W, T2W, and STIR images, combined with an understanding of a few basic principles, can markedly improve the diagnostic accuracy of MRI in this setting. Postcontrast imaging also may be beneficial in certain cases, as described subsequently.

A lack of increased signal intensity on T2W or STIR images is a strong predictor of no tumor recurrence because recurrent tumor usually shows high signal intensity on these images. There are other, non-neoplastic causes of increased signal intensity in these patients, however, which can mimic tumor, including radiation-induced edema and postoperative fluid collections such as hematoma, seroma, or abscess.[20] Certain features help to separate these entities.

Surgery and radiation therapy often result in edema or hemorrhage within tissues, but the absence of a discrete mass is strong evidence against tumor recurrence. This can be evaluated on T1W images by looking for loss of the normal fatty marbling within muscle or distortion of the intermuscular fascial planes. The presence of normal skeletal muscle architecture in these regions on T1W images (normal "texture sign") is highly predictive of no tumor recurrence, despite the presence of increased signal intensity on T2W images or enhancement after gadolinium administration (Fig. 7-4).[21]

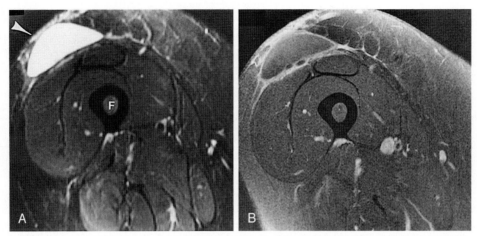

Figure 7-5   Postoperative seroma. **A,** STIR axial image of the proximal right thigh. There is a well-marginated, lenticular-shaped mass (*arrowhead*) showing homogeneous high signal intensity within the subcutaneous fat at the site of prior sarcoma resection. F, femur. **B,** T1 axial image with fat saturation of the proximal right thigh after the administration of IV gadolinium. There is enhancement of the periphery of the mass without central enhancement, confirming that this represents a postoperative fluid collection.

If a mass is discovered, administration of intravenous (IV) gadolinium may be helpful for further characterization. A postoperative lymphocele, seroma, or abscess appears as a high signal intensity mass on T2W images, but does not show internal enhancement on postgadolinium T1W images (Fig. 7-5). If an enhancing mass is identified, biopsy is indicated because recurrent tumor is likely (Fig. 7-6); however, post-therapy granulation tissue also can enhance and produce an identical appearance.

How to Image Tumors

Based on these principles, an imaging protocol can be designed that provides the information needed for accurate staging or post-therapy follow-up.

* *Coils and patient position:* In most cases, the patient is scanned in a supine position. Rarely, a prone position may allow for improved comfort and less motion artifact (eg, when scanning the sternum). We typi-

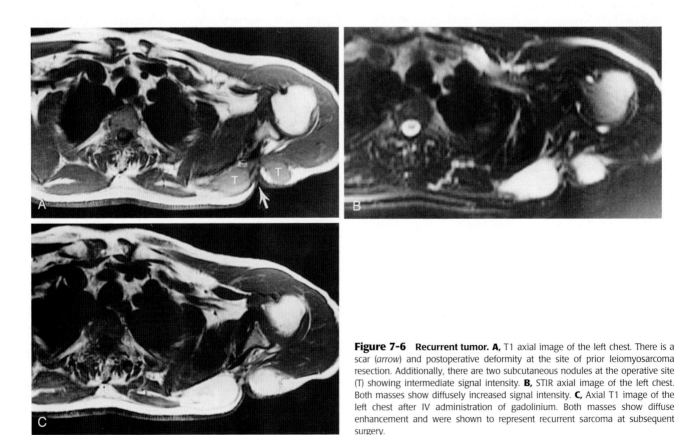

Figure 7-6   Recurrent tumor. **A,** T1 axial image of the left chest. There is a scar (*arrow*) and postoperative deformity at the site of prior leiomyosarcoma resection. Additionally, there are two subcutaneous nodules at the operative site (T) showing intermediate signal intensity. **B,** STIR axial image of the left chest. Both masses show diffusely increased signal intensity. **C,** Axial T1 image of the left chest after IV administration of gadolinium. Both masses show diffuse enhancement and were shown to represent recurrent sarcoma at subsequent surgery.

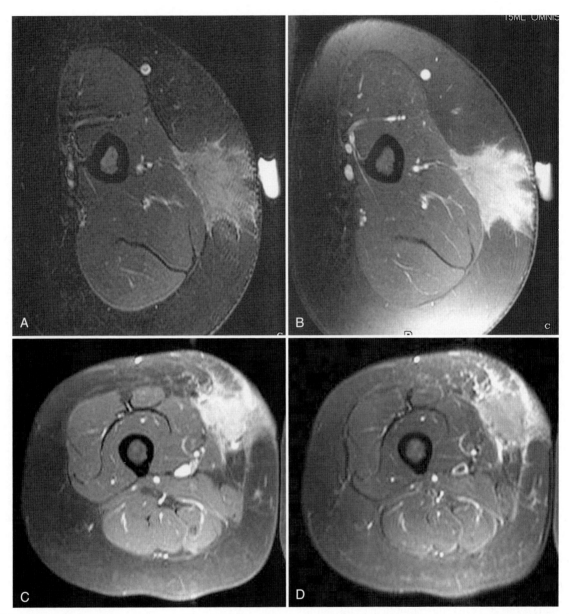

Figure 7-7 **Indeterminate soft tissue masses. A,** STIR axial image of the upper arm. An ill-defined mass within the lateral subcutaneous tissues shows very irregular margins and superficial invasion of the underlying musculature. **B,** T1 fat-saturated axial image of the upper arm after gadolinium administration. The mass shows intense, diffuse enhancement. Biopsy revealed this to be a focus of benign, inflammatory tissue containing non-necrosing granulomatous changes. **C,** STIR axial image of the thigh (different patient than in **A** and **B**). An infiltrative mass in the subcutaneous tissues displays a similar MRI appearance to the lesion in **A** and **B** with irregular margins and superficial involvement of the underlying musculature. **D,** T1 fat-saturated axial image of the thigh after gadolinium administration. Diffuse enhancement is seen throughout the mass, which was found to be follicular lymphoma on biopsy.

cally begin with a sequence using the body coil and a large field of view to ensure that all portions of the primary tumor are identified. This is important for surgical planning, identifying skip or metastatic lesions, and designing additional sequences. When the extent of the tumor has been documented, higher resolution images should be obtained, using a surface coil whenever possible. This provides for optimal assessment of tumor margins and involvement of neurovascular or joint structures.

- *Image orientation:* The initial large field-of-view sequence should be performed in a coronal or sagittal plane to display best the entire length of the lesion. Axial images

are obtained with a smaller field of view to delineate tumor margins and neurovascular or articular involvement. These should be supplemented with additional longitudinal images to produce images that are tangential, rather than en face, to the lesion. Sagittal images are most helpful for a mass involving the anterior or posterior tissues of an extremity, whereas coronal images are used for lesions that are primarily medial or lateral in location.

- *Pulse sequences and regions of interest:* A skin marker should be placed over the suspected mass to confirm that the tissues of interest have been covered. In a postoperative patient, the entire length of the scar should be imaged. STIR imaging is most helpful for the initial large field-of-view sequence because it is very sensitive to neoplastic tissue and associated edema or hemorrhage. It also is superb for detecting any skip or metastatic lesions. It may be difficult to differentiate tumor from edema in the medullary canal on STIR images alone, and an additional body coil coronal or sagittal T1W sequence is a useful adjunct because of the sharp contrast between tumor and fat on this sequence. T1W images also are useful for defining anatomy and detecting high signal fat or hemorrhage within a lesion. Axial T1W and STIR images are obtained, followed by T1 and fast spin echo–T2W or STIR images in a longitudinal plane, using a surface coil, if possible, to resolve tumor margins and involvement of adjacent structures better. A word of caution regarding fast spin echo–T2W sequences: The relatively bright signal intensity of fat on these images is similar to that of most pathologic processes, and this may mask an intramedullary lesion. Fat saturation should be used routinely with this sequence to improve lesion detection. Gradient echo sequences are not a part of our routine tumor protocol, although these can be used for evaluating flow within a lesion or adjacent vessels. This technique is also useful for detecting the presence of hemosiderin within a hematoma or within an area of pigmented villonodular synovitis.

- *Contrast enhancement:* We do not administer IV gadolinium as part of our standard tumor protocol, but use it when attempting to differentiate cystic from cystic-appearing solid lesions.

After surgical or radiation therapy, we use T1W and STIR sequences to image the area of interest and postgadolinium imaging to evaluate for any enhancing masses in the treatment area.

Approach to Image Interpretation

GENERAL PRINCIPLES

Many benign lesions generally show smooth margins, homogeneous signal intensity, and a lack of involvement of neurovascular structures. Conversely, malignant masses tend to display heterogeneous signal, irregular margins, associated edema, and invasion of neurovascular or osseous structures.

There is a large amount of overlap in the appearances of benign and malignant lesions using these characteristics, and it can be dangerous to attempt to determine conclusively whether a mass is benign or malignant based on its MRI appearance (Fig. 7-7).[22] Most lesions need to be classified as indeterminate and undergo biopsy for accurate characterization.[23]

Contrast enhancement using standard, T1W sequences has not been helpful in differentiating benign from malignant lesions, although gadolinium-enhanced imaging using rapid T1W gradient echo sequences can provide some information regarding the malignant potential of a tumor based on the rate of enhancement.[24] Benign tumors tend to enhance more slowly than malignant lesions, but in a given patient, we prefer to perform a biopsy of the lesion, rather than rely

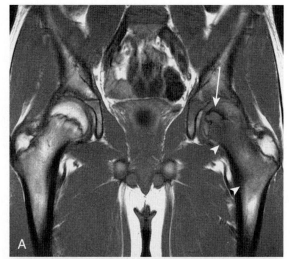
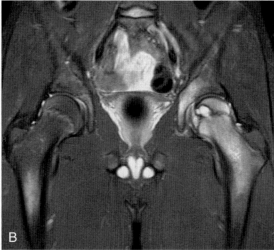

Figure 7-8 **Aggressive-appearing benign lesion. A,** T1 coronal image of the pelvis. A focal lesion (*arrow*) is present within the proximal femoral epiphysis in this child who presented with hip pain. Note also the ill-defined, low signal intensity edema throughout the femoral neck (*arrowheads*). **B,** STIR coronal image of the pelvis. The mass is hyperintense, and associated marrow edema is shown throughout the femoral neck and in the medial portion of the acetabulum. Biopsy revealed Langerhans cell histiocytosis.

on statistical probability, because of the large amount of overlap between benign and malignant lesions.

BONE LESIONS

A reasonable differential diagnosis can be developed for most osseous lesions using the patient's age and the location of the lesion (within the skeleton and within the particular bone) and its radiographic appearance. For most bone tumors, MRI is used for staging, rather than for arriving at a specific diagnosis, because the true nature and aggressiveness of a lesion are determined much more accurately with conventional radiographs. Consequently, recent radiographs always should be viewed in conjunction with MR images; this is also important because some benign osseous lesions display a very aggressive, potentially misleading appearance on MRI. These include osteoid osteoma, chondroblastoma, osteoblastoma, eosinophilic granuloma, and stress fracture (Fig. 7-8). The edema associated with

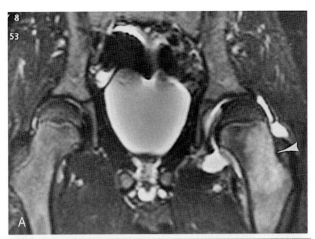

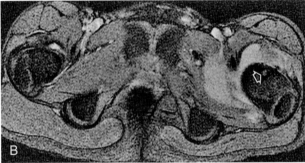

Figure 7-9 Marrow edema related to an osteoid osteoma. **A,** STIR coronal image of the pelvis. There is a geographic area of increased signal intensity within the left femoral neck (*arrowhead*), along with a moderate-sized left hip effusion. **B,** T2* (gradient echo) axial image of the proximal left femur. The tumor nidus is seen along the anterior left femoral neck as a small subcortical focus of increased signal intensity (*open arrow*).

these lesions often results in extensive signal abnormality in the medullary cavity and adjacent soft tissues, mimicking more aggressive lesions, such as osteomyelitis or malignant tumor.[25]

An osteoid osteoma is a cortically based lesion. The key to its diagnosis is to show a focal tumor nidus within the area of cortical/periosteal reaction. The tumor nidus typically shows low to intermediate signal intensity on T1W images, low or high signal on T2W images, and a variable degree of enhancement after gadolinium administration.[26] There is usually a significant amount of surrounding marrow or soft tissue edema that can obscure the nidus and lead to an erroneous diagnosis (Fig. 7-9).[27] In many cases, the nidus is more readily identified with CT scanning through the lesion.[28,29]

Chondroblastoma should be suspected when a lesion is found in a skeletally immature patient with its epicenter in

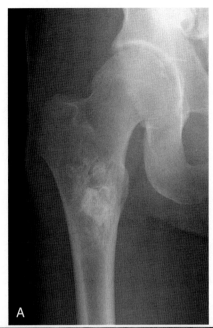

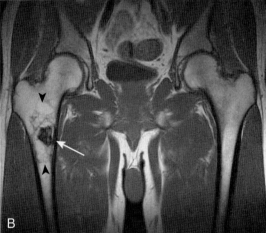

Figure 7-10 High signal intensity, T1: intraosseous lipoma affecting the femur. **A,** Frontal radiograph of the right hip. A mixed lytic and sclerotic lesion is seen in the proximal right femur. **B,** T1 coronal image of the pelvis. Extensive high signal intensity fat is seen within the lesion (*arrowheads*), along with a focus of low signal intensity centrally (*arrow*) corresponding to the dense calcification shown on the radiograph.

the epiphysis. Striking signal abnormality, corresponding to edema, often extends into the adjacent medullary cavity and overlying soft tissues.

In the case of a stress fracture, the presence of a linear fracture line within an area of marrow edema or cortical bone is diagnostic. In the absence of a fracture line, follow-up radiographs obtained 2 to 3 weeks later may be diagnostic. Biopsy should be avoided because the immature osteoid related to the healing process may be mistaken for malignancy at histology.

Differential Features

Although conventional radiographs provide the most specific information regarding the true nature of a bone tumor, there are some MRI features that can help to limit the differential diagnosis.

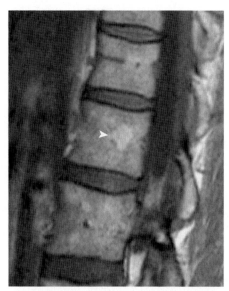

Figure 7-11 High signal intensity, T1: intraosseous hemangioma. T1 sagittal image of the lumbar spine. A rounded focus of high signal intensity is present in the L1 vertebra (*arrowhead*), indicating fat within this small hemangioma.

Increased Signal: T1W Images (Box 7-2)

Intraosseous Lipoma. Intraosseous lipomas most commonly occur in the calcaneus, proximal femur, and humerus. They sometimes are difficult to differentiate from other lytic lesions on conventional radiographs, but are easily recognized on MR images because of their predominantly fat signal on all sequences.[30] An intraosseous lipoma also may contain areas of increased or decreased signal intensity on T2W images, reflecting cystic degeneration or calcification (Fig. 7-10).

Intraosseous Hemangioma. Intraosseous hemangiomas are common in the spine. Simple hemangiomas display increased

BOX 7-3

Bone Lesions Containing Low Signal on T2W Images

• Sclerosis/calcification/matrix
• Some fibrous lesions
• Primary lymphoma of bone

signal intensity on T2W images, but are differentiated from other lesions by high signal intensity on T1W images caused by their fat content (Fig. 7-11). Alternatively, hypervascular (aggressive) intraosseous hemangiomas typically do not contain fat and are indistinguishable from other tumors.[31]

Medullary Bone Infarct. A medullary bone infarct is a geographic lesion with a serpentine, low signal intensity margin on T1W and T2W MR images. These usually contain fat centrally, interspersed with foci of mixed signal intensity, corresponding to areas of fibrosis, calcification, or edema (Fig. 7-12).

Paget's Disease. The MRI appearance of Paget's disease varies. Areas of fat commonly are found within involved areas, but more heterogeneous signal intensity, corresponding to hypervascular marrow, may be seen in the active stage of the disease (Fig. 7-13).[32] Other findings, such as cortical thickening, bone enlargement, and prominent, coarse trabeculae, often are better shown on conventional radiographs.

Decreased Signal: T2W Images (Box 7-3)

Sclerosis/Calcification/Matrix. The presence of extremely low signal intensity within an osseous lesion on T2W images suggests sclerotic bone, calcification, or osteoid/chondroid tumor matrix. These are better characterized with conventional radiographs or CT (Fig. 7-14).

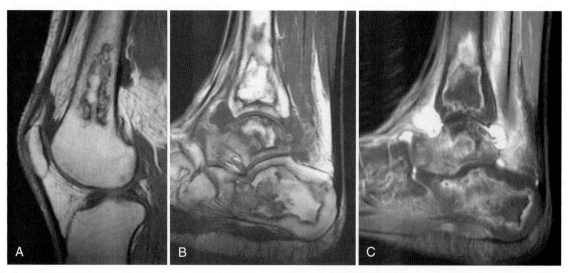

Figure 7-12 High signal intensity, T1: medullary bone infarcts. **A,** T1 sagittal image of the knee. An irregular, geographic area of abnormal signal intensity within the medullary cavity of the distal femoral shaft is compatible with a medullary infarct. Note the low signal intensity serpentine margins and the extensive fat signal intensity within the lesion. **B,** T1 sagittal image of the ankle (different patient than in **A**). Similar lesions are seen within multiple bones of the ankle and hindfoot in this patient who had a long history of steroid therapy. **C,** STIR sagittal image of the ankle. High and low signal intensity bands are seen along the margins of the infarcts ("double-line sign"). Note also the suppressed fat within the central portions of the lesions.

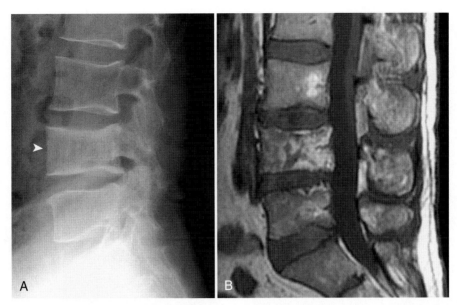

Figure 7-13 **High signal intensity, T1: Paget's disease. A,** Lateral radiograph of the lumbar spine. Classic features of Paget's disease are present within the L4 vertebra (*arrowhead*), including increased sclerosis, thickening of the end plates and trabeculae, and mild overall enlargement of the vertebra relative to adjacent vertebral bodies. **B,** T1 sagittal image of the lumbar spine. There is prominent fat signal intensity within the vertebral body, especially in its posterior portion.

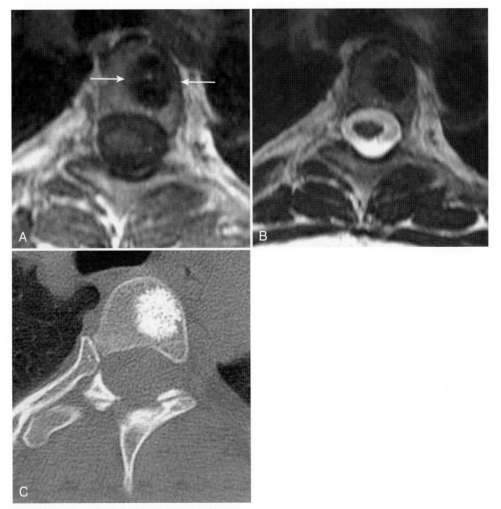

Figure 7-14 **Low signal intensity, T2: large bone island (enostosis). A,** T1 axial image of the thoracic spine. An ovoid focus of extremely low signal intensity is seen in the T4 vertebral body (*arrows*). **B,** Fast spin echo–T2 axial image of the thoracic spine. The lesion remains extremely low signal intensity, confirming its sclerotic nature. **C,** CT scan of the thoracic spine. The dense sclerosis and typical spiculated margins of this large bone island are better shown.

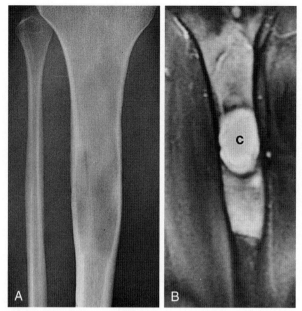

Figure 7-15 **Fibrous dysplasia.** **A,** Anteroposterior radiograph shows typical findings of fibrous dysplasia in the proximal tibia, with a long, mildly expansile lytic lesion that shows hazy internal matrix. **B,** STIR coronal image of the proximal tibia. Most of the lesion shows homogeneous, mildly increased signal intensity, with a focus of higher signal intensity cystic change centrally (C). (From Higgins CB, Hricak H, Helms CA [eds]. *Magnetic Resonance Imaging of the Body,* ed 3. Philadelphia: Lippincott-Raven; 1997.)

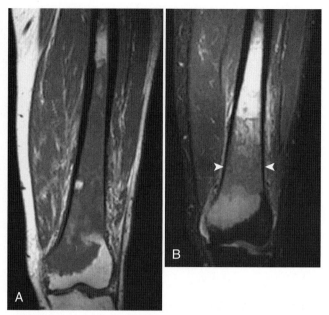

Figure 7-16 **Low signal intensity, T2: lymphoma of bone. A,** T1 coronal image of the distal femur. Extensive, abnormal low signal intensity is present throughout the mid to distal portion of the femur. **B,** STIR coronal image of the distal femur. Much of the lesion shows markedly increased signal intensity, but a broad, bandlike area of low signal intensity persists distally (*arrowheads*). Biopsy revealed B cell lymphoma.

Fibrous Lesions. Fibrous tissue is usually of low to intermediate signal intensity on T2W images, but fibrous lesions of bone often show variable MRI features.

A xanthofibroma (fibrous cortical defect, nonossifying fibroma) is a benign osseous lesion found in adolescents and young adults. These are readily diagnosed on conventional radiographs, but may be incidentally detected on MR images. They display intermediate to low signal intensity on T1W images and often show low to intermediate signal on T2W images because of their fibrous nature. Increased signal also may be seen on T2W images, however, along with variable degrees of enhancement after gadolinium administration. Their lobular contour, eccentric location, low signal intensity, and sclerotic margin are helpful distinguishing features.[33]

Similarly, it was suggested in the early MRI literature that fibrous dysplasia displays decreased signal intensity on T1W and T2W images because of its predominantly fibrous nature. This lesion does not have a characteristic appearance on MR images, however, and often shows heterogeneous signal intensity that may be high, low, or mixed on T2W images (Fig. 7-15).[34]

Primary Lymphoma of Bone. Primary lymphoma of bone is often of low signal intensity on T2W images, although its appearance varies (Fig. 7-16).[35-37] Some investigators have found that the low signal intensity tissue corresponds to areas of fibrosis on pathologic analysis.

Fluid-Fluid Levels. The classic MRI appearance of an aneurysmal bone cyst is that of an expansile, lobular mass that contains multiple cystlike collections and shows high signal intensity on T2W images. Fluid-fluid levels usually are present within these cavities and correspond to stagnant blood products within the cavernous spaces that make up

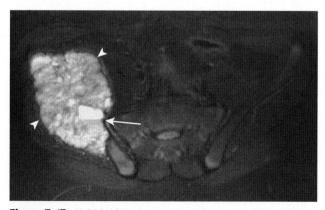

Figure 7-17 **Fluid-fluid levels: aneurysmal bone cyst.** STIR axial image of the pelvis. The markedly expansile lesion (*arrowheads*) in the right iliac bone of this 10-year-old boy shows diffusely increased signal intensity and a prominent fluid-fluid level (*arrow*). Subsequent biopsy revealed this to be an aneurysmal bone cyst.

BOX 7-4

MRI Features of Cartilage Tumors

- High signal lobules (cartilage) on T2 separated by thin, low signal septa
- Low signal intensity foci on T1W and T2W images (calcified cartilage matrix)
- Arcs and rings enhancement pattern
- Often impossible to distinguish enchondroma from low-grade chondrosarcoma
- Watch out for features suggesting chondrosarcoma
  - Endosteal scalloping greater than two thirds of cortex
  - Cortical destruction and soft tissue mass
  - Edema in adjacent marrow or soft tissues

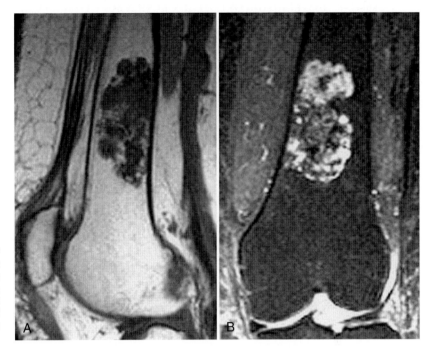

Figure 7-18 Enchondroma. **A,** T1 sagittal image of the distal femur. A lobular intramedullary mass is present in the distal femoral shaft. **B,** STIR coronal image of the distal femur. The lesion shows typical features of an enchondroma, including predominantly high signal intensity, lobular margins, thin internal septations, and low signal foci related to chondroid matrix. Note also the lack of surrounding marrow edema.

these lesions (Fig. 7-17).[38] Initially, fluid-fluid levels were thought to be specific for an aneurysmal bone cyst, but they are a nonspecific feature of many entities that contain collections of blood, including telangiectatic osteosarcoma, chondroblastoma, giant cell tumor of bone, fibrous dysplasia, malignant fibrous histiocytoma of bone, and others.[39] Also, because an aneurysmal bone cyst may arise within some of these lesions, such as telangiectatic osteosarcoma or giant cell tumor (secondary aneurysmal bone cyst), unless these cystic, nonenhancing spaces are seen to fill the entire mass, one of these other tumors must be suspected, and biopsy is indicated.

There is some evidence that the degree of involvement of a lesion with fluid-fluid levels may be helpful in differentiating benign from malignant lesions. In one investigation, if fluid-fluid levels made up more than two thirds of the lesion, it was found to be benign, most commonly an aneurysmal

bone cyst. Conversely, in most malignant lesions, fluid-fluid levels made up less than one third of the mass.[40]

Cartilaginous Tumors (Box 7-4)

Enchondroma/Chondrosarcoma. An enchondroma displays a distinctive MRI appearance. This benign tumor is composed of multiple lobules that show homogeneously high signal intensity on T2W or STIR images, usually separated by thin, low signal intensity septa (Fig. 7-18). The increased signal intensity corresponds to the high water content of the hyaline cartilage lobules that compose these lesions. Low signal intensity foci corresponding to calcified cartilage matrix also may be apparent. A pattern of enhancing rings and arcs is seen in cartilaginous tumors on postcontrast images, presumably caused by the presence of vessels within the fibrous septa and lack of cartilage enhancement. This MRI appearance, including the

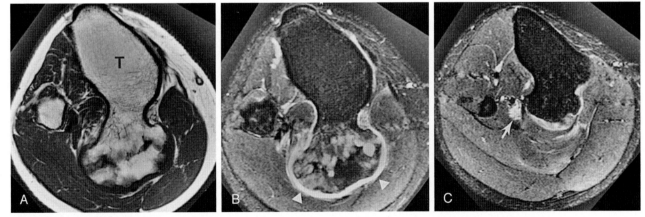

Figure 7-19 Osteochondroma causing neuritis. **A,** T1 axial image of the proximal tibia. A large, pedunculated osteochondroma arises from the posterior tibia (T). Note the continuity of cortical margins and medullary cavities of the lesion and parent bone and the normal marrow signal intensity within the proximal lesion and tibia. **B,** STIR axial image of the proximal tibia. The high signal intensity, thin cartilage cap is well shown (*arrowheads*), as are high signal cartilaginous foci within the lesion. **C,** STIR axial image of the tibia (4 cm distal to **B**). The tibial nerve is focally enlarged (*arrow*) and shows increased signal intensity where it abuts the osteochondroma. Mechanical irritation resulted in a focal neuritis.

Table 7-2　DISTRIBUTION OF COMMON BENIGN SOFT TISSUE TUMORS BY ANATOMIC LOCATION AND AGE
(Based on an Analysis of 18,677 Cases Seen in Consultation by the Department of Soft Tissue Pathology, AFIP, Over 10 Years)

Ages (yr)	Hand and Wrist	No. (%)	Upper Extremity	No. (%)
0-5	Hemangioma	15 (15)*	Fibrous hamartoma infancy	15 (16)
	Granuloma annulare	14 (14)	Granuloma annulare	15 (16)
	Infantile fibromatosis	13 (13)	Hemangioma	14 (15)
	Infantile digital fibroma	8 (8)	Infantile fibromatosis	12 (13)
	Fibromatosis	8 (8)	Fibrous histiocytoma	6 (6)
	Aponeurotic fibroma	7 (7)	Juvenile xanthogranuloma	6 (6)
	Fibrous histiocytoma	5 (5)	Myofibromatosis	6 (6)
	Other	27 (28)	Other	20 (21)
6-15	Fibrous histiocytoma	32 (14)	Fibrous histiocytoma	41 (23)
	Hemangioma	31 (13)	Nodular fasciitis	39 (21)
	Aponeurotic fibroma	25 (11)	Hemangioma	24 (13)
	Fibroma tendon sheath	22 (9)	Granuloma annulare	12 (7)
	GCT tendon sheath	17 (7)	Fibromatosis	11 (6)
	Fibromatosis	13 (6)	Neurofibroma	7 (4)
	Lipoma	9 (4)	Neurothekeoma	6 (3)
	Other	86 (37)	Other	42 (23)
16-25	GCT tendon sheath	84 (20)	Nodular fasciitis	130 (35)
	Fibrous histiocytoma	57 (14)	Fibrous histiocytoma	87 (23)
	Hemangioma	40 (10)	Hemangioma	36 (10)
	Fibroma tendon sheath	40 (10)	Neurofibroma	24 (6)
	Nodular fasciitis	26 (6)	Granuloma annulare	20 (5)
	Granuloma annulare	21 (5)	Granular cell tumor	17 (5)
	Ganglion	20 (5)	Schwannoma	11 (3)
	Other	132 (31)	Other	51 (14)
26-45	Fibrous histiocytoma	167 (18)	Nodular fasciitis	309 (38)
	GCT tendon sheath	148 (16)	Fibrous histiocytoma	145 (18)
	Fibroma tendon sheath	106 (11)	Angiolipoma	48 (6)
	Hemangioma	86 (10)	Hemangioma	43 (5)
	Nodular fasciitis	79 (8)	Schwannoma	43 (5)
	Fibromatosis	46 (5)	Neurofibroma	37 (5)
	Chondroma	42 (4)	Lipoma	32 (4)
	Other	269 (29)	Other	3 (19)
46-65	GCT tendon sheath	143 (23)	Nodular fasciitis	86 (20)
	Fibrous histiocytoma	63 (10)	Lipoma	80 (19)
	Hemangioma	61 (10)	Fibrous histiocytoma	44 (10)
	Lipoma	59 (9)	Schwannoma	30 (7)
	Chondroma	52 (8)	Neurofibroma	24 (6)
	Fibromatosis	43 (7)	Myxoma	24 (6)
	Fibroma tendon sheath	37 (6)	Hemangioma	19 (4)
	Other	172 (27)	Other	125 (29)
≥66	GCT tendon sheath	51 (21)	Lipoma	39 (22)
	Hemangioma	24 (10)	Myxoma	19 (11)
	Schwannoma	24 (10)	Nodular fasciitis	18 (10)
	Chondroma	24 (10)	Schwannoma	17 (9)
	Neurofibroma	21 (9)	Glomus tumor	12 (7)
	Fibromatosis	14 (6)	Neurofibroma	10 (6)
	Lipoma	13 (5)	Angiolipoma	10 (6)
	Other	71 (29)	Other	55 (31)

Ages (yr)	Hip, Groin, and Buttocks	No. (%)	Head and Neck	No. (%)
0-5	Fibrous hamartoma infancy	14 (20)	Nodular fasciitis	47 (20)
	Lipoblastoma	14 (20)	Hemangioma	43 (18)
	Myofibromatosis	8 (11)	Myofibromatosis	27 (11)
	Lymphangioma	7 (10)	Fibromatosis	17 (7)
	Fibrous histiocytoma	5 (7)	Granuloma annulare	14 (6)
	Nodular fasciitis	4 (6)	Fibrous histiocytoma	13 (5)
	Infantile fibromatosis	4 (6)	Infantile fibromatosis	13 (5)
	Other	14 (20)	Other	63 (27)
6-15	Nodular fasciitis	15 (27)	Nodular fasciitis	75 (33)
	Fibroma	7 (13)	Fibrous histiocytoma	34 (15)
	Fibrous histiocytoma	6 (11)	Neurofibroma	23 (10)
	Fibromatosis	5 (9)	Hemangioma	21 (9)
	Lipoma	5 (9)	Myofibromatosis	14 (6)
	Lipoblastoma	3 (5)	Fibromatosis	12 (5)
	Neurofibroma	3 (5)	Lipoma	6 (3)
	Other	11 (20)	Other	43 (19)

Axilla and Shoulder	No. (%)	Foot and Ankle	No. (%)	Lower Extremity	No. (%)
Fibrous hamartoma infancy	23 (29)	Granuloma annulare	23 (30)	Granuloma annulare	42 (23)
Hemangioma	12 (15)	Infantile fibromatosis	11 (14)	Hemangioma	26 (14)
Lipoblastoma	11 (14)	Hemangioma	8 (11)	Myofibromatosis	16 (9)
Fibrous hamartoma	7 (9)	Fibromatosis	8 (11)	Fibrous histiocytoma	15 (8)
Myofibromatosis	6 (8)	Infantile digital fibroma	7 (9)	Lipoblastoma	13 (7)
Lymphangioma	5 (6)	Lipoblastoma	6 (8)	Lymphangioma	10 (6)
Nodular fasciitis	4 (5)	Lipoma	4 (5)	Juvenile xanthogranuloma	10 (6)
Other	12 (15)	Other	9 (12)	Other	48 (27)
Fibrous histiocytoma	25 (34)	Fibromatosis	35 (22)	Hemangioma	47 (22)
Nodular fasciitis	18 (25)	Granuloma annulare	21 (13)	Fibrous histiocytoma	34 (16)
Hemangioma	7 (10)	Hemangioma	21 (13)	Nodular fasciitis	22 (10)
Granular cell tumor	4 (5)	Fibrous histiocytoma	14 (9)	Granuloma annulare	20 (9)
Neurofibroma	3 (4)	GCT tendon sheath	13 (8)	Fibromatosis	14 (6)
Lymphangioma	2 (3)	Chondroma	11 (7)	Lipoma	13 (6)
Myofibromatosis	2 (3)	Lipoma	9 (6)	Neurofibroma	8 (4)
Other	12 (16)	Other	37 (23)	Other	58 (27)
Fibrous histiocytoma	62 (36)	Fibromatosis	46 (22)	Fibrous histiocytoma	118 (24)
Nodular fasciitis	35 (20)	GCT tendon sheath	29 (14)	Nodular fasciitis	61 (13)
Fibromatosis	16 (9)	Granuloma annulare	25 (12)	Hemangioma	55 (11)
Lipoma	14 (8)	Fibrous histiocytoma	24 (12)	Neurofibroma	48 (10)
Neurofibroma	12 (7)	Hemangioma	13 (6)	Fibromatosis	38 (8)
Hemangioma	4 (2)	PVNS	12 (6)	Lipoma	22 (5)
Schwannoma	4 (2)	Neurofibroma	11 (5)	Schwannoma	20 (4)
Other	25 (15)	Other	45 (22)	Other	122 (25)
Lipoma	105 (28)	Fibromatosis	99 (21)	Fibrous histiocytoma	245 (25)
Fibrous histiocytoma	92 (24)	Fibrous histiocytoma	74 (16)	Nodular fasciitis	229 (23)
Nodular fasciitis	55 (14)	GCT tendon sheath	41 (9)	Lipoma	101 (10)
Fibromatosis	29 (8)	Hemangioma	36 (8)	Neurofibroma	71 (7)
Hemangioma	17 (4)	Schwannoma	30 (6)	Schwannoma	59 (6)
Neurofibroma	13 (3)	Neurofibroma	24 (5)	Myxoma	53 (5)
Schwannoma	12 (3)	Chondroma	23 (5)	Hemangioma	52 (5)
Other	57 (15)	Other	135 (29)	Other	185 (19)
Lipoma	189 (58)	Fibromatosis	83 (25)	Lipoma	7 (23)
Fibrous histiocytoma	28 (9)	Fibrous histiocytoma	43 (13)	Myxoma	109 (16)
Myxoma	16 (5)	Lipoma	35 (11)	Fibrous histiocytoma	93 (14)
Fibromatosis	14 (4)	Schwannoma	25 (8)	Nodular fasciitis	40 (6)
Nodular fasciitis	13 (4)	GCT tendon sheath	21 (6)	Schwannoma	39 (6)
Schwannoma	12 (4)	Chondroma	21 (6)	Neurofibroma	31 (5)
Granular cell tumor	12 (4)	Hemangioma	16 (5)	Proliferative fasciitis	28 (4)
Other	44 (13)	Other	89 (27)	Other	186 (27)
Lipoma	83 (58)	Fibromatosis	16 (14)	Lipoma	68 (26)
Myxoma	14 (10)	Schwannoma	15 (13)	Myxoma	44 (17)
Schwannoma	6 (4)	Fibrous histiocytoma	13 (11)	Fibrous histiocytoma	33 (13)
Fibromatosis	5 (3)	Chondroma	11 (9)	Schwannoma	31 (12)
Fibrous histiocytoma	5 (3)	Lipoma	10 (8)	Hemangiopericytoma	10 (4)
Proliferative fasciitis	5 (3)	Granuloma annulare	8 (7)	Neurofibroma	9 (4)
Hemangioma	4 (3)	GCT tendon sheath	6 (5)	Hemangioma	8 (3)
Other	22 (15)	Other	39 (33)	Other	56 (22)

Trunk	No. (%)	Retroperitoneum	No. (%)
Hemangioma	36 (18)	Lipoblastoma	7 (37)
Juvenile xanthogranuloma	24 (12)	Lymphangioma	5 (26)
Myofibromatosis	24 (12)	Hemangioma	4 (21)
Nodular fasciitis	17 (8)	Ganglioneuroma	2 (11)
Lipoblastoma	17 (8)	Fibrous hamartoma infancy	1 (5)
Infantile fibromatosis	15 (7)		
Fibrous hamartoma infancy	15 (7)		
Other	55 (27)		
Nodular fasciitis	54 (28)	Lymphangioma	7 (37)
Fibrous histiocytoma	43 (22)	Ganglioneuroma	4 (21)
Hemangioma	25 (13)	Schwannoma	2 (11)
Lipoma	9 (5)	Fibromatosis	2 (11)
Neurofibroma	7 (4)	Paraganglioma	1 (5)
Fibromatosis	6 (3)	Hemangioma	1 (5)
Granular cell tumor	6 (3)	Inflammatory pseudotumor	1 (5)
Other	45 (23)	Other	1 (5)

Continued on following page

Table 7-2 DISTRIBUTION OF COMMON BENIGN SOFT TISSUE TUMORS BY ANATOMIC LOCATION AND AGE (Continued)
(Based on an Analysis of 18,677 Cases Seen in Consultation by the Department of Soft Tissue Pathology, AFIP, Over 10 Years)

Ages (yr)	Hip, Groin, and Buttocks	No. (%)	Head and Neck	No. (%)
16-25	Neurofibroma	20 (16)	Nodular fasciitis	61 (21)
	Fibromatosis	18 (15)	Hemangioma	48 (17)
	Fibrous histiocytoma	18 (15)	Fibrous histiocytoma	45 (16)
	Nodular fasciitis	12 (10)	Neurofibroma	37 (13)
	Hemangioma	9 (7)	Schwannoma	19 (7)
	Lipoma	8 (7)	Fibromatosis	11 (4)
	Hemangiopericytoma	8 (7)	Lipoma	10 (4)
	Other	29 (24)	Other	56 (19)
26-45	Lipoma	57 (17)	Lipoma	168 (22)
	Neurofibroma	38 (12)	Nodular fasciitis	145 (19)
	Fibrous histiocytoma	37 (11)	Fibrous histiocytoma	137 (18)
	Fibromatosis	36 (11)	Hemangioma	97 (13)
	Nodular fasciitis	31 (9)	Neurofibroma	57 (8)
	Hemangiopericytoma	24 (7)	Hemangiopericytoma	37 (5)
	Myxoma	22 (7)	Schwannoma	27 (4)
	Other	83 (25)	Other	91 (12)
46-65	Lipoma	76 (35)	Lipoma	306 (46)
	Myxoma	36 (17)	Nodular fasciitis	66 (10)
	Fibrous histiocytoma	17 (8)	Hemangioma	55 (8)
	Schwannoma	17 (8)	Fibrous histiocytoma	42 (6)
	Nodular fasciitis	11 (5)	Neurofibroma	30 (4)
	Hemangiopericytoma	11 (5)	Schwannoma	25 (4)
	Hemangioma	9 (4)	Myxoma	23 (3)
	Other	40 (18)	Other	120 (18)
≥66	Lipoma	22 (21)	Lipoma	8 (50)
	Myxoma	16 (15)	Hemangioma	22 (7)
	Neurofibroma	13 (12)	Schwannoma	18 (6)
	Schwannoma	10 (9)	Fibrous histiocytoma	17 (5)
	Hemangiopericytoma	10 (9)	Neurofibroma	16 (5)
	Hemangioma	8 (8)	Nodular fasciitis	13 (4)
	Nodular fasciitis	4 (4)	Myxoma	12 (4)
	Other	23 (22)	Other	58 (18)

*15 (15) indicates there were 15 hemangiomas in the hand and wrist of patients 0-5 years, and this represents 15% of all benign tumors in this location and age group.
GCT, giant cell tumor; PVNS, pigmented villonodular synovitis.
From Kransdorf MJ. Benign soft-tissue tumors in a large referral population: distribution of specific diagnoses by age, sex, and location. *AJR Am J Roentgenol* 1995; 164:395-402.

enhancement pattern, can be seen in enchondromas and low-grade chondrosarcomas.[41,42]

Imaging findings suggestive of chondrosarcoma, rather than a benign enchondroma, include deep endosteal scalloping (greater than two thirds of the cortex), cortical destruction with or without an associated soft tissue mass, and edema-like signal intensity in the adjacent marrow cavity and overlying soft tissues on STIR images.[43,44] Even so, it is often difficult, if not impossible, to distinguish between benign and low-grade malignant cartilaginous tumors based on MRI features alone.

Chondroid Tumor Versus Medullary Bone Infarct. Differentiation of a cartilaginous tumor from a medullary bone infarct can be challenging on conventional radiographs because chondroid matrix can appear similar to the dystrophic calcifications present within an area of infarction. These can be distinguished easily using MRI. In contrast to the cartilaginous lobules that make up the chondroid tumor, a medullary infarct is seen as a flame-shaped region of heterogeneous signal intensity, often containing fat, that is surrounded by a serpentine margin of low signal intensity on all sequences.

Osteochondroma. Osteochondroma is the most common benign tumor of bone and usually is diagnosed on conven-

tional radiographs. MRI can differentiate an osteochondroma from other juxtacortical lesions by showing contiguity of the lesion's medullary cavity and cortex with those of the bone of origin. The marrow fat within the lesion should be isointense with the medullary fat of the host bone on all sequences. The cartilage cap of the lesion is detected easily because of its high signal intensity on T2W or STIR images (Fig. 7-19). Although the relationship between the thickness of the cap and malignancy is controversial, a thickness of greater than 2 cm should be viewed as suspicious for neoplastic degeneration.[45]

MRI also can show other symptomatic complications of these tumors, such as neurovascular impingement, bursal formation, or fracture (see Fig. 7-19).[46]

BOX 7-5

Soft Tissue Masses Containing High Signal on T1W Images

- Lipoma
- Liposarcoma
- Hematoma (subacute)
- Hemangioma
- Melanoma

Trunk	No. (%)	Retroperitoneum	No. (%)
Nodular fasciitis	112 (24)	Fibromatosis	14 (20)
Fibromatosis	72 (16)	Schwannoma	10 (14)
Fibrous histiocytoma	71 (15)	Neurofibroma	9 (13)
Hemangioma	52 (11)	Hemangiopericytoma	8 (11)
Neurofibroma	38 (8)	Lymphangioma	8 (11)
Lipoma	21 (5)	Ganglioneuroma	6 (8)
Schwannoma	17 (4)	Hemangioma	4 (6)
Other	79 (17)	Other	12 (17)
Lipoma	178 (19)	Schwannoma	38 (23)
Nodular fasciitis	0 (16)	Fibromatosis	30 (18)
Fibromatosis	148 (16)	Hemangiopericytoma	25 (15)
Fibrous histiocytoma	98 (10)	Neurofibroma	13 (8)
Hemangioma	78 (8)	Angiomyolipoma	10 (6)
Neurofibroma	65 (7)	Hemangioma	9 (5)
Schwannoma	51 (5)	Sclerosing retroperitonitis	7 (4)
Other	180 (19)	Other	34 (20)
Lipoma	290 (44)	Schwannoma	33 (19)
Fibromatosis	63 (9)	Fibromatosis	25 (14)
Nodular fasciitis	44 (7)	Sclerosing retroperitonitis	25 (14)
Hemangioma	31 (5)	Hemangiopericytoma	21 (12)
Fibrous histiocytoma	29 (4)	Angiomyolipoma	12 (7)
Neurofibroma	28 (4)	Lipoma	10 (6)
Schwannoma	28 (4)	Paraganglioma	9 (5)
Other	1 (23)	Other	40 (23)
Lipoma	124 (42)	Schwannoma	19 (26)
Fibromatosis	26 (9)	Hemangiopericytoma	14 (19)
Neurofibroma	20 (7)	Lipoma	6 (8)
Schwannoma	18 (6)	Mesothelioma	6 (8)
Elastofibroma	17 (6)	Sclerosing retroperitonitis	5 (7)
Myxoma	16 (5)	Fibromatosis	4 (6)
Hemangioma	14 (5)	Paraganglioma	4 (6)
Other	61 (21)	Other	14 (19)

SOFT TISSUE TUMORS

General Principles

Some soft tissue tumors can be diagnosed with certainty based on their MRI signal characteristics; helpful differential MRI features are discussed subsequently. There is a large degree of overlap, however, in the MRI appearance of many benign and malignant soft tissue masses. For masses that have a nonspecific, indeterminate MRI appearance, a differential diagnosis can be generated using the patient's age, the location of the mass, and the information found in Tables 7-2 and 7-3.[47,48] For most lesions, a reasonable differential diagnosis would include the top three benign and malignant tumors listed in Tables 7-2 and 7-3 for a given age and location, but most indeterminate soft tissue masses should be biopsied.

Differential Features

High Signal on T1W Images (Box 7-5). The differential diagnosis for lesions that contain areas of high signal

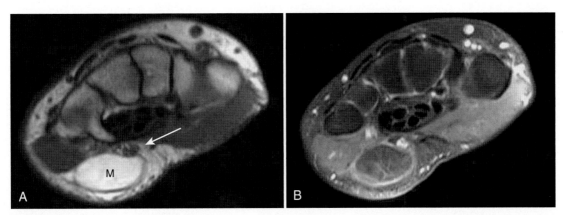

Figure 7-20 **High signal intensity, T1: soft tissue lipoma. A,** T1 axial image of the wrist. A sharply circumscribed, high signal intensity mass (M) abuts and slightly compresses the ulnar neurovascular bundle (*arrow*) in this patient who presented with an ulnar neuropathy. **B,** T2 axial image with fat suppression of the wrist. With the exception of the thin internal septations, there is excellent suppression of the signal intensity from this mass, confirming its lipomatous nature. Subsequent resection revealed a benign lipoma.

Table 7-3 DISTRIBUTION OF COMMON MALIGNANT SOFT TISSUE TUMORS BY ANATOMIC LOCATION AND AGE

(Based on an Analysis of 12,370 Cases Seen in Consultation by the Department of Soft Tissue Pathology, AFIP, Over 10 Years)

Ages (yr)	Hand and Wrist	No. (%)	Upper Extremity	No. (%)
0-5	Fibrosarcoma	5 (45)*	Fibrosarcoma	9 (29)
	Angiosarcoma	1 (9)	Rhabdomyosarcoma	7 (23)
	Epithelioid sarcoma	1 (9)	Angiomatoid MFH	3 (10)
	Malignant GCT tendon sheath	1 (9)	DFSP	2 (6)
	DFSP	1 (9)	Giant cell fibroblastoma	2 (6)
	MPNST	1 (9)	MPNST	2 (6)
	Rhabdomyosarcoma	1 (9)	MFH	2 (6)
			Other	4 (13)
6-15	Epithelioid sarcoma	9 (21)	Angiomatoid MFH	30 (33)
	Angiomatoid MFH	7 (16)	Synovial sarcoma	14 (15)
	Synovial sarcoma	5 (12)	Fibrosarcoma	8 (9)
	MFH	4 (9)	MPNST	7 (8)
	Angiosarcoma	3 (7)	MFH	7 (8)
	Rhabdomyosarcoma	3 (7)	Rhabdomyosarcoma	7 (8)
	Clear cell sarcoma	2 (5)	Epithelioid sarcoma	4 (4)
	Other	10 (23)	Other	15 (16)
16-25	Epithelioid sarcoma	25 (29)	Synovial sarcoma	32 (23)
	MFH	11 (13)	MFH	19 (14)
	DFSP	7 (8)	MPNST	16 (12)
	Synovial sarcoma	7 (8)	Fibrosarcoma	12 (9)
	Rhabdomyosarcoma	7 (8)	Angiomatoid MFH	10 (7)
	Angiomatoid MFH	5 (6)	Epithelioid sarcoma	9 (7)
	Hemangioendothelioma	5 (6)	Hemangioendothelioma	6 (4)
	Other	19 (22)	Other	34 (25)
26-45	MFH	26 (18)	MFH	65 (28)
	Epithelioid sarcoma	24 (16)	MPNST	29 (12)
	Synovial sarcoma	21 (14)	Fibrosarcoma	25 (11)
	Fibrosarcoma	17 (12)	Synovial sarcoma	23 (10)
	Clear cell sarcoma	9 (6)	Liposarcoma	20 (8)
	Liposarcoma	9 (6)	DFSP	18 (8)
	MPNST	7 (5)	Epithelioid sarcoma	13 (6)
	Other	33 (23)	Other	43 (18)
46-65	MFH	16 (19)	MFH	133 (46)
	Synovial sarcoma	12 (14)	Liposarcoma	34 (12)
	Fibrosarcoma	8 (10)	Leiomyosarcoma	22 (8)
	Epithelioid sarcoma	7 (8)	Fibrosarcoma	18 (6)
	Liposarcoma	7 (8)	MPNST	17 (6)
	Chondrosarcoma	7 (8)	Synovial sarcoma	16 (5)
	Clear cell sarcoma	5 (6)	Hemangioendothelioma	9 (3)
	Other	22 (26)	Other	43 (15)
≥66	MFH	28 (35)	MFH	183 (60)
	Leiomyosarcoma	8 (10)	Liposarcoma	25 (8)
	Synovial sarcoma	6 (8)	Leiomyosarcoma	23 (8)
	Kaposi's sarcoma	5 (6)	MPNST	20 (7)
	DFSP	4 (5)	Kaposi's sarcoma	10 (3)
	MPNST	4 (5)	Fibrosarcoma	8 (3)
	Clear cell sarcoma	3 (4)	Angiosarcoma	6 (2)
	Other	21 (27)	Other	29 (10)

Ages (yr)	Hip, Groin, and Buttocks	No. (%)	Head and Neck	No. (%)
0-5	Fibrosarcoma	7 (32)	Fibrosarcoma	22 (37)
	Giant cell fibroblastoma	3 (14)	Rhabdomyosarcoma	20 (33)
	Rhabdomyosarcoma	3 (14)	Malignant hemangiopericytoma	3 (5)
	DFSP	2 (9)	Alveolar soft part sarcoma	2 (3)
	MFH	2 (9)	DFSP	2 (3)
	Leiomyosarcoma	1 (5)	MPNST	2 (3)
	Synovial sarcoma	1 (5)	Giant cell fibroblastoma	2 (3)
	Other	3 (14)	Other	7 (12)
6-15	Angiomatoid MFH	8 (21)	Rhabdomyosarcoma	17 (26)
	Synovial sarcoma	7 (19)	Fibrosarcoma	13 (20)
	Rhabdomyosarcoma	6 (16)	Synovial sarcoma	7 (11)
	MFH	4 (11)	MPNST	6 (9)
	Epithelioid sarcoma	2 (5)	MFH	6 (9)
	Fibrosarcoma	2 (5)	Angiomatoid MFH	4 (6)
	MPNST	2 (5)	DFSP	2 (3)
	Other	7 (18)	Other	10 (15)

Axilla and Shoulder	No. (%)
Fibrosarcoma	9 (56)
Rhabdomyosarcoma	4 (25)
Angiomatoid MFH	1 (6)
Chondrosarcoma	1 (6)
MPNST	1 (6)
Angiomatoid MFH	8 (21)
MFH	5 (13)
Ewing's sarcoma	4 (10)
MPNST	4 (10)
Rhabdomyosarcoma	4 (10)
Fibrosarcoma	3 (8)
Synovial sarcoma	3 (8)
Other	8 (21)
Synovial sarcoma	13 (18)
DFSP	12 (16)
MPNST	11 (15)
Fibrosarcoma	8 (11)
MFH	8 (11)
Rhabdomyosarcoma	4 (5)
Angiomatoid MFH	3 (4)
Other	15 (20)
DFSP	55 (33)
MFH	30 (18)
Liposarcoma	22 (13)
MPNST	21 (12)
Fibrosarcoma	10 (6)
Synovial sarcoma	7 (4)
Chondrosarcoma	6 (4)
Other	18 (11)
MFH	66 (35)
Liposarcoma	39 (21)
DFSP	22 (12)
MPNST	20 (11)
Leiomyosarcoma	14 (7)
Fibrosarcoma	8 (4)
Synovial sarcoma	4 (2)
Other	15 (8)
MFH	67 (50)
Liposarcoma	30 (23)
MPNST	12 (9)
DFSP	6 (5)
Fibrosarcoma	4 (3)
Leiomyosarcoma	3 (2)
Chondrosarcoma	2 (2)
Other	9 (7)

Foot and Ankle	No. (%)
Fibrosarcoma	5 (45)
DFSP	2 (18)
MPNST	2 (18)
Rhabdomyosarcoma	2 (18)
Synovial sarcoma	11 (21)
DFSP	9 (17)
Rhabdomyosarcoma	5 (9)
Angiosarcoma	4 (8)
Clear cell sarcoma	4 (8)
Fibrosarcoma	4 (8)
Chondrosarcoma	3 (6)
Other	13 (25)
Synovial sarcoma	27 (30)
Clear cell sarcoma	10 (11)
Fibrosarcoma	7 (8)
DFSP	7 (8)
MFH	6 (7)
Hemangioendothelioma	6 (7)
MPNST	5 (6)
Other	22 (24)
Synovial sarcoma	50 (26)
Clear cell sarcoma	25 (13)
MFH	25 (13)
Hemangioendothelioma	14 (7)
DFSP	13 (7)
Liposarcoma	1 (7)
MPNST	11 (6)
Other	38 (20)
MFH	39 (25)
Synovial sarcoma	27 (17)
Leiomyosarcoma	19 (12)
Kaposi's sarcoma	14 (9)
Liposarcoma	9 (6)
Fibrosarcoma	8 (5)
Clear cell sarcoma	7 (5)
Other	32 (21)
Kaposi's sarcoma	49 (37)
MFH	26 (19)
Leiomyosarcoma	20 (15)
Fibrosarcoma	9 (7)
Chondrosarcoma	6 (4)
MPNST	5 (4)
Liposarcoma	3 (2)
Other	16 (12)

Lower Extremity	No. (%)
Fibrosarcoma	24 (45)
Rhabdomyosarcoma	8 (15)
Giant cell fibroblastoma	5 (9)
MPNST	5 (9)
Angiomatoid MFH	3 (6)
DFSP	3 (6)
Angiosarcoma	2 (4)
Other	3 (6)
Synovial sarcoma	28 (22)
Angiomatoid MFH	22 (17)
MFH	13 (10)
Liposarcoma	11 (9)
MPNST	9 (7)
DFSP	8 (6)
Rhabdomyosarcoma	6 (5)
Other	31 (24)
Synovial sarcoma	76 (22)
Liposarcoma	45 (13)
MPNST	44 (13)
MFH	36 (11)
Fibrosarcoma	24 (7)
DFSP	18 (5)
Angiomatoid MFH	15 (4)
Other	80 (24)
Liposarcoma	196 (28)
MFH	1 (21)
Synovial sarcoma	78 (11)
MPNST	70 (10)
DFSP	47 (7)
Leiomyosarcoma	35 (5)
Fibrosarcoma	33 (5)
Other	98 (14)
MFH	399 (43)
Liposarcoma	232 (25)
Leiomyosarcoma	63 (7)
Synovial sarcoma	40 (4)
MPNST	38 (4)
Chondrosarcoma	37 (4)
Fibrosarcoma	24 (3)
Other	87 (9)
MFH	455 (55)
Liposarcoma	178 (22)
Leiomyosarcoma	86 (10)
Fibrosarcoma	22 (3)
Chondrosarcoma	16 (2)
MPNST	15 (2)
Synovial sarcoma	11 (1)
Other	43 (5)

Trunk	No. (%)
Fibrosarcoma	13 (26)
Giant cell fibroblastoma	8 (16)
Rhabdomyosarcoma	8 (16)
Angiomatoid MFH	6 (12)
DFSP	4 (8)
Ewing's sarcoma	3 (6)
Neuroblastoma	3 (6)
Other	5 (10)
Angiomatoid MFH	14 (15)
Fibrosarcoma	13 (14)
Ewing's sarcoma	12 (13)
DFSP	12 (13)
MPNST	9 (10)
Rhabdomyosarcoma	8 (9)
MFH	3 (3)
Other	20 (22)

Retroperitoneum	No. (%)
Fibrosarcoma	4 (20)
Neuroblastoma	4 (20)
Rhabdomyosarcoma	4 (20)
Ganglioneuroblastoma	3 (15)
Angiosarcoma	2 (10)
Leiomyosarcoma	2 (10)
Alveolar soft part sarcoma	1 (5)
Rhabdomyosarcoma	9 (31)
MPNST	5 (17)
Neuroblastoma	4 (14)
Ewing's sarcoma	2 (7)
Fibrosarcoma	2 (7)
MFH	2 (7)
Malignant hemangiopericytoma	2 (7)
Other	3 (10)

Continued on following page

Table 7-3   DISTRIBUTION OF COMMON MALIGNANT SOFT TISSUE TUMORS BY ANATOMIC LOCATION AND AGE (Continued)
(Based on an Analysis of 12,370 Cases Seen in Consultation by the Department of Soft Tissue Pathology, AFIP, Over 10 Years)

Ages (yr)	Hip, Groin, and Buttocks	No. (%)	Head and Neck	No. (%)
16-25	Synovial sarcoma	15 (18)	Fibrosarcoma	15 (17)
	MPNST	13 (16)	DFSP	14 (16)
	Liposarcoma	8 (10)	MPNST	8 (9)
	DFSP	6 (7)	Synovial sarcoma	8 (9)
	MFH	6 (7)	Rhabdomyosarcoma	8 (9)
	Rhabdomyosarcoma	5 (6)	MFH	7 (8)
	Leiomyosarcoma	4 (5)	Angiomatoid MFH	6 (7)
	Other	26 (31)	Other	23 (26)
26-45	Liposarcoma	45 (18)	DFSP	59 (30)
	DFSP	42 (17)	MPNST	27 (14)
	MFH	38 (16)	Liposarcoma	18 (9)
	Leiomyosarcoma	26 (11)	MFH	15 (8)
	MPNST	15 (6)	Fibrosarcoma	14 (7)
	Synovial sarcoma	13 (5)	Synovial sarcoma	10 (5)
	Fibrosarcoma	12 (5)	Angiosarcoma	9 (4)
	Other	53 (22)	Other	42 (22)
46-65	Liposarcoma	67 (24)	MFH	54 (28)
	MFH	66 (23)	DFSP	28 (15)
	Leiomyosarcoma	40 (14)	MPNST	23 (12)
	DFSP	20 (7)	Liposarcoma	22 (12)
	Fibrosarcoma	16 (6)	Angiosarcoma	16 (8)
	Synovial sarcoma	14 (5)	Atypical fibroxanthoma	12 (6)
	Chondrosarcoma	14 (5)	Leiomyosarcoma	11 (6)
	Other	46 (16)	Other	24 (13)
≥66	MFH	111 (46)	MFH	82 (34)
	Liposarcoma	49 (20)	Atypical fibroxanthoma	41 (17)
	Leiomyosarcoma	24 (10)	Angiosarcoma	27 (11)
	Angiosarcoma	11 (5)	Liposarcoma	20 (8)
	MPNST	11 (5)	MPNST	16 (7)
	Fibrosarcoma	10 (4)	Leiomyosarcoma	13 (5)
	Chondrosarcoma	7 (3)	Fibrosarcoma	10 (4)
	Other	20 (8)	Other	31 (13)

*5 (45) indicates there were 5 fibrosarcomas in the hand and wrist of patients 0-5 years, and this represents 45% of all malignant tumors in this location and age group.
DFSP, dermatofibrosarcoma protuberans; GCT, giant cell tumor; MFH, malignant fibrous histiocytoma; MPNST, malignant peripheral nerve sheath tumor.
From Kransdorf MJ. Malignant soft-tissue tumors in a large referral population: distribution by age, sex, and location. *AJR Am J Roentgenol* 1995; 164:129-134.

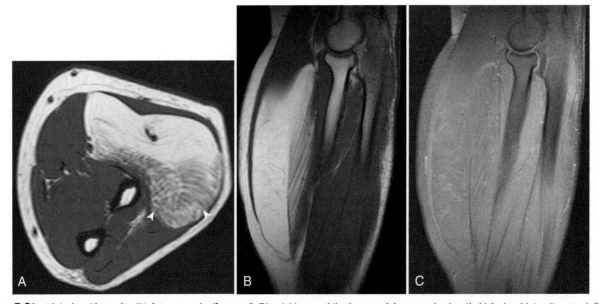

Figure 7-21   High signal intensity, T1: intramuscular lipoma. **A,** T1 axial image of the forearm. A large, predominantly high signal intensity mass infiltrates the musculature of the mid forearm. Note the feathery, intermediate signal intensity muscle fibers within the mass (*arrowheads*). **B,** T1 sagittal image of the forearm. The infiltration of muscle fibers is seen to better advantage in this plane. **C,** T1 fat-saturated sagittal image after gadolinium administration. There is complete saturation of the signal from the mass with the exception of some thin enhancing septations, compatible with an intramuscular lipoma.

Trunk	No. (%)	Retroperitoneum	No. (%)
DFSP	37 (23)	MPNST	9 (20)
MFH	21 (13)	Ewing's sarcoma	8 (18)
MPNST	19 (12)	Leiomyosarcoma	6 (14)
Fibrosarcoma	15 (9)	Ganglioneuroblastoma	4 (9)
Synovial sarcoma	13 (8)	Neuroblastoma	4 (9)
Ewing's sarcoma	12 (7)	Rhabdomyosarcoma	3 (7)
Angiomatoid MFH	6 (4)	Malignant hemangiopericytoma	2 (5)
Other	38 (24)	Other	8 (18)
DFSP	129 (30)	Leiomyosarcoma	57 (32)
MFH	77 (18)	Liposarcoma	52 (29)
MPNST	45 (10)	MFH	22 (12)
Liposarcoma	41 (9)	MPNST	11 (6)
Fibrosarcoma	36 (8)	Fibrosarcoma	7 (4)
Synovial sarcoma	20 (5)	Malignant hemangiopericytoma	7 (4)
Angiosarcoma	15 (3)	Ewing's sarcoma	3 (2)
Other	70 (16)	Other	20 (11)
MFH	131 (31)	Liposarcoma	170 (33)
Liposarcoma	80 (19)	Leiomyosarcoma	4 (30)
DFSP	60 (14)	MFH	111 (22)
MPNST	35 (8)	MPNST	23 (5)
Leiomyosarcoma	27 (6)	Malignant mesenchymoma	10 (2)
Fibrosarcoma	24 (6)	Fibrosarcoma	9 (2)
Angiosarcoma	15 (4)	Malignant hemangiopericytoma	7 (1)
Other	50 (12)	Other	27 (5)
MFH	137 (44)	Liposarcoma	164 (39)
Liposarcoma	56 (18)	Leiomyosarcoma	118 (28)
Leiomyosarcoma	23 (7)	MFH	93 (22)
MPNST	20 (6)	MPNST	13 (3)
DFSP	17 (5)	Fibrosarcoma	8 (2)
Fibrosarcoma	12 (4)	Osteosarcoma	6 (1)
Chondrosarcoma	11 (4)	Malignant mesenchymoma	5 (1)
Other	35 (11)	Other	9 (2)

intensity on T1W images is limited. This finding usually indicates fat or subacute blood products within the mass.

Lipomatous Masses. A lipoma is a benign fatty tumor that displays a characteristic MRI appearance, allowing for a confident diagnosis. These generally are well-defined, lobular masses that show homogeneous signal intensity that parallels subcutaneous fat on all sequences (high signal intensity on T1W images and intermediate to high signal intensity on T2W images) (Fig. 7-20). Thin, curvilinear septations often course through the fatty mass and may enhance mildly after gadolinium administration.[49] Most superficial lesions are well circumscribed, whereas deeper lesions may arise within muscle and appear more infiltrative (Fig. 7-21).[50,51]

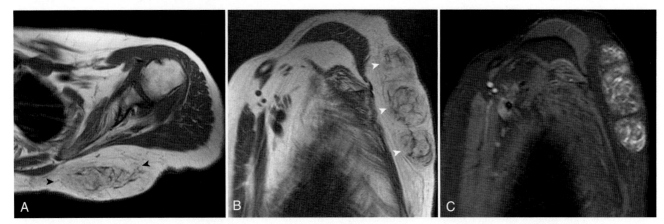

Figure 7-22 High signal intensity, T1: atypical lipoma (well-differentiated liposarcoma). **A,** T1 axial image of the posterior chest wall. There is an ovoid mass of predominantly fat signal intensity within the soft tissues of the upper back (*arrowheads*). Note the hazy intermediate signal intensity and mildly thickened septa in the central portion of the mass. **B,** T1 sagittal image of the chest wall and axilla. There are at least three lobules within the mass showing similar architecture and signal intensity with areas of fat and nonlipomatous tissue (*arrowheads*). **C,** STIR sagittal image of the chest wall and axilla. There is heterogeneous signal intensity throughout the mass. Subsequent biopsy revealed an atypical lipoma.

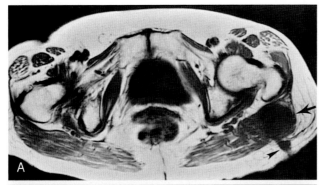

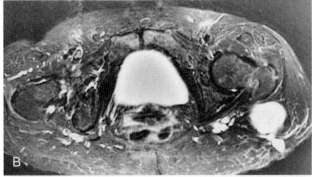

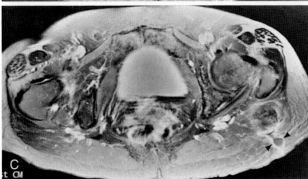

Figure 7-23 Liposarcoma without fat evident. **A,** T1 axial image of the pelvis. There is a very low signal intensity, rounded mass in the left gluteal musculature (*arrow*). The low signal intensity within the subcutaneous fat (*arrowhead*) is related to a prior biopsy. **B,** STIR axial image of the pelvis. The mass shows homogeneously increased signal intensity and smooth margins. **C,** T1 axial image with fat saturation of the pelvis, after administration of IV gadolinium. The mass shows poorly defined, heterogeneous enhancement. Note the enhancement along the margins of the biopsy track and lack of enhancement of the central fluid within it (*arrowheads*).

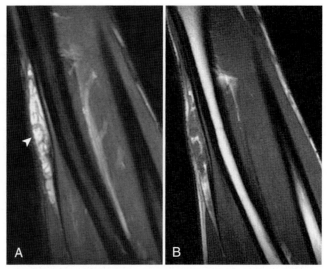

Figure 7-24 High signal intensity, T1: soft tissue hemangioma. **A,** STIR coronal image of the forearm. There is an elongated mass in the superficial soft tissues of the mid forearm (*arrowhead*), which shows lobules of increased signal and numerous septations. **B,** T1 coronal image of the forearm. The mass contains extensive fat between the lobular vascular channels, an appearance compatible with a soft tissue hemangioma.

appearance that is indistinguishable from other myxomatous tumors or even a simple cyst (Fig. 7-23). High-grade liposarcomas often contain no recognizable fat and are indistinguishable from other malignant soft tissue tumors.[52]

Vascular Malformations. Vascular malformations are benign lesions that lie along a pathologic spectrum ranging from capillary and cavernous hemangiomas (containing variable amounts of nonvascular tissue, such as fat, smooth muscle, or fibrous tissue) to true arteriovenous malformations that are composed of larger vessels. Regardless of the specific type of malformation, it is most important to recognize these as benign vascular lesions and to describe their extent and what anatomic structures they involve.

Cavernous hemangiomas usually display well-defined, lobular contours, although they may appear infiltrative. On T1W images, they are predominantly isointense to muscle, but often show variable amounts of increased signal intensity related to fat content. Their very high signal intensity on T2W images reflects the stagnant blood within their cavernous spaces (Fig. 7-24). Scattered foci of decreased signal intensity corresponding to calcified phleboliths, thrombosed channels, or septa seen on end also may be seen on T2W images.[55]

Arteriovenous malformations are composed of large, high-flow vessels, which result in dark intraluminal flow voids on T1W and T2W images and increased signal intensity on "flow-sensitive" gradient echo images (Fig. 7-25).[56] Large feeding arteries and draining veins also may be evident in the adjacent soft tissues.

Hematoma. Hemorrhage into soft tissues usually displays a heterogeneous, often laminated appearance. The signal characteristics of extracranial hemorrhage are less

An atypical lipoma (well-differentiated liposarcoma) is considered a low-grade malignant tumor that tends to recur locally after surgery, but does not metastasize.[52] Histologically, these tumors are composed of mature adipose tissue and other nonfatty elements, often contained in thick, irregular septa. The MRI appearance of these lesions parallels their histology. They typically show predominantly fat signal with coarse, thickened septa or scattered areas of nonfatty tissue. The nonlipomatous elements show low signal intensity on T1W images and high signal or enhancement on T2W or postgadolinium T1W images (Fig. 7-22).[53,54]

There are several subtypes of liposarcomas. Myxoid liposarcoma is the most common and may appear benign on MR images. These gelatinous lesions often show a cystic

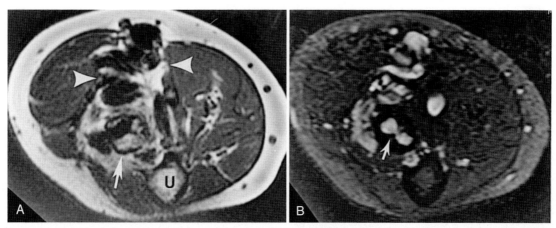

Figure 7-25   **High signal intensity, T1: arteriovenous malformation. A,** T1 axial image of the proximal forearm. A palpable mass in the volar soft tissues of the proximal forearm (*arrowheads*) is shown to be made up of large, low signal intensity tubular structures interspersed with high signal intensity fat. U, ulna. *Arrow* points to radius. **B,** T2* (gradient echo) axial image of the proximal forearm. Flow-related high signal intensity is seen within the large vessels making up this arteriovenous malformation on this "flow-sensitive" sequence. Note the direct extension into the proximal radius (*arrow*). (From Higgins CB, Hricak H, Helms CA [eds]. *Magnetic Resonance Imaging of the Body,* ed 3. Philadelphia: Lippincott-Raven; 1997.)

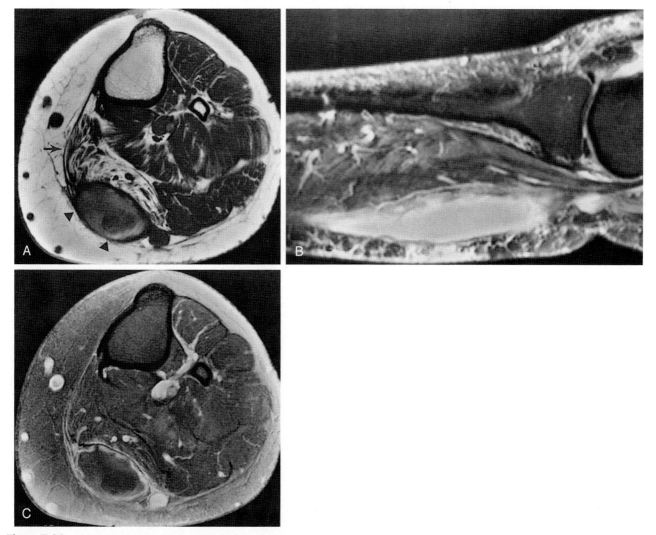

Figure 7-26   **High signal intensity, T1: hematoma. A,** T1 axial image of the proximal calf. This well-circumscribed mass (*arrowheads*) shows mildly increased signal intensity compatible with subacute blood products, surrounded by a low signal intensity rim. This hematoma could be traced back to the posteromedial knee joint, where it was seen to represent a hemorrhage within a Baker cyst. Note also the fatty atrophy within the medial head of the gastrocnemius muscle (*arrow*). **B,** STIR sagittal image of the calf. The hematoma shows diffusely increased signal intensity. **C,** T1 axial image with fat saturation of the proximal calf. There is peripheral enhancement, but compared with the precontrast image, there is no significant enhancement centrally, indicating its cystic nature.

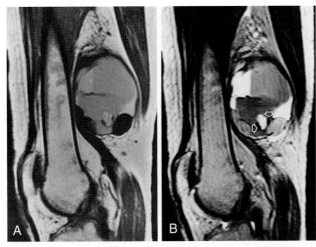

Figure 7-27 **High signal intensity, T1: hemorrhagic tumor. A,** T1 sagittal image of the distal thigh. A large, heterogeneous mass is seen in the posterior compartment of the distal thigh. Note the multiple fluid-fluid levels and areas of high signal intensity compatible with subacute hemorrhage. **B,** T2 sagittal image of the distal thigh. The peripheral rim and internal foci (*open arrows*) of persistent low signal intensity are compatible with hemosiderin. Biopsy revealed hemorrhagic synovial sarcoma.

predictable than with intracranial bleeding, but an acute hematoma (roughly up to 1 week old) is typically isointense to skeletal muscle on T1W images and of lower signal intensity than muscle on T2W images. In subacute and chronic hematomas, areas of high signal intensity usually are evident on T1W images somewhere within the mass (Fig. 7-26). These areas may display increased or decreased signal intensity on T2W images. In more chronic hematomas, areas of hemosiderin deposition, typically along the periphery, show decreased signal intensity on T1W and T2W images.[57]

A hemorrhagic neoplasm can be indistinguishable from a hematoma related to other causes (Fig. 7-27). At a minimum,

---

any hematoma detected with MRI must be followed to resolution, either clinically or with serial imaging. Gadolinium administration may reveal an enhancing tumor mass; however, this must be interpreted with caution because fibrovascular tissue within an organizing hematoma also may enhance.[19] In questionable cases, image-guided biopsy should be considered.

Melanoma. Malignant melanoma may show increased signal intensity on T1W images, presumably caused by the presence of paramagnetic compounds within the lesion. For the same reason, these tumors may display low signal intensity on T2W images (Fig. 7-28).

Low Signal on T2W Images (Box 7-6)
Pigmented Villonodular Synovitis. Pigmented villonodular synovitis is a synovial disease of unknown cause that most commonly affects the knee and results in an abnormal proliferation of histiocytes and giant cells, which usually contain hemosiderin. The most distinctive MRI features of this entity are masslike areas of synovial proliferation that show foci of low signal intensity on T1W and T2W images, related to the hemosiderin (Fig. 7-29).[58] A similar appearance may be seen with chronic hemarthrosis, chronic rheumatoid arthritis, chronic infectious arthritis (eg, tuberculosis), amyloidosis, or gout.

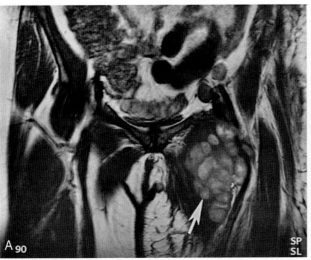
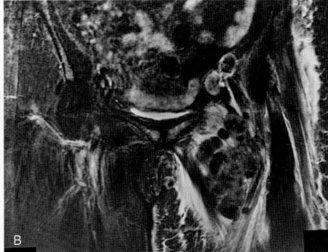

Figure 7-28 **High signal intensity, T1: melanoma. A,** T1 coronal image of the pelvis. There is a large, lobular melanoma metastasis in the proximal adductor muscles of the left thigh, showing extensive, increased signal intensity (*arrow*). **B,** STIR coronal image of the pelvis. Note the large foci of low signal intensity within the mass, presumably related to paramagnetic compounds.

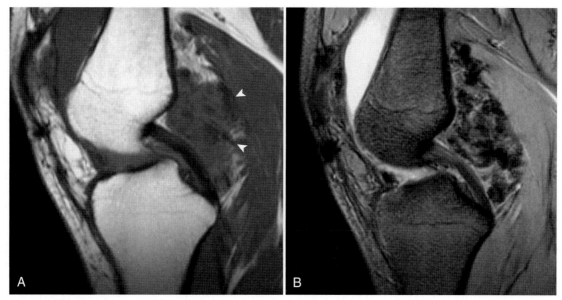

Figure 7-29 **Low signal intensity, T2: pigmented villonodular synovitis. A,** T1 sagittal image of the knee. Extensive intermediate signal intensity fluid or tissue distends the knee joint, most prominently posteriorly (*arrowheads*) where numerous low signal intensity foci are present within it. **B,** T2*−gradient echo sagittal image of the knee. The masses remain of low signal intensity and show prominent "blooming" secondary to susceptibility effects of hemosiderin, compatible with pigmented villonodular synovitis.

Giant Cell Tumor of the Tendon Sheath. An extra-articular form of pigmented villonodular synovitis is called *giant cell tumor of the tendon sheath.* This is typically a focal mass arising in proximity to a tendon and most commonly is found in the hand and wrist. Because of their similar histol-

ogy to pigmented villonodular synovitis, these lesions display intermediate to low signal intensity on T1W images and heterogeneous signal intensity on T2W images, with areas of decreased signal related to hemosiderin (Fig. 7-30).[59]

Fibrous Lesions. Soft tissue lesions containing predominantly fibrous tissue often show intermediate to low signal intensity on T2W images, at least in some portion of the mass (Fig. 7-31). Common entities include plantar fibroma

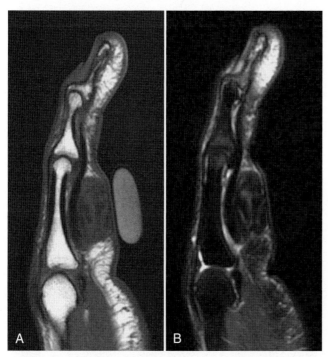

Figure 7-30 **Low signal intensity, T2: giant cell tumor of the tendon sheath. A,** T1 sagittal image of the finger. An ovoid, predominantly low signal intensity mass abuts and slightly deforms the underlying flexor tendons. **B,** Fat-saturated T2 sagittal image of the finger. The mass remains of low signal intensity and contains areas of darker signal intensity that are more prominent on this sequence, related to hemosiderin in this giant cell tumor of the tendon sheath (extra-articular pigmented villonodular synovitis).

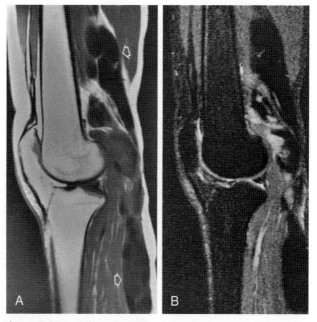

Figure 7-31 **Low signal intensity, T2: fibromatosis. A,** Sagittal T1 image of the knee. Large, lobular, low signal intensity masses are seen in the soft tissues of the posterior distal thigh and proximal calf (*arrows*). **B,** STIR sagittal image of the knee. The masses remain of diffusely low signal intensity and were shown on subsequent biopsy to represent fibromatosis.

Cystic-Appearing Masses

- Cyst/ganglion
- Intramuscular myxoma
- Myxoid malignancy
  - Liposarcoma
  - Chondrosarcoma
  - Malignant fibrous histiocytoma
- Synovial sarcoma
- Nerve sheath tumor
- IV gadolinium can differentiate cystic/solid lesions

(arising within the plantar aponeurosis), Morton's neuroma (a mass of perineural fibrosis surrounding a plantar digital nerve, most commonly between the third and fourth metatarsal heads), and desmoid tumors (benign but locally aggressive fibrotic lesions).

Amyloid. Amyloid is a protein-like substance that is deposited throughout musculoskeletal tissues as part of a primary disorder or related to other chronic diseases (secondary amyloidosis). The secondary form is most common in patients with end-stage renal disease who are undergoing hemodialysis. Amyloid deposition can occur in bone, intervertebral disk, or other soft tissues, with the hip and shoulder being the most commonly affected joints (Fig. 7-32). The tissue shows low to intermediate signal intensity on T1W and T2W images, probably caused by its collagen-like composition.[60]

Gout. Gouty tophi also may show low to intermediate signal intensity on T1W and T2W images, with or without associated bone erosions. These signal characteristics may be related to fibrous tissue, hemosiderin deposition, or calcification.[61]

Melanoma. Malignant melanoma shows variable signal intensities on MRI, but may display low signal intensity on T2W images, probably because of paramagnetic compounds within the tumor (see Fig. 7-28).

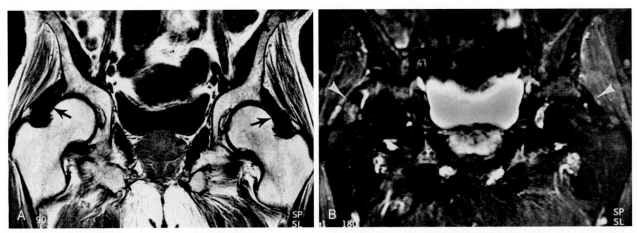

Figure 7-32 **Low signal intensity, T2: amyloid. A,** T1 coronal image of the pelvis. Prominent low signal intensity tissue is seen within both hip joints (*arrows*). **B,** STIR coronal image of the pelvis. The tissue remains of relatively low signal intensity and is outlined by small bilateral joint effusions (*arrowheads*). The patient has a history of end-stage renal disease.

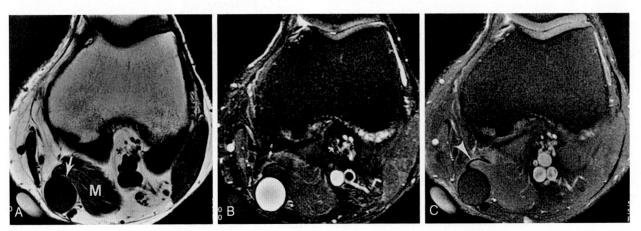

Figure 7-33 **Cyst. A,** T1 axial image of the knee. There is a well-circumscribed mass in the posteromedial soft tissues (*arrow*), distorting the adjacent semimembranosus muscle (M). Note the homogeneous internal signal intensity, which is lower than that of the adjacent muscle. **B,** STIR axial image of the knee. The mass shows homogeneously increased signal intensity. **C,** T1 fat-suppressed axial image of the knee after administration of IV gadolinium. There is no enhancement of the mass, confirming the cystic nature of this ganglion, which appears to arise from the semimembranosus tendon (*arrowhead*).

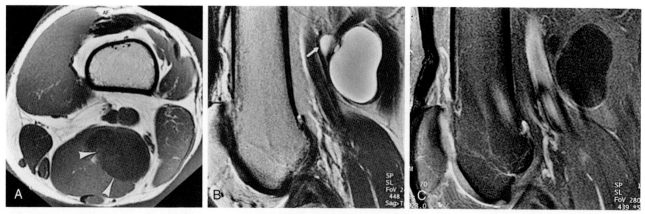

Figure 7-34 **Cystic-appearing lesion: myxoma. A,** T1 axial image of the distal thigh. A low signal intensity mass (*arrowheads*) is arising within the semimembranosus muscle. Its internal signal intensity is lower than that of the surrounding muscle. **B,** Sagittal turbo spin echo–T2 image of the distal thigh. The mass shows homogeneously increased signal intensity. Note the anterior lobulation (*small arrow*). **C,** T1 fat-suppressed sagittal image of the knee after administration of IV gadolinium. There is no internal enhancement within this intramuscular myxoma.

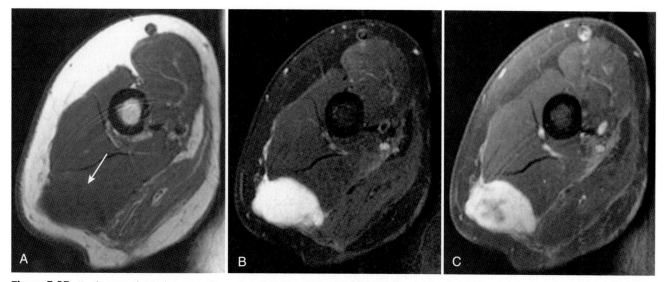

Figure 7-35 **Cystic-appearing lesion: myxofibrosarcoma. A,** T1 axial image of the upper arm. An ovoid intermediate signal intensity mass is seen within the posterior soft tissues of the upper arm (*arrow*). **B,** STIR axial image of the upper arm. The mass shows homogeneous increased signal, suggesting a possible cystic mass. **C,** T1 fat-suppressed axial image of the upper arm after administration of IV gadolinium. The mass shows diffuse enhancement, confirming the noncystic nature of this recurrent myxofibrosarcoma.

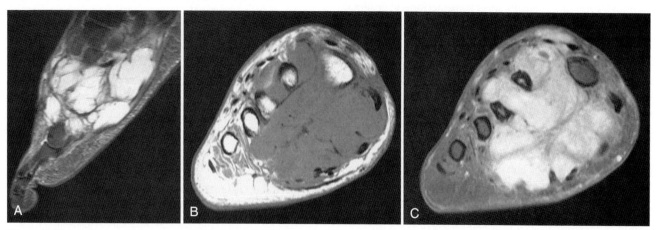

Figure 7-36 **Cystic-appearing lesion: synovial sarcoma. A,** STIR sagittal image of the foot. A multilobular, high signal intensity mass extends throughout the midfoot. The homogeneous increased signal suggests a possible cystic mass. **B,** T1 axial image of the foot. The mass shows intermediate signal intensity, higher than expected for simple fluid. **C,** T1 fat-suppressed axial image of the foot after administration of IV gadolinium. The mass shows diffuse enhancement, compatible with a solid mass, in this case a synovial sarcoma.

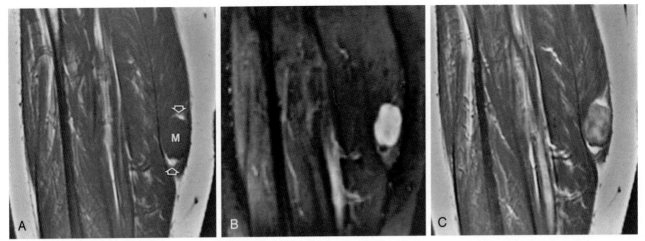

Figure 7-37   **Cystic-appearing lesion: nerve sheath tumor. A,** T1 sagittal image. There is an ovoid, low signal intensity mass (M) within the gastrocnemius muscle (*arrows*). **B,** STIR sagittal image of the proximal calf. The mass shows mildly heterogeneous, increased signal intensity with low signal intensity centrally (target sign). **C,** T1 sagittal image of the proximal calf after administration of IV gadolinium. The mass shows heterogeneous enhancement, proving it is not a cystic lesion.

Cystic-Appearing Masses (Box 7-7)

Cyst. Cystic lesions, such as fluid-filled bursae, synovial cysts, or ganglia, are common musculoskeletal masses. These often occur in typical locations such as the popliteal fossa or along the dorsum of the wrist, but may arise in unusual locations. A purely cystic mass shows homogeneous low signal intensity, hypointense to muscle, on T1W images, and diffusely high signal on T2W images. Thin, low signal intensity septa commonly are present within ganglion cysts on T2W images. After IV gadolinium administration, there is enhancement of the thin, peripheral wall and internal septa, if present, with a lack of central enhancement otherwise (Fig. 7-33).

Intramuscular Myxoma. These tumors are related to ganglion cysts and contain thick, gelatinous material that accounts for their cystic appearance on MRI. They are typically well-circumscribed lesions that are homogeneously hypointense to muscle on T1W images and diffusely hyperintense to fat on T2W images (Fig. 7-34). After gadolinium administration, these usually show some peripheral or septal enhancement, although heterogeneous internal enhancement may be seen.[62]

Cystic-Appearing Malignant Tumors. Solid tumors that contain myxoid elements (myxoid liposarcoma, chondrosarcoma, malignant fibrous histiocytoma) or synovial sarcoma may show a cystic, or predominantly cystic, appearance (Figs. 7-35 and 7-36).[63,64] When a cystic-appearing lesion is identified in an atypical location, evaluation with contrast enhancement is indicated. Unless the classic MRI features of a pure cyst are identified (thin wall, homogeneous low signal intensity on T1W images, high signal on T2W images, lack of central enhancement), aspiration or biopsy should be done to differentiate a benign cyst or intramuscular myxoma from a malignant lesion.

Nerve Sheath Tumors. Peripheral nerve sheath tumors (schwannoma, neurofibroma) may have a cystic appearance because of their well-circumscribed margins and homogeneous high signal intensity on T2W images. MRI features suggesting the diagnosis of a nerve sheath tumor rather than a cyst include identification of the tubular-shaped nerve entering and exiting the mass (best seen on longitudinal images), the split-fat sign (a peripheral rim of fat surrounding the lesion), multiple small nerve fascicles within the lesion on T2W images, and the target sign on T2W images (higher signal in the periphery surrounding central lower signal intensity) (Fig. 7-37).[65,66] These also typically show diffuse enhancement after IV administration of gadolinium.

REFERENCES

1. Ilaslan H, Sundaram M. Advances in musculoskeletal tumor imaging. *Orthop Clin North Am* 2006; 37:375-391.
2. Bloem JL, Taminiau AHM, Eulderink F, et al. Radiologic staging of primary bone sarcoma: MR imaging, scintigraphy, angiography and CT correlated with pathologic examination. *Radiology* 1988; 169:805-810.
3. Massengill AD, Seeger LL, Eckardt JJ. The role of plain radiography, computed tomography and magnetic resonance imaging in sarcoma evaluation. *Hematol Oncol Clin North Am* 1995; 9:571-604.
4. Enneking WF. Staging of musculoskeletal neoplasms. *Skeletal Radiol* 1985; 13:183-194.
5. Peabody TD, Gibbs CP, Simon MA. Current concepts review: evaluation and staging of musculoskeletal neoplasms. *J Bone Joint Surg [Am]* 1998; 80:1204-1218.
6. Peabody TD, Simon MA. Principles of staging of soft-tissue sarcomas. *Clin Orthop Relat Res* 1993; 289:19-31.
7. Lecouvet FE, Geukens D, Stainier A. Magnetic resonance imaging of the axial skeleton for detecting bone metastases in patients with high-risk prostate cancer: diagnostic and cost-effectiveness and comparison with current detection strategies. *J Oncol* 2007; 25:3281-3287.
8. Schmidt GP, Kramer H, Reiser MF, Glaser C. Whole-body magnetic resonance imaging and positron emission tomography-computed

tomography in oncology. *Top Magn Reson Imaging* 2007; 18:193-202.

9. Schmidt GP, Schoenberg SO, Schmid R, et al. Screening for bone metastases: whole-body MRI using a 32 channel system versus dual-modality PET-CT. *Eur Radiol* 2007; 17:939-949.

10. Sundaram M, McGuire MH, Herbold DR, et al. Magnetic resonance imaging in planning limb-salvage surgery for primary malignant tumors of bone. *J Bone Joint Surg [Am]* 1986; 68:809-819.

11. Frank JA, Ling A, Patronas NJ, et al. Detection of malignant bone tumors: MR imaging vs scintigraphy. *AJR Am J Roentgenol* 1990; 155:1043-1048.

12. Onikul E, Fletcher BD, Parham DM, Chen G. Accuracy of MR imaging for estimating intraosseous extent of osteosarcoma. *AJR Am J Roentgenol* 1996; 167:1211-1215.

13. Wetzel LH, Schweiger GD, Levine E. MR imaging of transarticular skip metastases from distal femoral osteosarcoma. *J Comput Assist Tomogr* 1990; 14:315-317.

14. Hanna SL, Fletcher BD, Parham DM, Bugg MF. Muscle edema in musculoskeletal tumors: MR imaging characteristics and clinical significance. *J Magn Reson Imaging* 1991; 1:441-449.

15. van Trommel MF, Kroon HM, Bloem JL, et al. MR imaging based strategies in limb salvage surgery for osteosarcoma of the distal femur. *Skeletal Radiol* 1997; 26:636-641.

16. Schima W, Amann G, Stiglbauer R, et al. Preoperative staging of osteosarcoma: efficacy of MR imaging in detecting joint involvement. *AJR Am J Roentgenol* 1994; 163:1171-1175.

17. Fletcher BD. Response of osteosarcoma and Ewing sarcoma to chemotherapy: imaging evaluation. *AJR Am J Roentgenol* 1991; 157:825-833.

18. Hanna SL, Parham DM, Fairclough DL, et al. Assessment of osteosarcoma response to preoperative chemotherapy using dynamic FLASH gadolinium-DTPA magnetic resonance mapping. *Invest Radiol* 1992; 27:367-373.

19. Kransdorf MJ, Murphey MD. The use of gadolinium in the MR evaluation of soft tissue tumors. *Semin Ultrasound CT MRI* 1997; 18:251-268.

20. Vanel D, Shapeero LG, DeBaere T, et al. MR imaging in the follow-up of malignant and aggressive soft-tissue tumors: results of 511 examinations. *Radiology* 1994; 190:263-268.

21. Biondetti PR, Ehman RL. Soft-tissue sarcomas: use of textural patterns in skeletal muscle as a diagnostic feature in postoperative MR imaging. *Radiology* 1992; 183:845-848.

22. Crim JR, Seeger LL, Yoo L, et al. Diagnosis of soft-tissue masses with MR imaging: can benign masses be differentiated from malignant ones? *Radiology* 1992; 185:581-586.

23. Papp DF, Khanna AJ, McCarthy EF, et al. Magnetic resonance imaging of soft-tissue tumors: determinate and indeterminate lesions. *J Bone Joint Surg [Am]* 2007; 89(Suppl 3):103-115.

24. Erlemann R, Reiser MF, Peters PE, et al. Musculoskeletal neoplasms: static and dynamic Gd-DTPA-enhanced MR imaging. *Radiology* 1989; 171:767-773.

25. Hayes CW, Conway WF, Sundaram M. Misleading aggressive MR imaging appearance of some benign musculoskeletal lesions. *Radio-Graphics* 1992; 12:1119-1134.

26. Assoun J, Richardi G, Railhac JJ, et al. Osteoid osteoma: MR imaging versus CT. *Radiology* 1994; 191:217-223.

27. Hosalkar HS, Garg BA, Moroz BA, et al. The diagnostic accuracy of MRI versus CT imaging for osteoid osteoma in children. *Clin Orthop Relat Res* 2005; 433:171-177.

28. Allen SD, Saifuddin A. Imaging of intra-articular osteoid osteoma. *Clin Radiol* 2003; 58:845-852.

29. Harish S, Saifuddin A. Imaging features of spinal osteoid osteoma with emphasis on MRI findings. *Eur Radiol* 2005; 15:2396-2403.

30. Campbell RSD, Grainger AJ, Mangham DC, et al. Intraosseous lipoma: report of 35 new cases and a review of the literature. *Skeletal Radiol* 2003; 32:209-222.

31. Laredo J-D, Assouline E, Gelbert F, et al. Vertebral hemangiomas: fat content as a sign of aggressiveness. *Radiology* 1990; 177:467-472.

32. Roberts MC, Kressel HY, Fallon MD, et al. Paget disease: MR imaging findings. *Radiology* 1989; 173:341-345.

33. Jee WH, Choe BY, Kang HS, et al. Nonossifying fibroma: characteristics at MR imaging with pathologic correlation. *Radiology* 1998; 209:197-202.

34. Norris MA, Kaplan PA, Pathria M, Greenway G. Fibrous dysplasia: magnetic resonance imaging appearance at 1.5 Tesla. *Clin Imaging* 1990; 14:211-215.

35. Vincent JM, Ng YY, Norton AJ, Armstrong P. Case report: primary lymphoma of bone—MRI appearances with pathological correlation. *Clin Radiol* 1992; 45:407-409.

36. Stiglbauer R, Augustin I, Kramer J, et al. MRI in the diagnosis of primary lymphoma of bone: correlation with histopathology. *J Comput Assist Tomogr* 1992; 16:248-253.

37. White LM, Schweitzer ME, Khalili K, et al. MR imaging of primary lymphoma of bone: variability of T2-weighted signal intensity. *AJR Am J Roentgenol* 1998; 170:1243-1247.

38. Beltran J, Simon DC, Levey M, et al. Aneurysmal bone cysts: MR imaging at 1.5T. *Radiology* 1986; 158:689-690.

39. Tsai JC, Dalinka MK, Fallon MD, et al. Fluid-fluid level: a nonspecific finding in tumors of bone and soft tissue. *Radiology* 1990; 175:779-782.

40. O'Donnell P, Saifuddin A. The prevalence and diagnostic significance of fluid-fluid levels in focal lesions of bone. *Skeletal Radiol* 2004; 33:330-336.

41. Cohen EK, Kressel HY, Frank TS, et al. Hyaline cartilage-origin bone and soft tissue neoplasms: MR appearance and histologic correlation. *Radiology* 1988; 167:477-481.

42. Aoki J, Sone S, Fujioka F, et al. MR of enchondroma and chondrosarcoma: rings and arcs of Gd-DTPA enhancement. *J Comput Assist Tomogr* 1991; 15:1011-1016.

43. Janzen L, Logan PM, O'Connell JX, et al. Intramedullary chondroid tumors of bone: correlation of abnormal peritumoral marrow and soft tissue MRI signal with tumor type. *Skeletal Radiol* 1997; 26:100-106.

44. Murphey MD, Flemming DJ, Boyea SR, et al. Enchondroma versus chondrosarcoma in the appendicular skeleton: differentiating features. *RadioGraphics* 1998; 18:1213-1237.

45. Lee JK, Yao L, Wirth CR. MR imaging of solitary osteochondromas: report of eight cases. *AJR Am J Roentgenol* 1987; 149:557-560.

46. Mehta M, White LM, Knapp T, et al. MR imaging of symptomatic osteochondromas with pathological correlation. *Skeletal Radiol* 1998; 27:427-433.

47. Kransdorf MJ. Benign soft-tissue tumors in a large referral population: distribution of specific diagnoses by age, sex and location. *AJR Am J Roentgenol* 1995; 164:395-402.

48. Kransdorf MJ. Malignant soft-tissue tumors in a large referral population: distribution of diagnoses by age, sex, and location. *AJR Am J Roentgenol* 1995; 164:129-134.

49. Hosono M, Kobayashi H, Fujimoto R, et al. Septum-like structures in lipoma and liposarcoma: MR imaging and pathologic correlation. *Skeletal Radiol* 1997; 26:150-154.

50. Matsumoto K, Hukuda S, Ishizawa M, et al. MRI findings in intramuscular lipomas. *Skeletal Radiol* 1999; 28:145-152.

51. Bush CH, Spanier SS, Gillespy T III. Imaging of atypical lipomas of the extremities: report of three cases. *Skeletal Radiol* 1988; 17:472-475.

52. Einarsdottir H, Soderlund V, Larson O, et al. MR imaging of lipoma and liposarcoma. *Acta Radiol* 1999; 40:64-68.

53. Gaskin CM, Helms CA. Lipomas, lipoma variants, and well-differentiated liposarcomas (atypical lipomas): results of MRI evaluations of 126 consecutive fatty masses. *AJR Am J Roentgenol* 2004; 182:733-739.

54. Kransdorf MJ, Bancroft LW, Peterson JJ, et al. Imaging of fatty tumors: distinction of lipoma and well-differentiated liposarcoma. *Radiology* 2002; 224:99-104.

55. Cohen EK, Kressel HY, Perosio T, et al. MR imaging of soft-tissue hemangiomas: correlation with pathologic findings. *AJR Am J Roentgenol* 1988; 150:1079-1081.

56. Cohen JM, Weinreb JC, Redman HC. Arteriovenous malformations of the extremities: MR imaging. *Radiology* 1986; 158:475-479.

57. Rubin JI, Gomori JM, Grossman RI, et al. High-field MR imaging of extracranial hematomas. *AJR Am J Roentgenol* 1987; 148:813-817.

58. Hughes TH, Sartoris DJ, Schweitzer ME, Resnick DL. Pigmented villonodular synovitis: MRI characteristics. *Skeletal Radiol* 1995; 24:7-12.

59. Jelinek JS, Kransdorf MJ, Shmookler BM, et al. Giant cell tumor of the tendon sheath: MR findings in nine cases. *AJR Am J Roentgenol* 1994; 162:919-922.

60. Otake S, Tsuruta Y, Yamana D, et al. Amyloid arthropathy of the hip joint: MR demonstration of presumed amyloid lesions in 152 patients with long-term hemodialysis. *Eur Radiol* 1998; 8:1352-1356.

61. Chen KHC, Yeh LR, Pan B-H, et al. Intra-articular gouty tophi of the knee: CT and MR imaging in 12 patients. *Skeletal Radiol* 1999; 28:75-80.

62. Peterson KK, Renfrew DL, Feddersen RM, et al. Magnetic resonance imaging of myxoid containing tumors. *Skeletal Radiol* 1991; 20:245-250.

63. Kransdorf MJ, Murphey MD. *Imaging of Soft Tissue Tumors.* Philadelphia: Saunders; 1997.

64. Morton MJ, Berquist TH, McLeod RA, et al. MR imaging of synovial sarcoma. *AJR Am J Roentgenol* 1991; 156:337-340.

65. Stull M, Moser RP, Kransdorf MJ, et al. Magnetic resonance appearance of peripheral nerve sheath tumors. *Skeletal Radiol* 1991; 20:9-14.

66. Suh JS, Abernoza P, Galloway HR, et al. Peripheral (extracranial) nerve tumors: correlation of MR imaging and histologic findings. *Radiology* 1992; 183:341-346.

Osseous Trauma

8

How to Image Osseous Trauma

- *Coils and patient position:* The patient should be placed in a comfortable position with passive restraints, such as tape or Velcro straps, applied to the region of interest to minimize motion. Pain medication also may be required in cases of acute trauma to improve patient comfort. Although the body coil may be used in cases where a large field of view is needed, whenever possible a smaller coil, such as a phased array pelvic coil or an appropriate surface coil, should be used.
- *Image orientation:* Images should be obtained in the axial plane and the sagittal or coronal planes, depending on the area of interest. The coronal plane is best for imaging the hips and proximal femora; sagittal images are most useful for the spine.
- *Pulse sequences:* Inversion recovery (STIR) sequences are the most sensitive for detecting abnormal marrow signal intensity that results from skeletal trauma and should be used in all cases. A fast spin echo–T2W sequence with fat saturation also is quite sensitive, but the incomplete fat saturation that sometimes occurs with this technique can produce areas of artifactually increased signal intensity, which can mimic marrow edema when none is present. T1W images should be obtained in at least one plane because they provide an excellent depiction of overall anatomy, and are reasonably sensitive for detecting osseous injuries, although they are less sensitive than STIR sequences. Gradient echo sequences should not be used when imaging osseous trauma with a high field strength magnet (>1T), because marrow pathology is obscured by susceptibility artifacts related to trabecular bone. With mid and low field strength magnets, however, some gradient echo sequences are quite sensitive for detecting traumatic injuries because susceptibility artifacts are less pronounced at these field strengths. Because of the exquisite sensitivity of MRI for detecting osseous injuries, a streamlined screening protocol may be used to provide a rapid diagnosis, minimize costs, and enhance patient throughput. For this purpose, we employ a three-sequence trauma protocol using T1 and STIR sequences to show osseous abnormalities optimally.
- *Contrast:* We do not use intravenous contrast material in cases of trauma.

ANATOMY

A familiarity with basic skeletal anatomy helps in understanding the MRI findings in osseous trauma. Cortical (compact) bone is found along the periphery of flat and tubular bones. The subchondral plate, the layer of cortical bone at the articular end of a long bone, plays an important role in providing support for the overlying articular cartilage.

Trabecular (cancellous) bone is composed of a meshwork of osseous struts that support the overlying cortex. Trabecular bone is found primarily in the axial skeleton and near the

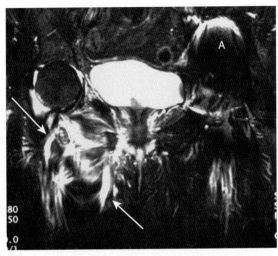

Figure 8-1   Soft tissue injury. Coronal STIR image of the pelvis. This patient presented with right hip pain after a fall. Note the high signal edema or hemorrhage within the adductor muscles of the right hip (*arrows*); there was no evidence of injury in the proximal right femur. Note also the prominent artifact related to a left hip prosthesis (A).

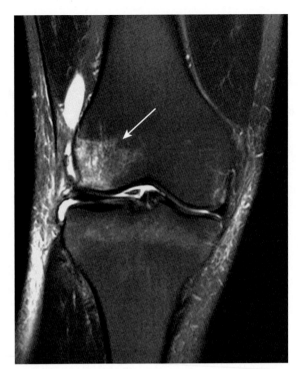

Figure 8-2   Bone contusion. T2 fat-saturated coronal image of the knee. Note the high signal intensity reticular contusion within the lateral femoral condyle (*arrow*).

ends of long bones, where it plays an important role in absorbing dynamic stresses. Because of its elastic compliance, cancellous bone has a load-bearing capacity 10 times that of compact, cortical bone.[1] This shock-absorbing capability is especially important around joints, where the trabecular bone dissipates axial forces away from the subchondral plate and overlying articular cartilage.

In a developing long bone, the physis (growth plate) allows for lengthening of the bone through enchondral ossification. Before closure, the growth plate constitutes the weak link in the muscle-tendon-bone and bone-ligament-bone units.[2] As such, it is particularly vulnerable to traumatic injuries at epiphyses (at the ends of long bones) and apophyses (growth centers not involved in longitudinal bone growth, such as the trochanter of the hip.)

OVERVIEW OF OSSEOUS TRAUMA

Osseous injury may result from a single traumatic event, or may occur over time as a result of repetitive stresses that lead to the gradual breakdown and ultimate mechanical failure of the bone. Acute trauma may result in impaction injuries (ranging from bone contusions to complete fractures) or avulsion fractures in which a tendon or ligament pulls off a piece of bone, cartilage, or both. Chronic injuries, resulting from less intense, repetitive trauma, range from a focal stress reaction to a frank fatigue or insufficiency fracture.

IMAGING OPTIONS

Conventional radiographs should be the first modality used for evaluating osseous trauma, but many acute and chronic osseous injuries are not detectable on radiographs. Most of these radiographically occult injuries can be detected with radionuclide bone scanning, but this technique has several limitations. The examination requires 4 to 6 hours, delaying diagnosis in these patients, who often are awaiting triage in the emergency department and the scan may be falsely nega-

tive for 24 to 72 hours after the injury, especially in elderly patients.[3] Finally, a positive scan is nonspecific because the images are of extremely low spatial resolution, and a wide variety of osseous pathology can result in abnormal uptake.[4] This can be especially problematic in older patients, in whom insufficiency fractures and neoplasms are common.

MRI is exquisitely sensitive for detecting osseous injuries that result from either acute or chronic repetitive trauma. By using streamlined protocols, MRI can be cost-competitive with a bone scan, while providing a more rapid and specific diagnosis.[5] As a result, we use MRI as the next study in a patient who has normal radiographs and a suspected osseous injury. A normal MR image essentially excludes the presence of an osseous injury. An additional strength of MRI is its ability to show soft tissue injuries that may mimic a fracture clinically in cases in which no osseous injury is present (Fig. 8-1).[6]

Acute Osseous Trauma

IMPACTION INJURIES

Contusion

Trabecular injuries that result from impaction forces are known as *bone contusions*, *bone bruises*, or *microtrabecular fractures*. Pathologic studies of these injuries reveal trabecular fractures and edema and hemorrhage in the adjacent marrow fat.[7] MRI findings become evident within hours of the injury,[8] and their detection is important for several reasons. An isolated bone contusion on an MR image may explain a patient's symptoms and avoid an unnecessary arthroscopic procedure. The sites of contusion also may provide clues about the mechanism of injury and associated soft tissue abnormalities that may be present.

Additionally, although most contusions resolve without complications, there is evidence that focal contusions involving the subchondral bone are associated with damage to the overlying cartilage.[9] Some investigators believe that this may place the patient at increased risk for collapse of the articular surface in the short term, or the development of osteoarthritis later.[10] Detection of a subchondral contusion may result in a more conservative treatment plan, including a longer delay before returning to a normal activity level, to allow for trabecular healing and to minimize the potential for collapse of the overlying articular surface.[11]

Bone contusions are most conspicuous on STIR or fat-saturated T2W images, where they appear as focal areas of increased signal intensity, usually with poorly defined margins, presumably secondary to the hemorrhage and edema related to the trabecular fractures (Fig. 8-2).[12,13] Contusions are typically of intermediate signal intensity on T1W images (lower than fat, higher than muscle) because marrow fat is intermixed with the hemorrhage and edema. Contusions are easily missed on non–fat-saturated fast spin echo–T2W images because the trauma-related edema and surrounding marrow fat display similar signal intensities.[13]

Contusion Patterns

By analyzing the locations of osseous contusions, the mechanism of injury often can be inferred, and associated soft tissue abnormalities can be predicted and carefully searched for. Two commonly encountered patterns are discussed here (Box 8-1).

Anterior Cruciate Ligament Tear. Osseous contusions are evident on MRI studies in approximately 80% of patients with acute anterior cruciate ligament tears.[14] The most common mechanism of injury that results in a complete tear of the anterior cruciate ligament involves a twisting force combined with a valgus stress. The ensuing impaction of the mid to anterior aspect of the lateral femoral condyle against the posterolateral tibial plateau results in typical contusions at these sites (Fig. 8-3).[15] Another contusion pattern often is seen concurrently in the medial compartment of the knee after an anterior cruciate ligament tear.[16] These contusions involve the mid to anterior medial femoral condyle and posteromedial tibial plateau. These contusions probably arise

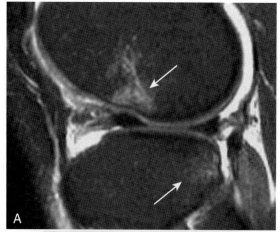

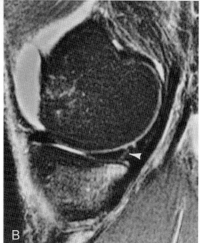

Figure 8-3 **Bone contusions associated with anterior cruciate ligament tear. A,** STIR sagittal image of the knee. Focal contusions are present in the lateral femoral condyle and posterolateral tibial plateau (*arrows*) in this patient who sustained an anterior cruciate ligament tear. **B,** STIR sagittal image of the knee. A contusion is seen in the posteromedial tibial plateau along with a vertical, peripheral tear at the posterior horn of the medial meniscus (*arrowhead*).

from a medial impaction force that results from the unstable knee rebounding after the anterior cruciate ligament tear and lateral injuries have occurred (see Fig. 8-3).

Lateral Patellar Dislocation. The typical contusions that result from patellar dislocation involve the medial patellar facet and the lateral femoral condyle, and are explained by the mechanism of injury. The patella dislocates in a lateral direction. As it relocates, the medial facet of the patella impacts against the anterolateral margin of the lateral femoral condyle, resulting in contusions at these sites (Fig. 8-4). Common associated findings include a tear of the medial patellar retinaculum, a large joint effusion, and a chondral or osteochondral injury to the medial patella or lateral trochlear groove.[17] Less commonly, the osteochondral injury may involve the weight-bearing surface of the lateral femoral condyle.[18,19]

Radiographically Occult Fracture

In the case of a radiographically occult fracture, in addition to marrow edema, a fracture line is present. The fracture line

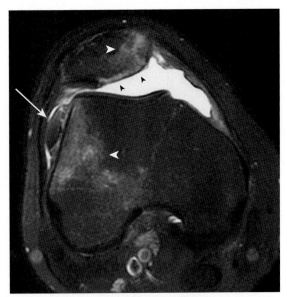

Figure 8-4 Bone contusions associated with patellar dissociation. STIR axial image of the knee. There are focal contusions in the lateral femoral condyle and medial patella (*large arrowheads*). Note the loss of cartilage on the medial facet of the patella (*small arrowheads*), and displaced cartilage fragment in the lateral patellofemoral gutter (*arrow*).

occasionally may be obscured by adjacent marrow edema, but usually is identified as a linear or curvilinear focus of low signal intensity on T1W images that may show either low or high signal intensity on STIR images (Figs. 8-5 to 8-7).[20] Marrow signal intensity returns to normal with healing.

It has been well established that MRI is able to show radiographically occult fractures in a rapid, cost-effective manner, allowing for optimal patient management.[21,22] This is possible because the associated marrow edema and hemorrhage are present on MR images from the time of injury. Even if a fracture is evident on conventional radiographs, MRI may provide additional useful information regarding the true extent of the fracture, the presence of additional fractures or contusions, and associated soft tissue injuries.

AVULSION INJURIES

Avulsion fractures occur when excessive tensile forces result in a piece of bone or cartilage being pulled away from the host bone by ligament, tendon, or capsular structures. These injuries may occur with a single, acute event or may result from repetitive avulsive stresses.

Although these injuries can occur at any age, they are most common in the developing skeleton (children and especially adolescents) because of the imbalance between muscle strength and the weak, unfused apophysis. Avulsion fractures occur less frequently in adults, in whom the musculotendinous junction is the site that is most vulnerable to injuries from excessive tensile forces.

Common Sites (Table 8-1)

Avulsion fractures are most common in the pelvis. Frequent sites include the anterior superior iliac spine (sartorius and tensor fascia lata tendons), the anterior inferior iliac spine

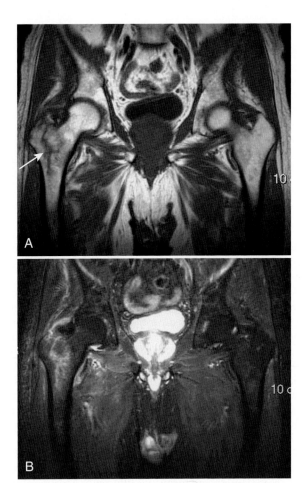

Figure 8-5 Radiographically occult right hip fracture. **A,** T1 coronal image of the pelvis. A nondisplaced right intertrochanteric fracture is identified by the low signal intensity fracture line (*arrow*). **B,** STIR coronal image of the pelvis. Note the high signal intensity fracture line and adjacent edema.

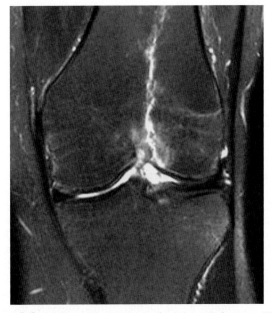

Figure 8-6 Radiographically occult distal femoral fracture. T2 fat-saturated image of the knee. There is a high signal intensity nondisplaced fracture line in the intercondylar region of the distal femur in this elderly patient who had fallen 6 weeks previously.

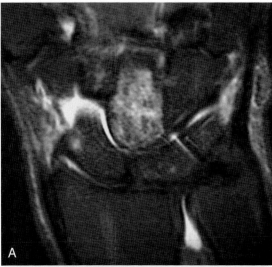

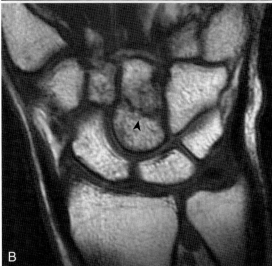

Figure 8-7 Radiographically occult fracture of the capitate. **A,** STIR coronal image of the wrist. There is diffuse edema within the capitate. **B,** T1 coronal image of the wrist. A nondisplaced low signal intensity fracture line in the mid capitate is shown to better advantage (*arrowhead*).

Table 8-1   COMMON SITES OF AVULSION INJURIES

	Site	Tendon or Ligament
Pelvis	Ischial tuberosity	Hamstrings
	Anterior superior iliac spine	Sartorius/tensor fascia lata
	Anterior inferior iliac spine	Rectus femoris
	Symphysis/inferior pubic ramus	Adductors/gracilis
Femur	Greater trochanter	Gluteus medius, minimus/hip rotators
	Lesser trochanter	Iliopsoas (young person) (older patient = metastasis)
Knee	Lateral tibial plateau (Segond fracture)	Lateral capsular ligament (mid third)
	Fibular head	Lateral collateral ligament
		Biceps femoris—long head
	Tibial eminence	Anterior cruciate ligament
	Posterior tibial plateau	Posterior cruciate ligament
	Inferior pole of patella	Patellar tendon (Sinding-Larsen-Johansson syndrome)
	Tibial tubercle	Patellar tendon (Osgood-Schlatter disease)
Ankle/foot	Calcaneus	Achilles
	Posterior margin—distal tibia	Posterior ankle joint capsule
	Dorsal margin, neck of talus	Anterior ankle joint capsule
	Base fifth metatarsal	Peroneus brevis
Humerus	Greater tubercle	Supraspinatus, infraspinatus, teres minor
	Lesser tubercle	Subscapularis
	Proximal shaft	Pectoralis major or latissimus dorsi
Elbow	Medial epicondyle	Flexor/pronator tendon
	Ulnar (sublime) tubercle	Ulnar collateral ligament

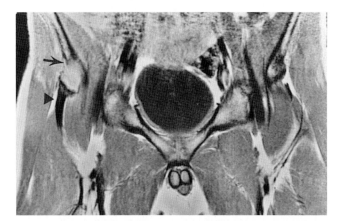

Figure 8-8 Avulsion fracture: right anterior inferior iliac spine. T1 coronal image of the pelvis. The right rectus femoris tendon (*arrowhead*) has avulsed a portion of the anterior inferior iliac spine (*arrow*).

(rectus femoris tendon) (Fig. 8-8), ischial tuberosity (hamstring tendon), iliac crest (abdominal muscles), symphysis pubis, and inferior pubic rami (adductor muscles and gracilis tendon). In the proximal femur, the greater trochanter may be affected (hip rotators, including the gluteus minimus and medius tendons).[23] The lesser trochanter may rarely avulse in a young patient (iliopsoas tendon), but in an adult this injury is virtually always secondary to metastatic disease in the trochanter.

Common sites for avulsion fractures around the knee include the lateral tibial plateau (Segond fracture at the attachment of the lateral capsular ligament) (Fig. 8-9), the fibular head (biceps femoris tendon, lateral collateral ligament), the tibial eminence (anterior cruciate ligament), posterior tibial plateau (posterior cruciate ligament) and tibial tubercle (patellar tendon) (Fig. 8-10).[23] Avulsion of the inferior pole of the patella can occur in children secondary to chronic avulsive forces (Sinding-Larsen-Johansson syn-

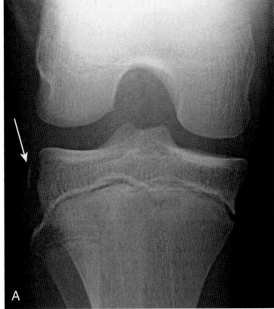

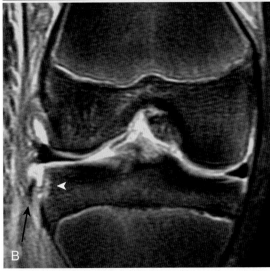

Figure 8-9 **Avulsion fracture: lateral tibial plateau. A,** Posteroanterior flexed radiograph of the knee. A small avulsion fracture (*arrow*) is seen adjacent to the lateral tibial plateau (Segond fracture) in this patient who had sustained a tear of the anterior cruciate ligament. **B,** STIR coronal image of the knee. The low signal intensity avulsed fragment is shown (*arrow*) as is high signal intensity edema within the adjacent soft tissues. Note the relative lack of marrow edema at the site of the avulsion (*arrowhead*).

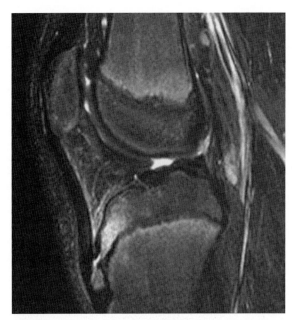

Figure 8-10 **Avulsion injury: tibial tubercle.** STIR sagittal image of the knee. Focal high signal intensity at the tibial tubercle apophysis in this skeletally immature patient is compatible with avulsive injury (Osgood-Schlatter disease).

pronator tendon) in children. The avulsed fragment may become entrapped in the humeral–ulnar joint space. Other sites in the upper extremity include the greater and lesser tuberosities (rotator cuff tendons), deltoid insertion on the lateral humeral shaft, and the insertion sites of the pectoralis major and latissimus dorsi tendons along the intertubercular sulcus.[23]

MRI Appearance

Avulsion fractures typically show abnormal marrow signal at the site of the injury, but the extent of the marrow abnormality generally is limited, and significantly less than what is seen with an impaction mechanism of injury. Prominent signal abnormality often is seen in the adjacent soft tissues, and the appearance may mimic a neoplasm or infection if a history of trauma is not obtained.[23] In these cases, correlation with conventional radiographs generally is useful because the injuries often have a typical radiographic appearance.

Repetitive Trauma

Stress injuries of bone typically are divided into two categories: insufficiency and fatigue fractures. Insufficiency fractures result from normal stresses applied to abnormal bone, whereas fatigue fractures occur when abnormal or unaccustomed stresses are applied to normal bone (Box 8-2).

INSUFFICIENCY FRACTURES

Several conditions weaken the elastic resistance of bone and predispose it to insufficiency fractures. The most common is osteoporosis, but others include Paget's disease, osteoma-

drome),[24] or as an acute cartilaginous avulsion fracture (patellar sleeve fracture).[25]

Avulsion of the posterior tuberosity of the calcaneus by the Achilles tendon (calcaneal insufficiency avulsion fracture) is seen almost exclusively in diabetics. Avulsion fractures also may be seen along the dorsal surface of the neck of the talus or posterior margin of the distal tibia secondary to pull of the anterior and posterior portions of the ankle joint capsule. The base of the fifth metatarsal is another common site for an avulsion fracture (peroneus brevis tendon).[23]

The most common avulsion fracture in the upper limb involves the medial epicondyle apophysis (common flexor/

Chronic Repetitive Injuries (Stress Fractures)

Insufficiency Fracture
- Normal stresses → abnormal bone
- Causes
  - Osteoporosis
  - Osteomalacia
  - Steroids
  - Paget's disease
  - Hyperparathyroidism
  - Rheumatoid arthritis
  - Radiation

Fatigue Fracture
- Abnormal stresses → normal bone
- Causes
  - New activity
  - ↑ Activity level (↑ exertion or duration)
  - Poor equipment (eg, worn-out shoes)
  - Abnormal biomechanics (eg, excessive pronation)

lacia, and irradiation. Clinical diagnosis often is challenging because the onset of symptoms may be insidious.

MRI Appearance

Radiographic findings of insufficiency fractures often are subtle and difficult to appreciate because of the osteopenia associated with most of these conditions (Fig. 8-11). MRI is able to detect these injuries with a very high degree of sensitivity, however. Insufficiency fractures appear as amorphous or linear foci of decreased signal intensity on T1W images. High signal intensity edema is seen on STIR sequences, classically surrounding a low signal intensity fracture line.[26] Their appearance may mimic neoplasm, but a specific diagnosis of insufficiency fracture usually can be provided based on the MRI morphology and location of the lesions.

With regard to morphology, a linear component (corresponding to a fracture line) within the area of marrow signal abnormality indicates an insufficiency fracture (Fig. 8-12).[26] In many locations, the orientation of the fracture line also is typical. In the sacrum, the fracture lines usually extend vertically through the sacral alae,[27] whereas in the supra-acetabular region, they often parallel the curvature of the acetabular roof, forming the "arched eyebrow" appearance (Fig. 8-13).[28] Generally, insufficiency fractures typically lie perpendicular to the long axis and major trabeculae of the affected bone (with the exception of the uncommon longitudinal fractures of the tibial and femoral shafts).

Any bone can be affected, but most insufficiency fractures occur in certain predictable locations (Table 8-2). In the pelvis, common sites include the sacrum, pubic rami, symphysis, and supra-acetabular regions. Pelvic insufficiency fractures frequently develop in patients who have undergone prior radiation therapy for a pelvic neoplasm, often within 12 months of completing the therapy.[29]

Common sites in the lower extremity include the femoral head and neck, the supracondylar region of the distal femur, the proximal and distal tibial metaphyses, the distal fibular shaft, the calcaneus, and the talus. The upper extremities are not usually affected by insufficiency fractures.

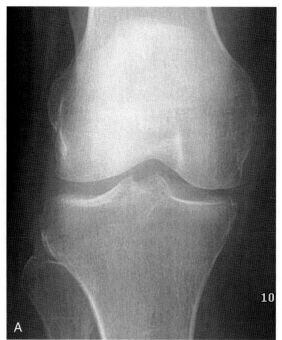

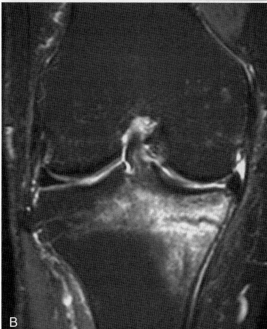

Figure 8-11 **Radiographically occult insufficiency fracture. A,** Antero-posterior radiograph of the knee. Diffuse osteopenia is noted without other abnormality in this elderly patient presenting with knee pain. **B,** Coronal STIR image of the knee. A low signal intensity fracture line with surrounding edema is present in the medial tibial plateau.

Amorphous foci of edema-like signal intensity, presumably representing insufficiency fractures, have been observed in the epiphyseal bone marrow of renal transplant recipients. These transient lesions all resolved within 1 year and could be distinguished from foci of avascular necrosis on the basis of their MRI appearance because truly necrotic areas showed more sharply circumscribed, low signal intensity margins, usually surrounding a focus of normal marrow fat.[30]

Insufficiency fractures are common in the spine. With an acute insufficiency fracture, the compressed vertebral body

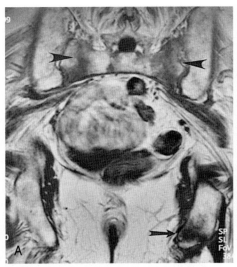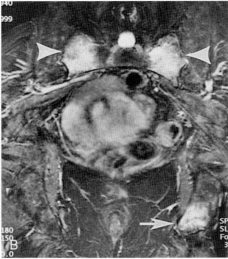

Figure 8-12 Pelvic insufficiency fractures. **A,** T1 coronal image of the posterior pelvis. Low signal intensity linear edema is seen in the sacral ala bilaterally and in the left ischium (*arrow*). Note the vertical orientation of the low signal intensity fracture lines within the sacral ala (*arrowheads*). **B,** STIR coronal image of the posterior pelvis. High signal intensity marrow edema within the sacral ala obscures the fracture lines (*arrowheads*). Note the low signal intensity fracture line in the left ischium surrounded by high signal edema (*arrow*).

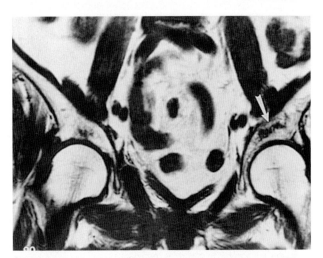

Figure 8-13 Supra-acetabular fractures. Low signal intensity fracture lines are seen in the supra-acetabular regions bilaterally. Note the curvilinear "arched eyebrow" morphology on the left (*arrow*).

shows intermediate to low signal intensity on T1W images and increased signal on T2W or STIR images, reflecting the associated marrow edema or hemorrhage. A fracture line usually is seen as well (Fig. 8-14). An old, healed compression fracture displays normal marrow signal intensity on all sequences.

It often is difficult to differentiate an acute osteoporotic compression fracture in the spine from a pathologic fracture

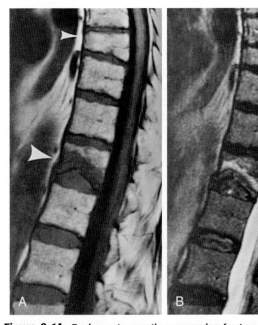

Figure 8-14 Benign, osteoporotic compression fracture of the spine. **A,** T1 sagittal image of the thoracolumbar junction. There is a compression fracture of the inferior end plate of T12 with bandlike, low signal intensity edema in the lower two thirds of the vertebra (*large arrowhead*). Note the normal fat within the superior third of the T12 vertebra and the old, healed compression fracture at T9 (*small arrowhead*). **B,** T2 sagittal image of the thoracolumbar junction. High signal edema clearly demarcates the fracture line in the T12 vertebra.

Table 8-2   COMMON SITES OF INSUFFICIENCY FRACTURES

Spine	Vertebral body (compression)
Pelvis	Parasymphyseal
	Pubic rami
	Supra-acetabular
	Sacrum
Proximal femur	Head
	Neck
	Basicervical region
Distal femur	Supracondylar region
Tibia	Proximal metaphysis
	Distal metaphysis
Fibula	Distal shaft
Calcaneus	Tuberosity

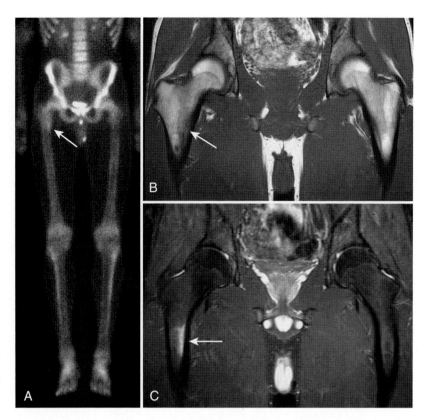

Figure 8-15 **Femoral stress reaction. A,** Bone scan, frontal view. Focus of faintly increased activity is present in the proximal right femur (*arrow*) in this young athlete with right hip pain. **B,** T1 coronal image of the pelvis. Vague area of asymmetric, decreased signal intensity is seen at that location (*arrow*). **C,** STIR coronal image of the pelvis. There is increased signal intensity at that site without a discrete fracture line (*arrow*). Findings are compatible with a focal stress reaction.

related to underlying tumor. Features that suggest a benign insufficiency fracture include abnormal signal intensity involving only a portion of the vertebral body marrow, a sharp linear margin between normal and abnormal marrow, lack of pedicle involvement, presence of a fluid-filled cleft within the vertebra on T2W images, the lack of a paraspinous mass, and a return to normal marrow signal intensity after gadolinium injection.[31,32] Some success using in-phase and opposed-phase imaging also has been reported.[33]

In indeterminate cases, an immediate biopsy or follow-up MRI examination in 6 to 8 weeks is indicated. With a benign compression fracture, there usually is some evidence of healing in that time, with vertebral marrow signal intensity returning to normal.

FATIGUE FRACTURES

Bone remodeling occurs in response to the mechanical stresses of normal, daily activities. Bone initially is resorbed in areas of activity-related microdamage, in preparation for reparative bone formation. Because bone formation is slower than resorption, however, this leaves the bone in a temporarily weakened state. This process usually is maintained in a physiologic balance, but becomes pathologic when the development of microdamage greatly exceeds the reparative capacity of the bone, such as when a new activity is attempted, or there is an abrupt increase in the level of activity or intensity of exertion.[34]

Accurate diagnosis is important because these injuries may progress to a displaced fracture if not treated promptly. The patient usually describes activity-related pain that abates

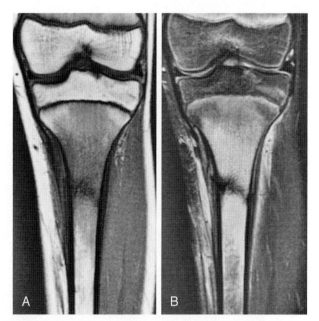

Figure 8-16 **Tibial stress fracture. A,** T1 coronal image of the tibia. There is a horizontal, low intensity fracture line surrounded by diffuse marrow edema. **B,** STIR coronal image of the tibia. The low intensity fracture line is more conspicuous because of the high signal intensity of the adjacent edema. Elevation of the low signal periosteum also is present medially and laterally.

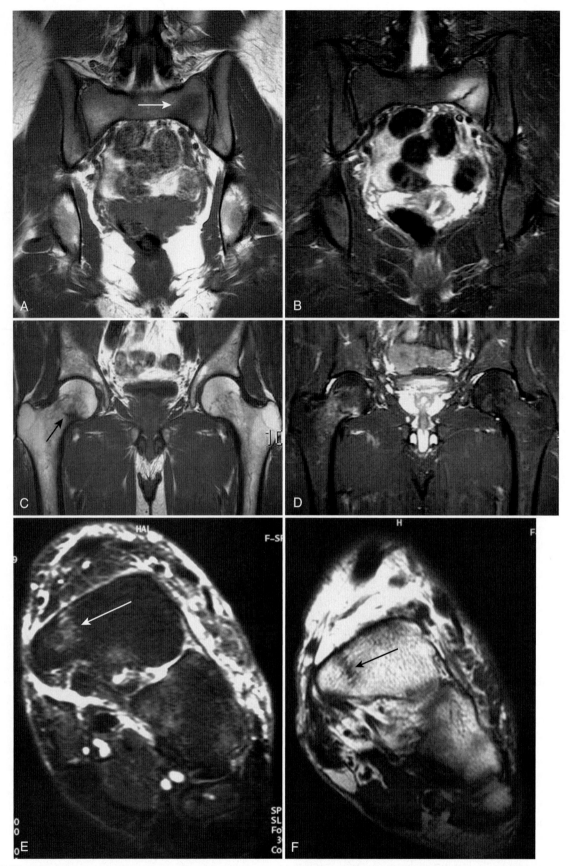

Figure 8-17 **Fatigue fractures: pelvis and lower extremities. A,** T1 coronal image of the pelvis. Low signal intensity edema is seen within the left sacral ala in this young long distance runner (*arrow*). **B,** STIR coronal image of the pelvis. A small, low signal intensity fracture line is seen within the edema. **C,** T1 coronal image of the pelvis. Low signal intensity fracture line is seen within the right femoral neck (*arrow*). **D,** STIR coronal image of the pelvis. A low signal fracture line is seen with mild adjacent edema. **E,** STIR coronal image of the foot. Focal increased signal intensity is present in the medial aspect of the navicular (*arrow*). **F,** T1 coronal image of the foot. A small, low signal fracture line is seen to better advantage at that site (*arrow*).

Table 8-3 COMMON SITES OF FATIGUE FRACTURES

Lower extremity	Tibia (especially posterior cortex, proximal shaft)
	Fibula (distal shaft)
	Metatarsal
	Calcaneus
	Navicular
	Femur (neck and shaft)
Pelvis	Sacrum
Spine	Pars interarticularis

Table 8-4 MRI GRADING SYSTEM FOR CHRONIC STRESS INJURIES

Grade	T1	STIR
0	Normal	Normal
1	Normal	↑ SI (periosteum)
2	Normal	↑ SI (marrow)
3	↓ SI (marrow)	↑ SI (marrow)
4	Fracture line	Fracture line

SI, signal intensity.

with rest, but the symptoms may be quite insidious. If the activity is curtailed, the damage often heals before the development of a true fracture, and this probably explains why many stress-related bone injuries are never radiographically apparent. The sensitivity of early radiographs may be as low as 15%, and follow-up films are positive in only 50% of cases.[36,37] Even so, radiographs should always be obtained in a patient with a suspected fatigue fracture because classic radiographic findings, if present, allow for a specific diagnosis.

MRI Appearance

MRI is exquisitely sensitive for detecting fatigue injuries in bone and is typically more specific than a radionuclide bone scan. In areas of osseous stress reaction, MRI findings include marrow edema on T1 and STIR images (Fig. 8-15). Increased signal intensity also may be observed on STIR images in the juxtacortical/subperiosteal region, which likely corresponds to periosteal buttressing, and a fracture line eventually may

be detectable within the marrow or overlying cortex (Fig. 8-16).[22,35] The imaging findings must be closely correlated with the clinical examination, however, because 42% of asymptomatic distance runners were shown to have MRI findings compatible with tibial stress reactions in one study.[38] The abnormal signal intensity resolves as the injury heals, usually within 6 months. Persistence of signal abnormality beyond this point most likely represents recurrent injury.[39]

Fatigue fractures most often involve the pelvis and lower extremity (Fig. 8-17). Common sites include the posterior aspect of the proximal tibia (running), the anterior midshaft of the tibia (jumping sports, dancing), the metatarsals (running, marching), the distal fibular shaft (running), the femoral neck (running, ballet), and the sacrum (running, aerobics). Within the spine, the pars interarticularis in the vertebrae also may be affected (ballet, running, gymnastics) (Table 8-3). Fatigue fractures are uncommon in the upper extremities, but can involve the humerus, ulna, clavicle, and first ribs.[40] Fatigue fractures occurring at certain locations are considered "high risk" because of their propensity for delayed union or progression to a complete fracture (Box 8-3).[41]

MRI Grading System

Because fatigue damage occurs along a spectrum from accelerated remodeling to frank fracture, the degree of signal

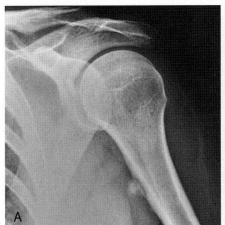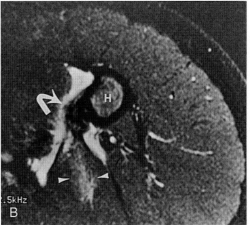

Figure 8-18 Chronic avulsion injury: proximal humerus. A, Anteroposterior radiograph of the left humerus in internal rotation. A rounded calcific focus along the anteromedial surface of the proximal humeral shaft was thought to represent a possible surface tumor. **B,** STIR axial image of the proximal upper arm. Extensive fluid or hemorrhage is seen around the avulsion injury at the origin of the latissimus dorsi (*curved arrow*) along the proximal humerus (H). Note also the edema or hemorrhage within the muscle compatible with strain or partial tear (*arrowheads*).

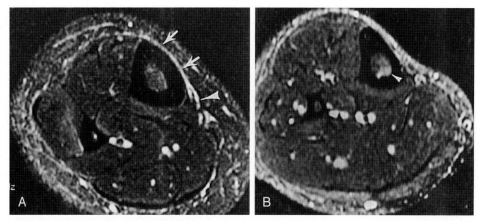

Figure 8-19 **Shin splints. A,** STIR axial image of the mid tibia. There is high signal intensity periosteal fluid or edema along the anterior tibia (*arrows*), with some extension medially along the insertion of the soleus (*arrowhead*). This appearance is analogous to a grade I stress reaction. **B,** STIR axial image of the mid tibia (different patient than in **A**). In addition to high signal intensity periosteal fluid or edema along the anterior tibia, there is focal intramedullary edema (*arrowhead*) in this patient who presented with symptoms of acute shin splints.

abnormality on MRI also varies. A grading system has been established to help quantitate the degree of injury (Table 8-4)[42]:

> *Grade 0:* A normal MRI study
> *Grade 1:* Periosteal edema or fluid on STIR images
> *Grade 2:* High signal intensity within the marrow on STIR images, but normal-appearing marrow on T1W images
> *Grade 3:* Marrow signal abnormality on T1 and STIR images
> *Grade 4:* Either cortical signal abnormality or a discrete fracture line

CHRONIC AVULSIVE INJURIES

Chronic avulsive injuries of bone and periosteum result from repetitive forces at the sites of tendon insertions. These injuries tend to occur at the usual sites of avulsion fractures described previously. Radiographic findings include periosteal reaction and cortical irregularity that may mimic a malignancy. MRI can assist in arriving at a correct diagnosis (and avoiding a potentially confusing biopsy) by localizing the abnormality to the site of a tendon insertion, where it shows cortical thickening, a lack of abnormal marrow signal intensity, and the absence of an associated soft tissue mass (Fig. 8-18).[43]

Shin Splints

Shin splints is a nonspecific term used to describe pain and tenderness in the lower leg that worsens with activity and abates with rest. The symptoms typically are localized along the posteromedial aspect of the tibia in the region of the soleus muscle origin. The pain is thought to be secondary to tears of Sharpey's fibers at the interface between muscle and bone,

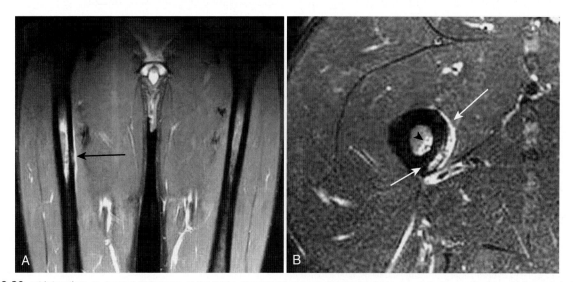

Figure 8-20 **Thigh splints. A,** Coronal STIR image of the thighs. Elongated increased signal intensity is present in the proximal to mid femoral shaft (*arrow*). **B,** STIR axial image of the right thigh. Abnormal increased signal is seen along the periosteal (*long arrow*) and endosteal (*arrowhead*) surfaces of the femur along with similar abnormal signal within the posteromedial cortex (*short arrow*). Findings are compatible with a developing stress fracture.

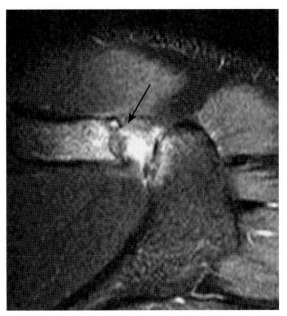

Figure 8-21   Stress-related osteolysis in the left clavicle. STIR axial image of the left shoulder. This young football player had high signal intensity edema and fluid in and around the left acromioclavicular joint and osteolysis of the distal left clavicle (*arrow*).

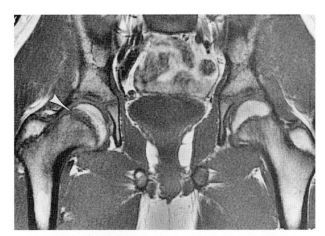

Figure 8-22   Epiphysiolysis: right hip. T1 coronal image of the hips. There is low signal intensity edema within the right femoral neck, with widening of the lateral capital femoral physis (*arrowhead*) and malalignment of the capital femoral epiphysis.

Thigh Splints

Similar to shin splints in the lower leg, a clinical syndrome has been described in the thigh known as *adductor insertion avulsion syndrome* ("thigh splints"). Thought to be secondary to the pull of the adductor muscles along the anteromedial border of the femur, abnormal linear activity at the adductor insertions was observed on bone scans in an early study.[46] MRI findings, including increased signal intensity on STIR images involving the medial periosteum and adjacent marrow of the proximal to mid femoral shaft, suggest that this syndrome represents a stress reaction of the femoral shaft that could lead to a true stress fracture. In more advanced cases, abnormal signal intensity also may involve

resulting in a traction periostitis, but the exact cause of this syndrome is unclear. In some cases, the pain also may be related to osseous fatigue damage. MRI findings in patients with clinical evidence of acute shin splints include periosteal fluid or edema along the anteromedial or posteromedial aspects of the tibia, abnormal marrow signal intensity within the tibia and, in some cases, discrete fractures (Fig. 8-19).[44,45]

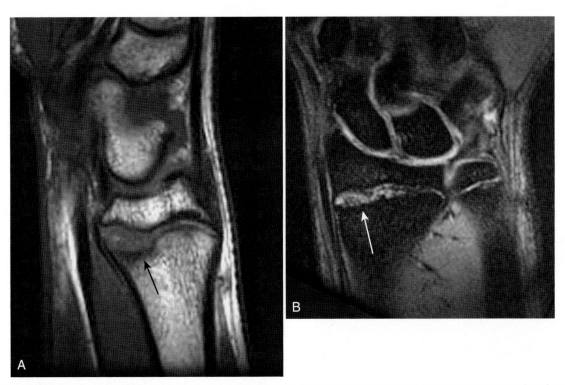

Figure 8-23   Epiphysiolysis: right wrist. **A,** T1 sagittal image of the wrist. There is widening of the volar aspect of the distal radial physis (*arrow*) in this young gymnast. **B,** Gradient echo–T2* coronal image of the wrist. The widening is seen along the radial aspect of the physis in this plane (*arrow*).

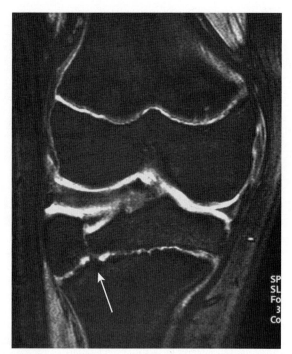

Figure 8-24 **Physeal bridge.** Gradient echo–T2* coronal image of the knee. A low signal intensity osseous bar (*arrow*) is seen crossing the high signal intensity proximal tibial physis in this patient who had sustained a prior physeal fracture. Note the residual incongruity of the proximal tibial epiphysis at that site.

the medial femoral cortex.[47,48] Because these typically athletic patients often present with vague groin pain, a large field of view should be used in these cases to include the hips and as much of the femoral shafts as possible to allow for accurate diagnosis (Fig. 8-20).

Post-traumatic Osteolysis

Post-traumatic osteolysis affects joints that sustain vertical stresses, such as the symphysis pubis, acromioclavicular, and

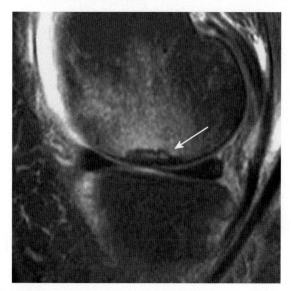

Figure 8-25 **Spontaneous osteonecrosis of the knee.** STIR sagittal image of the knee. Extensive marrow edema is present throughout the medial femoral condyle with a small subchondral fracture line (*arrow*).

sacroiliac joints. These stresses result in hyperemia, synovitis, and subchondral bone resorption in the affected joint. MRI findings include erosions and marrow edema related to the osteolysis and joint fluid and synovial hypertrophy caused by the synovitis (Fig. 8-21).[49]

TRAUMA TO THE IMMATURE SKELETON

Epiphysiolysis

Epiphysiolysis refers to traumatic injury to the growth plate secondary to compression and shear forces that result in a Salter I injury. This injury most commonly occurs in the proximal femur (slipped capital femoral epiphysis), distal radius in gymnasts, and proximal humerus and medial epicondyle of the elbow in baseball pitchers.[50-52] The MRI findings in epiphysiolysis include joint effusion, physeal widening, bone marrow edema mainly involving the metaphysis, metaphyseal fractures, and abnormal angulation of the epiphysis relative to the metaphysis (Figs. 8-22 and 8-23).[53] Premature closure of the epiphysis may occur.

Post-traumatic Physeal Bridges

Fractures involving the developing growth plate may result in premature closure of a portion of the physis. These osseous bridges cause differential growth across the physis with resulting angular deformities. Diagnosis on conventional radiographs can be challenging; however, these bridges are readily diagnosed with MRI.[54] Gradient echo–T2*W images are excellent for identifying the presence, extent, and location of the osseous bridge. The low signal bone bridge is easily seen as it crosses the bright cartilage in the normal portions of the growth plate (Fig. 8-24). On T1W images, these are seen as areas of bridging marrow fat across the dark physis.

Avulsion Fractures

Before closure of the physis, tendons and ligaments are stronger than the growth plate. This accounts for the high

Table 8-5 **COMMON LOCATIONS OF OSTEOCHONDRITIS DISSECANS**

Knee	Medial femoral condyle (non–weight-bearing surface)
Elbow	Capitellum
Ankle	Talar dome (anterolateral or posteromedial) (currently referred to as *osteochondral lesions*)

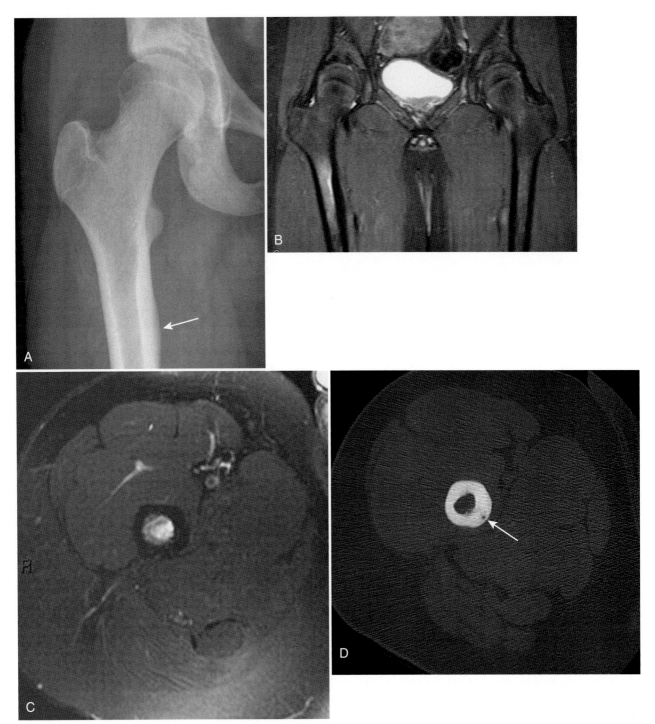

Figure 8-26 **Stress fracture versus tumor. A,** Anteroposterior radiograph of the right hip. Prominent cortical thickening is present along the medial aspect of the proximal femoral shaft (*arrow*) in this adolescent with right hip pain. Differential considerations include osteoid osteoma versus stress injury. **B,** STIR coronal image of the pelvis. Thickening of the proximal femoral cortex is again noted, as is nonspecific edema-like signal intensity within the adjacent medullary cavity. **C,** STIR axial image of the thigh. Nonspecific signal abnormality is present within the femoral shaft. The differential diagnosis remains the same. **D,** Axial computed tomography scan of the thigh. A small, rounded lucent nidus is seen within the thickened cortex (*arrow*), compatible with an osteoid osteoma (as was subsequently proved on biopsy).

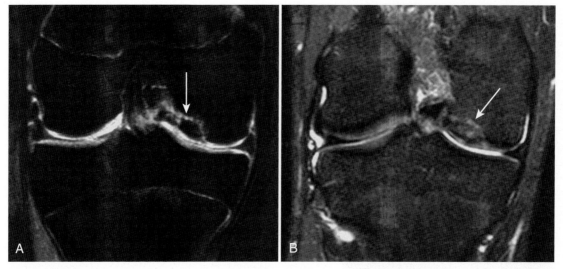

Figure 8-27 Osteochondritis dissecans: knee. **A,** STIR coronal image of the knee. A small ossific fragment is present along the lateral, non–weight-bearing aspect of the medial femoral condyle. Note the high signal fluid extending between the fragment and underlying bone (*arrow*), suggesting at least a partially unstable fragment. **B,** STIR coronal image of the knee (different patient than in **A**). No fluid is seen between this fragment and the underlying bone (*arrow*), compatible with a stable fragment. The overlying articular cartilage is intact as well.

incidence of apophyseal avulsions in skeletally immature patients. This topic is discussed more fully in the section on avulsion injuries.

Differential Diagnosis

EPIPHYSEAL MARROW EDEMA (Box 8-4)

Conditions other than trauma can cause marrow signal abnormalities that may be indistinguishable from trauma-related changes, especially in the epiphysis. These include degenerative arthritis, transient osteoporosis, early avascular necrosis, infection, altered weight bearing, and fatigue or insufficiency fractures (including "spontaneous osteonecrosis" of the knee).

Degenerative arthritis can result in chronic subchondral edema, but other signs of osteoarthritis, such as articular cartilage loss and osteophytes, also are present. Transient bone marrow edema ("transient osteoporosis") most commonly affects the hips and may mimic contusion, but its typical involvement of the entire femoral head and neck and a history of a gradual onset of symptoms aid in its diagnosis. This syndrome also has been observed in the knee and foot.[55] Early avascular necrosis initially may result in MRI findings of epiphyseal marrow edema.

Spontaneous osteonecrosis of the knee is a misnomer because it has been shown to represent a subchondral insufficiency fracture.[56] A history of an abrupt onset of pain without a traumatic event in an elderly individual is often reported. This condition most commonly involves the weight-bearing surface of the medial femoral condyle, and results in extensive epiphyseal bone marrow edema. Close inspection also usually reveals a small, low signal fracture line paralleling the subchondral plate, confirming the diagnosis (Fig. 8-25). Infection can mimic traumatic marrow edema, but usually can be differentiated on the basis of the clinical presentation.

Patchy, edema-like signal intensity may be present within the marrow of asymptomatic individuals, secondary to altered weight bearing or a recent change in activity level.[57] It also is often seen in asymptomatic pediatric patients up to 16 years of age.[58]

FATIGUE FRACTURE VERSUS TUMOR

Perhaps the most difficult problem is differentiating a developing fatigue fracture from tumor because both may manifest with similar radiographic and MRI findings. Caution should be exercised because biopsy of a stress fracture may result in a mistaken diagnosis of neoplasm, caused by the immature osteoid formed as part of the healing process. If a stress fracture is suspected, follow-up radiographs in 1 to 2 weeks or a repeat MRI examination may reveal signs of healing or a discrete fracture line, allowing for accurate diagnosis. Additionally, because of its ability to delineate cortical and periosteal changes better, computed tomography is often useful in these cases and may provide a definitive answer (Fig. 8-26).

Osteochondritis Dissecans

Osteochondritis dissecans refers to fragmentation or separation of a portion of subchondral bone along an articular surface. Two forms have been described: juvenile, occurring before physeal closure, and adult. Most juvenile lesions heal with conservative therapy, whereas the prognosis for adult osteochondritis dissecans is poorer. The knee, ankle, and elbow joints most frequently are involved, but the shoulder and hip also may be affected (Table 8-5).[59]

In the knee, the most common site of involvement is the lateral aspect of the medial femoral condyle (Fig. 8-27), along its non–weight-bearing surface. In the elbow, the lesion involves the capitellum along its convex anterior surface (Fig. 8-28). The exact etiology at these sites is

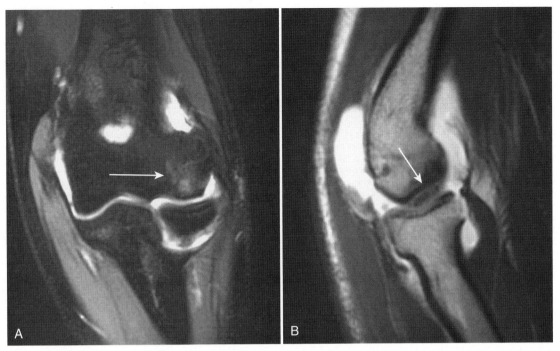

Figure 8-28 **Osteochondritis dissecans: capitellum. A,** STIR coronal image of the elbow (MR arthrogram). Focal subchondral edema is present in the capitellum (*arrow*). **B,** T1 sagittal image of the elbow. The subchondral fragment (*arrow*) is seen to better advantage and appears stable with no contrast extending between it and the underlying bone.

unknown, but repetitive trauma or acute shear forces are likely involved in most cases.

In the ankle, these subchondral abnormalities are found in the anterolateral or posteromedial aspects of the talar dome (Fig. 8-29) and are typically referred to as *osteochondral lesions,* rather than osteochondritis dissecans, probably because of their common association with a prior traumatic episode. Additionally, lesions at this site may resolve over time, calling into question some of the staging systems that have been proposed.[60]

Noninvasive assessment of the stability of the fragment is important because it may help direct further therapy. Fragments are considered stable if they are attached to the host bone and generally are treated nonoperatively. If the fragment is unstable (loose) or displaced from its site of origin, operative therapy is indicated.

Conventional radiographs may show a displaced osseous fragment, but are otherwise unreliable for assessing lesion stability. MRI is able to show the fragment, the overlying cartilage, and the interface between the fragment and parent bone. MRI signs of an unstable fragment include one or more of the following findings on T2W or STIR images (Box 8-5; see Figs. 8-27 to 8-29)[61]:

1. Linear high signal intensity (equivalent to fluid) surrounding the fragment
2. 5 mm or larger cystic changes between the fragment and host bone
3. A high signal intensity linear defect in the overlying cartilage
4. A focal, 5 mm or larger, associated cartilage defect

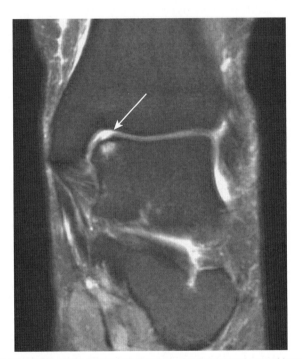

Figure 8-29 **Osteochondral lesion: talus.** T2 fat-saturated coronal image of the ankle. A small subchondral focus of increased signal intensity in the medial talar dome is compatible with an osteochondral lesion. Note the small defect in the overlying cartilage (*arrow*).

BOX 8-5

Osteochondritis Dissecans: MRI Signs of an Unstable Fragment

On STIR or T2W images:
- Linear high signal intensity surrounding the fragment
- ≥5 mm cystic foci between fragment and host bone
- High signal intensity linear focus in overlying cartilage
- ≥5 mm defect in overlying cartilage

REFERENCES

1. Radin E, Paul I, Lowy M. A comparison of the dynamic force transmitting properties of subchondral bone and articular cartilage. *J Bone Joint Surg [Am]* 1970; 52:444-456.
2. El-Khoury GY, Brandser EA, Kathol MH, et al. Imaging of muscle injuries. *Skeletal Radiol* 1996; 25:3-11.
3. Rizzo PF, Gould ES, Lyden JP, Asnis SE. Diagnosis of occult fractures about the hip: magnetic resonance imaging compared with bone-scanning. *J Bone Joint Surg [Am]* 1993; 75:395-401.
4. Shin AY, Morin WD, Gorman JD, et al. The superiority of magnetic resonance imaging in differentiating the cause of hip pain in endurance athletes. *Am J Sports Med* 1996; 24:168-176.
5. Rubin SJ, Marquardt JD, Gottlieb RH, et al. Magnetic resonance imaging: a cost-effective alternative to bone scintigraphy in the evaluation of patients with suspected hip fractures. *Skeletal Radiol* 1998; 27:199-204.
6. Bogost GA, Lizerbram EK, Crues JV III. MR imaging in evaluation of suspected hip fracture: frequency of unsuspected bone and soft-tissue injury. *Radiology* 1995; 197:263-267.
7. Rangger C, Kathrein A, Freund MC, et al. Bone bruise of the knee: histology and cryosections in 5 cases. *Acta Orthop Scand* 1998; 69:291-294.
8. Blankenbaker DG, De Smet AA, Benderby R, et al. MRI of acute bone bruises: timing of the appearance of findings in a swine model. *AJR Am J Roentgenol* 2008; 190:W1-7.
9. Johnson DL, Urban WP, Caborn DNM, et al. Articular cartilage changes seen with magnetic resonance imaging-detected bone bruises associated with acute anterior cruciate ligament rupture. *Am J Sports Med* 1998; 26:409-414.
10. Faber K, Dill J, Thain L, et al. Intermediate follow-up of occult osteochondral lesions following ACL reconstruction [abstract]. *Arthroscopy* 1996; 12:370-371.
11. Nakamae A, Engebretsen L, Bahr R, et al. Natural history of bone bruises after acute knee injury: clinical outcome and histopathological findings. *Knee Surg Sports Traumatol Arthrosc* 2006; 14:1252-1258.
12. Vellet AD, Marks PH, Fowler PJ, Munro TG. Occult posttraumatic osteochondral lesions of the knee: prevalence, classification and short-term sequelae evaluated with MR imaging. *Radiology* 1991; 178:271-276.
13. Kapelov SR, Teresi LM, Bradley WG, et al. Bone contusions of the knee: increased lesion detection with fast spin-echo MR imaging with spectroscopic fat saturation. *Radiology* 1993; 189:901-904.
14. Spindler KP, Schils P, Bergfled JA, et al. Prospective study of osseous, articular, and meniscal lesions in recent anterior cruciate ligament tears by magnetic resonance imaging and arthroscopy. *Am J Sports Med* 1993; 21:551-557.
15. Kaplan PA, Walker CW, Kilcoyne RF, et al. Occult fracture patterns of the knee associated with anterior cruciate ligament tears: assessment with MR imaging. *Radiology* 1992; 183:835-838.
16. Kaplan PA, Gehl RH, Dussault RG, et al. Bone contusions of the posterior lip of the medial tibial plateau (contrecoup injury) and associated internal derangements of the knee at MR imaging. *Radiology* 1999; 211:747-753.
17. Kirsch MD, Fitzgerald SW, Friedman H, Rogers LF. Transient lateral patellar dislocation: diagnosis with MR imaging. *AJR Am J Roentgenol* 1993; 161:109-113.
18. Mashoof AA, Scholl MD, Lahav A, et al. Osteochondral injury to the mid-lateral weight-bearing portion of the lateral femoral condyle associated with patella dislocation. *Arthroscopy* 2005; 21:228-232.
19. Sanders TG, Paruchuri NB, Zlatkin MB. MRI of osteochondral defects of the lateral femoral condyle: incidence and pattern of injury after transient lateral dislocation of the patella. *AJR Am J Roentgenol* 2006; 187:1332-1337.
20. Meyers SP, Wiener SN. Magnetic resonance imaging features of fractures using the short tau inversion recovery (STIR) sequence: correlation with radiographic findings. *Skeletal Radiol* 1991; 20:499-507.
21. Fowler C, Sullivan B, Williams LA, et al. A comparison of bone scintigraphy and MRI in the early diagnosis of the occult scaphoid waist fracture. *Skeletal Radiol* 1998; 27:683-687.
22. Haramati N, Staron RB, Barax C, Feldman F. Magnetic resonance imaging of occult fractures of the proximal femur. *Skeletal Radiol* 1994; 23:19-22.
23. Stevens MA, El-Khoury GY, Kathol MH, et al. Imaging features of avulsion injuries. *RadioGraphics* 1999; 19:655-672.
24. Donnelly LF, Bisset GS, Helms CA, Squire DL. Chronic avulsive injuries of childhood. *Skeletal Radiol* 1999; 28:138-144.
25. Bates GD, Hresko MT, Jaramillo D. Patellar sleeve fracture: demonstration with MR imaging. *Radiology* 1994; 193:825-827.
26. Crangier C, Garcia J, Howarth NR, et al. Role of MRI in the diagnosis of insufficiency fractures of the sacrum and acetabular roof. *Skeletal Radiol* 1997; 26:517-524.
27. Brahme SK, Cervilla V, Vint V, et al. Magnetic resonance appearance of sacral insufficiency fractures. *Skeletal Radiol* 1990; 19:489-493.
28. Otte MT, Helms CA, Fritz RC. MR imaging of supra-acetabular insufficiency fractures. *Skeletal Radiol* 1997; 26:279-283.
29. Blomlie V, Rofstad EK, Talle K, et al. Incidence of radiation-induced insufficiency fractures of the female pelvis: evaluation with MR imaging. *AJR Am J Roentgenol* 1996;167:1205-1210.
30. Van de Berg BC, Malghem J, Goffin EJ, et al. Transient epiphyseal lesions in renal transplant recipients: presumed insufficiency stress fractures. *Radiology* 1994; 191:403-407.
31. An HS, Andershak TG, Nguyen C, et al. Can we distinguish between benign versus malignant compression fractures of the spine by magnetic resonance imaging? *Spine* 1995; 20:1776-1782.
32. Moulopoulos LA, Yoshimitsu K, Johnston DA, et al. MR prediction of benign and malignant vertebral compression fractures. *J Magn Reson Imaging* 1996; 6:667-674.
33. Erly WK, Oh ES, Outwater EK. The utility of in-phase/opposed-phase imaging in differentiating malignancy from acute benign compression fractures of the spine. *AJNR Am J Neuroradiol* 2006; 27:1183-1188.
35. Anderson MW, Greenspan A. Stress fractures. *Radiology* 1996; 199:1-12.
36. Greaney RB, Gerber FH, Laughlin RL, et al. Distribution and natural history of stress fractures in U.S. Marine recruits. *Radiology* 1983; 146:339-346.
37. Nielsen MB, Hansen K, Holmes P, Dyrbye M. Tibial periosteal reactions in soldiers: a scintigraphic study of 29 cases of lower leg pain. *Acta Orthop Scand* 1991; 62:531-534.
38. Bergman AG, Fredericson M, Ho C, Matheson GO. Asymptomatic tibial stress reactions: MRI detection and clinical follow-up in distance runners. *AJR Am J Roentgenol* 2004; 183:635-638.
39. Slocum KA, Gorman JD, Puckett ML, Jones SB. Resolution of abnormal MR signal intensity in patients with stress fractures of the femoral neck. *AJR Am J Roentgenol* 1997; 168:1295-1299.
40. Daffner RH, Pavlov H. Stress fractures: current concepts. *AJR Am J Roentgenol* 1992; 159:245-252.
41. Boden BP, Osbahr DC. High-risk stress fractures: evaluation and treatment. *J Am Acad Orthop Surg* 2000; 8:344-353.
42. Fredericson M, Bergman AG, Hoffman KL, Dillingham MS. Tibial stress reaction in runners: correlation of clinical symptoms and scintigraphy with a new magnetic resonance grading system. *Am J Sports Med* 1995; 23:472-481.
43. Donnelly LF, Helms CA, Bisset GS III. Chronic avulsive injury of the deltoid insertion in adolescents: imaging findings in three cases. *Radiology* 1999; 211:233-236.
44. Anderson MW, Ugalde V, Batt ME, Gaycayan J. Shin splints: MR appearance in a preliminary study. *Radiology* 1997; 204:177-180.
45. Aoki Y, Yasuda K, Tohyama H, et al. Magnetic resonance imaging in stress fractures and shin splints. *Clin Orthop Relat Res* 2004; 421:260-267.
46. Charkes ND, Siddhivarn N, Schneck CD. Bone scanning in the adductor insertion avulsion syndrome ("thigh splints"). *J Nucl Med* 1987; 28:1835-1838.
47. Anderson MW, Kaplan PA, Dussault RG. Adductor insertion avulsion syndrome (thigh splints): spectrum of MR imaging features. *AJR Am J Roentgenol* 2001; 177:673-675.
48. Lawande MA, Sankhe S, Pungavkar SA, Patkar DP. Adductor insertion avulsion syndrome with stress fracture of femoral shaft: MRI findings. *Australas Radiol* 2007; 51:B104-B106.
49. De la Puente R, Boutin RD, Theodorou DJ, et al. Post-traumatic and stress-induced osteolysis of the distal clavicle: MR imaging findings in 17 patients. *Skeletal Radiol* 1999; 28:202-208.
50. Umans H, Liebling MS, Moy L, et al. Slipped capital femoral epiphysis: a physeal lesion diagnosed by MRI with radiographic and CT correlation. *Skeletal Radiol* 1998; 27:139-144.

51. Shih C, Chang C-Y, Penn I-W, et al. Chronically stressed wrists in adolescent gymnasts: MR imaging appearance. *Radiology* 1995; 195:855-859.

52. Obembe OO, Gaskin CM, Taffoni MJ, Anderson MW. Little Leaguer's shoulder (proximal humeral epiphysiolysis): MRI findings in four boys. *Pediatr Radiol* 2007; 37:885-889.

53. Laor T, Hartman AL, Jamarillo D. Local physeal widening on MR imaging: an incidental finding suggesting prior metaphyseal insult. *Pediatr Radiol* 1997; 27:654-662.

54. Craig JG, Cramer KE, Cody DD, et al. Premature partial closure and other deformities of the growth plate: MR imaging and three-dimensional modeling. *Radiology* 1999; 210:835-843.

55. Gigena LM, Chung CB, Lektrakul N, et al. Transient bone marrow edema of the talus: MR imaging findings in five patients. *Skeletal Radiol* 2002; 31:202-207.

56. Yamamoto T, Bullough PG. Spontaneous osteonecrosis of the knee: the result of subchondral insufficiency fracture. *J Bone Joint Surg [Am]* 2000; 82:858-866.

57. Schweitzer ME, White LM. Does altered biomechanics cause marrow edema? *Radiology* 1996; 198:851-853.

58. Shabshin N, Schweitzer ME, Morrison WB, et al. High-signal T2 changes of the bone marrow of the foot and ankle in children: red marrow or traumatic changes? *Pediatr Radiol* 2006; 36:670-676.

59. Schenck RC, Goodnight JM. Osteochondritis dissecans. *J Bone Joint Surg [Am]* 1996; 78:439-456.

60. Elias I, Jung JW, Jaikin SM, et al. Osteochondral lesions of the talus: change in MRI findings over time in talar lesions without operative intervention and implications for staging systems. *Foot Ankle Int* 2006; 27:157-166.

61. DeSmet AA, Ilahi OA, Graf BK. Reassessment of the MR criteria for stability of osteochondritis dissecans in the knee and ankle. *Skeletal Radiol* 1996; 25:159-163.

Temporomandibular Joint

9

How to Image the Temporomandibular Joint

See the temporomandibular joint (TMJ) protocols at the end of the chapter.

- *Coils and patient position:* Small surface coils are used, generally with a diameter of about 3 inches. Bilateral simultaneous examinations of the TMJs can be done with coupled surface coils. The patient is supine in the bore of the magnet, with the coils centered over the TMJs by centering the coils just anterior to the tragus of the ear. Images are obtained through the joints with the mouth closed. Images also can be obtained with the mouth open, which is done with a special device that holds the mouth open, or for the more innovative (cheap) among us, gauze can be wrapped around a syringe and placed in the mouth for the patient to bite down on. The size of the syringe is determined by the extent that the mouth can open.
- *Image orientation:* An axial localizer image through the TMJ condyles is obtained first. Using the axial scout image, a line is drawn between the anterior aspects of the two condyles, then sagittal images are obtained perpendicular to this line. This is essentially always the sagittal plane relative to the bore of the magnet, but is a sagittal oblique image of the TMJs. These images are obtained first with the mouth closed, and then the sagittal sequence can be repeated with the mouth open if one wishes to know if the TMJ disk reduces with mouth opening. Coronal oblique images through the TMJs are obtained as an optional sequence in some patients to show the condyles well in another plane and to show the disk in the rare event that it may displace in exclusively a medial or lateral direction relative to the condyle. These images are obtained parallel to the long axis of the condyles based on the axial scout view. Coronal oblique images are done only with the mouth closed. Our only indication for obtaining coronal oblique images is that the referring physician asks for them.

- *Pulse sequences and regions of interest:* T1W images show the pertinent anatomy well. The section thickness is 3 mm with no gap; a 6-cm field of view is used. Both TMJs generally are imaged, mainly because we have the coupled coils that allow it to be done easily, and because bilateral abnormalities are common. It is necessary only to image the symptomatic joint, however. T2W images are not necessary for evaluation of routine internal derangement, but may be valuable in patients who have had recent trauma to the joint because they may show abnormalities in the muscles surrounding the joint.
- *Contrast:* Contrast enhancement is of no value for diagnosing routine internal derangements of the TMJ.

Normal Temporomandibular Joint

OSSEOUS STRUCTURES

The osseous components of the TMJ are the mandibular condyle and the temporal bone at the base of the skull (Figs. 9-1 and 9-2). The relevant portions of the temporal bone that articulate with the condyle are the glenoid fossa and the articular eminence. The condyle should be concentrically positioned in the glenoid fossa with the mouth closed. With the mouth open, the condyle translates anteriorly so that the condyle is positioned directly underneath the apex of the articular eminence. The articular surfaces of the TMJ are covered with a thin layer of fibrocartilage.[1]

DISK

The soft tissue structure of interest in the TMJ is the articular meniscus or disk. The disk is interposed between the condyle and the temporal bone, completely separating the joint into superior and inferior recesses. The TMJ disk is made of fibrous tissue and has an asymmetric biconcave configuration. The disk is thicker peripherally than it is centrally. The thin central portion of the disk is called the *intermediate*

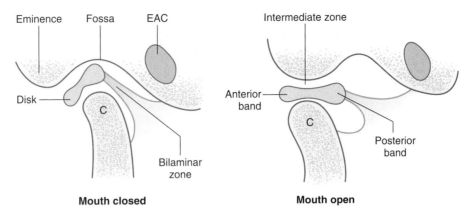

Figure 9-1 Normal temporomandibular joint anatomy (sagittal view). Mouth closed (*left*) and open (*right*); anterior is to the left of each figure. The relationship of the disk to the osseous structures is depicted, with the intermediate zone interposed between the eminence and condyle wherever they are closest to each other. The posterior band is located at the 12-o'clock position on the condyle. C, condyle; EAC, external auditory canal.

zone. The thicker periphery of the disk is divided into anterior and posterior bands (see Figs. 9-1 and 9-2). The anterior band of the disk is usually smaller than the posterior band. The disk attaches to the joint capsule, pterygoid muscle, and bone. Posteriorly, the disk is continuous with collagen fibers and loose fibroelastic tissue known as the bilaminar zone or posterior attachment. The bilaminar zone functions as a rubber band, allowing the meniscus to move forward with the condyle during mouth opening, and then recoils back to its original position, bringing the disk with it, as the mouth closes.

The normal position of the TMJ disk, regardless of whether or not the mouth is open or closed, is with the thin intermediate zone interposed between the condyle and the adjacent temporal bone, wherever the two bones are most closely apposed to one another.[1]

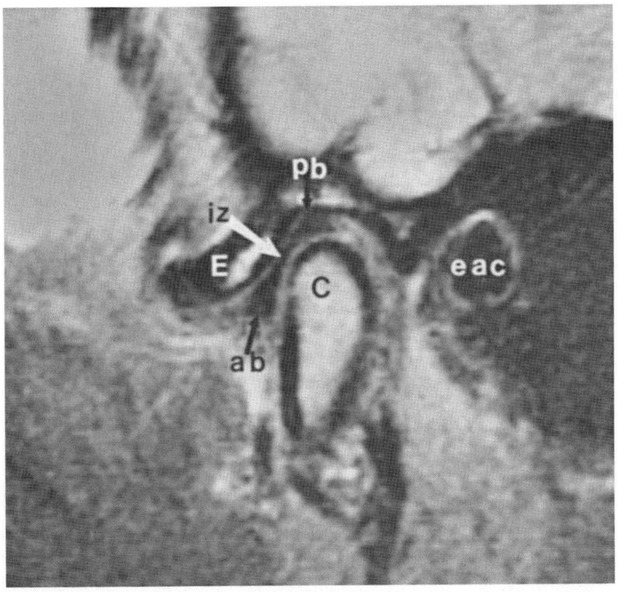

MRI of the normal TMJ in the sagittal plane shows the biconcave disk as an asymmetric bow-tie configuration. The thin intermediate zone can be seen between the two most closely apposed cortical bone surfaces of the condyle and eminence with any degree of mouth opening and with the mouth completely closed. Normally, the posterior band is located at the 12-o'clock position, directly on top of the condyle, with the mouth closed. The posterior band may not always be evident when the mouth is closed because its signal blends with the adjacent low signal intensity cortical bone of the condyle and glenoid fossa. The posterior band becomes more obvious with the mouth open, as it displaces away from adjacent bone (Fig. 9-3). The disk is overall low signal intensity on all pulse sequences, but careful scrutiny shows intermediate signal intensity centrally in the anterior or posterior bands.

Abnormal Temporomandibular Joint (Box 9-1)

The TMJ is undoubtedly the dullest joint radiologists image. It performs only two tricks that relate to MRI diagnosis: The disk can become displaced (internal derangement), and degenerative joint disease can occur as a consequence of chronic disk displacement. Trauma and inflammatory arthritides also affect the TMJ, but we essentially never image with MRI for those indications. Some clinicians believe that avascular necrosis of the mandibular condyle occurs. With such a limited repertoire, it is hard for clinicians to misdiagnose a patient with TMJ symptoms. Still, we are asked a few times a year to image the TMJ to look for internal derangements in patients who do not respond to therapy as expected, or who have unusual symptoms. Radiologists need to know how to evaluate images of the TMJ.

INTERNAL DERANGEMENTS

Internal derangements of the TMJ occur in women more often than men, and young adults generally are affected.

Figure 9-2 Normal temporomandibular joint. Mouth closed (sagittal T1 image). Osseous structures: C, condyle; E, articular eminence; EAC, external auditory canal. Disk: ab, anterior band; pb, posterior band; iz, intermediate zone. Note the posterior band at the 12-o'clock position relative to the condyle, and the intermediate zone between the condyle and the eminence, where they are most closely apposed.

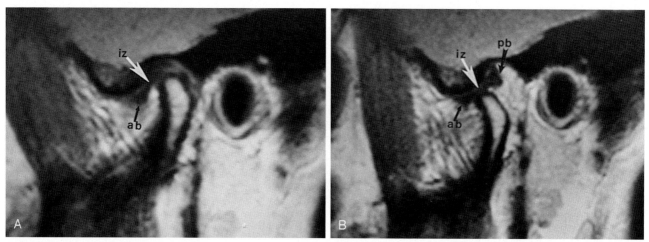

Figure 9-3 **Normal temporomandibular joint. A,** Mouth closed (sagittal T1 image). Disk is in normal position, but the posterior band is difficult to identify because it blends with adjacent cortical bone. The intermediate zone (iz) and anterior band (ab) are easy to see and confirm the normal disk position. **B,** Mouth partially open (sagittal T1 image). The entire disk, including the posterior band (pb), becomes obvious as it displaces away from adjacent bones. The intermediate zone (iz) remains in its normal position, interposed between the condyle and eminence wherever they are closest together, and the anterior band (ab) remains obvious.

BOX 9-1

Temporomandibular Joint: All You Really Need to Know

Normal Disk

- Biconcave structure with thin intermediate zone articulating between the condyle and the eminence wherever they are most closely apposed on sagittal images

Abnormal Disk

- Disk displaced anteriorly from normal closed-mouth position. Intermediate zone no longer interposed between the closest contact point of condyle and eminence
- Disk may reduce to normal position with mouth opening (anterior displacement with reduction)
- Disk may remain displaced with mouth opening (anterior displacement without reduction)
- Disk degenerates with loss of internal intermediate signal and biconcave shape
- Joint degenerates
  - Subchondral cyst, subchondral sclerosis, osteophytes of condyle
  - Osteonecrosis

Symptoms may include headache, earache, pain and tenderness over the joint, joint noise ("snap, crackle, pop"), and a limited ability to open the mouth.

Internal derangements of the TMJ may be classified into three different categories, and frequently a patient progresses in sequence from one category to the next.[1] The forms of internal derangement, in increasing order of severity, are listed:

1. Anterior displacement of the disk, *with* reduction to normal position with mouth opening
2. Anterior displacement of the disk, *without* reduction to normal position with mouth opening
3. Anterior displacement of the disk with a perforation

An internally deranged disk is always in an abnormal position when the mouth is closed, but may or may not be in an abnormal position when the mouth is open (Fig. 9-4). Although we evaluate as to whether or not the disk reduces to normal position with mouth opening, this can change

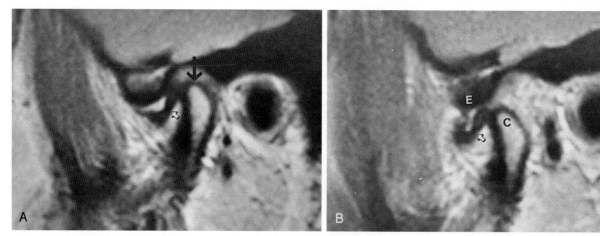

Figure 9-4 **Anterior disk displacement without reduction. A,** Closed mouth (sagittal T1 image). The posterior band is located anterior to the 12-o'clock position (*solid arrow*) of the condyle. The intermediate zone (*open arrow*) is not positioned between the condyle and eminence, where they are closest together. **B,** Open mouth image (sagittal T1 image) shows limited anterior translation, with the condyle (C) not reaching the apex of the articular eminence (E). The disk remains anteriorly displaced and folded at the intermediate zone (*open arrow*).

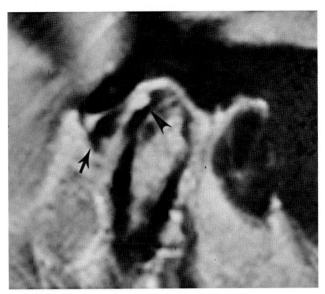

Figure 9-5 **Degenerative erosion of the temporomandibular joint.** Closed mouth (sagittal T1 image). Erosion of the condyle (*arrowhead*) from degenerative joint disease secondary to a chronically displaced disk (*arrow*).

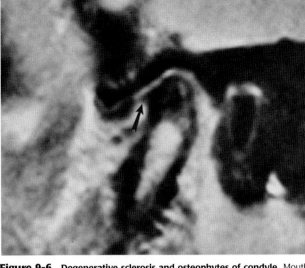

Figure 9-6 **Degenerative sclerosis and osteophytes of condyle.** Mouth open (sagittal T1 image). Severe degenerative joint disease with low signal sclerosis of the condyle and an anterior osteophyte (hammer-and-nail deformity) (*arrow*), along with limited anterior translation of the condyle from long-standing internal derangement of the joint with disk displacement.

from day to day, is usually an easy clinical diagnosis, and generally does not contribute to the type of therapy chosen. Limited mouth opening occurs with internal derangements as the result of a displaced disk that does not reduce to normal position with mouth opening; the disk acts as a physical barrier to anterior translation of the condyle (see Fig. 9-4). The disk is less likely to reduce to a normal position as the bilaminar zone becomes progressively stretched and dysfunctional.

Finally, a disk perforation can occur, or the disk may become thickened and fibrotic. Degenerative joint disease generally occurs with this most advanced stage of internal derangement.

MRI OF INTERNAL DERANGEMENTS AND DEGENERATION

Sagittal MR images of internal derangements of the TMJ show the disk in an abnormal anterior position relative to the condyle with the mouth closed. The posterior band is not positioned directly on top of the condyle, and the intermediate zone does not articulate directly between the condyle and eminence where they are most closely apposed to one another. Perforations of the disk cannot be detected by MRI. A thickened disk that has lost its biconcave configuration and intermediate signal intensity should be mentioned because it may affect treatment.

Sagittal images with the mouth open show the disk in normal position (anterior displacement with reduction), or the disk remains displaced anterior to the condyle (anterior displacement without reduction). The key to diagnosis is the

position of the thin intermediate zone relative to the adjacent osseous structures. The displaced disk may have a crumpled, folded, or globular appearance (see Fig. 9-4). The joint shows limited anterior translation if the apex of the condyle does not progress as far anterior as the apex of the articular eminence of the temporal bone.

An erosion of the condyle may be the earliest osseous manifestation of degenerative changes of the TMJ (Fig. 9-5). This erosion has the appearance of a subchondral, rounded area of low signal intensity on the T1W sagittal images. More advanced degenerative changes may be seen as areas of low signal intensity sclerosis in the subchondral medullary bone of the condyle; anterior osteophytes also may be present, resembling a "hammer-and-nail" deformity (especially for radiologists who are not accurate with the hammer) (Fig. 9-6).

Certain abnormalities in signal intensity in the marrow of the condyle are considered by some clinicians to be the result of avascular necrosis; others believe they are simply degenerative changes. Biopsy or surgical specimens of subchondral bone obtained from patients with degenerative joint disease show areas of osteonecrosis histologically, so the differentiation is probably impossible to make with certainty, and it probably makes no difference to the treatment or outcome of the TMJ patient.

REFERENCE

1. Kaplan PA, Helms CA. Current status of temporomandibular joint imaging for diagnosis of internal derangements. *AJR Am J Roentgenol* 1989; 152:697-705.

Temporomandibular Protocols

This is one set of suggested protocols; there are many variations that would work equally well.

Sequence No.	1	2	3
Sequence Type	T1	T1	Optional T1
Orientation	Closed mouth sagittal	Open mouth sagittal	Coronal
Field of View (cm)	6	6	6
Slice Thickness (mm)	3	3	3
Contrast	No	No	No

Scout

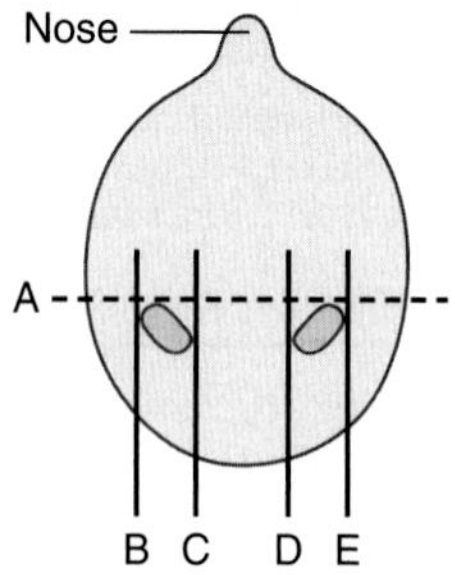

Final Image

Axial scout

Obtain sagittal images perpendicular to a line connecting mandibular condyles* (line A)

Cover entire mandibular condyle between lines B and C and lines D and E

Sagittal

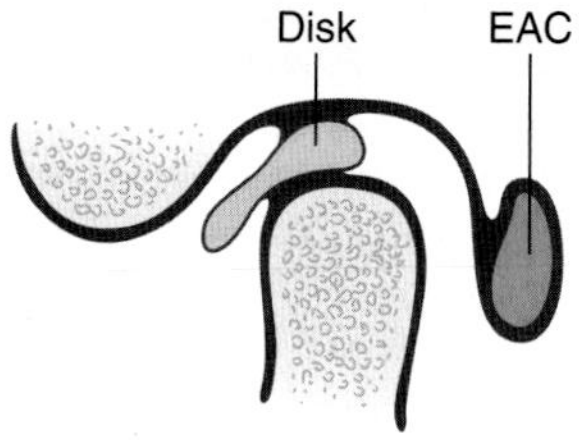

*Image both joints.

Scout

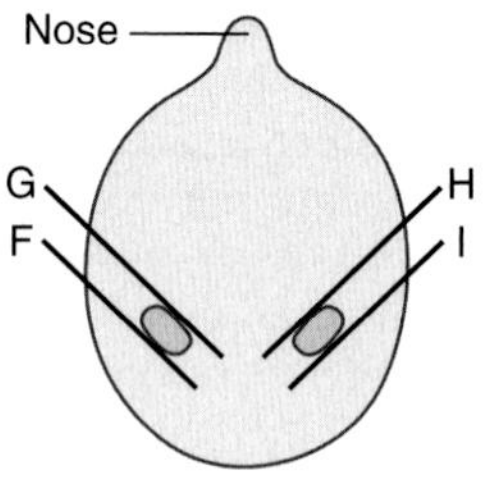

Final Image

Axial scout

Obtain coronal oblique images parallel to long axis of mandibular condyles*

Cover between lines F and G and lines H and I

Coronal oblique

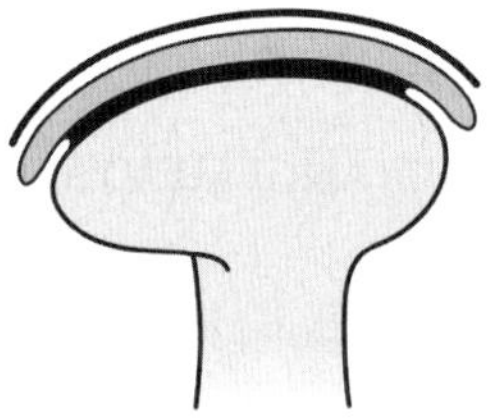

*Image both joints.

Shoulder

How to Image the Shoulder

See the shoulder protocols at the end of the chapter.

- *Coils and patient position:* A surface coil is required to obtain high-resolution, detailed images. The patient is positioned supine with the arm at the side in neutral position or slight external rotation for a standard examination. The arm position influences how well different structures can be identified on MRI.[1,2]
- *Image orientation (Box 10-1):* A small field of view (12 cm) and 3- to 4-mm-thick slices are obtained in three imaging planes: (1) coronal oblique, (2) axial, and (3) sagittal oblique. The coronal oblique images are acquired with cuts made parallel to the supraspinatus tendon, which is seen on an axial cut through the superior portion of the shoulder; alternatively, they may be acquired in a plane perpendicular to the articular surface of the glenoid, as seen on axial images. The axial images are obtained from the top of the acromion to the bottom of the glenohumeral joint using a coronal scout image as a localizer. The sagittal oblique images are acquired with cuts parallel to the articular surface of the glenoid as seen on axial images, from the scapular neck through the lateral margin of the humerus.

**Shoulder Structures to Evaluate
in Different Planes**

Coronal Oblique

Infraspinatus muscle and tendon: *Longitudinally*
Supraspinatus muscle and tendon: *Longitudinally*
Acromioclavicular joint
Acromion
Glenohumeral joint
Subacromial/subdeltoid bursa
Labrum (superior and inferior portions)

Sagittal Oblique

Supraspinatus muscle and tendon: *In cross section*
Infraspinatus muscle and tendon: *In cross section*
Teres minor muscle and tendon: *In cross section*
Long head of biceps tendon (proximal portion): *In cross section*
Subscapularis muscle and tendon: *In cross section*
Rotator interval
Acromion
Coracoacromial ligament
Coracoacromial arch
Glenohumeral ligaments

Axial

Long head of biceps tendon: *In cross section through bicipital groove*
Subscapularis muscle and tendon: *Longitudinally*
Labrum (anterior and posterior portions)
Capsule
Glenohumeral joint
Glenohumeral ligaments

- *Pulse sequences and regions of interest:* Several different pulse sequences are used for the evaluation of internal derangements of the shoulder joint. They depend on whether the shoulder is imaged with or without intra-articular gadolinium. The pulse sequences we use for standard shoulder MRI are (1) sagittal oblique T1W and FSE T2 with fat suppression, (2) coronal oblique FSE T2 with fat suppression, and (3) axial FSE T2 with fat suppression and FSE proton density with fat suppression. The T1W sagittal oblique is used to assess the size of the cuff muscles and to look for fatty infiltration of the muscles. The FSE T2 sagittal oblique is used to look for muscle edema and fluid in the various bursae around the shoulder. The rotator cuff insertion onto the greater tuberosity also is nicely displayed, and partial-thickness or full-thickness cuff tears can be readily identified. The oblique coronal FSE T2 sequence confirms the cuff tears in the supraspinatus or infraspinatus tendons seen on the sagittal images. It also shows the superior labrum. The axial images show the anterior and posterior labrum, the long head of the biceps tendon, and the subscapularis tendon and muscle. The FSE T2 sequence seems to show the labrum better when there is a joint effusion, whereas the FSE proton density (or gradient echo) sequence shows the labrum better if there is no joint effusion. With gadolinium arthrography, we do three planes of T1W with fat suppression and oblique coronal and axial FSE T2 with fat suppression. We also do a non–fat-suppressed T1W oblique sagittal sequence.
- *Contrast:* We previously did standard shoulder MRI routinely without intra-articular gadolinium. We found

ourselves struggling to be certain in many cases, and correlations with arthroscopic or surgical findings were suboptimal. For this reason, we now do shoulder MR arthrography whenever possible. As more and more of our referring physicians learn to look at their patients' MRI studies, they realize, as we do, that pathology and normal anatomy are better visualized if fluid is distending the joint. Referring physicians soon begin ordering shoulder MRI studies with arthrography. Several of our orthopedic surgeons order 100% of their shoulder MRI studies with arthrograms. Shoulder MR arthrography is required in the evaluation of patients with instability. In our experience, it also is extremely useful in showing subtle and sometimes not so subtle full-thickness tears of the rotator cuff. Shoulder MR arthrography is performed after intra-articular injection of gadopentetate dimeglumine (gadolinium). The solution used for the arthrogram consists of 0.1 mL of gadolinium mixed with 20 mL of normal saline and 3 mL of iodinated contrast material. About 10 to 12 mL of the mixture is injected into the shoulder joint before MRI using fluoroscopic guidance and the same approach as for a conventional shoulder arthrogram.

Tendons and the Coracoacromial Arch

NORMAL ANATOMY

Tendons

The rotator cuff typically is considered to be composed of four tendons:

1. Supraspinatus
2. Infraspinatus
3. Teres minor
4. Subscapularis

The rotator cuff is a laminated structure formed by the joint capsule and the ligaments in addition to the four tendons listed. The four tendons of the rotator cuff have cylindrical and flat portions that fan out and interdigitate with each other to form a continuous tendinous hood at their insertions onto the tuberosities of the humerus. There are no synovial tendon sheaths or surrounding paratenon investing the rotator cuff tendons. The coracohumeral ligament extends from the coracoid process to insert onto the lesser and greater tuberosities and the intervening transverse humeral ligament on the humerus. The coracohumeral ligament is located superficial to the joint capsule and the supraspinatus and infraspinatus tendons. These structures constitute the multiple layers of the rotator cuff.[3]

The supraspinatus tendon runs between the undersurface of the acromion and the top of the humeral head. It inserts into fibrocartilage (not hyaline cartilage) on top of the greater tuberosity of the humerus. Located posteriorly on the greater tuberosity, from a superior to an inferior position, are the infraspinatus and the teres minor tendons; running anterior to the shoulder joint is the subscapularis tendon, which attaches to the lesser tuberosity. The supraspinatus muscle acts with the deltoid muscle to abduct the arm. The infraspinatus muscle and the teres minor muscle externally rotate the humerus, and contraction of the

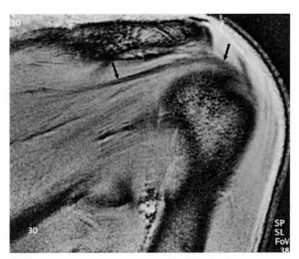

Figure 10-1 **Normal infraspinatus tendon.** T2* coronal oblique image of the shoulder. The low signal infraspinatus tendon runs obliquely (*arrows*) in a craniocaudal direction, attaching to the posterior and superior aspect of the greater tuberosity of the humerus.

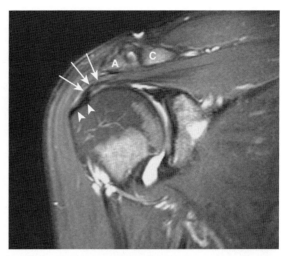

Figure 10-2 **Normal supraspinatus tendon.** FSE T2 coronal oblique image of the shoulder. The cigar-shaped supraspinatus muscle runs horizontally. The musculotendinous junction is located just lateral to the acromioclavicular joint. The tendon (*arrows*) is located between the acromion and the humerus, attaches to the top of the greater tuberosity, and is low signal. Note the broad footprint of the tendon insertion onto the greater tuberosity (*arrowheads*). A, acromion; C, clavicle.

subscapularis muscle results in internal rotation of the humerus.

The entire length of two of the rotator cuff tendons, the supraspinatus and infraspinatus, can be seen well in the coronal oblique plane. Posterior to the humeral head, the infraspinatus tendon can be seen coursing obliquely in a craniocaudal direction at about a 45-degree angle to attach to the posterior portion of the greater tuberosity (Fig. 10-1). On more anterior slices, the horizontally oriented supraspi-

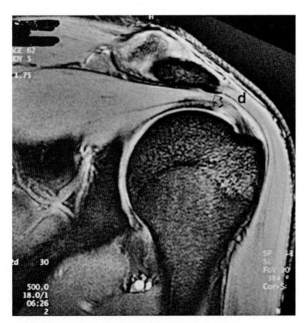

Figure 10-3 **Normal deltoid tendon.** T2* coronal oblique image of the shoulder. There is horizontal linear low signal (*open arrow*) that represents the tendon slip of the deltoid attaching to the acromion. This must not be confused with a subacromial spur. The deltoid muscle (d) is intermediate signal and located just lateral to the acromion and humerus.

natus muscle and tendon are always seen on the same cuts that best show the acromioclavicular joint. The musculotendinous junction of the supraspinatus normally is located just lateral to the acromioclavicular joint (Fig. 10-2). The supraspinatus runs at an angle of approximately 45 degrees relative to the coronal plane.

Other tendons that also can be evaluated well on coronal oblique images are the deltoid tendon slips that attach to the superior and inferior margins of the acromion (Fig. 10-3) and portions of the long head of the biceps tendon. The coracoacromial ligament is another low signal intensity structure that inserts on the lateral and inferior aspect of the acromion, appearing similar to the deltoid tendon attachment. The long head of the biceps tendon can be seen on far anterior cuts through the shoulder,[4] from its origin at the superior labrum (the so-called biceps anchor) (Fig. 10-4A), and inferiorly in the bicipital groove. We have found that with internal rotation of the humerus, which is the position most patients assume, the bicipital groove is a good anatomic landmark to key on for inspecting the leading edge of the supraspinatus. The supraspinatus tendon inserts just lateral to the bicipital groove, and commonly tears begin or are isolated at this location and are frequently overlooked (see Fig. 10-4B).[5]

The subscapularis muscle runs anterior to the shoulder, and its tendon attaches to the lesser tuberosity. The length of the subscapularis tendon and muscle can be shown best on axial images (Fig. 10-5). Its attachment blends with the transverse humeral ligament, which bridges the lesser and greater tuberosities and holds the long head of the biceps tendon in the bicipital groove.

The portion of the long head of the biceps tendon that is located within the bicipital groove is cut transversely on axial images and is a round or oval structure. In some cases, it blends with the low signal intensity cortex of the humerus and may be difficult to identify. A small amount of fluid is seen in the dependent side of the long head of the biceps

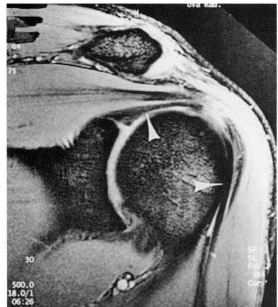

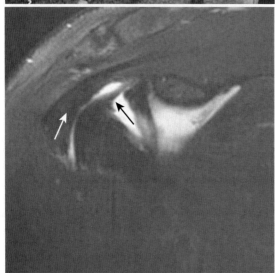

B

Figure 10-4   **Normal biceps tendon. A,** T2* coronal oblique image of the shoulder. The long head of the biceps tendon (*arrowheads*) runs vertically in the bicipital groove and attaches to the superior labrum (the biceps-labral anchor). The biceps is located far anterior in the shoulder and runs underneath the supraspinatus tendon. **B,** FSE T2 coronal oblique image of the shoulder. A far anterior image shows the biceps as it exits the bicipital groove and extends through the joint to insert onto the superior labrum (*black arrow*). The anterior edge of the supraspinatus tendon can be seen inserting onto the greater tuberosity just lateral to the bicipital groove (*white arrow*).

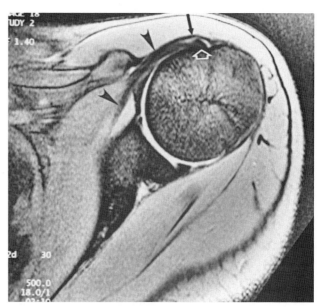

Figure 10-5   **Normal subscapularis tendon.** T2* axial image of the shoulder. The subscapularis tendon (*arrowheads*) runs anterior to the shoulder beneath the coracoid process and blends with the transverse humeral ligament (*solid arrow*) that spans the bicipital groove and holds the biceps tendon (*open arrow*) in place.

of imaging is valuable for confirming the status of tendons when abnormalities are seen or suspected in the other planes of imaging, where the tendons are viewed longitudinally. The space between the supraspinatus tendon and the subscapularis tendon, which also is seen well on sagittal oblique images, is known as the rotator interval.

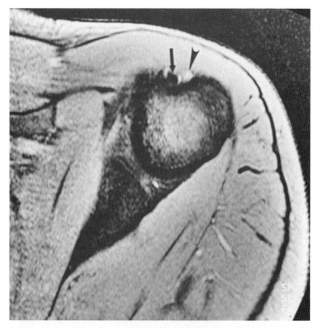

Figure 10-6   **Biceps tendon and adjacent vessels.** T2* axial image of the shoulder. The biceps tendon (*arrow*) is imaged transversely in the bicipital groove. A small amount of fluid is seen on either side of the tendon in its sheath. The round, high signal structure lateral to the tendon is the anterior circumflex humeral artery/vein (*arrowhead*) and does not represent tenosynovitis.

tendon sheath normally; with a shoulder joint effusion, fluid may encircle the biceps tendon because the tendon sheath is in direct communication with the shoulder joint. One or two rounded fluid collections may be seen lateral to the biceps tendon, which represent the anterolateral branch of the anterior circumflex artery and vein (Fig. 10-6).

On sagittal oblique images, the tendons of the supraspinatus, infraspinatus, teres minor, and most proximal portion of the long head of the biceps, and the multiple tendon slips of the subscapularis all are imaged in cross section, surrounded by their associated muscles (Fig. 10-7). This plane

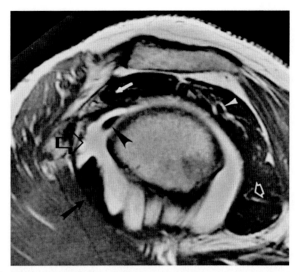

Figure 10-7 **Normal shoulder: sagittal plane.** T1 sagittal oblique image of the shoulder, MR arthrogram. Beneath the acromion is the supraspinatus tendon (*white arrow*) and infraspinatus tendon (*white arrowhead*) with their surrounding muscles. Posteroinferiorly is the teres minor tendon (*open white arrow*) and muscle. The biceps tendon (*black arrowhead*) is located inferior to the supraspinatus tendon. The multiple slips of the subscapularis are seen anteriorly (*black arrow*). The space between the supraspinatus and subscapularis tendons is the rotator interval (*open black arrow*). The acromion is flat (type I acromion).

Tendons are normally low signal intensity on all pulse sequences; however, increased signal intensity in normal tendons may be caused by the magic angle phenomenon.[6,7] The magic angle phenomenon occurs when collagen fibers are oriented at about 55 degrees to the constant magnetic induction field.[8] This orientation results in an intermediate signal intensity within the otherwise low signal intensity tendon on TE sequences such as T1W, proton density, and gradient echo (T2*) images. In the shoulder, this phenomenon occurs commonly about 1 cm proximal to the insertion

of the supraspinatus tendon on the greater tuberosity, which is the hypovascular region of the tendon, also known as the critical zone.[6,7]

The intermediate signal intensity from the magic angle phenomenon disappears with long TE sequences, such as T2W images, making it possible to differentiate magic angle from an abnormal tendon.[8] A good rule to distinguish the magic angle phenomenon from a tear on T2* images is that the signal intensity within the tendon is never higher than the signal intensity within the adjacent muscle if it is from the magic angle phenomenon (see Fig. 10-2), whereas with a tendon tear, the signal intensity is higher than that of muscle. Other potential causes of increased signal intensity in a normal supraspinatus tendon besides the magic angle phenomenon include the presence of connective tissue between tendon fascicles, partial volume averaging effect, and overlap of the supraspinatus and infraspinatus tendons from imaging with the arm in internal rotation (Box 10-2).

Coracoacromial Arch

The coracoacromial arch is formed by the humeral head posteriorly, the acromion superiorly, and the coracoid process and the intervening coracoacromial ligament anteriorly.[9] Located within the coracoacromial arch, from superior to inferior, are the subacromial/subdeltoid bursa, the

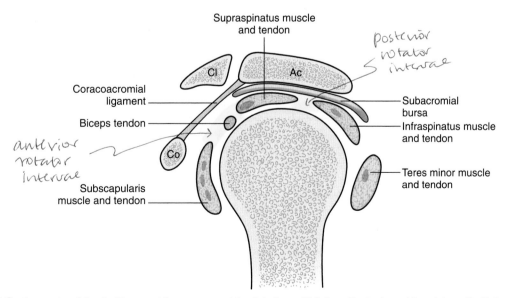

Figure 10-8 **Coracoacromial arch.** Diagram of the coracoacromial arch in the sagittal plane. The tendons of the rotator cuff with their surrounding muscles are arranged around the humeral head. The biceps tendon is inferior to the supraspinatus tendon. The coracoacromial ligament forms the anterior margin of the arch. Ac, acromion; Cl, clavicle; Co, coracoid process.

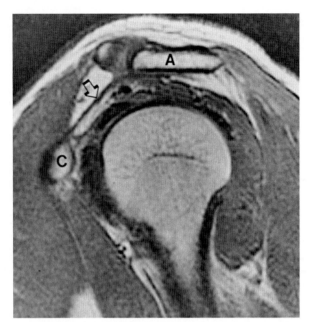

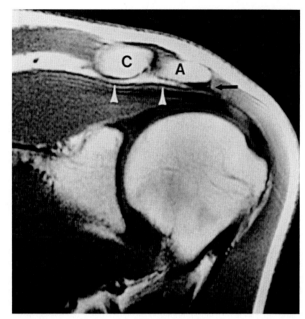

Figure 10-9 **Coracoacromial arch; type I acromion.** T1 sagittal oblique image of the shoulder. The coracoacromial ligament (*open arrow*) anterior to the shoulder is a taut, low signal band between its attachments on the acromion (A) and the coracoid process (C). The muscles and tendons of the rotator cuff and the long head of the biceps, are seen well in cross section. The undersurface of the acromion is flat (type I acromion).

Figure 10-10 **Normal acromiohumeral interval.** T1 coronal oblique image of the shoulder. There is a normal orientation of the acromion (A) with the clavicle (C), with a flat undersurface oriented horizontally. The intact fat plane (*arrowheads*) between the acromioclavicular joint and the underlying supraspinatus tendon indicates no signs of impingement. The linear low signal (*arrow*) on the undersurface of the acromion is the deltoid tendon slip/coracoacromial ligament attachment, and not a subacromial spur.

supraspinatus tendon and muscle, and the long head of the biceps tendon. The coracoacromial ligament restricts anterior and superior motion of the humeral head and overlying tendons (Fig. 10-8; see Fig. 10-7). Anything that decreases the space within the coracoacromial arch could lead to symptoms of impingement. Structures that form or are contained by the coracoacromial arch must be evaluated carefully in the different planes of imaging.

On sagittal oblique images, the coracoacromial ligament is seen as a taut, thin band with parallel margins. Typical of all ligaments, it has low signal intensity on all pulse sequences (Fig. 10-9).

The configuration and the orientation of the acromion are evaluated in the coronal and the sagittal oblique planes. Normally, the anterior and the most posterior aspects of the inferior black cortical line of the acromion on a sagittal oblique view should be nearly horizontal or else curved, paralleling the humeral head (see Fig. 10-9). On coronal oblique images, the anterior aspect of the acromion should be horizontal and at the same level as the clavicle (Fig. 10-10). The normal acromioclavicular joint has a smooth undersurface, with both bones running in a smooth horizontal plane. Similarly, the undersurface of the acromion should be smooth and without spurs.

A boomerang-shaped fat plane surrounding the subacromial/subdeltoid bursa is evident between the acromioclavicular joint and the underlying supraspinatus tendon and muscle on coronal oblique images (Fig. 10-11). The subacromial/subdeltoid bursa normally is evident only because it is outlined by fat. The bursa should have no fluid, or only a small wisp of fluid; it should not be distended with fluid. Another fat plane that is separate from that of the subacro-

mial/subdeltoid bursa normally is evident, separating the supraspinatus muscle and tendon from the undersurfaces of the overlying acromion and acromioclavicular joint (see Fig. 10-10).

SHOULDER IMPINGEMENT

In 1972, Neer, an orthopedic surgeon, proposed the concept that tears of the supraspinatus tendon are related to impingement on the tendon by the structures that form the coracoacromial arch. Any condition that limits the space within the coracoacromial arch can produce impingement on the subacromial bursa, the supraspinatus tendon, and the long head of the biceps tendon. Neer proposed surgical decompression to treat this impingement syndrome, consisting of an anteroinferior acromioplasty and resection of the coracoacromial ligament, decompressing and creating more room for the supraspinatus tendon and other affected structures.[10] Abnormalities from impingement that affect the supraspinatus tendon and surrounding structures range from edema to full-thickness tendon tears. All of these abnormalities are associated with symptoms of pain and collectively are referred to as the *impingement syndrome*. The syndrome is characterized clinically by acute or chronic shoulder pain induced by movements of abduction and external rotation or by elevation and internal rotation of the shoulder. It can occur in young athletes involved with repetitive movements of elevation and abduction of the shoulder, or in elderly individuals from degenerative changes of the acromioclavicular joint and formation of subacromial spurs. Generally, impingement is more common with increasing age (Box 10-3).

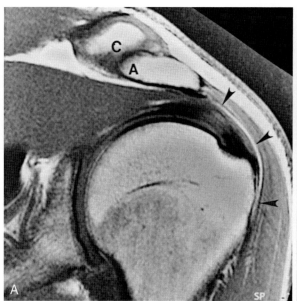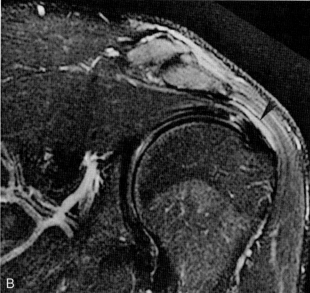

Figure 10-11 **Subacromial/subdeltoid bursal fat; low-lying acromion. A,** T1 coronal oblique image of the shoulder. The boomerang-shaped, thin, high signal fat (*arrowheads*) is associated with the subacromial/subdeltoid bursa. The fat of the bursa may appear normal on T1W images, even in the presence of bursitis. The acromion (A) is low-lying compared with the clavicle (C), which predisposes to impingement syndrome. **B,** Fast T2 with fat suppression coronal oblique image of the shoulder. There is a small amount of fluid in the subacromial/subdeltoid bursa (*arrowhead*) from bursitis.

Causes

The supraspinatus tendon is reportedly predisposed to impingement from several sources that can be identified with MRI[11,12]:

BOX 10-3

Shoulder Impingement Syndrome

Symptoms
- Pain
  - Abduction and external rotation
  - Elevation and internal rotation

Causes (Anything Decreasing Size of Coracoacromial Arch)
- Acromial shape
  - Type III: Inferiorly projecting hook (sagittal oblique)
- Acromial orientation
  - Anterior down-sloping (sagittal oblique)
  - Inferolateral tilt (coronal oblique)
  - Low-lying (coronal oblique)
- Acromioclavicular degenerative joint disease
- Os acromiale
- Thick coracoacromial ligament
- Post-traumatic osseous deformity
- Instability
- Muscle overdevelopment

Potential Consequences

Tendons
- Supraspinatus tendon
  - Degeneration, partial tear, complete tear
- Proximal long head, biceps brachii tendon
  - Degeneration, partial tear, complete tear

Bones
- Degenerative cysts, sclerosis of greater tuberosity or humeral head or both

Bursa
- Subacromial/subdeltoid bursitis

1. Abnormal configuration of the anterior acromion
2. Anterior downsloping of the acromion
3. Low-lying acromion
4. Inferolateral tilt of the acromion
5. Os acromiale
6. Acromioclavicular degenerative joint disease
7. Thickening of the coracoacromial ligament
8. Post-traumatic osseous deformity
9. Instability
10. Muscle overdevelopment

Several of these believed causes have been discredited and are not considered to be predisposing factors for cuff pathology. They are discussed individually.

Acromial Configuration. Bigliani and colleagues[13] described three predominant shapes of the acromion based on scapular Y view radiographs of the shoulder and believed the shape was an important factor contributing to impingement. A *type I* acromion has a flat undersurface. *Type II* acromion has a concave undersurface with the inferior acromial cortex parallel to the cortex of the underlying humeral head. *Type III* acromion has an inferiorly projecting anterior hook that narrows the space between the acromion and the humerus.[13] It was thought that type II and III acromions had an increased incidence of cuff pathology, but this has not borne out in practice. Our surgeons do not inquire about the shape of the acromion, and acromion type is no longer considered to be an important factor relating to cuff pathology.

Acromial Slope. The slope of the acromion can be evaluated on sagittal and coronal oblique images. Normally, the lateral aspect of the acromion is oriented nearly horizontal or slopes downward posteriorly on sagittal oblique images. An anteriorly downsloping acromion occurs when the inferior cortex of the anterior acromion is located more caudally than the inferior cortex of the posterior aspect of the acro-

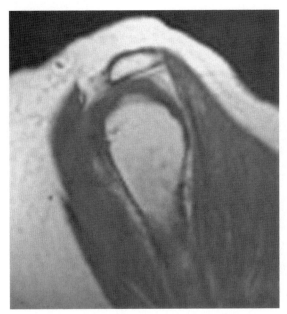

Figure 10-12 **Anterior-sloping acromion.** T1 sagittal oblique image of the shoulder. The acromion is downward sloping anteriorly (anterior is to the left), which is believed by many to be a cause of impingement.

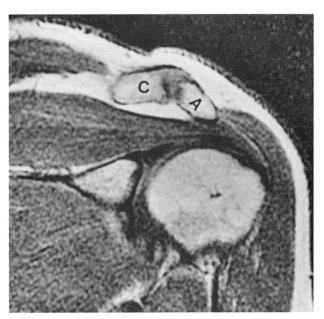

Figure 10-13 **Acromial slope: inferolateral tilt.** T1 coronal oblique image of the shoulder. The acromion (A) tilts inferiorly relative to the horizontal clavicle (C). This narrows the space between the humeral head and the acromion where the supraspinatus tendon and the subacromial/subdeltoid bursa exist, increasing the risk of impingement.

mion (Fig. 10-12). Another abnormal slope to the acromion consists of an inferolateral tilt, which can be detected on coronal oblique images. An inferolateral tilt or slope occurs when the most lateral portion of the acromion is tilted inferiorly relative to the clavicle (Fig. 10-13). Sloping of the acromion in either direction increases the risk for impingement from mechanical trauma to the underlying distal supraspinatus tendon (Fig. 10-14).

Acromial Position. Normally, the inferior cortex of the acromion is in line with the inferior cortex of the clavicle on coronal oblique views. A low-lying acromion exists when its inferior cortex is positioned below the inferior cortex of the clavicle (see Fig. 10-11). This positioning causes narrowing of the acromiohumeral space, which may predispose to impingement.

Os Acromiale. Os acromiale is an accessory ossification center of the acromion that is normally fused by 25 years of age. An unfused os acromiale after this age may be seen in 15% of the population; its presence is associated with an increased incidence of impingement and rotator cuff tears, presumably because the os is mobile and decreases the space in the coracoacromial arch with motion.[14] The os acromiale is best identified on axial images, although it can be seen in all imaging planes (Fig. 10-15).

Acromioclavicular Joint Degenerative Changes. Degenerative joint disease of the acromioclavicular joint may manifest as inferiorly projecting osteophytes, fibrous overgrowth of the capsule, or both (Fig. 10-16).[15,16] On radiographs, osteophytes are underestimated, and fibrous overgrowth is not depicted at all; MRI directly shows the presence, severity, and extent of these structures that may cause impingement.

Obliteration of the fat between the supraspinatus muscle or tendon and the overlying acromioclavicular joint and indentation of the supraspinatus tendon or muscle by abnormalities of the acromioclavicular joint are indications that the degenerative changes are considerable and may contribute to impingement.

Coracoacromial Ligament. Focal thickening of the coracoacromial ligament may be observed on sagittal oblique MRI, but has never been shown to be related to impingement. Evaluation of the coracoacromial ligament is not part of our interpretation of shoulder MRI.

Post-traumatic Deformity. As a result of hypertrophic callus formation or malalignment of fracture fragments that involve the bones adjacent to the coracoacromial arch, there may be narrowing of the coracoacromial arch with resultant impingement, although this is uncommon.

Instability. Glenohumeral degenerative changes can be caused by shoulder instability, and instability can be a contributing factor to impingement. Instability and impingement are two conditions that often coexist; this is discussed later in this chapter.

Muscle Overdevelopment. Supraspinatus muscle enlargement, as seen in weightlifters, swimmers, and other athletes, may induce impingement even if the coracoacromial arch and acromiohumeral intervals are normal because the large muscle decreases the space available for the tendon to glide between the structures of the coracoacromial arch. A deformity (indentation) of the superior surface of the supraspinatus muscle caused by the acromioclavicular joint is the only abnormality seen with MRI.

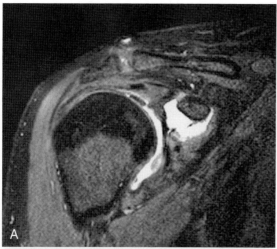

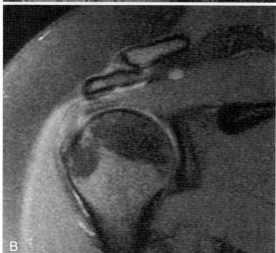

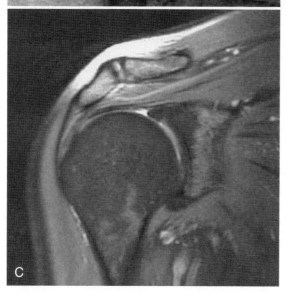

Figure 10-14 Acromial orientation. FSE T2 oblique coronal images showing the relationship of the acromion to the distal clavicle in three different shoulders. **A,** Horizontal; this is the normal orientation. **B,** Low-lying; the acromion is inferior to the distal clavicle. **C,** Inferolateral; the acromion is laterally sloping in relation to the clavicle. The low-lying and inferolateral positions are thought to be associated with impingement.

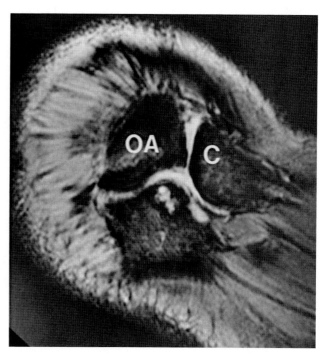

Figure 10-15 Os acromiale. T2* axial image of the shoulder. A cut through the level of the acromioclavicular joint shows a separate os acromiale (OA) that did not fuse in this patient. This predisposes to impingement. There are degenerative, high signal cysts between the os and the adjacent scapula.

Effects of Impingement (Box 10-4)

Tendons. The supraspinatus tendon is affected far more commonly than other tendons in the shoulder. Impingement on the supraspinatus tendon from any source can cause tendon degeneration and partial-thickness or full-thickness tears. Conversely, the same tendon abnormalities may exist without evidence of structural or mechanical causes of impingement. Most partial-thickness tears of the supraspinatus tendon occur on the undersurface (articular) aspect of the tendon, rather than on the superior (bursal) surface where abnormalities in the coracoacromial arch would logically be expected to cause early partial tears. The proximal long head of the biceps tendon may be affected by impingement in the same ways as the supraspinatus tendon because of its similar location and course just beneath the supraspinatus tendon within the shoulder joint.

Degenerative Osseous Cysts. Although the supraspinatus tendon is the structure most often affected by impingement,

BOX 10-4

MRI of Shoulder Impingement

- Identification of mechanical causes
- Evaluation of tendon integrity
  - Abnormal high signal intensity (degeneration/partial tears)
  - Abnormal shape: Thin, thick, irregular (partial tears)
  - Discontinuity (complete tears)
- Subacromial/subdeltoid bursal fluid
- Glenohumeral degenerative joint disease

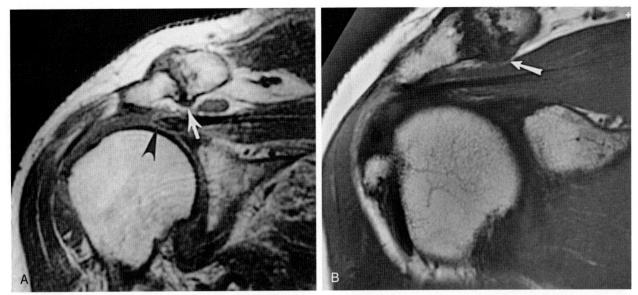

Figure 10-16 Acromioclavicular joint degenerative changes. **A,** T1 coronal oblique image of the shoulder. There is degenerative joint disease of the acromioclavicular joint with osteophytes projecting inferiorly (*arrow*). The supraspinatus is completely torn, with the tendon (*arrowhead*) retracted medially. **B,** T1 coronal oblique image of the shoulder (different patient than in **A**). There is fibrous overgrowth of the capsule and osteophytes of the acromioclavicular joint, impinging on and indenting the top of the supraspinatus muscle and tendon (*arrow*). The distal tendon is mildly abnormal with high signal and thickening from degeneration and partial tears.

certain associated osseous findings are very common as well. Cortical hypertrophy, sclerosis, and small degenerative cysts in the greater tuberosity often are present and may precede MRI evidence of abnormalities within the tendons. The osseous degenerative changes have been found histologically to be associated with microtears of the adjacent tendon.

Subacromial/Subdeltoid Bursitis. Irritation of the subacromial/subdeltoid bursa can occur from impingement. When this occurs, the bursa becomes distended with fluid and is painful (see Fig. 10-11). Normally, there is no fluid, or only a trace of detectable fluid, in this bursa. Bursal fluid is common in the presence of rotator cuff tears. Bursal fluid cannot be seen without a T2W sequence, so this sequence is needed even when an MR arthrogram is performed.

TENDON TEARS, DEGENERATION, AND DISLOCATION

Supraspinatus (Box 10-5)

Degeneration and Partial Tendon Tears. Degeneration and partial tendon tears generally are indistinguishable from one another on T1W images, where they appear as focal or diffuse regions of intratendinous intermediate signal intensity, which is one of the reasons we no longer acquire T1W images in the coronal plane. If these areas maintain the same signal intensity as muscle on T2W images, they are most consistent with tendon degeneration; if these areas become high signal intensity, similar to fluid on T2W images, they represent partial tendon tears. It frequently is difficult to distinguish between degeneration or partial tendon tears,

and in such a situation the general term tendinopathy may be used to describe the abnormalities. Tendon degeneration and partial tears often coexist.

Magic angle phenomenon has similar signal characteristics as tendon partial tears or degeneration on short TE images. The findings, however, are focal instead of diffuse, are at a specific location (1 cm from the insertion of the supraspinatus tendon on the greater tuberosity) and, most importantly, disappear on long TE images.[17,18] In addition, the signal changes are not associated with thinning, thickening, or irregularity of the tendon.

A partial tear on the undersurface (joint surface) of the tendon fills with high signal intensity gadolinium solution on MR arthrograms (Fig. 10-17). Partial-thickness tears on the upper (bursal) surface of the tendon need to be evaluated

---

BOX 10-5

Rotator Cuff Tendon Pathology

Full-Thickness Tear
- Direct signs
  - Tendon discontinuity
  - Fluid signal in tendon gap
  - Retraction of musculotendinous junction
- Associated findings
  - Subacromial/subdeltoid bursal fluid
  - Muscle atrophy

Partial-Thickness Tear
- Increased signal T1 and T2, joint or bursal surface
  - Higher signal than muscle on T2 (similar to joint fluid)

Degeneration
- Intrasubstance increased signal T1 and T2
  - Not as high signal as joint fluid

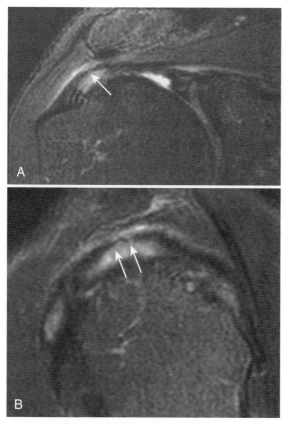

Figure 10-17 **Partial supraspinatus tear. A** and **B**, FSE T2 coronal oblique (**A**) and FSE sagittal oblique (**B**) images of the shoulder. Thinning of the under-surface of the supraspinatus tendon can be seen in both planes (*arrows*), indicative of a partial articular-sided cuff tear.

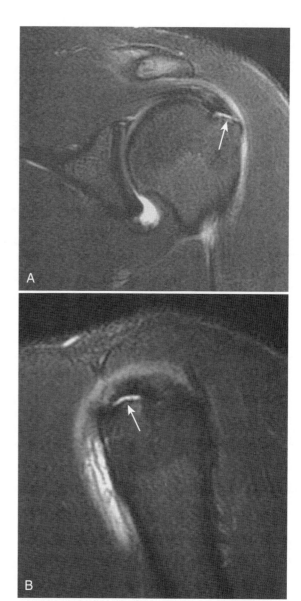

Figure 10-18 **Partial supraspinatus tear (rim rent tear). A**, T1 fat-suppressed, coronal oblique image of the shoulder. The broad footprint of the normal insertion of the supraspinatus tendon onto the greater tuberosity is interrupted with fluid (*arrow*), which indicates a partial articular-sided cuff tear. **B**, T1 fat-suppressed, sagittal oblique image of the shoulder. Sagittal image confirms fluid disrupting the cuff insertion (*arrow*).

similar to regular shoulder MRI without arthrography because gadolinium cannot enter the tear in that location. Partial-thickness tears generally start on the undersurface of the distal end of the supraspinatus tendon; the inferior layers may retract medially, whereas the superior layers remain intact.

The most common partial tear, which is the most common cuff tear of all kinds, is one in which the insertional fibers of the cuff on the greater tuberosity are disrupted from the bone (Fig. 10-18). This has been termed a *rim rent* tear. It was first described by an orthopedic surgeon, Codman, in 1934.[19] It was found in about 10% of cases by Tuite and coworkers,[20] but we believe it is seen more commonly in our practice. In a series of 200 consecutive shoulder MRI studies, we found 117 cuff tears, 70 (60%) of which were partial cuff tears.[5] Only 2 of the 70 were bursal-sided tears. Bursal-sided tears are much less common than joint-sided tears. Of the 70 partial tears, 49 (42%) were rim rent tears.

We had overlooked many of these tears on our original interpretations primarily because we did not appreciate the significance of internal rotation of the humerus. The ante-riormost fibers of the supraspinatus tendon insert just lateral to the bicipital groove and can be overlooked easily on the oblique coronal images if the shoulder is internally rotated (Fig. 10-19). If one finds the biceps on the most anterior coronal images, the more anterior fibers of the cuff can be

seen just adjacent to the bicipital groove (Fig. 10-20). When these fibers are disrupted, the tear can be seen as an inter-ruption of the normal tissue adjacent to the bicipital groove (Fig. 10-21). The tear can be confirmed on sagittal oblique images, but because the biceps is so close to the tear it is often difficult to tell if fluid in the cuff is from partial volume averaging with fluid in the bicipital groove (see Fig. 10-21C).

We believe that the most common cuff tear is a partial-thickness tear at the insertion of the cuff fibers onto the greater tuberosity, many of which progress to a full-thickness tear. These tears can occur anteriorly on the greater tuberosity involving the supraspinatus, or posteriorly on the greater tuberosity involving the infraspinatus. These joint-

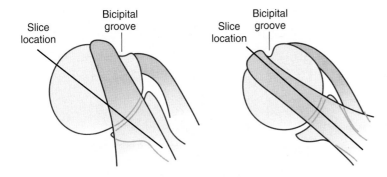

Figure 10-19 **Schematic showing effect of internal rotation.** This axial drawing shows how with external rotation (*right*) an oblique coronal image goes through the length of the supraspinatus and shows the insertion of the tendon just lateral to the bicipital groove, whereas if the patient is internally rotated (*left*), the same oblique coronal slice misses the anterior portion of the supraspinatus adjacent to the bicipital groove.

sided or articular-sided tears are much more common than bursal-sided partial tears. Tears at the so-called critical zone, 1 to 1.5 cm proximal to the tendon insertion, are not as common as previously believed.

Detection of tendon abnormalities before the development of a full-thickness tear is important because the process may be arrested with conservative therapy, débridement, and decompression surgery. A full-thickness tear, in addition to pain, results in limited active movements of abduction and requires more involved surgery than that performed for a partial tear. MRI is reportedly less sensitive for detecting partial-thickness tears of the supraspinatus tendon than full-thickness tears. The specificity is in the range of 90%, but the sensitivity of standard MRI for detecting partial-thickness tears is reported to be 35% to 90%; these figures are significantly improved with MR arthrography.

Full-Thickness Tears. Direct evidence of a full-thickness tear by conventional MRI (not MR arthrography) consists

of discontinuity of the tendon with high signal intensity fluid traversing the gap between the tendon fragments from the articular to the bursal surfaces of the tendon on T2W sequences (Fig. 10-22). MR arthrography shows high signal gadolinium on T1W images in the glenohumeral joint and in the subacromial/subdeltoid bursa with discontinuity of the tendon and gadolinium filling the gap between disrupted tendon fragments (Fig. 10-23). MRI also can show the size of the tear, the degree of retraction of fragments, the quality of the remaining tendon fragments, and if there is associated muscle atrophy or osseous abnormalities; these features should be commented on in the report. Muscle atrophy is seen as high signal intensity within the muscle on T1W images (Fig. 10-24), whether in the sagittal or the coronal plane.

A supraspinatus tendon tear usually is located distally in the supraspinatus tendon, either near its attachment to the greater tuberosity or in the critical zone of the tendon located about 1 cm proximal to its insertion. Tears usually start in

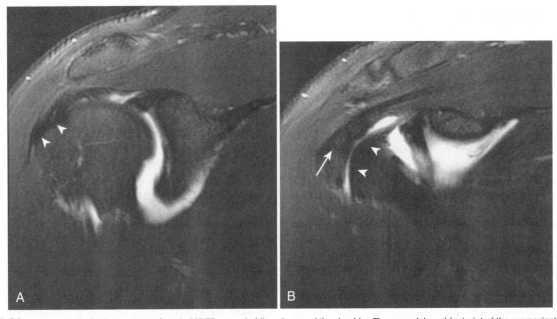

Figure 10-20 **Normal cuff with internal rotation. A,** FSE T2 coronal oblique image of the shoulder. The normal, broad footprint of the supraspinatus inserting onto the greater tuberosity appears normal on this image (*arrowheads*). **B,** FSE T2 coronal oblique image of the shoulder, just anterior to the image in **A**. The biceps can be seen exiting the bicipital groove (*arrowheads*), and the normal insertion of the leading edge of the supraspinatus tendon can be seen just lateral to the bicipital groove (*arrow*).

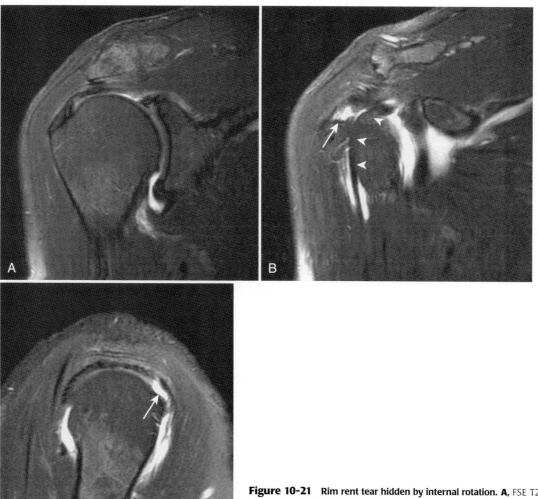

Figure 10-21 Rim rent tear hidden by internal rotation. A, FSE T2 coronal oblique image of the shoulder. The normal, broad footprint of the supraspinatus inserting onto the greater tuberosity appears normal on this image. **B,** Two images anterior to that, at the point where the biceps exits the bicipital groove (*arrowheads*), the greater tuberosity just lateral to the bicipital groove (*arrow*) is bare with no supraspinatus tendon fibers seen. At surgery, this was found to be a high-grade partial articular-sided tear. **C,** FSE T2 sagittal oblique image of the shoulder. Fluid can be seen on the anterior greater tuberosity where the anterior fibers of the supraspinatus tendon are lifted off (*arrow*). This can easily be mistaken for fluid in the adjacent bicipital groove, which is seen on this image just anterior to the humeral head.

the anterior portion of the distal supraspinatus tendon as rim rent tears and propagate posteriorly. Complete disruption of fibers in the craniocaudal direction with communication between the joint and bursa indicates a full-thickness tear, even if it has not separated the tendons completely in the anteroposterior direction.

Disruption of the supraspinatus tendon is not always clearly evident or easy to diagnose by standard MRI. Granulation tissue or debris may obscure the tear, the tear may be very small, or it may be located far anteriorly, all of which make the diagnosis much more difficult. These difficulties can be alleviated with MR arthrography, which provides much more information (see Fig. 10-23). It is unusual, however, for us to see gadolinium in the subacromial-subdeltoid bursa without seeing a gap in the tendon. One could propose not using gadolinium in the arthrogram

solution—only injecting saline for joint distention. We think this is a reasonable approach; it would shorten imaging time considerably and decrease cost, but this hypothesis needs to be tested because the current standard of care for MR shoulder arthrography entails gadolinium.

The sensitivity and specificity for full-thickness rotator cuff tears by MRI are greater than 90%. MR arthrography improves these figures and increases the confidence with which the diagnoses are made. The ability of MRI to show complete tears of the rotator cuff tendons is significantly better than its ability to show partial-thickness tears.

Long Head of the Biceps (Box 10-6)

Tears. The long head of the biceps tendon is completely torn in about 7% of patients with supraspinatus tendon tears and is abnormal (degeneration or partial tears) in about one

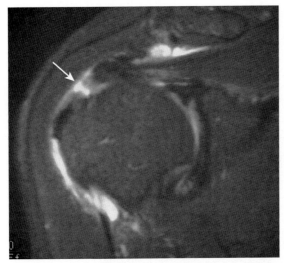

Figure 10-22 **Complete supraspinatus tear.** FSE T2 oblique coronal image of the shoulder. A full-thickness gap is seen in the supraspinatus tendon (*arrow*) at the critical zone.

third.[21] Its proximity to the supraspinatus tendon makes it vulnerable to forces of impingement identical to forces affecting the supraspinatus tendon. Long head of the biceps tendon tears associated with supraspinatus tendon tears involve the impingement zone just proximal to the bicipital groove, and usually occur in older individuals. The distal tendon fragment and the muscle may retract distally, and an empty bicipital groove may be shown on axial MRIs of the shoulder (Fig. 10-25). Acute tears of the long head of the biceps tendon may occur with severe trauma in young individuals or in older weekend athletes. Acute tears unrelated

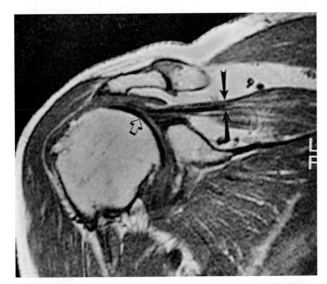

Figure 10-24 **Complete supraspinatus tear with secondary signs.** T1 coronal oblique image of the shoulder. The end of the torn supraspinatus tendon is seen (*open arrow*). There are secondary signs of a tendon tear with medial retraction of the musculotendinous junction (*solid arrows*), atrophy of the muscle with fatty infiltration, and a decreased acromiohumeral interval. There are degenerative changes of the acromioclavicular and glenohumeral joints and a subacromial spur.

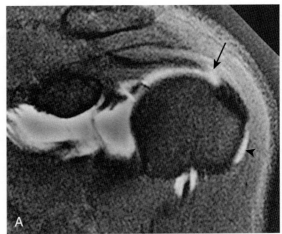

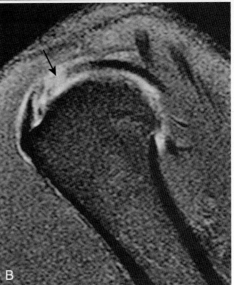

Figure 10-23 **Complete supraspinatus tear. A,** T1 fat-suppressed coronal oblique shoulder MR arthrogram. A small full-thickness tear (*arrow*) of the distal supraspinatus tendon is seen with contrast enhancement in the subacromial/subdeltoid bursa (*arrowhead*). **B,** T1 fat-suppressed sagittal oblique shoulder MR arthrogram. The defect in the supraspinatus tendon is easily seen (*arrow*); contrast enhancement also is noted in the overlying bursa.

to impingement generally occur distally in the tendon, near the musculotendinous junction.

Dislocation. Other abnormalities of the long head of the biceps tendon may occur, unassociated with impingement. Acute trauma can cause avulsion, subluxation, and dislocation of the tendon, all of which need to be repaired surgically. For subluxation or dislocation to exist, there must be disruption of the transverse humeral ligament that normally bridges the lesser and greater tuberosities and holds the long head of the biceps tendon in place. Usually, a tear of the subscapularis tendon also coexists. With dislocation, the long head of the biceps tendon may displace anteromedially, which may or may not be associated with an intact subscapularis tendon. It may dislocate medially within the shoulder joint, which is always associated with a tear of the subscapularis tendon at its attachment to the lesser tuberosity.[22,23] Biceps tendon subluxation and dislocation are shown

Long Head of Biceps Tendon

Tears/Degeneration

- Attachment to superior labrum
  - Associated with SLAP lesions
- Proximal to bicipital groove
  - Associated with impingement
  - Older population
- Musculotendinous junction
  - Acute, traumatic injuries
  - Younger population

Dislocation

- Associated disruptions
  - Transverse humeral ligament
  - Usually subscapularis tendon
- MRI
  - Empty bicipital groove (axial)
  - Tendon displaced medially, either anterior to or within the glenohumeral joint
  - Biceps tendon may be anterior to, posterior to, or within a torn subscapularis tendon
  - Subscapularis tendon avulsed from tuberosity (or may be intact)

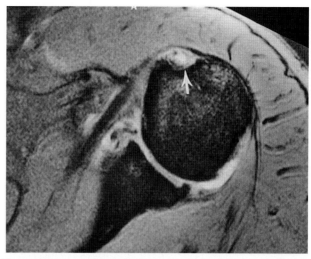

Figure 10-25   **Biceps tendon tear.** T2* axial image of the shoulder. The bicipital groove (*arrow*) is empty, without evidence of the oval, low signal long head of the biceps tendon, indicating a complete rupture.

best on axial MRIs, where the bicipital groove is empty, and the low signal round tendon is seen at variable distances medial to the groove, either deep or superficial to the subscapularis tendon (Fig. 10-26).

Infraspinatus

Infraspinatus tendon tears can be seen in isolation after acute trauma (although this is rare), can occur in association with massive tears of the supraspinatus tendon, or can be associated with posterosuperior impingement of the shoulder (Fig. 10-27). We have found isolated rim rent tears to be common[5]; however, because isolated full-thickness tears of the infraspinatus are rare, the rim rent tears must not progress to full-thickness tears as often as in the supraspinatus.

Posterosuperior Impingement (Box 10-7). Posterosuperior impingement refers to impingement of the supraspina-

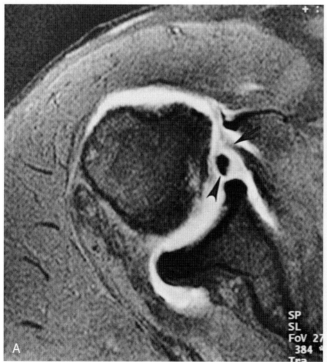

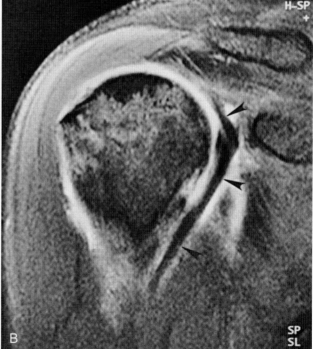

Figure 10-26   **Dislocated biceps tendon. A,** T1 fat-suppressed axial shoulder MR arthrogram. The bicipital groove is empty. The biceps tendon (*arrowhead*) is located over the anterior glenohumeral joint and posterior to the subscapularis tendon (*arrow*), which has been avulsed from its attachment to the lesser tuberosity of the humerus. **B,** T1 fat-suppressed coronal oblique shoulder MR arthrogram. The biceps tendon (*arrowheads*) is dislocated medially overlying the shoulder joint.

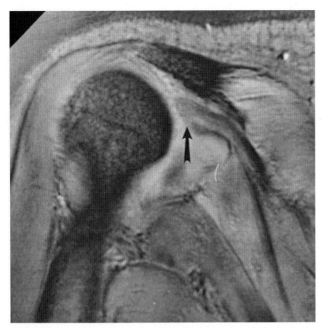

Figure 10-27 **Infraspinatus tendon tear.** T2* coronal oblique image of the shoulder. The end of the torn infraspinatus tendon (*arrow*) is seen retracted inferomedially to its normal attachment to the posterolateral humerus.

Clinical
• Impingement of infraspinatus and supraspinatus tendons between humeral head and posterosuperior labrum
• Occurs in late cocking phase of pitching
• Occurs with maximum abduction and external rotation
• Posterosuperior pain and anterior instability

MRI
• Humeral cysts adjacent to infraspinatus tendon insertion
• Infraspinatus (and supraspinatus) tendon undersurface tears
• Posterosuperior labral tear

tus tendon, and mainly of the infraspinatus tendon, between the humeral head and the posterior glenoid rim during overhead movements with abduction and external rotation, such as pitching.[24,25] Posterosuperior impingement results in abnormalities affecting the rotator cuff, most commonly the infraspinatus tendon, the posterosuperior labrum, and the humeral head at the point of impaction with the posterosuperior glenoid. Patients present with posterior shoulder pain and may have associated anterior shoulder instability. MRI findings include degenerative cysts on the posterior aspect of the humeral head near the insertion of the infraspinatus

tendon; fraying, partial, or complete tears of the infraspinatus tendon or supraspinatus tendon; and fraying or tears of the posterior glenoid labrum (Fig. 10-28).

Subscapularis (Box 10-8)

Subscapularis tendon tears are common.[26] They can result from acute trauma on an adducted arm in hyperextension or in external rotation. They can result from an anterior shoulder dislocation, they can be associated with massive tears of the rotator cuff and with biceps tendon dislocations, or they can result from subcoracoid impingement. Subcoracoid impingement is caused by narrowing of the space between the tip of the coracoid process and the humerus, which may be congenital in origin or may result from a coracoid fracture or surgery. The narrowed space can result in impingement on, and resultant tears of, the subscapularis tendon (Fig. 10-29).[27,28]

Tears of the subscapularis tendon are best evaluated on axial MRIs, where the entire length of the tendon is evident (see Fig. 10-29), or on sagittal images. The tears are seen best on T2W images or on T1W images after intra-articular gadolinium injection. Tears may be seen as tendon discontinuity, contrast media entering into the tendon substance,

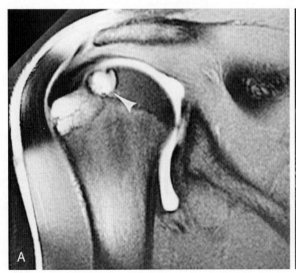

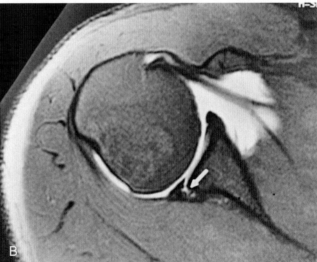

Figure 10-28 **Posterior impingement. A,** T1 fat-suppressed coronal oblique shoulder MR arthrogram. There is a large cyst in the posterolateral humeral head (*arrowhead*) that is filled with contrast material at the site of impaction between the humeral head and posterior labrum during overhead movements. There is incomplete fat suppression in this image, with fat remaining high signal laterally. **B,** T1 fat-suppressed axial shoulder MR arthrogram. The posterior labrum is detached from the adjacent glenoid (*arrow*).

intrasubstance abnormal tendon signal, abnormal caliber of the tendon, and abnormal position of the tendon. Other helpful accessory signs are the leakage of intra-articular contrast material under the insertion of the subscapularis tendon onto the lesser tuberosity and fatty atrophy of the subscapularis muscle, usually localized at the cranial aspect of the muscle and seen as high signal intensity streaks on T1W images. Abnormalities in the course of the long head of the biceps tendon (subluxation or dislocation) usually are associated with subscapularis tendon tears.[29] They often extend into the subscapularis muscle.

Massive Cuff Tears

Massive rotator cuff tears usually are seen in older patients with either marked tendon degeneration or with predisposing factors, such as an associated inflammatory arthritis or diabetes, or who have been on long-term steroid therapy. These massive tears affect multiple tendons of the rotator cuff, with full-thickness tears, musculotendinous retraction, and muscle atrophy (Fig. 10-30). There is a large communication between the glenohumeral joint and the subacromial/

subdeltoid bursa, and a synovial cyst develops in some patients that extends through the acromioclavicular joint and forms a soft tissue mass on the superior aspect of the shoulder, which may be large. Associated bone changes consist of superior migration of the humeral head with associated subacromial degenerative changes and severe degenerative joint disease of the glenohumeral joint with osteophyte formation and subchondral cysts.

ROTATOR INTERVAL ABNORMALITIES
(Box 10-9)

The rotator cuff interval is a triangular space between the supraspinatus tendon and the subscapularis tendon (Fig.

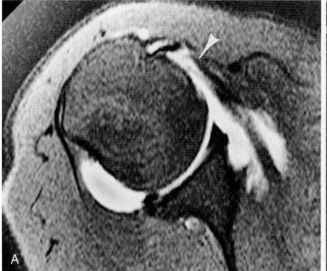
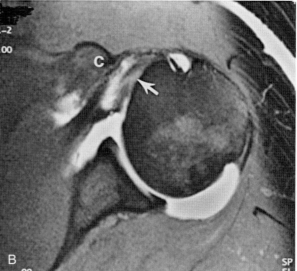

Figure 10-29 Subscapularis tendon tears; subcoracoid impingement. **A,** T1 fat-suppressed axial shoulder MR arthrogram. The subscapularis has been detached from the lesser tuberosity (*arrowhead*). The biceps tendon is subluxed medially from the bicipital groove. Contrast material covers the lesser tuberosity. **B,** T1 fat-suppressed axial shoulder MR arthrogram (different patient than in **A**). The coracoid process (C) was excessively long in this patient, causing narrowing of the space between it and the humerus (subcoracoid impingement). This is associated with tears of the subscapularis tendon, as was evident in this case (*arrow*). The tendon is thickened, longitudinally split, and filled with contrast material.

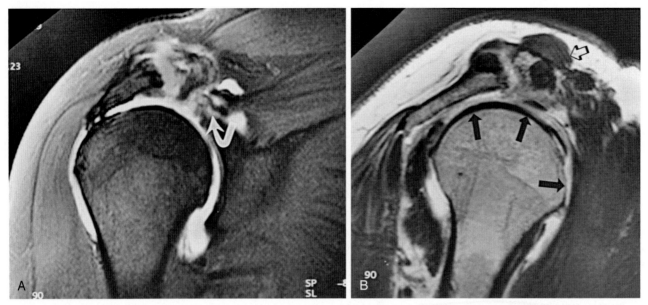

Figure 10-30   **Massive rotator cuff tear. A,** T1 fat-suppressed coronal oblique shoulder MR arthrogram. The supraspinatus tendon is torn and retracted a long distance medially (*curved arrow*). There is narrowing between the acromion and humeral head because of absence of the tendon. The acromioclavicular joint is degenerated, and high signal contrast material fills it from the glenohumeral joint injection. **B,** T1 sagittal oblique shoulder MR arthrogram. The superior mass (*open arrow*) is a small synovial cyst arising from the acromioclavicular joint. The absence of tendons overlying the humeral head indicates multiple tendon tears with retraction. *Solid arrows* point to the sites where the infraspinatus, supraspinatus, and subscapularis tendons (from left [posterior] to right [anterior]) should be seen, but are absent. The biceps tendon remains intact (*middle arrow*), but no supraspinatus is seen above it.

10-31).[30] The base of the triangle is at the coracoid process, which separates the supraspinatus and subscapularis tendons. The apex of the triangular rotator interval is at the transverse humeral ligament, which forms the roof of the bicipital groove. The superior and inferior margins of the interval are formed by the supraspinatus and subscapularis tendons. The anterior aspect of the interval is formed by the capsule and coracohumeral ligament.[31] The long biceps tendon courses

through the rotator interval. This is the site on the anterior shoulder where arthroscopists enter the shoulder joint to avoid damaging tendons.

Rotator cuff interval tears may occur secondary to anterior glenohumeral dislocations or glenohumeral instability, or may represent a surgical defect from arthroscopy (see Fig. 10-31B). The tears are shown best on T2W or postcontrast T1W sagittal oblique images. When torn, the rotator interval

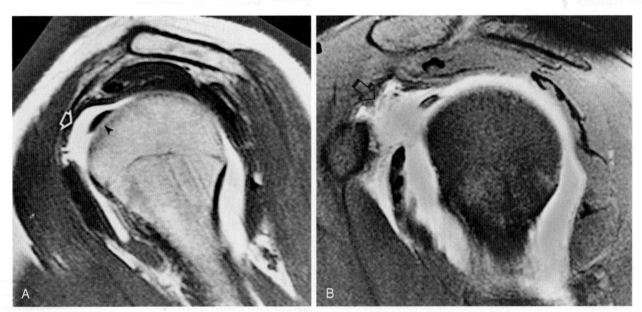

Figure 10-31   **Rotator interval: normal and abnormal. A,** T1 sagittal oblique shoulder MR arthrogram. The normal rotator interval is seen (*open arrow*) between the supraspinatus tendon superiorly and the subscapularis tendon inferiorly. The biceps tendon runs through the interval (*arrowhead*). **B,** T1 fat-suppressed sagittal oblique shoulder MR arthrogram (different patient than in **A**). The rotator interval (*open arrow*) is patulous and irregular owing to a previous anterior shoulder dislocation.

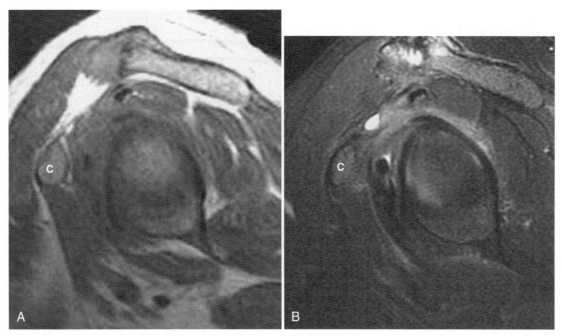

Figure 10-32   **Rotator interval in adhesive capsulitis. A,** T1 sagittal oblique shoulder MR arthrogram. The subcoracoid fat is replaced with scar in this patient with adhesive capsulitis. **B,** FSE T2 sagittal oblique shoulder MR arthrogram. Note the intermediate signal scar in the rotator interval and posterosuperior joint. **C,** coracoid process.

may become patulous, and contrast material is identified extending anterosuperiorly through the coracohumeral ligament and the capsule (superior glenohumeral ligament). These tears may communicate with the subacromial/subdeltoid bursa, mimicking a rotator cuff tear on a shoulder MR arthrogram, without a distinct tendon tear of the rotator cuff being identified.

The rotator interval is characteristically involved in adhesive capsulitis. Scar tissue forms around the superior glenohumeral ligament and the coracohumeral ligament in the rotator interval and obliterates the subcoracoid fat (Fig. 10-32). This was found to be a highly specific sign in a recent publication,[32] although it lacked sensitivity (meaning some of the patients with adhesive capsulitis did not have obliteration of the subcoracoid fat). We believe absence of subcoracoid fat on the T1W sagittal images to be a reliable indicator of adhesive capsulitis. A large joint effusion also can replace the subcoracoid fat, but patients with adhesive capsulitis have little or no joint fluid.

Instability

After rotator cuff disease, instability is the major abnormality that affects the shoulder. Glenohumeral instability and cuff disorders often coexist. Instability of the shoulder refers to subluxation or dislocation of the glenohumeral joint, which may be traumatic or atraumatic in origin. It is a painful disorder that, with the exception of an acute episode of dislocation, may be difficult to diagnose.

Stability of the shoulder joint depends on a combination of soft tissue and osseous structures surrounding and forming the glenohumeral joint. There is no isolated abnormality

that accounts for instability, but rather a combination of different factors interacting with one another. Contributing factors to glenohumeral instability include labral abnormalities, a lax or torn joint capsule, deficient or torn glenohumeral ligaments, shallow or abnormal glenoid version, and Hill-Sachs and Bankart fractures from previous dislocations.

Shoulder instability can be separated clinically into two groups: functional and anatomic. With functional instability, the joint is stable on physical examination, but the patient has symptoms of clicking, pain, intermittent locking, and a subjective feeling of an unstable joint. These patients often have labral abnormalities that cause pain without clinical evidence of instability. With anatomic instability, the patient usually has recurrent episodes of subluxation or dislocation, is symptomatic, and has signs of instability on physical examination.

The different types of instabilities are (1) anterior, (2) posterior, (3) multidirectional, and (4) superior. The most common type of unstable joint subluxes or dislocates anteriorly (95%). Posterior and multidirectional instability account for most of the other 5% of all instabilities of the shoulder. Superior instability generally is associated with multidirectional instability, and superior subluxation of the humeral head may create impingement when the supraspinatus tendon is repeatedly trapped between the coracoacromial arch and the humeral head. As a consequence of any of the different types of instabilities, hypertrophy of the greater tuberosity, subacromial spur formation, and thickening of the coracoacromial ligament associated with glenohumeral osteophyte formation may develop and lead to a secondary impingement syndrome involving the rotator cuff (Box 10-10).

Glenohumeral Instability

- Subluxation or dislocation of joint
- Often coexists with impingement
  - May cause secondary impingement
- Multiple structures responsible
  - Bones, labrum, capsule, ligaments
- Clinical
  - *Functional:* Subjective instability; clinically stable; labral tears often are present
  - *Anatomic:* Subjective instability; instability on examination
- Types
  - Anterior (95%)
  - Posterior, superior, multidirectional (5%)
- Causes
  - Acute traumatic dislocation (causes disruption of several structures crucial to stability that predispose to subsequent instability)
  - Chronic, repetitive overhead motions (throwing), without an acute injury
  - Congenital
    Osseous: Dysplastic glenoid
    Far medial (type III) anterior capsular attachment
    Capsular/ligamentous laxity

Many patients have instability secondary to a recognized previous traumatic dislocation. Many others have no history of a specific inciting event. Athletes engaged in repetitive throwing or overhead activities, such as baseball pitchers, football quarterbacks, tennis players, and swimmers (throwing oneself on the couch generally is not a risk factor), commonly have instability but no acute traumatic event that caused it. These athletes acquire an increased laxity of the anterior supporting structures of the shoulder to allow an increased range of motion, in particular in external rotation.

In addition to overuse and abuse, congenital abnormalities may contribute to shoulder instability. These congenital predisposing factors include osseous abnormalities, such as congenital deficiency of the depth and radius of curvature of the glenoid fossa (referred to as *glenoid dysplasia*),[33] and abnormal version angle of the glenoid, or soft tissue abnormalities, such as a medial (type III) capsular insertion, congenitally small or absent glenohumeral ligaments, and congenital capsular and ligamentous laxity. Regardless of the type of abnormality present, or which instability pattern exists, MR arthrography is undoubtedly the best imaging study to evaluate for them.

ANATOMY RELATING TO INSTABILITY

Capsule

The joint capsule attaches laterally on the anatomic neck of the humerus. Medially, the capsule usually attaches to the labrum or to the adjacent periosteum of the glenoid. Three types of anterior capsular insertions have been described: Type I consists of a medial attachment on or very near the labrum, a type II insertion is found within 1 cm medial to the labrum, and a type III capsular attachment is more than 1 cm medial to the labrum. It is believed that a type III anterior capsular insertion may either predispose to instability or represent the sequelae of a previous dislocation with stripping of the anterior capsule and periosteum off the glenoid. This belief is not widely acknowledged, however. We do not routinely comment on the capsular insertion. The posterior capsule attaches directly on the posterior glenoid labrum.

Glenohumeral Ligaments (Box 10-11)

The glenohumeral ligaments represent thickenings of the anterior joint capsule. The three ligaments are the superior, middle, and inferior glenohumeral ligaments. They extend from the anterior aspect of the glenoid to the lesser tuberosity of the humerus. When viewed en face, the three ligaments form a Z configuration (Fig. 10-33). Numerous variations of size and position have been described. The superior glenohumeral ligament originates from the region of the superior glenoid tubercle anterior to the origin of the long head of the biceps tendon and inserts on the superior aspect of the lesser tuberosity, blending with fibers of the coracohumeral ligament. The middle glenohumeral ligament is the most variable of the three glenohumeral ligaments and is absent in about 30% of shoulders, but its absence does not seem to increase the incidence of instability. It arises most frequently below the superior glenohumeral ligament on the anterosuperior aspect of the labrum and inserts onto the medial aspect of the lesser tuberosity of the humerus. The inferior glenohumeral ligament is the main stabilizing ligament of the shoulder. It is composed of an anterior and a posterior band, with an intervening axillary pouch or recess. The anterior and posterior bands arise from the inferior two thirds of the anterior and posterior portions of the labrum, and they extend laterally to attach to the surgical neck of the humerus.[34-37]

The superior glenohumeral ligament is seen at the level of the body of the coracoid process on axial MRIs and parallels this osseous structure (Fig. 10-34). The middle glenohumeral ligament is seen at and just inferior to the level of the tip of the coracoid process on axial cuts and lies deep to the subscapularis tendon and adjacent to the anterior labrum, where it can mimic a torn labral fragment (see Fig. 10-34). The inferior glenohumeral ligament is seen on axial images through the inferior aspect of the glenoid, attaching to the anterior and posterior labrum. The glenohumeral ligaments also can be identified well on sagittal oblique images (see Fig. 10-34).

Glenohumeral Ligaments

Superior
- From supraglenoid tubercle to lesser tuberosity
- At body of coracoid on axial MRI
- Limits inferior subluxation

Middle
- From supraglenoid tubercle to lesser tuberosity
- At inferior tip of coracoid, behind subscapularis tendon on axial MRI
- Variable to absent in 30%

Inferior
- From inferior glenoid labrum to anatomic neck of humerus
- Anterior and posterior bands
- Provides anterior and posterior stability
- Seen on inferior halves of labrum on sagittal oblique and axial MRI

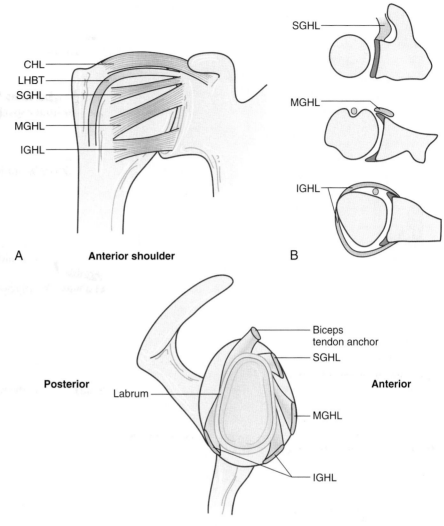

Figure 10-33 **Normal superior, middle, and inferior glenohumeral ligaments. A,** Diagram of the superior, middle, and inferior glenohumeral ligaments (SGHL, MGHL, and IGHL) en face from a coronal perspective, forming the Z configuration. The coracohumeral ligament (CHL) and long head of the biceps tendon (LHBT) also are shown. **B,** Diagram of the SGHL, MGHL, and IGHL from an axial perspective. The SGHL parallels the coracoid process. The MGHL runs anterior to the anterior labrum at the level of the subscapularis tendon. The anterior and posterior limbs of the IGHL attach to the anterior and posterior labrum. **C,** Diagram of the SGHL, MGHL, and IGHL from a sagittal perspective. The ligaments attach to the labrum and are a thickening of the joint capsule.

The glenohumeral ligaments contribute to the stability of the shoulder joint in several ways. The superior glenohumeral ligament prevents inferior displacement of the humerus when the shoulder is abducted. The middle glenohumeral ligament contributes to anterior stability in concert with the subscapularis tendon. The inferior glenohumeral ligament is the most important of the glenohumeral ligaments for anterior and posterior joint stabilization. It limits anterior translation of the humeral head with abduction and external rotation of the arm and limits posterior translation with the shoulder in internal rotation.

The glenohumeral labroligamentous complex (the glenohumeral ligaments in combination with the labrum) to some extent passively stabilizes the glenohumeral joint. Although the labrum deepens the concavity of the glenoid fossa, its function as a mechanical barrier against humeral subluxation is much less important than its function as an attachment site for the glenohumeral ligaments. Because the labrum and ligamentous collagen fibers intertwine to form a strong histologic bond, injury is more likely to occur between the labrum and osseous glenoid (labral detachment) than at the labroligamentous junction.

The position of the shoulder and rotation of the humeral head at the time of injury determines which glenohumeral ligament develops excessive tension and where the labral abnormality develops. The injury most likely to lead to anterior instability of the shoulder occurs with the shoulder abducted and externally rotated, which places stress on the anterior limb of the inferior glenohumeral ligament. The ligament is taut in this position, and excessive stress leads to detachment or tear of the anterior labrum or the anterior band of the inferior glenohumeral ligament. It has been shown that imaging the shoulder in the ABER position (abduction and external rotation) tightens the inferior glenohumeral labroligamentous complex, rendering labral tears more conspicuous.[38] We rarely use this position, however, as it considerably increases the length of time to perform an examination because of the need to reposition the patient and change surface coils, and we have not found it increased our accuracy for labral or cuff tears.

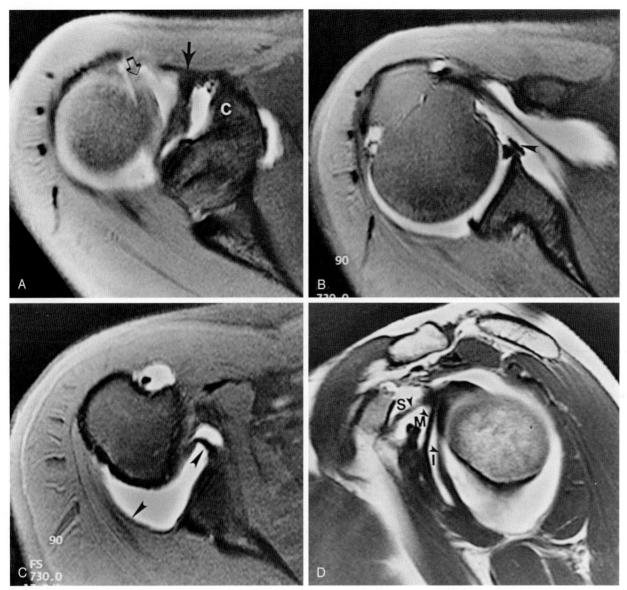

Figure 10-34 **Normal glenohumeral ligaments. A,** T1 fat-suppressed axial shoulder MR arthrogram. The low signal superior glenohumeral ligament (*solid arrow*) parallels the coracoid process (C) from the capsule to attach to the superior aspect of the anterior labrum. The biceps tendon (*open arrow*) also passes through the superior joint to anchor to the superior labrum. **B,** T1 fat-suppressed axial shoulder MR arthrogram. The linear, low signal middle glenohumeral ligament (*arrowhead*) is located just anterior to the anterior labrum at the level of the subscapularis tendon. It may mimic a torn labrum. **C,** T1 fat-suppressed axial shoulder MR arthrogram. The anterior and posterior limbs of the inferior glenohumeral ligaments (*arrowheads*) extend from the humerus to the anterior and posterior glenoid labrum in the inferior shoulder joint. **D,** T1 sagittal oblique shoulder MR arthrogram. The glenohumeral ligaments are outlined by contrast material in the anterior joint, extending from the anterior labrum to the joint capsule. S, M, I, superior, middle, inferior glenohumeral ligaments.

Labrum

The labrum is a redundant fold of the joint capsule made of fibrocartilaginous tissue that attaches to the rim of the glenoid of the scapula. It deepens the glenoid fossa and is the attachment site for the long head of the biceps tendon and of the glenohumeral ligaments. The glenohumeral ligaments, together with the labrum, constitute the glenohumeral labroligamentous complex. Frequently, there is a rim of hyaline cartilage interposed between the labrum and the underlying osseous glenoid, which is seen as a line of high signal intensity (the same signal as hyaline cartilage) partially separating the labrum from the glenoid (Fig. 10-35). This

line should not be mistaken for an avulsion or a tear of the labrum. The labrum is normally low signal intensity on all pulse sequences. It may be affected by the magic angle phenomenon, and it may develop myxoid degeneration with aging; in both instances, there is intrasubstance globular intermediate signal intensity on MRIs. The anterior and posterior portions of the labrum are seen best on axial images (Fig. 10-36), whereas the superior labrum is depicted optimally on coronal oblique images (see Fig. 10-35). The labrum may have a wide variety of shapes on MRI in asymptomatic individuals (see Fig. 10-36). The most common labral shapes are triangular, followed by rounded, flat, and absent, in decreasing order of frequency.[39,40]

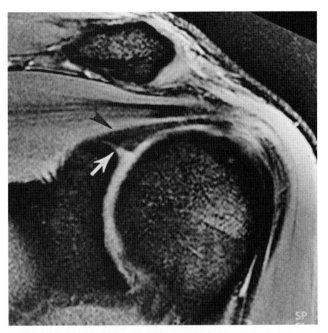

Figure 10-35 Normal superior labrum. T2* coronal oblique image of the shoulder. The superior labrum (*arrowhead*) is seen best in this plane. The biceps tendon is seen in continuity with the labrum, where it forms its anchor. There is undercutting of hyaline cartilage on the glenoid deep to the labrum, which creates linear high signal (*arrow*) that is normal and must not be misinterpreted as a labral detachment. A portion of the labrum is clearly attached to the osseous glenoid.

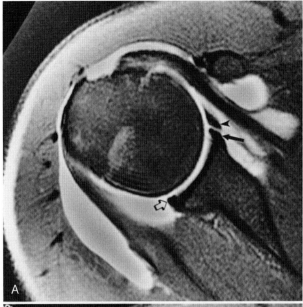

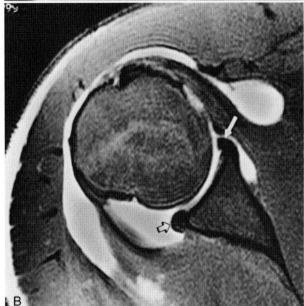

Figure 10-36 Normal anterior and posterior glenoid labrum. A, T1 fat-suppressed axial shoulder MR arthrogram. The anterior labrum (*solid arrow*) and posterior labrum (*open arrow*) have a triangular, low signal appearance. The middle glenohumeral ligament (*arrowhead*) is seen anterior to the anterior labrum. **B,** T1 fat-suppressed axial shoulder MR arthrogram (different patient than in **A**). The anterior labrum is triangular (*solid white arrow*), but the posterior labrum is rounded (*open arrow*), which is one of several normal variations in labral configuration.

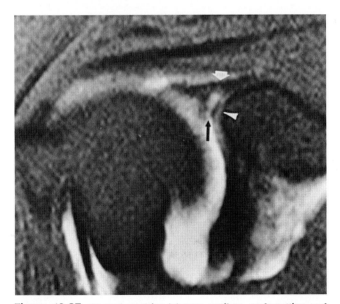

Figure 10-37 Normal superior labrum: cartilage undercutting and sulcus pitfalls. T1 fat-suppressed coronal oblique shoulder MR arthrogram. The triangular superior labrum is attached to the glenoid (*white arrow*). The normal hyaline cartilage (*arrowhead*) that is interposed between the labrum and the glenoid is lower signal than the gadolinium solution and must not be confused with a detached or torn labrum. Just lateral to the cartilage is the normal sulcus (*black arrow*), which is interposed between the labrum and the hyaline cartilage and filled with contrast material. The sulcus and the undercutting of the cartilage are following the contour of the glenoid, pointing medially. Labral tears diverge from the glenoid (are directed laterally).

BOX 10-12

Anterosuperior Labral Normal Variants

- Sublabral foramen
  - Anterosuperior labrum not attached to glenoid
- Buford complex
  - Anterosuperior labrum congenitally absent, thick middle glenohumeral ligament
- Sublabral recess versus SLAP
  - Sublabral recess does not extend posterior to the biceps attachment, whereas SLAP does

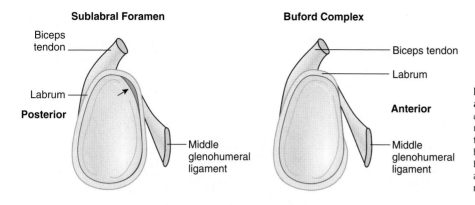

Figure 10-38 Anterosuperior labral variants. *Left,* Diagram of the sublabral foramen. The *arrow* points to the gap between the anterosuperior labrum and the glenoid (the sublabral foramen), which does not extend posterior to the biceps tendon anchor. *Right,* Diagram of the Buford complex—congenital absence of the anterosuperior labrum with a larger-than-usual middle glenohumeral ligament.

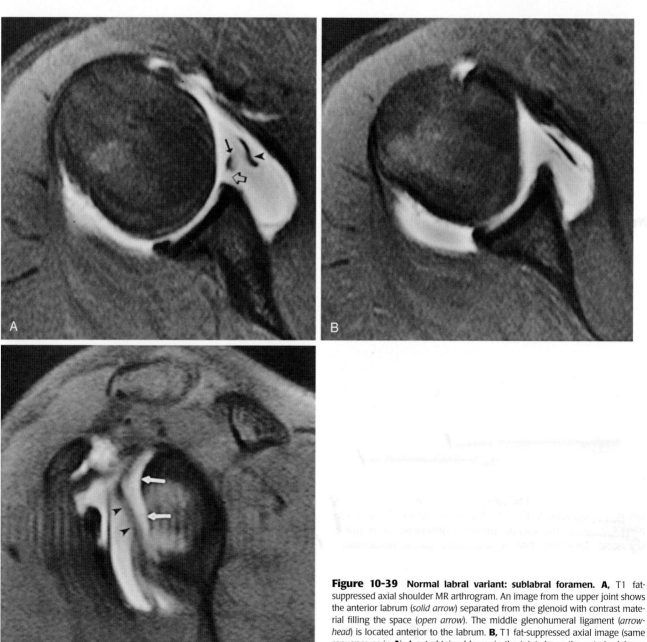

Figure 10-39 Normal labral variant: sublabral foramen. A, T1 fat-suppressed axial shoulder MR arthrogram. An image from the upper joint shows the anterior labrum (*solid arrow*) separated from the glenoid with contrast material filling the space (*open arrow*). The middle glenohumeral ligament (*arrowhead*) is located anterior to the labrum. **B,** T1 fat-suppressed axial image (same sequence as in **A**). A cut obtained lower in the joint shows the anterior labrum is present and solidly attached to the glenoid. **C,** T1 fat-suppressed sagittal shoulder MR arthrogram. The anterosuperior labrum (*arrowheads*) is separated from the anterior margin of the glenoid (*arrows*), with contrast material between the two structures.

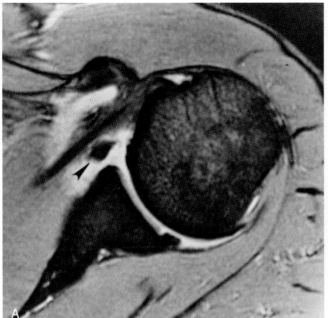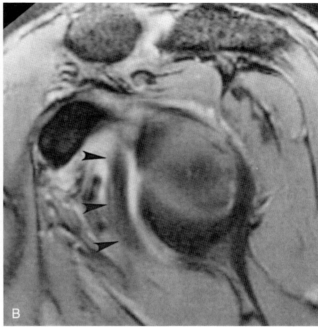

Figure 10-40   Normal labral variant: Buford complex. **A,** T1 fat-suppressed axial shoulder MR arthrogram. No labrum is attached to the anterosuperior portion of the glenoid. The round, low signal structure anterior to the glenoid (*arrowhead*) blended with the anterior joint capsule on lower images through the joint. This is an enlarged middle glenohumeral ligament with absence of the anterosuperior labrum. **B,** T1 fat-suppressed sagittal shoulder MR arthrogram. The large middle glenohumeral ligament (*arrowheads*) parallels the anterior glenoid, but merges with the anterior capsule distally. Contrast material is interposed between the ligament and the glenoid.

Normal Variants of the Labrum (Box 10-12). In addition to the variations in the normal shape of the labrum, there are two normal structures that may mimic tears of the superior labrum. Undercutting of articular cartilage between the labrum and the glenoid cortex or the presence of a synovial recess (sulcus) interposed between the glenoid rim and the labrum may mimic labral tears. These two normal variants follow the contour of the glenoid (go with the flow of the glenoid) (Fig. 10-37), whereas tears of the superior labrum are oriented laterally into the labrum (go against the flow or do not follow the contour of the glenoid) on coronal oblique images. Other normal variants occur at the anterosuperior aspect of the glenoid, including labral detachment from the glenoid (sublabral foramen) or congenital absence of the labrum (Buford complex) (Fig. 10-38).[41-44]

A detached anterosuperior labrum, which is of no clinical significance, is referred to as a *sublabral foramen* or *hole.* The anterior labrum is separated from the osseous glenoid superiorly, but reattaches to the glenoid in its mid to inferior portion (Fig. 10-39). The labrum must not be detached at any point posterior to the attachment of the long head of the biceps tendon (the biceps anchor); otherwise, it is not a sublabral foramen, but a traumatic labral detachment instead, although this has been shown to not be a hard and fast rule.[45]

Another normal labral variant is a congenitally absent anterosuperior labrum, which is associated with a markedly thickened middle glenohumeral ligament; this combination of findings is known as the Buford complex (Fig. 10-40).[43] Distinguishing between a sublabral foramen and a Buford complex with a thick middle glenohumeral ligament occasionally may be difficult. The thick middle glenohumeral

ligament in the Buford complex can be seen to blend with the anterior joint capsule as the axial images progress inferiorly. Conversely, with a sublabral foramen, the labrum attaches to the glenoid, rather than anteriorly to the joint capsule. These variants are important to recognize on MRI to avoid confusing them with significant pathology, but they are of no clinical significance.

INSTABILITY LESIONS

Lesions associated with instability are depicted best with shoulder MR arthrography. They may involve the labrum, the capsule, the glenohumeral ligaments, and the bones in various combinations.[46,47] Many acronyms and eponyms have been used to name the different abnormalities, and these may Drive You Nuts (DYN) (Boxes 10-13 and 10-14).

Capsule

A type III anterior capsular attachment, patulous anterior capsule, thickening and irregularity of the capsule, and capsular shearing or stripping from the scapula can be seen on MRI and indicate anterior instability. MR arthrography with capsular distention may mimic a type III insertion. Traumatic anterior glenohumeral joint dislocation also may be associated with subscapularis tendon tears and enlargement of the subscapularis recess of the joint. The posterior capsule also may show sequelae of a posterior dislocation in the same manner as with the anterior capsule. Capsular abnormalities are best seen on MRI when fluid is present in the joint, as is usually the case with an acute injury. In other circumstances, distention of the joint with MR arthrography is the only

BOX 10-13

Acronyms and Eponyms Related to the Shoulder

ALPSA: Anterior *l*abroligamentous *p*eriosteal *s*leeve *a*vulsion. A variation of the Bankart lesion with injury to the anteroinferior labrum, but the anterior scapular periosteum is intact.

Bankart lesion: Tear of the anteroinferior glenoid labrum with torn anterior scapular periosteum. May have an associated fracture of the anteroinferior glenoid rim.

Bennett lesion: Mineralization of the posterior band of the inferior glenohumeral ligament and posterior capsule from chronic traction forces.

BHAGL lesion: *B*ony *HAGL* lesion (see further on).

Buford complex: Congenital absence of the anterosuperior glenoid labrum associated with a thickened middle glenohumeral ligament.

DYN: *D*rives *y*ou *n*uts.

GLAD lesion: *G*leno*l*abral *a*rticular *d*isruption is a tear of the anteroinferior labrum with a glenoid chondral defect.

HAGL lesion: *H*umeral *a*vulsion of the *g*lenohumeral *l*igament occurs from shoulder dislocation with avulsion of the inferior glenohumeral ligament from the anatomic neck of the humerus.

Hill-Sachs lesion: Impaction fracture of the posterolateral aspect of the humeral head from anterior shoulder dislocation.

SLAP lesion: *S*uperior *l*abrum tear propagating *a*nterior and *p*osterior to the biceps anchor.

BOX 10-15

Bennett Lesion

Clinical

- Baseball pitchers during decelerating phase of throwing
- Traction of posterior limb, inferior glenohumeral ligament on labrum
- Pain and eventually instability

MRI

- Thickened low signal posteroinferior capsule (mineralization)
- May be associated with posterior labral tear

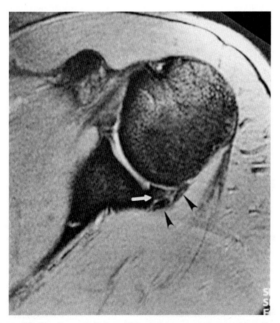

Figure 10-41 **Bennett lesion.** T2* axial image of the shoulder. There is thickening and low signal (calcification) in the posterior capsule/posterior limb of the inferior glenohumeral ligament (*arrowheads*). The adjacent posterior labrum (*arrow*) is normal. This is a traction injury to the capsule from the deceleration phase of pitching. Linear calcification was present on an axillary view radiograph.

BOX 10-14

Instability: MRI Evidence (Axial Images Are Best)

Osseous

- Subluxed glenohumeral joint
- Steep, shallow glenoid
- Hill-Sachs fracture
  - Concave posterolateral defect on superior two axial cuts through humeral head (anterior dislocation)
- Bankart fracture
  - Fracture of anteroinferior glenoid rim (anterior dislocation)
- Trough sign
  - Impaction fracture, anteromedial humeral head (posterior dislocation)
- Reverse Bankart
  - Fracture of posterior rim of glenoid (posterior dislocation)

Capsule

- Type III anterior attachment (>1 cm medial to labrum)
- Patulous capsule and stripping from scapula
- Thickened, irregular capsule
- Mineralization posteriorly (Bennett lesion)

Glenohumeral Ligaments

- Torn, thickened, absent, or avulsed
- Inferior ligament most important
  - Avulsion from humerus (HAGL lesion)
  - Avulsion from labrum

Labrum

- Tears, detachment from glenoid, crushed
  - Linear or diffuse increased signal in labrum (tears, crush)
  - Increased signal between labrum and glenoid (detachment)
  - Absent or small labral remnant
- Bankart lesion
  - Detachment of anteroinferior labrum and tear of anterior scapular periosteum, with or without glenoid rim fracture
- ALPSA lesion (anterior labroligamentous periosteal sleeve avulsion)
  - Same as Bankart, but scapular periosteum is not torn

Tendons

- Subscapularis
  - Tears, or detaches from tuberosity
- Biceps, long head
  - Dislocates medially

reliable means to show the glenohumeral labroligamentous complex and the joint capsule.

A Bennett lesion is an extra-articular posterior capsular avulsive injury associated with a posterior labral injury (Box 10-15).[48] This injury is seen most commonly in pitchers and occurs from traction of the posterior band of the inferior glenohumeral ligament during the decelerating phase of pitching. A crescent of mineralization can be identified on an axillary radiographic view or, even better, on computed tomography. On MRI, this mineralization appears as a low signal intensity band posterior to the posterior labrum on axial images (Fig. 10-41). If left untreated, patients progress from functional to anatomic instability.

Glenohumeral Ligaments

Torn, thickened, or absent glenohumeral ligaments are a manifestation of instability on MRI. The inferior glenohumeral ligament is the most important stabilizer of the glenohumeral joint and is the most frequently affected with instability. It may be affected at its labral or its humeral attachment. Avulsion of the inferior glenohumeral ligament from the humerus, called a *HAGL lesion* (humeral avulsion

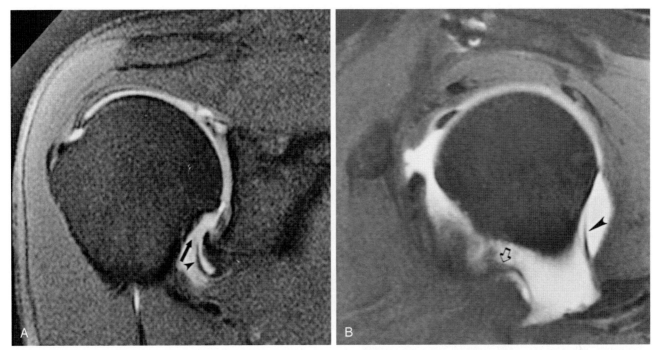

Figure 10-42   **Humeral avulsion of the glenohumeral ligament (HAGL). A,** T1 fat-suppressed coronal oblique shoulder MR arthrogram. The anterior limb of the inferior glenohumeral ligament (*arrowhead*) is detached from the humerus (*arrow*) in this patient with a previous anterior dislocation. There also is a bucket-handle superior labral anterior and posterior (SLAP) tear of the superior labrum. **B,** T1 fat-suppressed sagittal oblique shoulder MR arthrogram (different patient than in **A**). The anterior limb of the inferior glenohumeral ligament (*open arrow*) is avulsed from its humeral attachment, is thickened, and is drooping inferiorly (compare with normal posteroinferior glenohumeral ligament [*arrowhead*]). The patient had several prior dislocations.

of the glenohumeral ligament), may result from shoulder dislocation.[49] It often is associated with a tear of the subscapularis tendon. A *BHAGL lesion* (bony humeral avulsion of the glenohumeral ligament) also can occur.

HAGL lesions can be identified on axial, coronal, or sagittal MRIs (Fig. 10-42). The inferior glenohumeral ligament may show high signal intensity on T2 images, and may show morphologic disruption at its insertion on the anatomic neck of the humerus and wavy contours of the residual ligament, and the ligament may be displaced inferiorly. The diagnosis also can be inferred on MR arthrography when extravasation of contrast material from the joint occurs in the region of the ligament insertion on the humerus.

Bones

The osseous abnormalities associated with instability can be either of developmental origin or acquired. A congenitally steep, retroverted, or shallow glenoid may predispose to instability (Fig. 10-43). This condition is known as glenoid dysplasia and has an increased incidence of posterior labral tears or detachments.[33] This is because of the absence of the bony posterior lip of the inferior glenoid, which is replaced by labral tissue that is easily injured with posterior forces or stress, such as heavy weights used in benchpressing. Glenoid dysplasia is common (reported in ~15% of shoulders).

An anterior dislocation may produce an acquired osseous abnormality from an impaction fracture on the posterolateral aspect of the humeral head, this is known as the Hill-Sachs defect. This fracture may be seen in any plane of imaging, but is seen best on axial MRIs on the two most superior images through the humeral head as a concave

defect in the posterolateral aspect of the humeral head (Fig. 10-44). The humeral head is normally round on these superior cuts (above the coracoid process), whereas below this level a posterior flattening of the humerus is a normal appearance.[50] Anterior dislocation of the humeral head also may create a fracture of the anteroinferior glenoid (Bankart

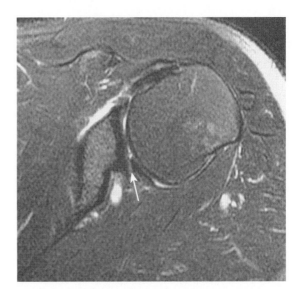

Figure 10-43   **Congenital osseous cause of instability: glenoid dysplasia.** FSE T2 axial image of the shoulder. The posterior aspect of the glenoid is retroverted and hypoplastic, predisposing to shoulder instability. Note the detached posterior labrum (*arrow*), which is found more frequently in glenoid dysplasia.

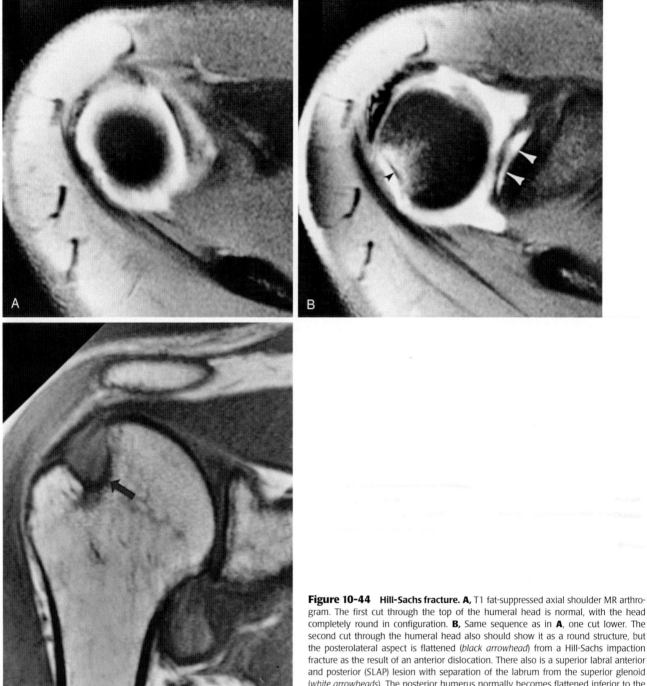

Figure 10-44 **Hill-Sachs fracture. A,** T1 fat-suppressed axial shoulder MR arthrogram. The first cut through the top of the humeral head is normal, with the head completely round in configuration. **B,** Same sequence as in **A,** one cut lower. The second cut through the humeral head also should show it as a round structure, but the posterolateral aspect is flattened (*black arrowhead*) from a Hill-Sachs impaction fracture as the result of an anterior dislocation. There also is a superior labral anterior and posterior (SLAP) lesion with separation of the labrum from the superior glenoid (*white arrowheads*). The posterior humerus normally becomes flattened inferior to the first two cuts through the humeral head and must not be mistaken for a Hill-Sachs impaction fracture. **C,** T1 coronal oblique image of the shoulder (different patient than in **A** and **B**). A large Hill-Sachs impaction fracture is evident (*arrow*) in the posterolateral humeral head.

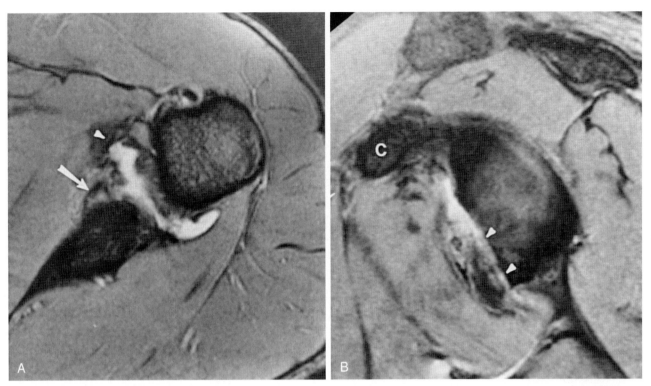

Figure 10-45 Bony Bankart lesion. **A,** T1 fat-suppressed axial shoulder MR arthrogram. The anterior capsule is thickened and irregular (*arrowhead*) from injury caused by an anterior shoulder dislocation. The anterior labrum is difficult to see because of fibrillation from tears (crushed). There also is a low-signal fracture fragment (*arrow*) off of the anteroinferior glenoid (a bony Bankart lesion). **B,** T1 fat-suppressed sagittal oblique shoulder MR arthrogram. The vertical fracture line (*arrowheads*) through the anterior glenoid is obvious. C, coracoid process.

fracture). This fracture can be shown best on axial and sagittal oblique images (Fig. 10-45). A posterior shoulder dislocation may result in an impaction fracture of the anteromedial aspect of the humeral head, called a *trough lesion,* and the posterior aspect of the glenoid, called a *reverse Bankart fracture* (Fig. 10-46).

Labrum

The labrum may have partial-thickness tears, have full-thickness tears, be avulsed (traumatically detached) from the glenoid, or be crushed or frayed.[51,52] The labral lesion definitely associated with shoulder instability is a Bankart (some of its variations, such as an ALPSA [anterior labroligamentous periosteal sleeve avulsion], are really just Bankart lesions with a twist).

The Bankart lesion is the most common injury following anterior dislocation of the glenohumeral joint. It is a detachment of the anteroinferior labrum (with or without labral tears) from the glenoid with a tear of the anterior scapular periosteum (Fig. 10-47). The Bankart lesion may or may not be associated with a fracture of the anteroinferior glenoid.

A variation of the Bankart lesion is the ALPSA lesion.[51] The ALPSA lesion is an avulsion of the anterior labrum from the anteroinferior glenoid with an intact anterior scapular periosteum that has been stripped from the bone (periosteal sleeve), but that remains attached to the labrum (Fig. 10-48). The stripped periosteum allows the anterior labroligamentous complex to displace medially and rotate inferiorly on the scapular neck. If not repaired, the ALPSA lesion can heal

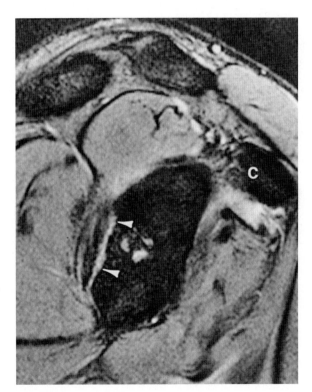

Figure 10-46 Reverse bony Bankart lesion. T1 fat-suppressed sagittal oblique shoulder MR arthrogram. There is a vertical fracture through the posterior margin of the glenoid (*arrowheads*) caused by a posterior shoulder dislocation. C, coracoid process.

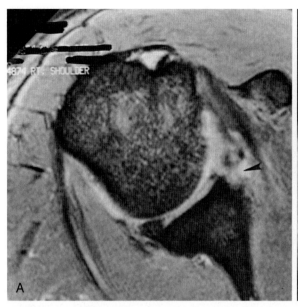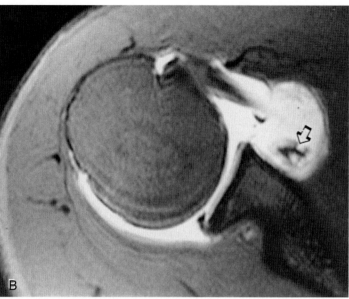

Figure 10-47 **Bankart lesions. A,** T1 fat-suppressed axial shoulder MR arthrogram. The anteroinferior labrum is detached from the glenoid (*arrowhead*) and is irregular in shape and high signal from tears. There is no linear periosteum seen attached to the labrum because it has been torn. The flat posterolateral humerus in the lower portion of the joint is normal and not from a Hill-Sachs impaction fracture. **B,** T1 fat-suppressed axial shoulder MR arthrogram (different patient than in **A**). The anteroinferior labrum is absent from its normal position adjacent to the glenoid; it has been completely detached and torn free of the scapular periosteum, coming to rest in the medial aspect of the joint (*open arrow*).

with a resultant deformed labrum that allows for joint instability. Surgical reduction of the labrum is thought by some experts to be desirable for an ALPSA lesion because it can heal in place. This is in contrast to Bankart lesions, which have no potential for healing and may be managed

differently from ALPSA lesions. These differences are not believed to be clinically relevant by many surgeons, however.

A reverse Bankart lesion may occur after a posterior dislocation as the result of excessive stress on the glenohumeral joint with the arm in abduction and internal rotation. A reverse Bankart lesion consists of a detachment of the posteroinferior labrum, which may or may not be associated with a fracture of the posterior glenoid.

The MRI criteria for diagnosing a labral abnormality includes linear high signal intensity (greater than hyaline cartilage) within the substance of the labrum that exists on a labral surface; diffuse high signal intensity of the labrum from a crush injury; absent or abnormally small labrum; and detachment and displacement of the labrum from the glenoid rim, with high signal intensity between the labrum and the glenoid (Fig. 10-49).[52,53] A traumatic detachment of the superior labrum can be difficult to distinguish from a sublabral recess, a normal variant of the labrum. Detachment of the labrum from the glenoid at any site other than the superior or the anterosuperior glenoid is a true abnormality.

NON-INSTABILITY LABRAL LESIONS

Lesions may affect the labrum, but not be associated with anatomic glenohumeral joint instability. These include SLAP lesions, labral cysts, and GLAD (glenolabral articular disruption) lesions (Box 10-16).

SLAP Lesions

SLAP lesion is a term applied to tears involving the superior labrum that are oriented in an anterior and posterior direction.[54] These labral tears occur at the attachment site of the long head of the biceps tendon to the superior labrum. SLAP

Figure 10-48 **Anterior labroligamentous periosteal sleeve avulsion (ALPSA) lesion.** T1 fat-suppressed axial shoulder MR arthrogram. The anteroinferior labrum is detached from the bone of the glenoid (*arrow*). The detached labrum is attached to a linear, low signal sleeve of intact periosteum (*arrowhead*) that has been stripped from the scapula. Had the periosteum been torn rather than stripped (and not evident on MR arthrography), this would be a Bankart lesion.

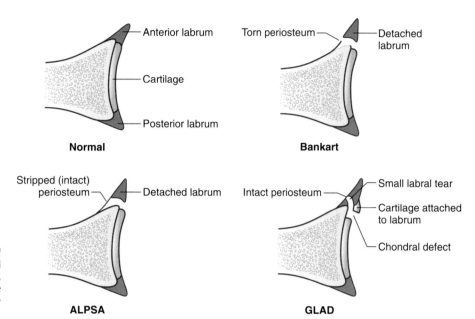

Figure 10-49 **Labral lesions.** Diagram of the normal anterior labrum from an axial perspective, and the key features of Bankart, anterior labroligamentous periosteal sleeve avulsion (ALPSA), and glenolabral articular disruption (GLAD) labral lesions.

lesions occur from compression or overhead movements that trap the labrum between the humeral head and the glenoid, or from traction on the biceps tendon that results in avulsion of the superior labrum. Patients with a SLAP lesion have pain, catching, popping, and a sensation of instability, although the joint is stable on physical examination. *"micro-instability"*

SLAP lesions initially were classified into four types:

Type I: Fraying of the free edge of the superior glenoid labrum

Type II: Detachment of the superior labrum from the glenoid

Type III: Bucket-handle tear of the superior labrum without involvement of the long head of the biceps tendon

Type IV: Bucket-handle tear of the labrum extending into the long head of the biceps tendon

At least 12 types of SLAP lesions have now been described. There may be many more SLAP lesions described in the future, owing to people's penchant for splitting hairs. Categorizing SLAP lesions into the different types with MRI has limited practical value and may be difficult to do. No large studies have evaluated the accuracy of MRI in staging SLAP lesions.

Although the treatment may vary for certain lesions, they usually are addressed arthroscopically, and differences in treatment are based on whether or not there is involvement of the biceps anchor. It is most important to assess the integrity of the biceps tendon on the MRIs and include that information in the report, rather than trying to determine which specific type of SLAP lesion exists. Generally, we determine if a SLAP lesion consists of a partial-thickness or full-thickness tear of the superior labrum versus detachment from the glenoid (Fig. 10-50), and whether or not the biceps tendon is torn—that is as complex a classification system as is necessary, and all that orthopedists expect from radiologists (Box 10-17).

Using T2, gradient echo, or T1W images after intra-articular gadolinium injection, the various features of SLAP lesions can be diagnosed on MRI. Fraying of the labrum is seen as irregularity of the margins and diffuse increased signal in the substance of the superior labrum.

Avulsion of the superior labrum manifests as linear high signal separating the labrum from the glenoid (Fig. 10-51). The abnormal signal extends anterior and posterior to the attachment of the biceps tendon to the labrum, which some believe distinguishes the SLAP lesion from a sublabral recess, where the labrum is separated only from the glenoid anterior to the biceps tendon anchor. Superior labral detachment resembles the normal labral recess and undercutting of hyaline cartilage between the labrum and glenoid on coronal oblique images. Detachment differs from normal anatomy, however, because the labrum is completely separated from the underlying glenoid by high signal fluid, and the separation extends posterior to the biceps anchor. This is controversial, however, because separation posterior to the biceps anchor has been shown to be an unreliable sign for a labral detachment.[45]

SLAP tears either extend partially through the substance of the superior labrum in a generally craniocaudal direction, extending to its inferior surface, or extend completely through the labrum, separating it into medial and lateral labral fragments. The latter situation is known as a

BOX 10-16

Glenoid Labrum Tears: Stable or Unstable

Associated With Instability
- Bankart lesions
- ALPSA lesions

Without Associated Instability
- SLAP lesions
- GLAD lesions

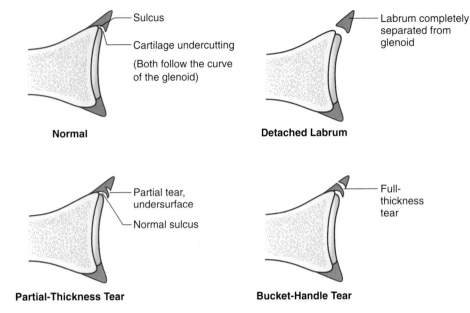

Figure 10-50 **Superior labrum anterior and posterior (SLAP) lesions.** Diagram of the normal superior labrum and SLAP lesions from a coronal perspective. The normal labrum has cartilage undercutting it and a normal sulcus between cartilage and labrum. The key features of SLAP lesions shown here include detachment, partial-thickness tears, and full-thickness (bucket-handle) tears.

bucket-handle tear of the labrum. In the first situation, we describe the tears as partial-thickness tears of the labrum, extending to the inferior surface of the superior labrum; others call these labral detachments.

Partial-thickness tears of the superior labrum may resemble the normal undercutting of hyaline cartilage between the labrum and the adjacent glenoid. The normal sulcus between the labrum and glenoid also may create confusion with labral tears. Tears and normal anatomy are distinguished by the fact that the linear high signal of a labral tear is oriented laterally, whereas the linear high signal from normal anatomy (sulcus or cartilage undercutting) is oriented in the opposite (medial) direction, following the normal curve (going with the flow) of the superior glenoid on coronal oblique images (Fig. 10-52). The bucket-handle tear of the labrum results in linear high signal traversing the entire substance of the superior labrum, separating it into medial and lateral halves (see Fig. 10-52C). The lateral labral fragment may displace inferiorly and be evident as a low signal intensity fragment within the glenohumeral joint on coronal oblique and axial images.

If high signal is present in the proximal biceps tendon, it indicates the tendon is abnormal and involved in the SLAP lesion. There is either diffuse high signal at the labral attachment or linear high signal from a longitudinal split of the tendon (Fig. 10-53). Determining the integrity of the biceps tendon is crucial when a SLAP lesion of the labrum is diagnosed.

Paralabral Cysts

Paralabral cysts occur next to the glenoid labrum, are similar to ganglion cysts, always are associated with labral tears, and may or may not be associated with instability. The cysts may be located anywhere, but most frequently are seen postero-superiorly in association with a posterior labral tear. These cysts form when joint fluid extravasates from the joint

through the labral tear, and if a ball-valve phenomenon exists, fluid accumulates. Water is reabsorbed from the cyst, and a thick proteinaceous material remains. MRIs show a multiloculated round or oval mass of low signal intensity on T1W images and high signal intensity on T2W images (Fig. 10-54). The labral tear associated with the cyst is inconsistently evident. These patients complain of pain more than instability. These cysts may cause symptoms of suprascapular nerve entrapment from their mass effect[55] if located in the appropriate site where the nerve passes.

GLAD Lesions

GLAD refers to a nondisplaced anteroinferior labral tear with an associated chondral injury (see Fig. 10-49).[56] This lesion results more from an impaction type of injury, rather than a shearing injury, as occurs with Bankart lesions. The labrum remains attached to the anterior scapular periosteum, distinguishing this from a Bankart lesion, which has a torn periosteum. On MR arthrography, contrast material extends into the cartilaginous defect (Fig. 10-55), but may or may not be seen in the small labral defect. The lesion results from impaction of the humeral head against the

---

BOX 10-17

SLAP Lesions

- At least 12 types described (at least 9 too many)
- Important features of SLAP lesions worth remembering
  - Labrum
    Detached from glenoid (extends posterior to biceps-labral anchor), *or*
    Partial-thickness tear, *or*
    Full-thickness (bucket-handle) tear
  - Biceps-labral anchor
    Torn, *or*
    Not torn

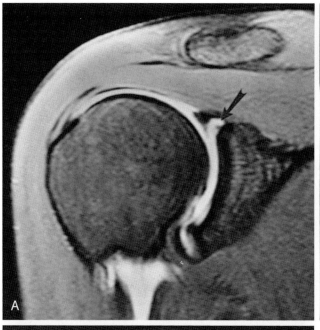

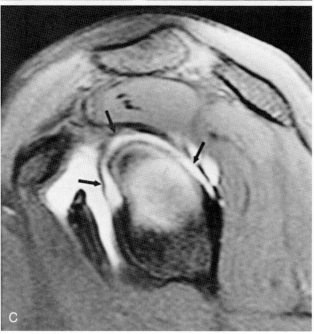

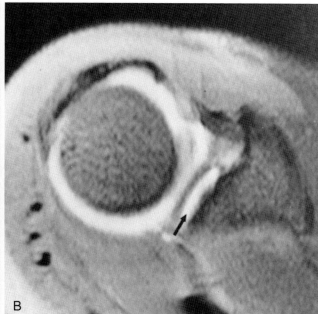

Figure 10-51 Superior labral tear propagating anterior and posterior (SLAP) lesion: detachment. **A,** T1 fat-suppressed coronal oblique shoulder MR arthrogram. The superior labrum is completely separated from the adjacent glenoid with no attachment identified (*arrow*). High signal contrast material fills the space between the glenoid and the detached labrum. If the labrum had an attachment to the glenoid, this high signal line would simply represent the normal sulcus between labrum and bone. **B,** T1 fat-suppressed axial shoulder MR arthrogram. The contrast material between the detached labrum and glenoid is seen (*arrow*) all the way across the top of the labrum, extending posterior to the predicted attachment site of the biceps tendon, which is located anterior on the superior labrum. **C,** T1 fat-suppressed sagittal oblique shoulder MR arthrogram. The separation between the labrum (*arrows*) and glenoid is filled with contrast material and involves the superior half of the glenoid.

articular surface of the glenoid with the arm in abduction and external rotation. These patients complain of pain rather than instability. The lesion can be treated with arthroscopic débridement without the need for a stabilization procedure.

Postoperative Shoulder

MRI of the postoperative shoulder ideally is performed after intra-articular injection of gadolinium. Gradient echo sequences should be avoided because of the blooming artifact created by hemosiderin or metal deposition that is present after surgery, which may prevent proper evaluation

of the joint. Knowledge of the surgical procedure performed is imperative. Postoperative MRIs show metallic and hemosiderin-related round foci of very low signal intensity along the surgical path on all imaging sequences. A band of scar tissue can be seen that is low signal intensity on T1W images and may be high signal intensity on T2W images during the first postoperative year, and low signal intensity after that.

IMPINGEMENT AND ROTATOR CUFF SURGERY

Acromioplasty is a common surgical treatment for mechanical impingement. This procedure is done either through an

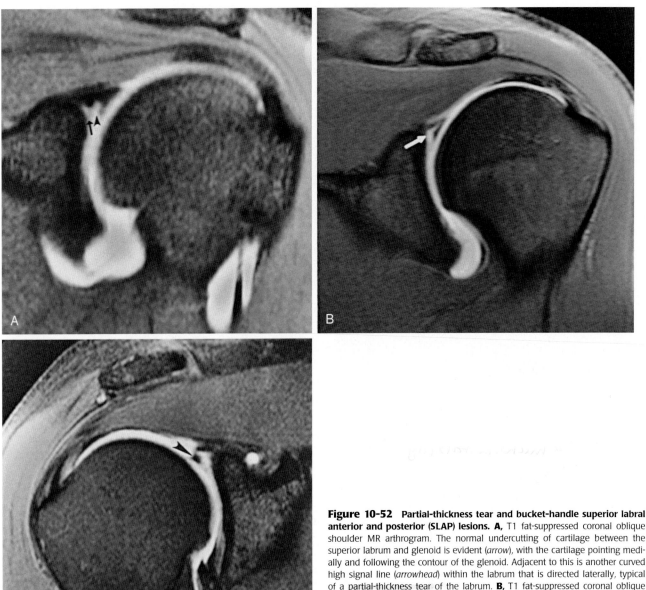

Figure 10-52 Partial-thickness tear and bucket-handle superior labral anterior and posterior (SLAP) lesions. A, T1 fat-suppressed coronal oblique shoulder MR arthrogram. The normal undercutting of cartilage between the superior labrum and glenoid is evident (*arrow*), with the cartilage pointing medially and following the contour of the glenoid. Adjacent to this is another curved high signal line (*arrowhead*) within the labrum that is directed laterally, typical of a partial-thickness tear of the labrum. **B,** T1 fat-suppressed coronal oblique shoulder MR arthrogram (different patient than in **A**). A high signal line in the labrum does not follow the contour of the glenoid and represents a larger partial-thickness SLAP tear than in **A**. **C,** T1 fat-suppressed coronal oblique shoulder MR arthrogram (different patient than in **A** or **B**). There is high signal in the superior labrum that separates the labrum into two pieces (full-thickness or bucket-handle tear). The lateral half of the labrum (*arrowhead*) is displaced inferiorly in the glenohumeral joint.

arthroscope or with open surgery. The acromioplasty consists of removing the anteroinferior acromion, which is the insertion site of the coracoacromial ligament, and excision of the subacromial/subdeltoid bursa, if inflamed. The undersurface of the acromion is smoothed with a burr; osteophytes on the undersurface of the acromioclavicular joint are removed, and, with severe degenerative joint disease of the acromioclavicular joint, the joint and the distal end of the clavicle are resected. MRI depicts the surgical changes and shows any persistent causes of impingement or the development of a full-thickness tear of the rotator cuff.

After surgery that involves tendons, detection of degeneration or of partial cuff tears by MRI is unreliable.[57] Full-thickness tears of the rotator cuff usually are repaired by open surgery via a superior approach through a split made in the deltoid muscle, although more surgeons are repairing full-thickness tears with arthroscopy. An anteroinferior acromioplasty is performed as part of the procedure; the cuff is treated with either a tendon-to-bone repair or a tendon-to-tendon anastomosis. With a tendon-to-bone repair, the surgical trough in the superolateral aspect of the greater tuberosity is seen as low signal intensity cortical irregularity.

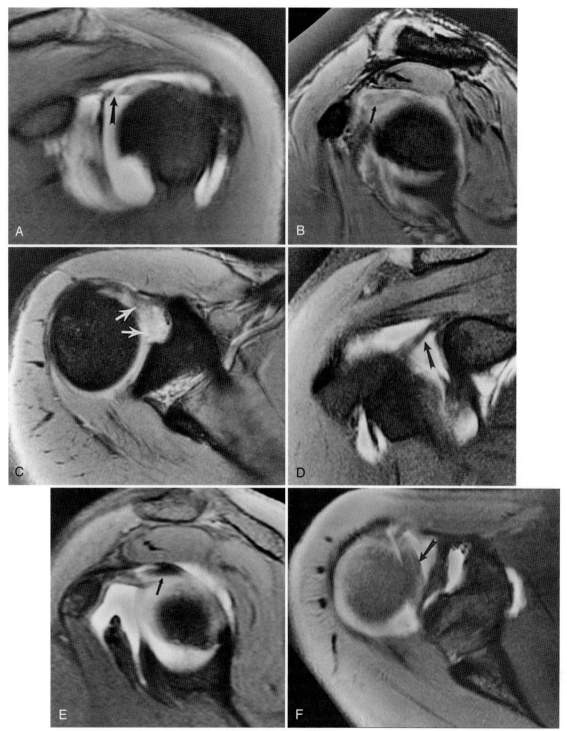

Figure 10-53   Superior labral anterior and posterior (SLAP) lesion with biceps anchor tears; normal biceps anchor for comparison. A-C, Biceps anchor tears. **A,** T1 fat-suppressed coronal oblique shoulder MR arthrogram. This patient has a bucket-handle SLAP tear of the superior labrum (not shown). The biceps anchor to the superior labrum also is torn, as manifested by high signal and irregularity in the proximal tendon (*arrow*). Compare with a normal biceps anchor in **D. B,** T1 fat-suppressed sagittal oblique shoulder MR arthrogram. The biceps anchor to the anterosuperior labrum is abnormally high signal (*arrow*) because of partial tears. Compare with normal biceps in **E. C,** T1 fat-suppressed axial shoulder MR arthrogram. The biceps anchor is high signal, difficult to identify, and wavy in appearance (*arrows*). The anterosuperior labrum is not evident on this image. Compare with normal biceps anchor in **F. D-F,** Normal biceps anchor (different patient than in **A-C**). **D,** T1 fat-suppressed coronal oblique shoulder MR arthrogram. The normal biceps anchor is taut and low signal (*arrow*). **E,** T1 fat-suppressed sagittal oblique shoulder MR arthrogram. The oval biceps tendon anchor (*arrow*) on the superior labrum is low signal. **F,** T1 fat-suppressed axial shoulder MR arthrogram. The normal biceps (*arrow*) courses obliquely in the anterior aspect of the upper shoulder to anchor to the superolateral labrum. It is taut, low signal, and easy to identify.

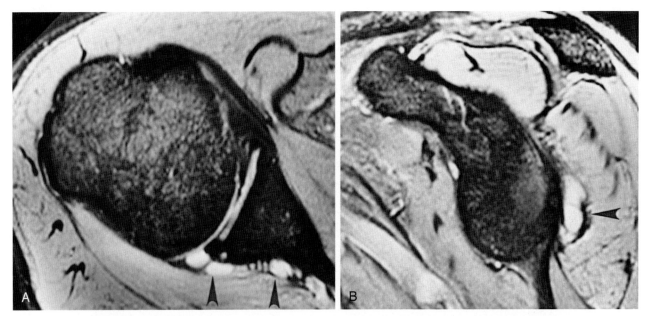

Figure 10-54 **Paralabral cysts. A,** T2* axial image of the shoulder. There are several high signal round structures (*arrowheads*) posterior to the glenoid with septations between them, typical of labral cysts. **B,** T2* sagittal oblique image of the shoulder. A portion of the paralabral cyst is seen posteroinferior to the glenoid (*arrowhead*) and adjacent to the labrum, which must be torn, even if the tear is not identified.

The tendon is usually of intermediate signal intensity, which may represent degeneration, postoperative granulation tissue, or partial tears. The diagnosis of a full-thickness tear is based on the presence of a high signal intensity gap in the tendon on T2W images, or on T1W images with intra-articular gadolinium, and retraction of the musculotendinous junction. The surgical repair may be incomplete, and the MR arthrogram may show filling of the subacromial/subdeltoid bursa, even if there is no recurrent tear.

SURGERY FOR INSTABILITY

The role of MRI in the postoperative evaluation of patients treated for instability is still unknown. No specific abnormalities after these surgical procedures have been described. The most accurate interpretation is obtained through a thorough understanding of the surgical procedure and in direct consultation with the referring surgeon.[58]

Miscellaneous Capsular, Bursal, and Tendon Abnormalities

ADHESIVE CAPSULITIS

Adhesive capsulitis, or frozen shoulder, is an inflammatory process that causes progressive capsular retraction. It affects women more frequently than men. Trauma, immobilization, hemiplegia, diabetes mellitus, and cervical disk disease are the most common predisposing factors. Clinically, adhesive capsulitis is characterized by shoulder pain at rest, at night, and with motion. These symptoms may mimic impingement and rotator cuff tears. Limitation of movement, mainly of abduction and external rotation, is progressive. The process is self-limited and usually lasts 12 to 18 months. Pain relief and improved range of motion can

be obtained with intra-articular injection of corticosteroids followed by physical therapy. The diagnosis can be confirmed with arthrography that shows a decreased joint capacity, small capsular recesses, and a serrated appearance of the capsular attachments. As discussed earlier, scar tissue preferentially involves the rotator interval in adhesive capsulitis and can be easily recognized on sagittal T1W images by obliteration of the subcoracoid fat (see Fig. 10-32).

SYNOVIAL CYSTS

Synovial cysts may occur at many different joints, but when they occur at the shoulder they tend to be quite large. Synovial cysts may occur as a consequence of rheumatoid arthritis, as a result of massive rotator cuff tears, or in the setting of a neuropathic arthropathy.

The shoulder is particularly predisposed to neuropathic changes in patients with a syrinx of the cervical spinal cord. Large synovial cysts may develop and dissect in the soft tissues a distance away from the shoulder joint and present a diagnostic dilemma on clinical grounds, with the masses usually being mistaken for soft tissue sarcomas. MRI is useful to show that the masses are cystic in nature and arise from the joint.

Massive rotator cuff tears (tears of more than one of the rotator cuff tendons) result in large joint effusions, which have access to the subacromial/subdeltoid bursa. The large fluid collections can protrude through the degenerated acromioclavicular joint and create a large soft tissue mass above the shoulder joint. The MRI features allow the diagnosis to be made by showing the communication of the mass with the acromioclavicular joint, and showing that the mass is cystic. The mass has low signal intensity on T1W images and becomes high signal intensity on any type of T2W image (Fig. 10-56). With intravenous gadolinium, only the periph-

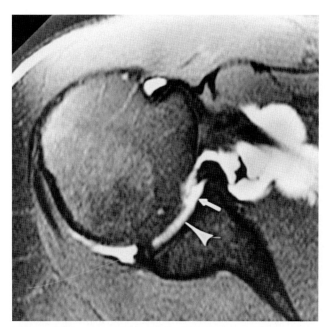

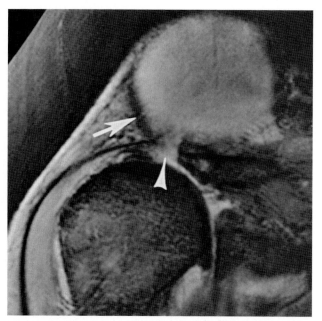

Figure 10-55 Glenolabral articular disruption (GLAD) lesion. T1 fat-suppressed axial shoulder MR arthrogram. The anterior glenoid has a chondral defect (*arrow*), which is filled with contrast material. The slightly lower signal hyaline cartilage (*arrowhead*) is seen posterior to the chondral defect. The anterior labrum appears normal on this image.

Figure 10-56 Synovial cyst secondary to a massive rotator cuff tear. T2* coronal image of the shoulder. This MRI study was done to evaluate a presumed sarcoma that was palpable above the shoulder. There is a large, round high signal mass (*arrow*) that is in direct communication with the acromioclavicular joint (*arrowhead*). There is absence of the supraspinatus tendon on this cut from a tear (subscapularis and infraspinatus tendons were torn on other images). There also is glenohumeral degenerative joint disease.

ery of the mass enhances showing a thin margin without irregular or thickened walls. The origin of synovial cysts that occur as a result of rheumatoid arthritis or other inflammatory arthritides should be obvious on MRI because of the concomitant findings of thickened synovium and osseous erosions within the joint.

CALCIFIC TENDINITIS AND BURSITIS

Calcium hydroxyapatite deposition disease occurs most commonly around the shoulder, with the supraspinatus tendon being the site most frequently involved. Many patients are asymptomatic; patients with symptoms present with pain at rest, at night, and with motion. They may have painful limitation of movement that mimics impingement syndrome. The calcification may develop in the tendon and progressively work its way from the tendon into the adjacent glenohumeral joint or into the adjacent subacromial/subdeltoid bursa.

These calcifications often are more easily recognized on radiographs than on MRIs, and, whenever possible, MRI studies should be correlated with the radiographs (or you will make a fool of yourself more often than you can afford). The calcifications are generally low signal intensity on all pulse sequences, similar to a normal tendon. They sometimes are lower signal intensity than normal tendons, in particular on T2* sequences (Fig. 10-57). There may be associated abnormalities in the involved tendon, such as thinning, thickening, and irregular margins. Calcific bursitis can be identified on MRIs as a distended subacromial/subdeltoid bursa filled with low signal intensity calcifications surrounded by high signal intensity fluid and synovitis on T2W

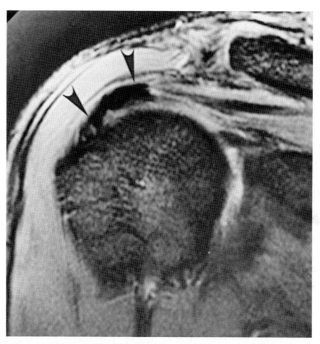

Figure 10-57 Calcific tendinitis. T2* coronal oblique image of the shoulder. There is very low signal (lower signal than tendon) in the distal 2 to 3 cm of the supraspinatus tendon (*arrowheads*) from calcium hydroxyapatite crystal deposition.

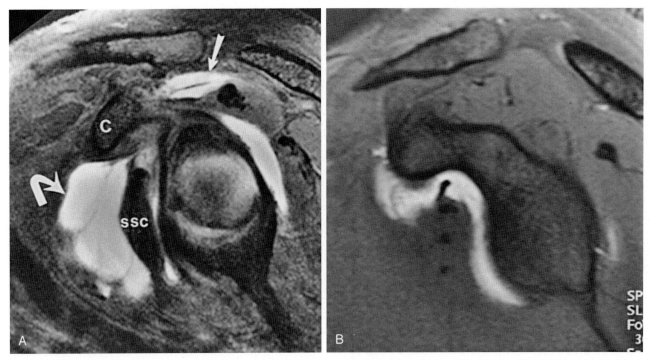

Figure 10-58 **Subcoracoid bursa and subscapularis recess. A,** T1 fat-suppressed sagittal oblique shoulder MR arthrogram. The shoulder joint was injected with contrast material, which filled the subacromial/subdeltoid bursa (*straight arrow*) owing to a rotator cuff tear. The subacromial bursa communicates with the subcoracoid bursa (*curved arrow*) in this patient, allowing filling of the bursa with contrast material. The subcoracoid bursa is located inferior to the coracoid process (C) and anterior to the subscapularis tendon/muscle (SSC). **B,** T1 fat-suppressed sagittal oblique shoulder MR arthrogram (different patient than in **A**). The subscapularis recess is filled with contrast material. It drapes over the top of the subscapularis tendon and muscle beneath the coracoid process. There is no high signal contrast material anterior to the subscapularis muscle because the subcoracoid bursa did not fill in this patient.

images. These findings usually are associated with an abnormal subjacent tendon.

SUBCORACOID BURSITIS

The subcoracoid bursa is a normal anatomic structure, located anterior to the subscapularis muscle and tendon. It may become inflamed and cause anterior shoulder pain. It does not communicate with the glenohumeral joint or the subscapularis recess of the shoulder joint. In about 20% of patients, the subcoracoid bursa communicates with the subacromial/subdeltoid bursa. It is positioned immediately anterior and inferior to the subscapularis recess of the shoulder joint, but is separated from it by a fibrous septum that should allow easy differentiation of the two structures should they both be distended with fluid. The subcoracoid bursa is bordered by the subscapularis posteriorly, and the coracoid process and the attached combined tendon of the short head of the biceps and the coracobrachialis superiorly and anteriorly.

On MRIs, this bursa is identified only if inflamed and filled with fluid (synovitis). It appears as an oblong soft tissue mass of low signal intensity on T1W and high signal intensity on T2W images in a characteristic location inferior to the coracoid process and anterior to the subscapularis muscle (Fig. 10-58), best seen on sagittal oblique images.[59] The subcoracoid bursa may be inadvertently injected during a shoulder MR arthrogram, mistaking it for the glenohumeral joint. If the subcoracoid bursa communicates with the subacromial/subdeltoid bursa, as it does in 20% of people,

there is contrast in the latter bursa that may mistakenly be interpreted as evidence of a rotator cuff tear. The key to the fact that no cuff tear is present is that no contrast material is evident in the glenohumeral joint, and the tendons are not disrupted, as well as the fact that no tear of the tendon is seen.

Nerve Abnormalities

SUPRASCAPULAR NERVE ENTRAPMENT
(Box 10-18)

Suprascapular nerve entrapment syndrome initially was described in male weightlifters who had shoulder pain and eventually weakness and muscle atrophy. These features were the result of compression of the suprascapular nerve, which runs superior to the scapula in an anteroposterior direction in the suprascapular notch. The suprascapular nerve provides sensory innervation to the acromioclavicular and glenohumeral joints. As the nerve courses through the suprascapular notch, it provides motor innervation to the supraspinatus and infraspinatus muscles, and as it extends distally into the spinoglenoid notch, it provides motor innervation only to the infraspinatus muscle (Fig. 10-59).[55]

The most common cause of suprascapular nerve compression is from a ganglion cyst, usually associated with a superior labral tear (Fig. 10-60), but other causes that affect the suprascapular notch, such as large veins (Fig. 10-61),[60] tumor, or fracture of the scapula, have been implicated.[61] If

Suprascapular Nerve Entrapment

- Mass in suprascapular or spinoglenoid notch compressing nerve
- Mass is usually a ganglion cyst arising from a labral tear
- Causes pain, weakness, and muscle atrophy in distribution of affected nerves
- Suprascapular notch: Nerve innervates supraspinatus and infraspinatus muscles
- Spinoglenoid notch: Nerve innervates infraspinatus only
- MRI
  - Shows the mass
  - Shows supraspinatus or infraspinatus muscle atrophy (increased signal intensity on T1 from fat infiltration of muscle)
  - Shows muscle edema in more subacute cases

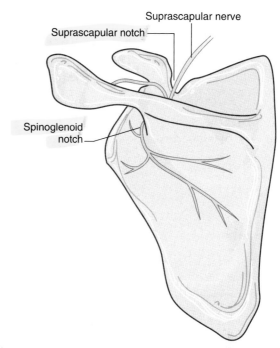

Figure 10-59 Suprascapular nerve. Diagram of the normal anatomy of the suprascapular nerve from a posterior perspective (innervates supraspinatus and infraspinatus) in the suprascapular notch on top of the scapula. Inferior to the suprascapular notch is the spinoglenoid notch, which contains only the nerve to the infraspinatus muscle.

the mass affects the suprascapular notch, the supraspinatus and the infraspinatus muscles are affected; if a mass is located in the spinoglenoid notch, only the infraspinatus muscle is affected. If entrapment is caused by a ganglion cyst, MRI shows a well-defined, round or oval septated mass of low signal intensity on T1W and high signal intensity on T2W images in the region of the suprascapular or spinoglenoid notch. If intravenous gadolinium is administered, the mass remains low signal intensity, with a thin line of peripheral enhancement on T1W images. The nerve compression is usually chronic and leads to fatty atrophy of the affected muscles, seen as high signal intensity on T1W images. Muscle edema can be seen as high signal on T2W1 in more subacute cases. Percutaneous drainage of the cyst and injection of corticosteroids in the lesion is an alternative to surgical removal, although the associated labral tear may need to be addressed surgically.

QUADRILATERAL SPACE SYNDROME
(Box 10-19)

Quadrilateral space syndrome results from compression of the axillary nerve that runs through this space. The quadri-

lateral space is located in the posterior aspect of the axilla. It is bounded by the humerus laterally, the long head of the triceps muscle medially, the teres minor muscle superiorly, and the teres major muscle inferiorly. The axillary nerve and the posterior humeral circumflex artery travel through this space (Fig. 10-62), and compression of the nerve may occur from fibrous bands, a mass, or a fracture of the scapula or proximal humerus. Pain and paresthesias involving the lateral aspect of the shoulder and the posterosuperior region

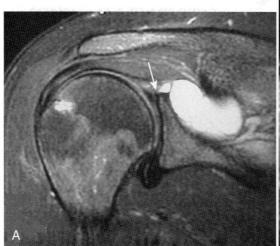
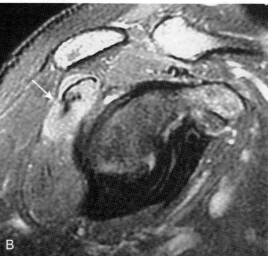

Figure 10-60 Suprascapular nerve compression from ganglion cyst. A, FSE T2 oblique coronal image of the shoulder. A large spinoglenoid notch cyst can be seen emanating from the posterosuperior labrum (*arrow*). **B,** FSE T2 sagittal oblique image of the shoulder. Atrophy and edema can be seen in the infraspinatus (*arrow*) owing to the cyst seen in **A** pressing on the suprascapular nerve.

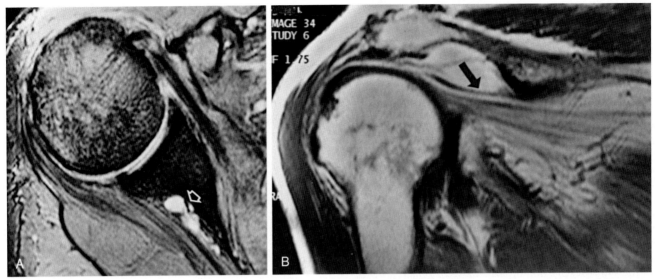

Figure 10-61   Spinoglenoid notch varices with nerve compression. A, T2* axial image of the shoulder. There are high signal varices (*open arrow*) in the spinoglenoid notch. The infraspinatus muscle posterior to the shoulder joint has a striated appearance caused by atrophy. **B,** T1 coronal oblique image of the shoulder. The infraspinatus muscle (*arrow*) is nearly totally replaced by fat because of atrophy from compression of the nerve by the varices in the spinoglenoid notch.

of the arm characterize the syndrome. The symptoms are exacerbated by abduction and external rotation. Eventually weakness and atrophy of the teres minor muscle may develop. It invariably spares the deltoid. On MRI, sagittal oblique images best show the fatty atrophy of these muscles, seen as high signal intensity on T1W images (Fig. 10-63).[62]

PARSONAGE-TURNER SYNDROME

Shoulder pain and weakness may be caused by acute brachial neuritis (Parsonage-Turner syndrome), which is probably the consequence of a viral inflammation of the nerves, although the exact etiology is unknown. The MRI findings of this acute neuromuscular disorder are initially those of muscle edema with high signal in muscle on T2W images (Fig. 10-64); later, muscle atrophy occurs with fatty infiltration that is high signal intensity within muscle on T1W images. The nerves (muscles) that have been reported to be involved with Parsonage-Turner include the suprascapular (supraspinatus and infraspinatus), axillary (teres minor and deltoid), subscapularis (subscapularis), and long thoracic (serratus anterior) (Box 10-20).[63,64] Although the etiology is unknown, precipitating factors include a recent viral infection, a recent vaccination, and general anesthesia.

MRI cannot distinguish between a brachial plexus or nerve injury and Parsonage-Turner syndrome, but the clinical presentation makes this an easy distinction. Parsonage-Turner syndrome has no trauma associated and has a sudden onset of pain with delayed weakness that follows the initial onset in 48 to 72 hours. Parsonage-Turner syndrome is seen in about 1% of our shoulder MRI studies.[64] It is self-limited, but can have a very prolonged course—sometimes a year or more in duration. It can be bilateral in 30% of cases. It was not described in the radiology literature until fat-suppressed imaging became routine, allowing the neurogenic edema to be identified.

Bone Abnormalities

POST-TRAUMATIC OSTEOLYSIS OF THE CLAVICLE

Post-traumatic osteolysis of the clavicle relates to bone resorption of the distal end of the clavicle after a single episode of severe trauma, or it may occur from repetitive trauma. Individuals who play contact sports, weightlifters, and swimmers are particularly prone to this problem. Clinically, patients present with localized pain increased by movement, with or without impingement, and swelling of the acromioclavicular joint.

MRI shows joint effusion or synovitis involving the acromioclavicular joint; loss of the black cortical line with resorption of the distal clavicle and, occasionally, of the medial end of the acromion; and bone marrow edema involving the distal end of the clavicle and acromion (Fig. 10-65).[65] In addition, signs of impingement may be present, such as loss

---

BOX 10-19
Quadrilateral Space Syndrome

Anatomic Boundaries of the Space
- Lateral: Humerus
- Medial: Long head, triceps
- Superior: Teres minor
- Inferior: Teres major

Clinical
- Compression of axillary nerve in quadrilateral space
  - Fibrous bands, mass, fracture fragments
- Pain, paresthesia, muscle atrophy

MRI
- Fatty atrophy of teres minor

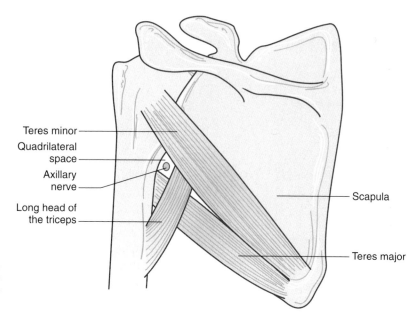

Figure 10-62 **Quadrilateral space anatomy.** Diagram of the quadrilateral space from a posterior perspective. The axillary nerve passes through the space formed by the humerus, teres major, triceps, and teres minor tendons.

or interruption of the fat plane separating the inferior aspect of the clavicle from the supraspinatus muscle, and swelling and synovial hypertrophy of the acromioclavicular joint indenting the supraspinatus muscle. A subchondral fracture line is often present suggesting these are sequela of trauma, or that an insufficiency fracture develops secondary to the osteoporosis.[66]

OCCULT FRACTURES

Fractures involving the proximal humerus or the glenoid may result from direct trauma or dislocation. These fractures may not be apparent on radiographs, but appear on MRI as either bone contusions or fractures. The characteristic sites of involvement after a shoulder dislocation have been described in the instability portion of this chapter. Another common site of occult fracture involves the greater tuberosity. Bone contusions are seen as poorly defined, heterogeneous, reticulated areas of intermediate to low signal intensity on T1W and high signal intensity on T2W images, which involves the cancellous bone. An acute, radiographically occult fracture is depicted by a linear or curvilinear line of low signal intensity, usually on T1W and T2W images, surrounded by poorly defined bone marrow edema of intermediate signal intensity on T1W and high signal intensity on T2W images (Fig. 10-66).

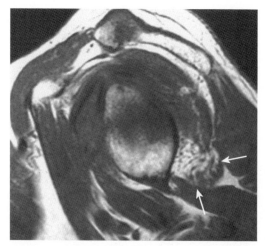

Figure 10-63 **Quadrilateral space syndrome: atrophy of teres minor.** T1 sagittal oblique image of the shoulder. The teres minor muscle (*arrows*) is atrophied and has fat infiltrating it, which creates a speckled appearance compared with the normal adjacent muscles. No mass was identified in the quadrilateral space, and this was presumed to be due to fibrous bands compressing the axillary nerve.

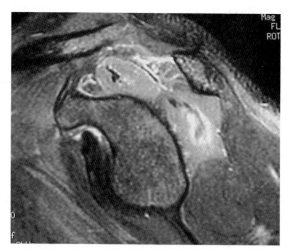

Figure 10-64 **Parsonage-Turner syndrome.** FSE T2 sagittal oblique image of the shoulder. Increased signal is seen throughout the supraspinatus and infraspinatus muscles in this patient with sudden onset of pain in the shoulder. This is neurogenic edema secondary to involvement of the suprascapular nerve in Parsonage-Turner syndrome.

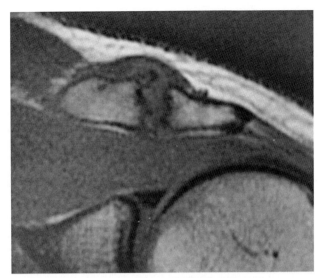

Figure 10-65 **Osteolysis of the distal clavicle.** T1 coronal oblique image of the shoulder. The distal end of the clavicle and, to a lesser extent, the medial acromion are irregular from bone resorption. There is synovitis of the acromio-clavicular joint, with a soft tissue mass centered at the joint. The synovitis impinges on the underlying supraspinatus muscle and obliterates the fat plane between the joint and muscle. This patient was a weightlifter.

AVASCULAR NECROSIS

The humeral head is the second most common site of osteo-necrosis after the femoral head. Osteonecrosis usually occurs secondary to a predisposing risk factor, such as corticoste-roids, marrow infiltrative disorders, or after a fracture of the anatomic neck of the humerus. MRI permits early detection of osteonecrosis in the shoulder, just as elsewhere in the skeleton. On T1W images, the area of necrosis is delineated by a well-defined, low signal intensity, serpiginous line or arc (Fig. 10-67). The center of the lesion is of variable signal intensity, depending on the pathologic alterations of the fragment, but most frequently the signal intensity is that of fat.

TUMORS (Box 10-21)

The shoulder girdle is not a site specific for any particular bone tumor. The most common primary bone tumor found incidentally on shoulder MRI is a benign enchondroma. It is a well-defined, lobular lesion of low signal intensity on T1W images and high signal intensity on T2W images, which may have stippled calcifications of low signal intensity (Fig. 10-68). Its malignant counterpart, chondrosarcoma, is the most common focal primary malignant tumor in the shoulder; the distinction from a benign enchondroma may be difficult to make unless there is destruction of the adjacent cortex, or a soft tissue mass.[67] Metastases and myeloma remain the most common malignant processes that affect the shoulder.

Soft Tissue Abnormalities

BENIGN AND MALIGNANT TUMORS

MRI is particularly helpful in detecting a soft tissue mass, defining its extent, and planning a biopsy. Lipoma and benign fibrous histiocytoma are the most common benign tumors that affect the shoulder girdle, whereas malignant fibrous histiocytoma and liposarcoma are the most common malignant soft tissue tumors in the shoulder. Elastofibromas are soft tissue masses that occur almost exclusively in the shoulder region, and their specific location may allow the diagnosis to be made by MRI.

Elastofibroma dorsi is a benign fibroelastic lesion that usually occurs in older women in a periscapular location. These lesions often are asymptomatic and bilateral. Elasto-

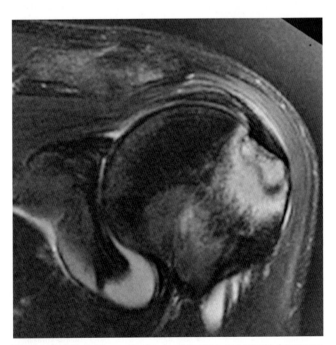

Figure 10-66 **Radiographically occult fracture.** Fast T2 with fat suppres-sion coronal oblique image of the shoulder. There is a nondisplaced fracture of the greater tuberosity with surrounding marrow edema. This was not evident radiographically.

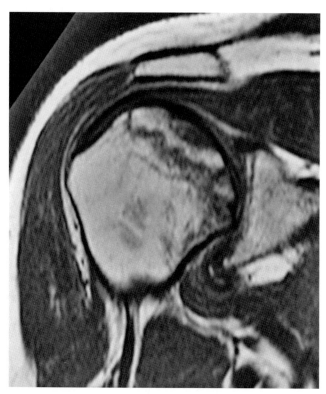

Figure 10-67   Avascular necrosis. T1 coronal oblique image of the shoulder. There is a serpiginous line in the humeral epiphysis, typical of avascular necrosis. A fracture could have a very similar appearance, but is rare in this location and should have lots of surrounding edema in the acute phase.

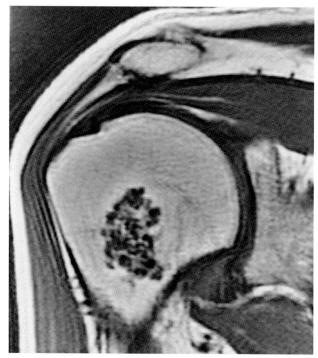

Figure 10-68   Enchondroma. T1 coronal oblique image of the shoulder. There are stippled, low signal calcifications in the humeral metaphysis from a benign enchondroma. There is no soft tissue mass, erosion of cortex, or other signs of an aggressive lesion to suggest a chondrosarcoma.

fibromas are located deep to the scapula or inferior to the tip of the scapula, usually involving the medial border. The MRI characteristics are of a mass with signal intensity similar to muscle on T1W and T2W images, with interspersed streaks of fat that are high signal on T1 (Fig. 10-69).[68]

MRI characteristics of soft tissue lesions usually are not sufficiently specific to permit a histologic diagnosis, or to differentiate between benign and malignant lesions, with the possible exceptions of lipomas, hemangiomas, paralabral ganglion cysts, and possibly elastofibromas.

PECTORALIS MUSCLE INJURIES

Tears of the pectoralis major muscle or tendon occasionally occur in athletes, especially in weightlifters as a result of bench-pressing. These tears result in pain and some loss of abduction strength. Treatment is either conservative or surgical, depending on precisely where the tear occurred. MRI can be valuable in making the diagnosis and in determining what type of therapy is optimal.[69]

The pectoralis major muscle is composed of two major heads, the clavicular and sternal, which converge laterally as they approach the humerus. The pectoralis major tendon attaches to the proximal shaft of the humerus at the bicipital groove.

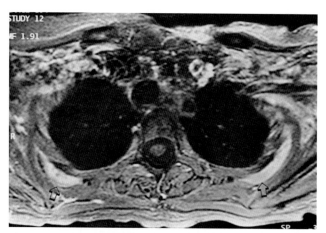

Figure 10-69   Elastofibromas. T1 axial fat-suppressed, contrast-enhanced image of the chest. There is diffuse contrast enhancement of bilateral periscapular masses (*open arrows*) in this elderly woman.

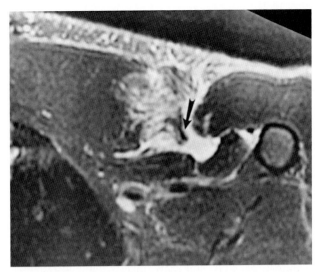

Figure 10-70 Pectoralis major muscle tear. Fast T2 with fat suppression axial image of the shoulder. There is edema on the medial side of the humerus, indicating avulsion of the pectoralis tendon attachment from the bone. The retracted tendon (*arrow*) is seen surrounded by high signal edema and hemorrhage in the muscle and fat planes. This patient was a weightlifter.

Pectoralis major tears are usually partial, but also may be complete. They may occur at different sites, such as the muscle belly, the musculotendinous junction, or the attachment of the tendon to the humerus. Surgery generally is the treatment for avulsions of the tendon from the humerus, whereas conservative treatment usually is warranted for injuries to the muscle or musculotendinous junction.

MRI in the axial and coronal oblique planes can show the muscle and tendon well. Tears have the same appearance as in all other muscles and depend on the age of the injury. Hemorrhage and edema (high signal on T2W images) can be seen in the lateral aspect of the muscle and surrounding the tendon (Fig. 10-70). High signal on T2W images around the humeral cortex is an important sign that the humeral periosteum has been stripped from the bone during an avulsion injury of the tendinous attachment to the bone.

REFERENCES

1. Kwak SM, Brown RR, Trudell D, et al. Glenohumeral joint: comparison of shoulder positions at MR arthrography. *Radiology* 1998; 208: 375-380.
2. Davis SJ, Teresi LM, Bradley WG, et al. Effect of arm rotation on MR imaging of the rotator cuff. *Radiology* 1991; 181:265-268.
3. Siebold CJ, Mallisee TA, Erickson SJ, et al. Rotator cuff: evaluation with US and MR imaging. *RadioGraphics* 1999; 19:685-705.
4. Vangsness CT Jr, Jorgenson SS, Watson T, et al. The origin of the long head of the biceps from the scapula and glenoid labrum: an anatomical study of 100 shoulders. *J Bone Joint Surg [Br]* 1994; 76:951-954.
5. Vinson EN, Helms CA, Higgins LD. Rim-rent tear of the rotator cuff: a common and easily overlooked partial tear. *AJR Am J Roentgenol* 2007; 189:943-946.
6. Kaplan PA, Bryans KC, Davick JP, et al. MR imaging of the normal shoulder: variants and pitfalls. *Radiology* 1992; 184:519-524.
7. Timins ME, Erickson SJ, Estkowski LD, et al. Increased signal in the normal supraspinatus tendon on MR imaging: diagnostic pitfall caused by the magic-angle effect. *AJR Am J Roentgenol* 1995; 165:109-114.
8. Erickson SJ, Cox IH, Hyde JS, et al. Effect of tendon orientation on MR imaging signal intensity: a manifestation of the "magic angle" phenomenon. *Radiology* 1991; 181:389-392.
9. Farley TE, Neumann CH, Steinbach LS, et al. The coraco-acromial arch: MR evaluation and correlation with rotator cuff pathology. *Skeletal Radiol* 1994; 23:641-645.
10. Rockwood CA Jr, Lyons FR. Shoulder impingement syndrome: diagnosis, radiographic evaluation and treatment with a modified Neer acromioplasty. *J Bone Joint Surg [Am]* 1993; 75:409-424.
11. Kieft GJ, Bloem JL, Rozing PM, et al. Rotator cuff impingement syndrome: MR imaging. *Radiology* 1988; 166:211-214.
12. Seeger LL, Gold RH, Bassett LW, et al. Shoulder impingement syndrome: MR findings in 53 shoulders. *AJR Am J Roentgenol* 1988; 150:343-347.
13. Bigliani LU, Ticker JB, Flatlow EL, et al. The relationship of the acromial architecture to rotator cuff disease. *Clin Sports Med* 1991; 10:823-838.
14. Park JG, Lee JK, Phelps CT. Os acromiale associated with rotator cuff impingement: MR imaging of the shoulder. *Radiology* 1994; 193:255-257.
15. Hijioka A, Suzuki K, Nakamura T, et al. Degenerative change and rotator cuff tears: an anatomical study in 160 shoulders of 80 cadavers. *Arch Orthop Trauma Surg* 1993; 112:61-64.
16. Getz JD, Recht MP, Piraino DW, et al. Acromial morphology: relation to sex, age, symmetry, and subacromial enthesophytes. *Radiology* 1996; 199:737-742.
17. Feller JF, Tirman PFJ, Steinbach LS, et al. Magnetic resonance imaging of the shoulder: review. *Semin Roentgenol* 1995; 30:224-239.
18. Rafii M, Hossein F, Sherman O, et al. Rotator cuff lesions: signal patterns at MR imaging. *Radiology* 1990; 177:817-823.
19. Codman E. *The Shoulder*. Boston: Thomas Todd Company; 1934.
20. Tuite MJ, Turnbull JR, Orwin JF. Anterior versus posterior, and rim-rent rotator cuff tears—prevalence and MR sensitivity. *Skeletal Radiol* 1998; 27:237-243.
21. Tuckman GA. Abnormalities of the long head of the biceps tendon of the shoulder: MR imaging findings. *AJR Am J Roentgenol* 1994; 163:1183-1188.
22. Cervilla V, Schweitzer ME, Ho C, et al. Medial dislocation of the biceps brachii tendon: appearance at MR imaging. *Radiology* 1991; 180: 523-526.
23. Chan TW, Dalinka MK, Kneeland JB, et al. Biceps tendon dislocation: evaluation with MR imaging. *Radiology* 1991; 179:649-652.
24. Tirman PFJ, Bost FW, Garvin GJ, et al. Posterosuperior glenoid impingement of the shoulder: findings at MR imaging and MR arthrography with arthroscopic correlation. *Radiology* 1994; 193:431-436.
25. Giaroli EL, Major NM, Higgins LD. MRI of internal impingement of the shoulder. *AJR Am J Roentgenol* 2005; 185:925-929.
26. Gerber C, Krushell RJ. Isolated rupture of the tendon of the subscapularis muscle: clinical features in 16 cases. *J Bone Joint Surg [Br]* 1991; 73:389-394.
27. Patte D. The subcoracoid impingement. *Clin Orthop Relat Res* 1990; 254:55-59.
28. Giaroli EL, Major NM, Lemley DE, et al. Coracohumeral interval imaging in subcoracoid impingement syndrome on MRI. *AJR Am J Roentgenol* 2006; 186:242-246.
29. Patten RM. Tears of the anterior portion of the rotator cuff (the subscapularis tendon): MR imaging findings. *AJR Am J Roentgenol* 1994; 162:351-354.
30. Harryman DT, Sidles JA, Harris SL, et al. The role of the rotator interval capsule in passive motion and stability of the shoulder. *J Bone Joint Surg [Am]* 1992; 74:53-66.
31. Morag Y, Jacobson JA, Shields G, et al. MR arthrography of rotator interval, long head of the biceps brachii, and biceps pulley of the shoulder. *Radiology* 2005; 235:21-30.
32. Mengiardi B, Pfirrmann CW, Gerber C, et al. Frozen shoulder: MR arthrographic findings. *Radiology* 2004; 233:486-492.
33. Harper KW, Helms CA, Haystead CM, et al. Glenoid dysplasia: incidence and association with posterior labral tears as evaluated on MRI. *AJR Am J Roentgenol* 2005; 184:984-988.
34. Massengill AD, Seeger LL, Yao L, et al. Labrocapsular ligamentous complex of the shoulder: normal anatomy, anatomic variation, and pitfalls of MR imaging and MR arthrography. *RadioGraphics* 1994; 14:1211-1223.
35. Palmer WE, Caslowitz PL, Chew FS. MR arthrography of the shoulder: normal intraarticular structures and common abnormalities. *AJR Am J Roentgenol* 1995; 164:141-146.

36. Chandnani VP, Gagliardi JA, Murnane TG, et al. Glenohumeral ligaments and shoulder capsular mechanism: evaluation with MR arthrography. *Radiology* 1995; 196:27-32.

37. Yeh LR, Kwak S, Kim Y-S, et al. Anterior labroligamentous structures of the glenohumeral joint: correlation of MR arthrography and anatomic dissection in cadavers. *AJR Am J Roentgenol* 1998; 171: 1229-1236.

38. Cvitanic O, Tirman PF, Feller JF, et al. Using abduction and external rotation of the shoulder to increase the sensitivity of MR arthrography in revealing tears of the anterior glenoid labrum. *AJR Am J Roentgenol* 1997; 169:837-844.

39. McCauley TR, Pope CF, Jokl P. Normal and abnormal glenoid labrum: assessment with multiplanar gradient-echo MR imaging. *Radiology* 1992; 183:35-37.

40. Loredo R, Longo C, Salonen D, et al. Glenoid labrum: MR imaging with histologic correlation. *Radiology* 1995; 196:33-41.

41. Kwak SM, Brown RR, Resnick D, et al. Anatomy, anatomic variations, and pathology of the 11- to 3-o'clock position of the glenoid labrum: findings on MR arthrography and anatomic sections. *AJR Am J Roentgenol* 1998; 171:235-238.

42. Tuite MJ, Orwin JF. Anterosuperior labral variants of the shoulder: appearance on gradient-recalled echo and fast spin-echo MR images. *Radiology* 1996; 199:537-540.

43. Tirman PFJ, Feller JF, Palmer WE, et al. The Buford complex—a variation of normal shoulder anatomy: MR arthrographic imaging features. *AJR Am J Roentgenol* 1996; 166:869-873.

44. Smith DK, Chopp TM, Aufdemorte TB, et al. Sublabral recess of the superior glenoid labrum: study of cadavers with conventional nonenhanced MR imaging, MR arthrography, anatomic dissection, and limited histologic examination. *Radiology* 1996; 201:251-256.

45. Jin W, Ryu KN, Kwon SH, et al. MR arthrography in the differential diagnosis of type II superior labral anteroposterior lesion and sublabral recess. *AJR Am J Roentgenol* 2006; 187:887-893.

46. Resnick D, Kang HS. Shoulder. In *Internal Derangements of Joints: Emphasis on MR Imaging*. Philadelphia: Saunders; 1997:163-333.

47. Beltran J, Rosenberg ZS, Chandnani VP, et al. Glenohumeral instability: evaluation with MR arthrography. *RadioGraphics* 1997; 17:657-673.

48. Ferrari JD, Ferrari DA, Coumas J, et al. Posterior ossification of the shoulder: the Bennett lesion. *Am J Sports Med* 1994; 22:171-175.

49. Tirman PFJ, Steinbach LS, Feller JF, et al. Humeral avulsion of the anterior shoulder stabilizing structures after anterior shoulder dislocation: demonstration by MRI and MR arthrography. *Skeletal Radiol* 1996; 25:743-748.

50. Richards RD, Sartoris DJ, Pathria MN, et al. Hill-Sachs lesion and normal humeral groove: MR imaging features allowing their differentiation. *Radiology* 1994; 190:665-668.

51. Neviaser TJ. The anterior labroligamentous periosteal sleeve avulsion lesion: a cause of anterior instability of the shoulder. *Arthroscopy* 1993; 9:17-21.

52. Chandnani VP, Yeager TD, DeBeradino T, et al. Glenoid labral tears: prospective evaluation with MR imaging, MR arthrography, and CT arthrography. *AJR Am J Roentgenol* 1993; 161:1229-1235.

53. Palmer WE, Caslowitz PL. Anterior shoulder instability: diagnostic criteria determined from prospective analysis of 121 MR arthrograms. *Radiology* 1995; 197:819-825.

54. Shankman S, Bencardino J, Beltran J. Glenohumeral instability: evaluation using MR arthrography of the shoulder. *Skeletal Radiol* 1999; 28:365-382.

55. Fritz RC, Helms CA, Steinbach LS, et al. Suprascapular nerve entrapment: evaluation with MR imaging. *Radiology* 1992; 182:437-444.

56. Saunders TG, Tirman PFJ, Linares R, et al. The glenolabral articular disruption lesion: MR arthrography with arthroscopic correlation. *AJR Am J Roentgenol* 1999; 172:171-175.

57. Gaenslen ES, Satterlee CC, Hinson GW. Magnetic resonance imaging for evaluation of failed repairs of the rotator cuff: relationship to operative findings. *J Bone Joint Surg [Am]* 1996; 78:1391-1396.

58. Haygood TM, Oxner KG, Kneeland JB, et al. Magnetic resonance imaging of the postoperative shoulder. *Magn Reson Imaging Clin N Am* 1993; 1:143-156.

59. Schraner AB, Major NM. MR imaging of the subcoracoid bursa. *AJR Am J Roentgenol* 1999; 172:1567-1571.

60. Carroll KW, Helms CA, Otte MT, et al. Enlarged spinoglenoid notch veins causing suprascapular nerve compression. *Skeletal Radiol* 2003; 32:72-77.

61. Tirman PFJ, Feller JF, Janzen DL, et al. Association of glenoid labral cysts with labral tears and glenohumeral instability: radiologic findings and clinical significance. *Radiology* 1994; 190:653-658.

62. Linker CS, Helms CA, Fritz RC. Quadrilateral space syndrome: findings at MR imaging. *Radiology* 1993; 188:675-676.

63. Helms CA, Martinez S, Speer KP. Acute brachial neuritis (Parsonage-Turner syndrome): MR imaging appearance—report of three cases. *Radiology* 1998; 207:255-259.

64. Gaskin CM, Helms CA. Parsonage-Turner syndrome: MR imaging findings and clinical information of 27 patients. *Radiology* 2006; 240:501-507.

65. De la Puente R, Boutin RD, Theodorou DJ, et al. Post-traumatic and stress-induced osteolysis of the distal clavicle: MR imaging findings in 17 patients. *Skeletal Radiol* 1999; 28:202-208.

66. Kassarjian A, Llopis E, Palmer WE. Distal clavicular osteolysis: MR evidence for subchondral fracture. *Skeletal Radiol* 2007; 36:17-22.

67. Murphey MD, Flemming DJ, Boyea SR, et al. Enchondroma versus chondrosarcoma in the appendicular skeleton: differentiating features. *RadioGraphics* 1998; 18:1213-1237.

68. Naylor MF, Nascimento AG, Sherrick AD, McLeod RA. Elastofibroma dorsi: radiologic findings in 12 patients. *AJR Am J Roentgenol* 1996; 167:683-687.

69. Connell DA, Potter HG, Sherman MF, Wickiewicz TL. Injuries of the pectoralis major muscle: evaluation with MR imaging. *Radiology* 1999; 210:785-791.

Shoulder Protocols

This is one set of suggested protocols; there are many variations that would work equally well.

SHOULDER MR ARTHROGRAM

Sequence No.	1	2	3 and 4	5
Sequence Type	T1 fat saturation	T2 fat saturation	T1 and T2 fat saturation	T1
Orientation	Coronal oblique	Coronal oblique	Axial	Sagittal oblique
Field of View (cm)	14	14	14	14
Slice Thickness (mm)	4	4	4	4
Contrast	Intra-articular			

Recipe for MR Arthrography

A. In a 20-mL syringe, draw up
- 3 mL iodinated contrast material
- 20 mL sterile saline

B. In a tuberculin syringe, draw up
- 0.1 mL gadolinium-DTPA

C. Inject gadolinium into the needle end of the 20-mL syringe in *A*. Mix the concoction (shaken, not stirred), and inject 10-12 mL

SHOULDER: WITHOUT ARTHROGRAPHY

Sequence No.	1	2	3	4	5
Sequence Type	T1	Fast T2 fat saturation	Fast T2 fat saturation	Fast T2 fat saturation	PD fat saturation
Orientation	Sagittal oblique	Sagittal oblique	Coronal oblique	Axial	Axial
Field of View (cm)	14	14	14	14	14
Slice Thickness (mm)	4	4	4	4	4
Contrast	No	No	No	No	No

SAMPLE STANDARD REPORT

Clinical Indications

Protocol

The routine protocol with multiple sequences and planes of imaging was used.

Discussion

1. **Joint effusion:** None

2. **Rotator cuff:** Tendons intact without evidence of tendinopathy or tears; normal muscles without evidence of atrophy, edema, or other abnormalities

3. **Long head of biceps tendon:** Normal in position, size, and signal

4. **Glenoid labrum:** No tear, detachment, or other abnormalities shown; no paralabral cysts

5. **Subacromial/subdeltoid bursa:** Normal without evidence for bursitis

6. **Acromioclavicular and glenohumeral joints:** No osteoarthritis or other abnormalities

7. **Osseous structures:** Normal

8. **Other abnormalities:** None

Opinion

Normal MRI of the (right/left) shoulder.

Scout		Final Image
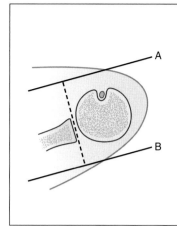	Axial scout Obtain coronal oblique images perpendicular to glenoid articular surface (dashed line) Cover from line A to B Film from posterior to anterior Obtain coronal plane first (most valuable)	Coronal oblique 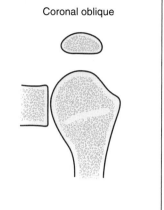

Scout		Final Image
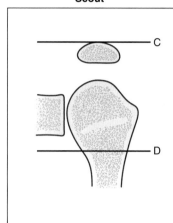	Coronal scout Obtain axial images Cover from line C at acromion to line D at inferior glenoid	Axial 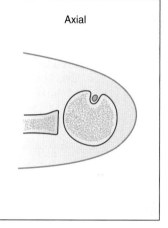

Scout		Final Image
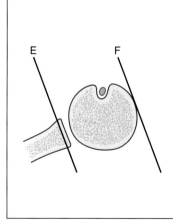	Axial scout Obtain sagittal images parallel to glenoid articular surface Cover from line E at glenohumeral joint to line F at edge of humeral head	Sagittal oblique 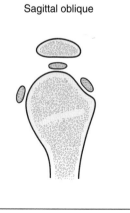

Elbow

11

How to Image the Elbow

- *Coils and patient position:* The elbow typically is scanned with the patient in a supine position with the arm at the side and palm up. A surface coil is imperative for obtaining high-quality images. Occasionally, the size of the patient precludes supine imaging because the surface coil would be too close to the magnet. These patients can be scanned prone with the arm overhead and the elbow as completely extended as possible. Patient comfort is most important for optimal imaging. Positioning the patient comfortably results in a higher yield of images not degraded by motion artifact. Using a vitamin E capsule to mark the area of the patient's pain or palpable mass is useful for assessing whether the area of concern has been evaluated in the field of view; this is especially important if the examination is normal.

- *Image orientation (Box 11-1):* The elbow should be scanned beginning about 10 cm above the elbow joint through the bicipital tuberosity distally. For convenience, the image should be oriented in the same way as in conventional radiography—the humerus at the top of the image. The axial images should be oriented with the volar surface superiorly.

- *Pulse sequence and regions of interest:* Axial imaging enables evaluation of tendons, ligaments, bone pathology, and neurovascular bundles. The axial images need to continue through the bicipital (radial) tuberosity to identify the biceps insertion. Coronal imaging is ideal for assessing the integrity of the collateral ligaments and the common flexor and extensor tendon origins. Sagittal images are useful to evaluate the biceps and triceps tendons. Additionally, loose bodies are often best seen on sagittal images. Generally, as with most joint imaging, a slice thickness of 3 mm is reasonable, with a 10% interslice gap (translation 0.3 mm). T1W images show anatomy, particularly in the axial plane, where nerves can be seen surrounded by fat. It is useful to apply fat suppression to T2W fast spin echo imaging because it makes the appearance of pathologic fluid more conspicuous. Because of the unique magnetic susceptibility properties of T2* imaging, this technique can be used when searching for loose bodies. This technique should not be used in a postsurgical elbow because of the amount of artifact created by micrometallic debris. The degree of artifact surrounding orthopedic hardware is most prominent on T2* sequences because of the lack of a 180-degree refocusing pulse, and is least prominent on fast spin echo sequences because of the presence of multiple 180-degree pulses.

• *Contrast:* Intravenous gadolinium may provide useful information in the assessment of synovial-based processes or to distinguish cystic from solid masses around the elbow. Intra-articular gadolinium is useful in patients without a joint effusion to detect loose bodies, capsular disruption, and partial tears of the ulnar collateral ligament or to assess the stability of an osteochondral fragment. The dilution is the same for shoulder arthrography (0.1 mL gadolinium mixed with 20-25 mL normal saline). The solution is injected to maximal distention of the joint as indicated by resistance to further injection. This usually occurs at about 10 mL of fluid injected.

Normal and Abnormal

Elbow abnormalities are increasing as the number of individuals participating in weightlifting and throwing and racquet sports increases. (Even couch potatoes are at risk from overuse of the elbow in consuming 12-oz. beverages.) The elbow is one of the most fascinating joints in the body to evaluate. It is the second most congruous joint in the body (knee), and allows for abnormalities to be present in more than one location in the joint. The understanding of elbow pathology is becoming more sophisticated with the advent of improved imaging techniques and the evolution of surface coils. MRI offers superior depiction of muscles, ligaments, and tendons, and the ability to visualize directly bone marrow, articular cartilage, and neurovascular structures.

BONES

Normal Relationships

The osseous anatomy of the elbow allows for two complex motions: flexion-extension and pronation-supination. The elbow is composed of three articulations contained within a common joint cavity. The radius articulates with the capitellum allowing for pronation and supination, and the ulna articulates with the trochlea of the humerus in a hinge fashion. The proximal radioulnar joint is composed of the radial head, which rotates within the radial (sigmoid) notch of the ulna, allowing supination and pronation. The radio-ulnar joint space also is responsible for one third of the stability of the elbow.

Osseous Disorders

Osteochondritis Dissecans and Panner's Disease (Box 11-2). Although osteochondritis dissecans can occur in throwers and in nonthrowers, in dominant and in nondominant elbows, and in the capitellum and in the radial head, it tends to occur in the capitellum of the dominant arm in throwers.[1-6] The exact cause is uncertain, but the leading hypothesis is that the lesion results from a combination of tenuous blood supply to the capitellum and repetitive trauma at the radiocapitellar joint, resulting in bone death.[7]

MRI can determine the stability of the osteochondral injury. Unstable lesions are characterized by high signal fluid that encircles the osteochondral fragment on T2W images. Round, cystic lesions may be seen beneath the osteochondral fragment, and abnormal high signal may be seen on the T2W images within the fragment of bone (Fig. 11-1). The overlying cartilage is not always damaged and should be closely inspected. The overlying cartilage is intact in stable lesions

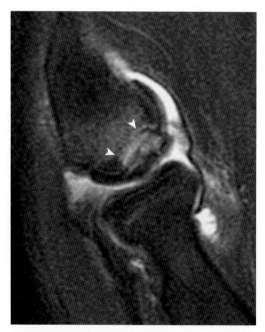

Figure 11-1 **Osteochondritis dissecans.** Sagittal T2W image shows irregularity to the capitellum with low signal bone marrow edema (*arrowheads*). This lesion is unstable by MRI criteria.

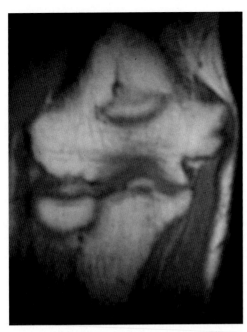

Figure 11-2   Pseudodefect of capitellum. Coronal T1W image located posteriorly shows irregularity of the capitellum without surrounding edema. Knowledge of this appearance prevents overdiagnosing osteochondritis dissecans of the capitellum.

and usually is treated with rest and splinting. Unstable lesions are either pinned or excised.

Osteochondritis dissecans has been replaced in the literature by the term *osteochondral lesion*. This entity should be distinguished from Panner's disease (an osteochondrosis of the capitellum), which coincidentally also occurs in throwers as a result of trauma. The MRI appearance, patient's age, and prognosis differ. An osteochondral lesion is seen in slightly older patients (12-16 years), whereas Panner's disease is in

patients 5 to 10 years old. Loose body formation usually is not seen with Panner's disease, and the entire capitellum generally is abnormal in signal (low signal on T1W images and high signal on T2W images) and may show irregular contour to the capitellum. Subsequent follow-up imaging in Panner's disease reveals normalization of these changes with little to no residual deformity at the articular surface. An osteochondral lesion can lead to intra-articular loose bodies and significant residual deformity of the capitellum.

A pitfall in diagnosing an osteochondral lesion is the pseudodefect of the capitellum. This pseudodefect occurs because the most posterior portion of the capitellum has an abrupt slope. A coronal image through the posterior capitellum mimics a defect. Examination of this area in another plane and the lack of edema support the pseudodefect as the cause of the irregularity of the capitellum (Fig. 11-2). Additionally, an osteochondral lesion generally begins on the anterior convex margin of the capitellum, whereas a pseudodefect is a finding in the posterior capitellum.

Unstable osteochondral lesions may fragment and migrate throughout the joint as loose bodies. Loose bodies also can occur from purely cartilaginous fragments breaking off in the joint from acute trauma or degenerative joint disease. Loose bodies can become large and cause mechanical symptoms, limiting mobility of the joint, or produce a synovitis that results in an effusion and stiff elbow (Fig. 11-3). Loose bodies may be identified in the posterior compartment in a throwing athlete and are easier to detect on MRI when joint fluid is present in the joint space; they appear as low to intermediate signal structures within high signal fluid. Occasionally, a loose body can have marrow within it. The signal characteristics follow that of fat, high in signal on T1W images. Axial and sagittal images aid in the diagnosis and location of loose bodies. Small fragments of cortical bone result in blooming on T2* sequences, which may make them more conspicuous than on other imaging sequences.

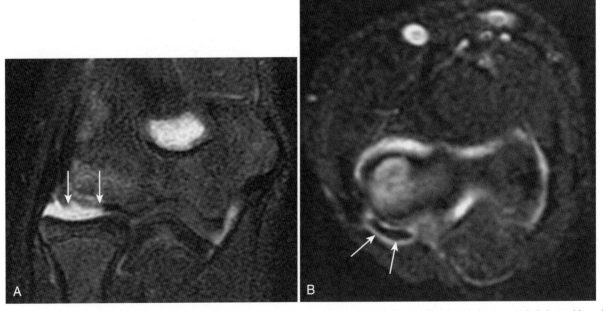

Figure 11-3   Loose body. A, Coronal T2W image of cartilage shows defect along capitellum (*arrows*). **B,** Axial T2W image shows posteriorly located loose body (*arrows*).

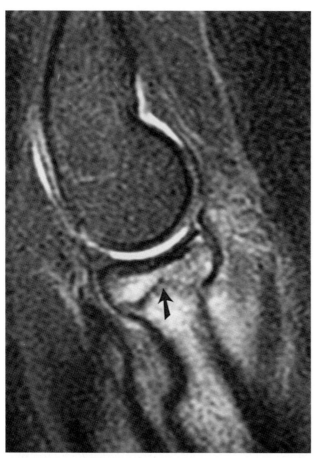

Figure 11-4 **Occult radial head fracture.** A female patient with a clinical diagnosis of biceps tendon tear. Sagittal FSE T2W fat-suppressed image shows a linear low signal fracture line along the radial head (*arrow*), with surrounding edema. There was no biceps tendon tear.

Fractures. MRI is useful in evaluating radiographically occult fractures when there is radiographic evidence of a joint effusion, but a fracture is not visualized. Marrow-sensitive sequences (T1W imaging, [fast] STIR, and fat-suppressed fast spin echo) are the most sensitive for assessing the fracture and edema associated with it (Fig. 11-4). Gradient echo is the least sensitive technique for evaluating the marrow. MRI is outstanding for evaluating stress fractures. One type of stress fracture diagnosis that is important in the elbow involves the middle third of the olecranon (Fig. 11-5). This type of fracture is seen in throwing athletes as a result of overload by the triceps mechanism. These fractures can displace and require surgical fixation. Similarly, nonunion of an injury through the olecranon physeal plate can be detected and may require surgical intervention. MRI can adequately assess fractures extending through the cartilage of the physis.

LIGAMENTS

The anterior and posterior portions of the joint capsule are thin. The medial and lateral portions are thickened to form the collateral ligaments. The ligaments of the elbow are divided into the radial and ulnar collateral ligament complexes.

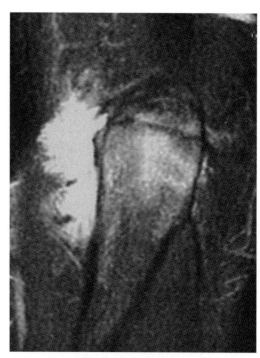

Figure 11-5 **Stress fracture of the olecranon.** Coronal T2W image with fat suppression shows bone marrow edema at middle third of olecranon.

Radial Collateral Ligament Complex (Box 11-3)

Normal Radial Collateral Ligaments. The radial collateral ligament complex provides varus stability. This complex consists of the radial collateral ligament, the annular ligament, the accessory collateral ligament, and the lateral ulnar collateral ligament (Fig. 11-6). The annular ligament surrounds the radial head, and originates and inserts onto the anterior and posterior margins of the lesser sigmoid notch of the ulna. It is the primary stabilizer of the proximal radioulnar joint and is best seen on axial images (Fig. 11-7). The radial collateral ligament proper arises from the anterior margin of the lateral epicondyle and inserts onto the annular ligament and fascia of the supinator muscle (Fig. 11-8). The lateral ulnar collateral ligament is more posterior and is absent in 10% of anatomic specimens; it is thought to provide the primary restraint to varus stress. It is a more superficial and posterior continuation of the radial collateral ligament, arising from the lateral epicondyle and extending along the lateral and posterior aspect of the proximal radius to insert on the ulna at the crista supinatoris (Fig. 11-9).

BOX 11-3

Radial Collateral Ligament Complex

- Restrains varus stress
- Lateral ulnar collateral ligament—most important
- Radial collateral ligament—less important
- Radial collateral ligament complex injury
  - MRI: increased T2 or complete disruption
  - Lateral ulnar collateral ligament insufficiency leads to posterolateral rotatory instability
- Associated with lateral epicondylosis (tennis elbow)

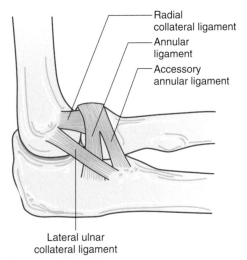

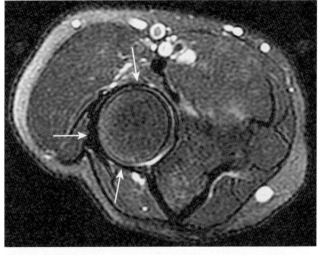

Figure 11-6. **Radial collateral ligament complex.** Diagram of the lateral side of the elbow showing components of the radial collateral ligament complex.

Figure 11-7 **Annular ligament.** Axial T2W image with fat suppression shows the annular ligament surrounding the radial head (*arrows*).

The origin of the three ligaments is immediately adjacent and deep to the common extensor tendon. Functionally, the lateral ulnar collateral ligament is more important because it is the primary posterolateral elbow stabilizer and maintains the support of the radial head and radioulnar articulation. The radial collateral ligament proper and the lateral ulnar collateral ligament are well seen on coronal images, and both should be evaluated as discrete structures because of their difference in functional significance. The lateral ulnar collateral ligament is often identified on the same coronal image as the pseudodefect.

Abnormal Radial Collateral Ligaments. Disruption of the lateral collateral ligament complex is more unusual than that of the ulnar collateral ligament complex. Job-related or sports-related injuries usually result in chronic, repetitive microtrauma that produces varus stress. Injury to the radial collateral ligament complex commonly is associated with lateral epicondylar soft tissue degeneration and tearing of the common extensor tendon (*lateral epicondylosis* or *tennis elbow*). Acute varus injury or elbow dislocation also can be associated with radial collateral ligament complex injury. Insufficiency of the lateral ulnar collateral ligament may

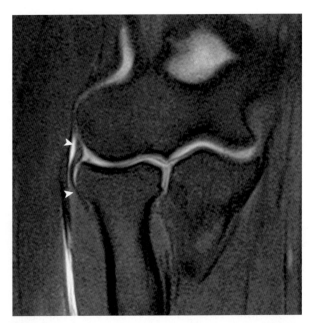

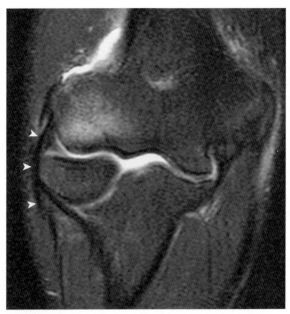

Figure 11-8 **Normal radial collateral ligament.** Coronal T2W image with fat suppression shows vertically oriented radial collateral ligament (*arrowheads*).

Figure 11-9 **Normal lateral ulnar collateral ligament.** Coronal T2W image with fat suppression shows obliquely oriented lateral ulnar collateral ligament (*arrowheads*).

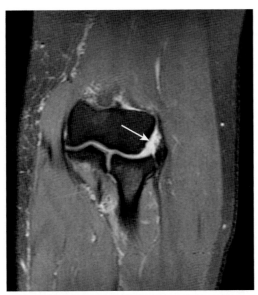

Figure 11-10   Radial collateral ligament tear. Coronal T2W image with fat suppression shows high signal at the origin of the proximal aspect of the radial collateral ligament (*arrow*). This appearance is compatible with a tear of the radial collateral ligament. Note also a partial tear of the extensor tendon.

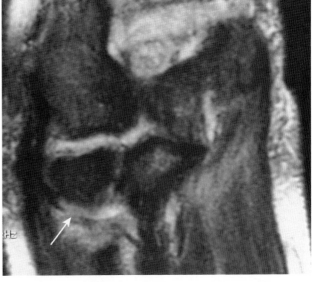

Figure 11-11   Lateral ulnar collateral ligament tear. Coronal T2W image with fat suppression shows high signal in midsubstance of lateral ulnar collateral ligament (*arrow*).

result in posterolateral rotatory instability, which allows transient rotatory subluxation of the ulnohumeral joint and secondary subluxation or dislocation of the radiohumeral joint. Rupture of this ligament occurs most commonly as a result of a posterior dislocation or varus stress.

Insufficiency of the lateral ulnar collateral ligament also may occur after a lateral extensor release for tennis elbow (because of the close proximity of the origin of the ligaments and tendons) or with resection of the radial head.[8] This injury most often is seen in patients who sustain a fall on an outstretched hand with resulting hyperextension and varus stress. Laxity of the lateral ulnar collateral ligament after surgical lateral extensor release for tennis elbow has been described as a result of extensive subperiosteal elevation of the common extensor tendon and radial collateral ligament complex during surgery, and as a result of unrecognized lateral ulnar collateral ligament insufficiency preoperatively.[8,9] Patients frequently complain of locking or snapping of the elbow. The physical examination may produce pain over the lateral aspect of the elbow, a subjective complaint

of laxity or instability with varus stress, and a positive lateral pivot shift maneuver.

At surgery, laxity or disruption of the lateral ulnar collateral ligament and the posterolateral portion of the capsule and possible radial collateral ligament laxity can be identified. Reconstruction or reattachment of the lateral ulnar collateral ligament on the lateral epicondyle is performed.

A sprain of the radial collateral ligament complex appears as a thickened or thinned ligament with high signal in and around it. A complete tear shows discontinuous fibers along the radial collateral ligament or lateral ulnar collateral ligament. Proximal detachment or avulsion of their common origin on the lateral epicondyle shows edema and hemorrhage extending into the defect and absence of the fibers of

BOX 11-4

Ulnar Collateral Ligament

Restrains Valgus Stress

- Bundles
  - Anterior (the important one)
  - Posterior
  - Transverse
- Best seen on coronal images
- Ulnar collateral ligament injury
  - MRI: increased T2, thickening (partial tear) or complete disruption
- Partial ulnar collateral ligament tear
  - Fluid between distal ligament and ulna (deep fibers disrupted)

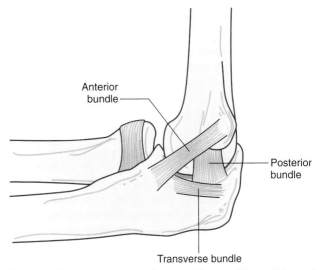

Figure 11-12   Medial collateral ligament. Diagram of the medial aspect of the elbow, showing components of the medial collateral ligament.

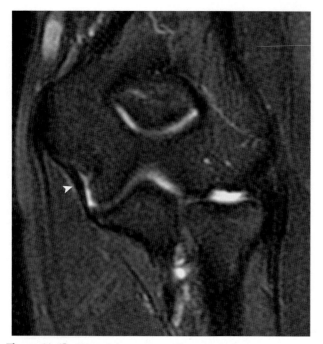

Figure 11-13 **Normal ulnar collateral ligament.** Coronal T2W image with fat suppression shows a normal ulnar collateral ligament (anterior bundle) (*arrowhead*). The ulnar collateral ligament adheres tightly to the olecranon.

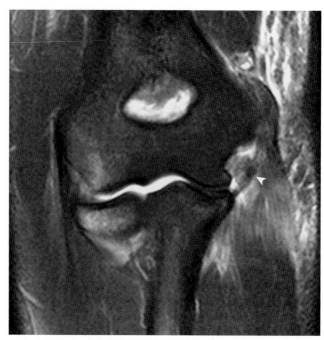

Figure 11-14 **Complete ulnar collateral ligament tear.** Coronal T2W image with fat suppression shows abnormal high signal through the disrupted ulnar collateral ligament (*arrowhead*). Increased signal also is noted in common flexor muscle groups.

the radial collateral ligament complex (Figs. 11-10 and 11-11).[10-12] When the lesion is seen in association with lateral epicondylosis, bone marrow edema in the lateral epicondyle and high signal in the extensor tendon group can be identified. If surgical release of the common extensor tendon is being considered, the integrity of the lateral ulnar collateral ligament must be assessed.

Ulnar Collateral Ligament Complex (Box 11-4)

Normal Ulnar Collateral Ligaments. The ulnar collateral ligament complex consists of three bundles: the anterior, posterior, and transverse bundles (Fig. 11-12). The anterior bundle is a thick, discrete ligament with parallel fibers arising from the medial epicondyle and inserting onto the medial coronoid process; it is the most important of the ligaments and is well seen on coronal images. The MRI appearance is that of a low signal linear structure that is flared proximally and tapers distally on all imaging sequences (Fig. 11-13). It is normal to see slight high signal in the proximally flared portion of the anterior bundle. The anterior bundle of the ulnar collateral ligament provides the primary restraint to valgus stress and commonly is damaged secondary to overuse in throwers.

The fan-shaped posterior bundle of the ulnar collateral ligament is a thickening of the capsule that is best defined with the elbow flexed at 90 degrees. The transverse bundle of the ulnar collateral ligament is formed from horizontally oriented capsule fibers joining the inferior margins of the anterior and posterior bundles. It stretches between the tip of the olecranon and the coronoid and does not contribute

to elbow stability because of ulna origin and insertion. The transverse and posterior bundles are located deep to the ulnar nerve and, in conjunction with the capsule, form the floor of the cubital tunnel. The posterior and transverse bundles are not well depicted on MRI, but their integrity is inferred based on the floor of the cubital tunnel; regardless, they are of limited importance and inconsistently present, and are not considered further here.

Abnormal Ulnar Collateral Ligaments. Ulnar collateral ligament injury commonly occurs in throwing athletes and may accompany an injury to the common flexor tendon group. Injury to these medial stabilizing structures is caused by chronic microtrauma from repetitive valgus stress during the acceleration phase of throwing.[13-15]

Complete rupture of the anterior bundle of the ulnar collateral ligament usually occurs suddenly. Patients with acute ulnar collateral ligament ruptures report sudden pain with or without a popping sensation that occurred with throwing, and they are unable to throw after the injury. These injuries are well seen on coronal MRIs. Abnormal signal is identified in the expected location of the linear, low signal structure of the ulnar collateral ligament (Fig. 11-14). The torn fragments also can be identified.

In a large series of throwing athletes, midsubstance ruptures of the anterior bundle of the ulnar collateral ligament accounted for 87% of ulnar collateral ligament tears, whereas distal and proximal avulsions were found in 10% and 3%, respectively.[16] Chronic degeneration of the ulnar collateral ligament is characterized by thickening of the ligament secondary to scarring, often accompanied by foci of calcifica-

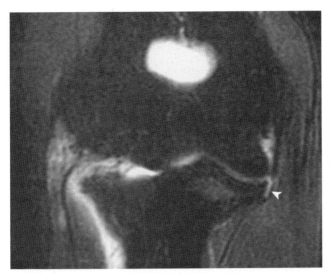

Figure 11-15 Partial ulnar collateral ligament tear. A javelin thrower with medial elbow pain. Coronal T2W image with fat suppression after intra-articular contrast (gadolinium) administration shows high signal deep to the fibers of the ulnar collateral ligament, separating bone from ligament (*arrowhead*). This has been referred to as the T sign. The ligament normally is tightly adherent to the ulna. Incidentally noted is contrast material in lateral soft tissues from a technical mishap during injection.

BOX 11-5

Anatomy of Muscles Around the Elbow

Anterior
- Biceps superficial to brachialis
- Bicipital aponeurosis
- Biceps tendon; extrasynovial paratenon

Posterior
- Triceps, anconeus

Medial
- Pronator teres, flexors of hand and wrist
- Common flexor tendon

Lateral
- Supinator, brachioradialis, extensors of hand and wrist

tion or heterotopic bone.[16] Treatment for acute ulnar collateral ligament tears is changing. Conservative treatment is recommended for non-elite athletes (mere mortals) because the flexor-pronator mass keeps the elbow functionally stable, although throwing is limited. Surgical reconstruction for competitive athletes has been recommended for many years.

Partial detachment of the deep undersurface fibers of the anterior bundle of the ulnar collateral ligament also may occur. These patients present with medial elbow pain. The diagnosis with routine MRI is difficult. This type of tear of the ulnar collateral ligament spares the superficial fibers of the anterior bundle and is invisible from an open surgical approach unless the undersurface of the ligament is inspected.[17,18] These tears are more easily identified after the injection of intra-articular contrast material (MR arthrography). The capsular fibers of the anterior bundle, which normally insert on the medial margin of the coronoid process, show fluid beneath the distal extension of the anterior bundle (Fig. 11-15).[18,19] This is often a very subtle finding, but can cause functional debilitation in a throwing athlete. Partial tears are treated with repair or reconstruction in athletes.

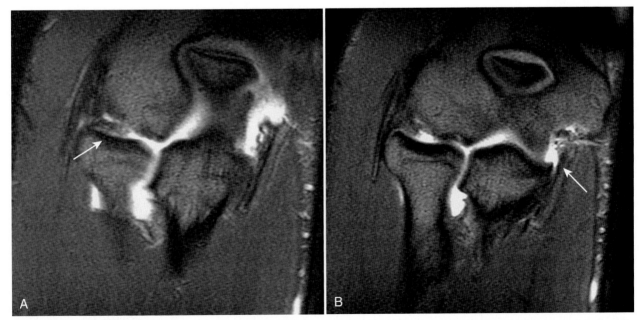

Figure 11-16 Synovial fringe. A, Coronal T2W image with fat suppression after intra-articular contrast administration shows thick intermediate signal tissue in the radiocapitellar joint space (*arrow*). **B,** Image of the same patient shows abnormal signal and morphology of ulnar collateral ligament (*arrow*) consistent with laxity and chronic injury.

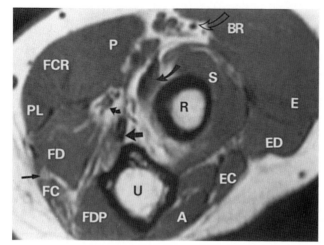

Figure 11-17 Normal muscle and nerve anatomy. T1W axial image just distal to the elbow joint. *Long curved black arrow* indicates biceps tendon. *Straight arrow* indicates brachialis tendon. *Short black arrow* indicates ulnar nerve. *Short curved arrow* indicates ulnar artery and median nerve. *Open arrow* indicates radial artery and superficial radial nerve. A, anconeus muscle; BR, brachioradialis muscle; E, extensor carpi radialis longus/brevis muscle; EC, extensor carpi ulnaris muscle; ED, extensor digitorum muscle; FC, flexor carpi ulnaris muscle; FCR, flexor carpi radialis muscle; FD, flexor digitorum superficialis muscle; FDP, flexor digitorum profundus muscle; P, pronator teres muscle; PL, palmaris longus muscle; R, radius; S, supinator muscle; U, ulna.

Synovial Fringe

A slip of tissue extends from posterior to anterior in the lateral aspect of the joint. It is mentioned here in the discussion of the ulnar collateral ligament because with an incompetent ulnar collateral ligament, this shelf of tissue can get impinged in the radiocapitellar portion of the joint. Although the patient may complain of pain on extension after throwing owing to the fringe being pinched, it is the incompetent ulnar collateral ligament that allowed for the development of impingement (Fig. 11-16).

MUSCLES AND TENDONS (Box 11-5)

The muscles around the elbow can be divided into anterior, posterior, medial, and lateral compartments.

Anterior Compartment

Normal Anatomy. The biceps and brachialis muscles are located anteriorly. These muscles and tendons are evaluated best on axial and sagittal images. The brachialis extends along the anterior joint capsule and inserts on the ulnar tuberosity. The tendon is surrounded by its muscle, and the brachialis tendon is much shorter than the adjacent biceps tendon. The biceps muscle lies superficial to the brachialis and has a long segment of tendon that is not surrounded by muscle, making it more susceptible to injury than the brachialis. The biceps tendon inserts on the radial tuberosity. The bicipital aponeurosis (or lacertus fibrosus) helps keep the biceps tendon located in proper position (Fig. 11-17). The distal aspect of the biceps tendon is covered by an extrasynovial paratenon and is separated from the radial tuberosity by the bicipital-radial bursa (normally not seen unless distended with fluid). There is no tendon sheath covering the distal biceps tendon.

Abnormal Anatomy (Box 11-6). Injuries to the brachialis muscle are less common than injuries to the biceps tendon. The brachialis can be injured in association with repetitive pull-ups, hyperextension, or repeated forceful supination, or, occasionally, from violent extension against a forceful extrinsic contraction overload (such as an arm-wrestling match that went bad).[20] *Climber's elbow* is defined as a strain of the brachialis tendon.[21] This musculotendinous unit is believed to be involved because climbing (when done correctly) involves the use of the forearms in a pronated and semiflexed position (Fig. 11-18).[21]

Distal biceps tendon rupture is uncommon, representing only 3% of all biceps ruptures.[22] Conversely, it is the most commonly (completely) torn tendon of the elbow. Most distal biceps tendon ruptures are complete, although partial tears have been reported.[23,24] The mechanism of injury of biceps rupture is a sudden, forceful overload with the elbow near mid flexion. The tendon typically tears from its attachment on the radial tuberosity as a result of resisted elbow flexion (Fig. 11-19)[25]; however, tears may be found anywhere along the length of the tendon. Partial tears often are associated with bicipitoradial bursitis; patients present with a painful mass in the antecubital fossa or median nerve symptoms because the bursa can have mass effect on the median nerve (Fig. 11-20). MRI is useful in evaluating these injuries

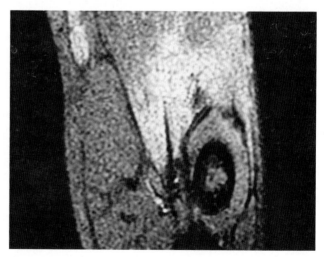

Figure 11-18 Brachialis strain. A football player injured while tackling an opponent. The clinical concern was a biceps tendon injury. Coronal (fast) STIR image shows high signal in the brachialis muscle.

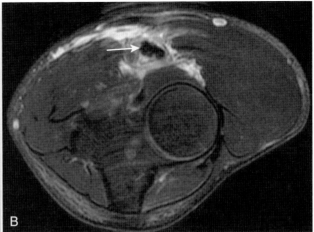

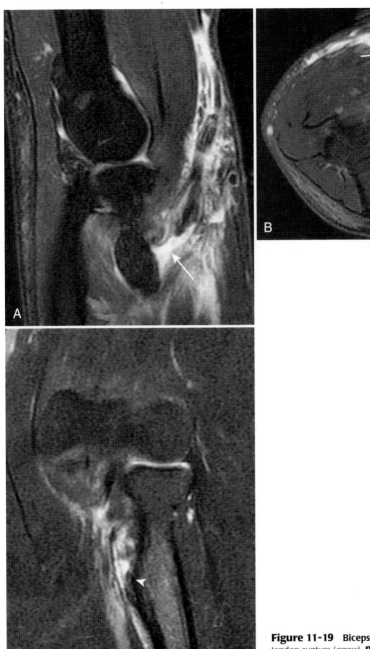

Figure 11-19   **Biceps tendon tear. A,** Sagittal T2W image with fat suppression shows biceps tendon rupture (*arrow*). **B,** Axial image shows retracted biceps tendon (*arrow*). **C,** Anterior coronal image shows biceps torn from radial tuberosity (*arrowhead*).

because tendinopathy, partial tears, and complete ruptures may be distinguished, and tearing of the aponeurosis can be identified.

Partial tears can be seen as alteration in signal and size of the tendon. These changes may be seen focally or more diffusely in the tendon. A full-thickness tear is identified as a gap that exists with the two ends of the tendon retracted from each other; assessing the size of the gap aids preoperative planning. The axial images must extend from the musculotendinous junction to the insertion of the tendon on the radial tuberosity.

Clinical diagnosis can be difficult because the bicipital aponeurosis (lacertus fibrosus) may remain intact, with minimal retraction of the muscle. The flexion strength at the elbow may be preserved if the aponeurosis remains intact, but supination of the forearm usually is weakened.

Current treatment is primary repair within a couple of weeks of the injury that allows for reinsertion of the biceps tendon to restore power, while reducing the risk of radial nerve injury. Nonoperative treatment can be expected to yield strength deficits of 30% to 40% in flexion and supination, whereas immediate repairs result in near-normal strength.[26]

Posterior Compartment

Normal Anatomy. Within the posterior compartment are the triceps and anconeus muscles. These muscles are best evaluated on axial and sagittal images. The triceps inserts on

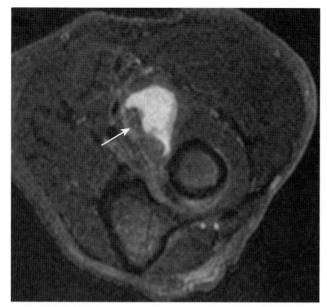

Figure 11-20 **Biceps tendon partial tear.** Axial T2W image with fat suppression shows abnormal signal in biceps tendon proximal to insertion (*arrow*). Note adjacent bursitis.

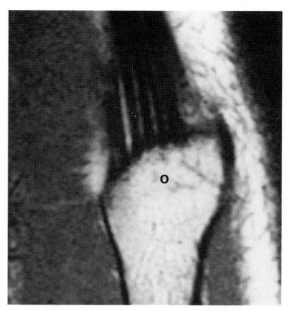

Figure 11-21 **Triceps tendon striations.** Coronal T1W image showing a striated appearance to the triceps tendon owing to fibrofatty tissue insinuating between the tendon slips. o, olecranon.

the proximal portion of the olecranon. At the insertion site, striated high signal can be identified on T1W and T2W images because of the fibrofatty slips between the tendon fibers (Fig. 11-21). This high signal should be noted so that an erroneous diagnosis of a partial tear of the triceps can be avoided. The anconeus arises from the posterior aspect of the lateral epicondyle and inserts more distally

on the olecranon. The anconeus provides dynamic support to the radial collateral ligament in resisting varus stress. Identification of the anconeus helps the radiologist become oriented regarding radial and ulnar aspects of the elbow on axial imaging—the anconeus is lateral (radial).

Abnormal Anatomy. Triceps tendon rupture is the least common of all tendon ruptures in the body and is an uncommon cause of posterior elbow pain.[26] Similarly, triceps tendinopathy is an uncommon cause of posterior elbow pain. The usual mechanisms of injury include a direct blow to the tendon or a decelerating counterforce during active extension.[27] The tendon also may undergo degeneration or erosion in association with olecranon bursitis.

Axial and sagittal imaging are necessary to evaluate the degree of tendinopathy, partial versus complete tear, and the size of the gap associated with the tear. This evaluation aids in preoperative planning. Abnormal signal may be seen in the tendon in a partial tear or tendinopathy, and discontinuous fibers are noted with a complete tear. Most tears occur at the insertion onto the olecranon (Fig. 11-22). There have been reports, however, of tears at the musculotendinous junction.[26-30] There is often associated distention of the olecranon bursa with injury to the triceps tendon. If there is

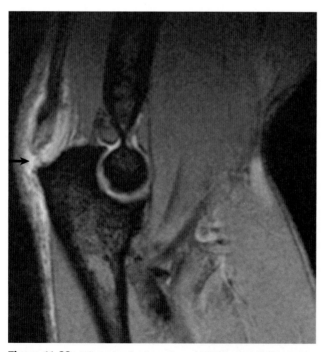

Figure 11-22 **Triceps tendon tear.** Coronal T2W image with fat suppression shows a completely torn and retracted triceps tendon (*arrow*).

BOX 11-7

Medial Tendon Pathology (Medial Epicondylosis)

- Repetitive valgus stress
- Tendon degeneration, partial tear, disruption
- MRI: Increased T1 and T2 signal or disruption, thickening or thinning of tendon, with or without marrow edema in adjacent epicondyle
- Best identified in axial and coronal planes

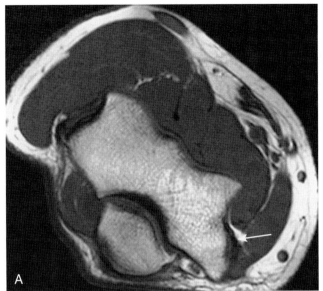

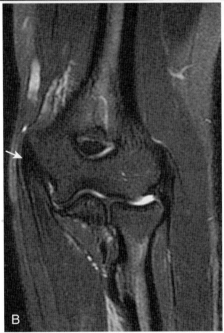

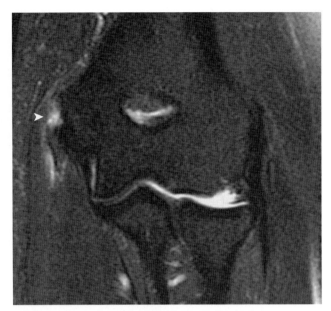

Figure 11-24 **Medial epicondylosis.** A male golfer presented with medial elbow pain. Coronal T2W image with fat suppression shows abnormal high signal at the insertion site of the flexor tendon group (*arrowhead*).

Figure 11-23 **Normal medial tendon. A,** Axial T1W image shows normal low signal structure inserting on medial epicondyle (*arrow*). **B,** Coronal T2W image with fat suppression shows low signal of flexor-pronator conjoined tendon as it inserts on the medial epicondyle (*arrow*).

distention of the olecranon bursa, a well-defined fluid collection is noted on the T2W image posterior to the triceps tendon.

These injuries should be treated as soon as possible with primary repair. The results are universally good.[26,31] Increased signal occasionally has been seen in patients with lateral epicondylosis. The cause may be due to the dynamic support the anconeus provides to the radial collateral ligament complex.[32]

Medial Compartment (Box 11-7)

Normal Anatomy. The medial compartment includes the pronator teres and the flexors of the hand and wrist that arise from the medial epicondyle as the common flexor tendon. The common flexor tendon provides dynamic support to the underlying ulnar collateral ligament in resisting valgus stress. These structures are best evaluated on axial and coronal images and are seen as uniformly low signal, round-to-oval structures inserting onto the medial epicondyle on T1W and T2W axial images (Fig. 11-23).

Abnormal Anatomy. Repetitive valgus stress injuries of the elbow are common overuse injuries seen in baseball pitchers (*Little Leaguer elbow*) and other sports that use a throwing motion. Medial epicondylosis is also known as *golfer's elbow* (associated with good and bad golf swings) or *medial tennis elbow*. It is caused by overload of the flexor-pronator muscle group, which has its origin at the medial epicondyle. Disruption of the flexor-pronator muscle group medially is more common than disruption of the extensor muscle group laterally, even though epicondylosis is more common on the lateral side.

The findings at MRI in medial epicondylosis include tendon degeneration, partial tear, tendon disruption, and muscle strain. Coronal and axial imaging is most useful for evaluating the flexor-pronator group. MRI shows abnormal signal with possible alteration in tendon thickness on T2W images in tendon degeneration and partial tear. Discontinuity of the fibers is seen with complete rupture (Fig. 11-24). MRI facilitates surgical planning by differentiating complete from partial tears and evaluating the underlying ulnar collateral ligament complex. The increased preoperative information may lessen the need for extensive surgical exploration.

Avulsion of the medial epicondylar apophysis may occur in a skeletally immature throwing athlete as a result of failure of the flexor muscle group. MRI may detect this injury before complete avulsion by showing abnormal high signal on the T2W image in the adjacent soft tissues and medial

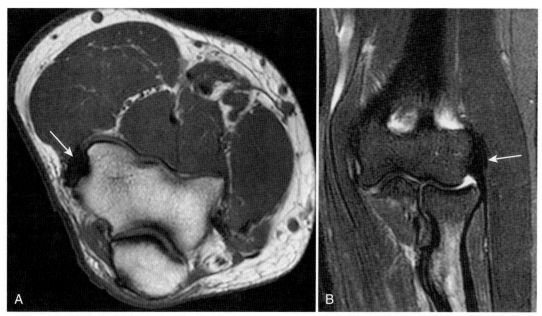

Figure 11-25   Normal lateral tendon. A, Axial T1W image shows low signal around a tendon inserting onto the lateral epicondyle (*arrow*). **B,** Coronal T2W image with fat suppression shows the extensor-supinator conjoined tendon as it inserts onto the lateral epicondyle (*arrow*).

apophysis. Additionally, the ulnar collateral ligament must be inspected for its integrity.

Lateral Compartment

Normal Anatomy. The lateral compartment structures consist of the supinator, the brachioradialis, and the extensors of the hand and wrist that arise from the lateral epicondyle as the common extensor tendon. As in the medial compartment, these structures are best evaluated on axial and coronal images (Fig. 11-25).

Abnormal Anatomy (Box 11-8). The lateral aspect of the elbow is the most common location of elbow pain in the general population. Lateral epicondylosis and lateral epicondylitis, or tennis elbow, occur 7 to 20 times more frequently than medial epicondylitis.[25] Lateral epicondylosis is a chronic tendinopathy of the extensor muscles, primarily the extensor carpi radialis brevis, caused by overuse (either increased intensity or duration). Degeneration and tearing of the common extensor tendon causes the symptoms of lateral epicondylitis. Typically, the extensor carpi radialis brevis tendon is partially avulsed from the lateral epicondyle (Fig. 11-26). Scar tissue forms in response to this partial avulsion, which is susceptible to further tearing with repeated trauma.

Lateral epicondylosis manifests as lateral elbow pain that has an insidious onset, beginning gradually after vigorous activity and progressing to pain with activity. Radiographs frequently are normal, although some patients have evidence of a spur at the lateral epicondyle or calcification of the common extensor tendon.

In patients refractory to conservative therapy, MRI is useful in assessing the degree of tendon damage and associated ligament abnormality. The axial and coronal planes are necessary for assessing the lateral tendons. Tendinopathy is characterized by thickening of tendon with intermediate signal within the substance of the tendon. Partial tears show

fluid signal within an enlarged or attenuated tendon. Complete tears may be diagnosed on MRI by identifying a fluid-filled gap separating the tendon from its adjacent bony attachment site (Fig. 11-27). MRI is useful in identifying high-grade partial tears and complete tears that are unlikely to respond to nonsurgical therapies. Additionally, MRI is useful in providing assessment of additional structures that may explain the lack of response to therapy. Rupture or injury to the radial collateral ligament may occur in association with tears of the common extensor tendon. The lack of significant abnormality involving the common extensor tendon on MRI may prompt consideration of an alternative diagnosis, such as radial nerve entrapment, which may occur with or mimic lateral epicondylosis.

NERVES (Box 11-9)

The nerves around the elbow are the ulnar, median, and radial nerves. They travel through numerous compartments and are subject to various entrapment syndromes. The nerves are small and are surrounded by fat.

MRI findings of neuropathies include increased signal of the nerve on T2W images, indistinct fascicles, enlargement of the nerve, and fluid (edema) surrounding the nerve.[33] Homogeneous high signal resembling a fluid collection on

---

BOX 11-8

Lateral Tendon Pathology (Lateral Epicondylosis)

- More common than medial tendon pathology
- Repetitive varus stress
- Extensor carpi radialis brevis partially avulsed from lateral epicondyle
- MRI: Increased T1 and T2 signal or disruption, thickening or thinning of tendon, with or without marrow edema
- Radial collateral ligament also may be disrupted
- Best identified in axial and coronal planes

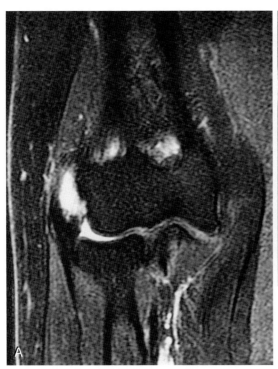
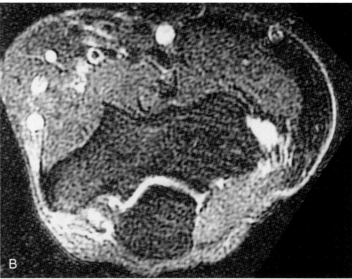

Figure 11-26 **Lateral epicondylosis.** A male patient with symptoms of tennis elbow. **A,** Coronal FSE T2W image shows high signal replacing the extensor tendon. **B,** Axial FSE T2W image shows high signal in the expected location of the extensor carpi radialis brevis tendon. The tendon was completely torn.

T2W images also can be seen. Nerve thickening can be focal or fusiform. The nerves are best evaluated on axial images. The amount of fat around a nerve increases the ability to identify it, particularly the radial and median nerves. MRI may be complementary to electromyography and nerve conduction studies in cases of nerve entrapment around the elbow.[33] Affected muscles in subacute denervation have prolongation of T1 and T2 relaxation times secondary to muscle fiber shrinkage and associated increase in extracellular water (Fig. 11-28).[34] Entrapment of a nerve around the elbow may cause increased signal within the muscles innervated by the nerve on T2W images. These changes may be followed to resolution or progress to atrophy and fatty infiltration with high signal in the muscle on T1W images.

Ulnar Nerve (Box 11-10)

Normal Ulnar Nerve. The ulnar nerve is most superficial, especially in the cubital tunnel. It is seen best on axial images. The roof of the cubital tunnel is formed by the flexor carpi ulnaris aponeurosis distally and the cubital tunnel retinaculum proximally (Fig. 11-29). The cubital tunnel retinaculum, also referred to as the arcuate ligament, is normally a thin fibrous structure that extends from the olecranon to the medial epicondyle; this structure may be complete, partial, or absent. The capsule of the elbow and the posterior and transverse portions of the ulnar collateral ligament form the floor of the cubital tunnel.

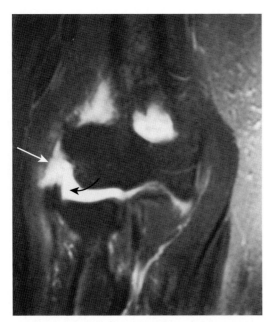

Figure 11-27 **Complete tear of the common extensor tendon.** A female patient with clinically suspected chronic lateral epicondylitis. Coronal FSE T2W, fat-suppressed image shows abnormal high signal in the expected location of the extensor tendon group (*straight arrow*). Note also disruption of the radial collateral ligament (*curved arrow*).

BOX 11-9

MRI of Neuropathy

- Increased T2 signal
- Indistinct fascicles
- Focal or diffuse thickening
- Best seen on axial images
- Neurogenic edema in muscles show increased signal on T2; late findings show atrophy of muscle

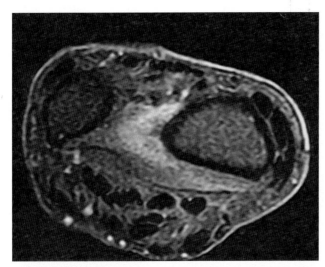

Figure 11-28   Neurogenic edema from anterior interosseous nerve syndrome. Axial FSE T2W fat-suppressed image shows high signal in the pronator quadratus muscle, which is innervated by the anterior interosseous nerve.

BOX 11-10

Ulnar Neuropathy

- Most frequent neuropathy
- Cubital tunnel most common (superficial)
- Thickened retinaculum, ulnar collateral ligament
- Bone spur
- Anconeus epitrochlearis
- Friction (absent retinaculum)
- Pressure (operating table, wheelchair)
- Masses

Treatment of ulnar neuropathy is conservative initially, with rest, removal of the causative agent, and steroid injection. Surgery should be performed if symptoms are not relieved after a few weeks of conservative management. Surgical procedures include arcuate ligament (cubital tunnel retinaculum) release, medial epicondylectomy, and anterior transposition of the nerve with or without the vascular bundle. Postsurgical ulnar nerve compression is avoided by releasing the arcade of Struthers (when present), the common aponeurosis for the humeral head, origin of the flexor carpi ulnaris, origin of the flexor digitorum superficialis, and the common intermuscular septum.

Median Nerve (Box 11-11)

Normal Median Nerve. As with the other nerves, the median nerve is best evaluated on axial imaging, but is best seen with prone positioning of the forearm. This position allows more fat to be present around the nerve, enabling easier identification of this tiny structure. The median nerve at the elbow is located superficially, behind the bicipital aponeurosis (lacertus fibrosus) and anterior to the brachialis muscle. As it leaves the cubital fossa (this fossa, not to be confused with

Abnormal Ulnar Nerve. The ulnar nerve is the most frequently injured nerve in the elbow. Anatomic and physiologic factors can result in abnormal nerve function and traction. The most common neuropathy is cubital tunnel syndrome (Fig. 11-30).

The ulnar nerve is well seen on axial MRIs because it is surrounded by fat, especially as it passes through the superficially located cubital tunnel. Anatomic variations of the cubital tunnel retinaculum may contribute to ulnar neuropathy. These variations in the retinaculum and the appearance of the ulnar nerve are well seen with MRI. The retinaculum may be thickened, resulting in dynamic compression of the ulnar nerve during flexion. Thickening of the ulnar collateral ligament and medial bone spurring from the ulna may undermine the floor of the cubital tunnel, resulting in ulnar neuropathy.[35,36] In 11% of the population, an anomalous muscle, the anconeus epitrochlearis, replaces the retinaculum, resulting in static compression of the ulnar nerve.[36] The cubital tunnel retinaculum may be absent in 10% of the population, allowing anterior subluxation of the nerve over the medial epicondyle with flexion, leading to a friction neuritis.

External compression on the ulnar nerve commonly is due to prolonged hospitalization; it occurs after surgery caused by pressure from the operating room table, and in bedridden or wheelchair-bound patients. Pressure from space-occupying lesions also can result in cubital tunnel syndrome. Such masses include ganglions, bursae, hematomas, tumors, osteophytes, and loose bodies.

Early symptoms of cubital tunnel syndrome are paresthesias in the ring and little fingers and varying degrees of sensory and motor loss in the muscles of the hand along the ulnar nerve distribution. Cubital tunnel syndrome should be differentiated clinically from other sites of ulnar nerve compression, such as the distal humerus (eg, supracondylar process syndrome), Guyon's canal in the wrist, and the palm of the hand (hypothenar hammer syndrome).

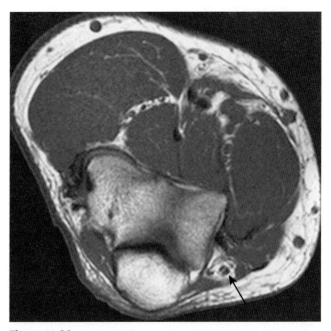

Figure 11-29   Normal cubital tunnel. Axial T1W image shows the normal ulnar nerve (*arrow*) surrounded by fat. The retinaculum (a portion of the flexor carpi ulnaris) is seen as a thin, linear, low signal structure containing the ulnar nerve.

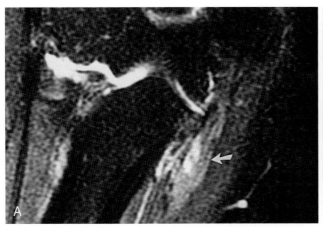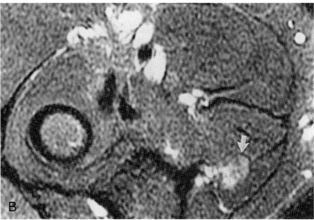

Figure 11-30 Ulnar neuropathy. A female patient with symptoms of ulnar neuritis. **A,** Sagittal FSE T2W image shows high signal with fusiform swelling in the ulnar nerve (*arrow*). **B,** Axial FSE T2W image shows fusiform swelling and abnormal high signal in the ulnar nerve (*arrow*).

the cubital tunnel, is ventral to the elbow joint), the median nerve passes between the ulnar and humeral heads of the pronator teres. The anterior interosseous nerve branches off the median nerve in close proximity to the bifurcation of the brachial artery, then courses over the interosseous membrane toward the wrist.

Abnormal Median Nerve. The most common cause of median nerve entrapment is the pronator syndrome, which can manifest as anterior elbow pain, with or without numbness and tingling in the distribution of the median nerve, and is a result of median nerve compression between the two heads of the pronator teres muscle with pronation, or the fibrous arch of the flexor digitorum superficialis muscle, the bicipital aponeurosis, or a supracondylar process (mass effect from bone spur or ligament). The most frequent cause is dynamic compression by the pronator teres muscle. The nerve gets trapped between the superficial humeral head and the deep, ulnar head.

The bicipital aponeurosis arises from the biceps tendon and courses obliquely over the flexor-pronator group of muscles to insert on the antebrachial fascia. An unusually thick bicipital aponeurosis can produce compression of the pronator muscle and median nerve. Bicipital-radial bursitis and partial tendon tears of the biceps may cause irritation

of the adjacent median nerve, complicating the clinical findings.

The initial course of treatment is conservative and includes rest, immobilization, and avoidance of exacerbating activities (pronation and finger flexion). If symptoms are severe, surgery is indicated. The region of the two heads of the pronator teres, the bicipital aponeurosis, and the fibrous arch of the flexor digitorum superficialis should be explored. A supracondylar spur can be identified on conventional radiographs.

The anterior interosseous syndrome (Kiloh-Nevin syndrome) is a rare compression neuropathy confined to the anterior interosseous nerve, which is purely a motor branch of the median nerve. The nerve courses along the interosseous membrane and ends in the pronator quadratus. Common causes of compression include masses, fibrous bands, accessory muscles, or an enlarged bicipital-radial bursa. Abnormal high signal can be seen in the pronator quadratus, flexor pollicis longus, and a part of flexor digitorum profundus (see Fig. 11-28).

Patients have pure motor loss and a characteristic type of pinch caused by the inability to flex the distal joints of the thumb and index fingers (such patients cannot pick dog or cat hair off clothing). Conservative treatment is warranted initially because the condition may be reversible. Surgery should be performed if no improvement is seen within 6 to 8 weeks.

Radial Nerve (Box 11-12)

Normal Radial Nerve. The radial nerve is located between the brachialis and brachioradialis muscles anterior to the lateral epicondyle. At the region of the capitellum, it divides into a deep motor branch (posterior interosseous nerve) and

---

BOX 11-11

Median Neuropathy

Pronator Syndrome Occurs From Compression by

- Two heads of pronator teres (most common)
- Fibrous arch of flexor digitorum superficialis
- Bicipital aponeurosis
- Supracondylar process
- Irritation secondary to bicipitoradial bursitis, biceps injury
- MRI: Increased T2 signal in anterior compartment of forearm, sparing flexor carpi ulnaris and ulnar half of flexor digitorum profundus

Anterior Interosseous Syndrome (Kiloh-Nevin)

- Motor branch of medial nerve
- Inability to flex distal joints of thumb and index finger
- MRI: Increased T2 in flexor pollicis longus, pronator quadratus, and a part of flexor digitorum profundus

---

BOX 11-12

Radial Neuropathy

- Above elbow: Secondary to trauma, fractures, cast, tourniquet, intramuscular injections
- Below elbow: Less common, thickening of arcade of Frohse
- Posterior interosseous nerve, purely motor
- MRI: Increased T2 in muscles of posterior compartment of forearm

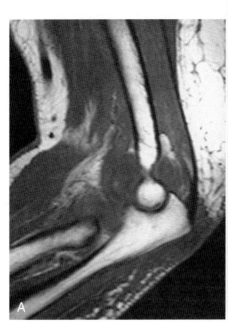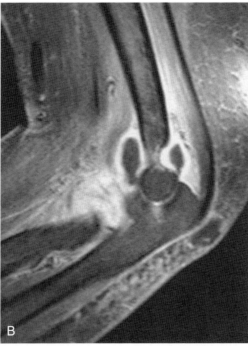

Figure 11-31 **Inflammatory arthritis. A,** Sagittal T1W image shows a low signal joint effusion. **B,** After contrast enhancement and fat suppression, synovial enhancement is present around the periphery of the effusion. Note the more uniformly enhancing pannus around the proximal radius.

a superficial branch (sensory). The posterior interosseous nerve gains access to the posterior compartment via the superficial and deep heads of the supinator muscle. Up to 35% of individuals have a fibrous arch, called the *arcade of Frohse.* The superficial branch of the radial nerve passes between the supinator and the brachioradialis muscles.

Abnormal Radial Nerve. Radial nerve injury above the elbow frequently is associated with trauma, such as displaced fracture of the humeral shaft, inappropriate use of crutches, prolonged tourniquet application, and lateral or posterior intramuscular injection. Pressure from a cast also may result in radial nerve injury. Nontraumatic radial neuropathy is much less common. Thickening of the arcade of Frohse (fibrous arch) along the proximal edge of the supinator muscle can lead to posterior interosseous nerve syndrome or supinator syndrome. The fibrous arch limits the space for the posterior interosseous nerve. Mass effect from fracture or dislocation of the proximal radius, neoplasms, or proliferative synovitis can compromise the tunnel further. Individuals who pursue occupations that require frequent pronation-supination or forceful extension, such as violinists, conductors, swimmers, basketball players who illegally "palm" the ball, and housewives who vigorously clean and make bread from scratch, are susceptible to this neuropathy. Abnormal high signal can be identified in the muscles of the posterior compartment of the forearm with a prolonged abnormality of the posterior interosseous nerve. Because posterior interosseous syndrome can coexist or mimic lateral epicondylosis, MRI becomes extremely valuable in making the diagnosis in refractory cases of tennis elbow.

Treatment of radial nerve compression is conservative and consists of rest, paraneural steroid injections, and physical therapy. Surgical decompression is recommended within 4 months of symptoms to avoid permanent nerve damage.

ARTICULAR DISORDERS

Because the distribution of articular findings is important in evaluating an arthropathy, plain films should be evaluated at the time of reviewing the MRIs. Some arthropathies have a propensity to affect the elbow, such as rheumatoid arthritis, crystal deposition diseases (gout and calcium pyrophos-

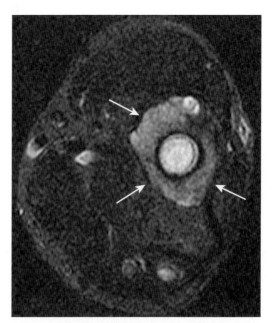

Figure 11-32 **Synovial chondromatosis.** Axial T2W image with fat suppression shows conglomerate intermediate signal loose bodies that are similar in size (*arrows*). This is consistent with primary synovial chondromatosis.

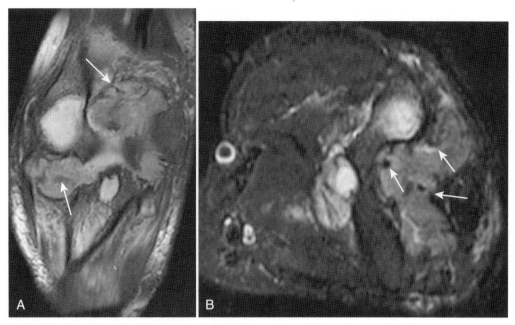

Figure 11-33 **Pigmented villonodular synovitis.** A male patient with elbow pain and fullness. **A,** Coronal T1W image shows erosions involving ulna and radius. Note low signal elements (*arrows*). **B,** Axial T2W image with fat suppression shows intermediate signal within joint and low signal areas compatible with hemosiderin (*arrows*).

phate deposition disease), septic arthritis, and synovial osteochondromatosis.

Rheumatoid arthritis, a pancompartmental process, has involvement of the wrist and hands if the elbow is involved (Fig. 11-31). It is a bilateral process, but can be asymmetric in symptoms and appearance. Synovial proliferation occurs in this arthropathy and in numerous arthritides. To assess for synovial proliferation, MRI can be used to monitor therapy by performing contrast-enhanced imaging. Subchondral cysts or erosions with bone marrow edema can occur with any of the arthritides.

Osteoarthritis typically affects a portion of the joint and, when present, has a predisposing factor, such as trauma, underlying rheumatoid arthritis, calcium pyrophosphate deposition, neuropathy, or infection. Usually, osteophytes can be identified. A joint effusion can be diagnosed by MRI if the fluid in the synovial recesses of the elbow has convex margins. An effusion is not specific for any type of arthropathy.

Gradient echo imaging can be valuable in identifying loose bodies. The magnetic susceptibility properties of gradient echo imaging cause blooming of the cortical portions of the loose bodies when present The loose bodies appear as low to intermediate signal structures within the high signal joint fluid. Primary synovial chondromatosis can ossify (similar size loose bodies) (Fig. 11-32). Degenerative joint changes also can be seen with secondary (post-traumatic) osteochondromatosis. In addition to evaluating for loose bodies, gradient echo imaging can identify the blooming property of hemosiderin, which is seen in pigmented villonodular synovitis and hemophilia (Fig. 11-33).

Masses

Masses described for other areas of the body also can occur around the elbow. A few warrant special mention because they can occur with increased frequency around the elbow.

Epitrochlear Adenopathy

Cat-scratch disease is characterized by local lymphadenitis within 1 or 2 weeks after being scratched by a cat. A soft tissue mass, representing swollen epitrochlear nodes, can be identified easily on MRI. The history is important to help distinguish this entity from a worrisome soft tissue mass, such as a sarcoma. The distribution of the mass along the nodal chain in the epitrochlear region also is helpful (Fig. 11-34). The nodes appear as high signal on T2W images, but their appearance is nonspecific. Hematogenous dissemination and spread from a contiguous contaminated source, such as a lymph node, represent potential mechanisms of osseous involvement. The responsible organism is reported to be *Bartonella henselae/B. clarridgeiae*.

Bursae

Two bursae can be identified at the biceps tendon insertion on the radial tuberosity—the bicipitoradial and the interosseous bursae. These bursae are located anterior to the biceps tendon. These bursae should be considered if a well-defined, isointense mass is identified on T1W images and becomes high signal on T2W images and is located anterior to the biceps tendon. Bursitis in either of these locations may impair flexion and extension. Posterior interosseous nerve compression can result from distention of the bicipitoradial bursa (Fig. 11-35). The median nerve can be affected by enlargement of the interosseous bursa. These bursae may communicate with each other, and both bursae may affect both nerves. Enlargement of either of these bursae occasionally may manifest as a nonspecific antecubital fossa mass. Intravenous administration of gadolinium may aid in recognition of this enlarged bursa and differentiates this benign entity from a solid neoplasm by showing peripheral enhance-

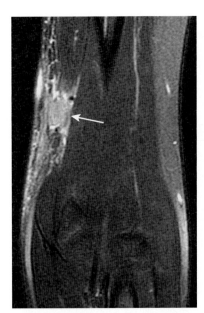

Figure 11-34   Cat-scratch disease. Coronal T2W image with fat suppression shows intermediate signal node in characteristic location for cat scratch (*arrow*). Note overlying changes in soft tissues consistent with inflammatory process.

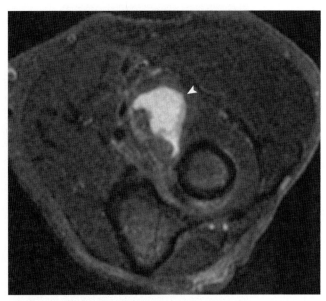

Figure 11-35   Bicipitoradial bursitis. Axial T2W image with fat suppression shows a fluid-filled mass in a patient with a partial tear of the biceps tendon (*arrowhead*).

ment around the bursa, whereas a solid neoplasm shows diffuse enhancement in the lesion.

Gout typically is extra-articular and affects the olecranon bursa. Fluid in the olecranon bursa is considered a bursitis, and any fluid in this bursa is considered abnormal. The most common causes for fluid in the olecranon bursa are gout, trauma (hemorrhage), and infection.

Septic olecranon bursitis usually is clinically apparent, and MRI has limited application in evaluating uncomplicated cases. MRI is useful to exclude osteomyelitis in patients refractory to therapy. Many of the arthritides can mimic infection by MRI appearance. Superimposed infection also can exist with arthritis. Aspiration of the joint remains the most efficacious diagnostic study to exclude infection.

REFERENCES

1. Aronen J. Problems of the upper extremity in gymnastics. *Clin Sports Med* 1985; 4:61-71.
2. Ellman H. Unusual affections of the preadolescent elbow. *J Bone Joint Surg [Am]* 1967; 49:203.
3. Fixsen J, Maffulli N. Bilateral intra-articular loose bodies of the elbow in an adolescent BMX rider. *Injury* 1989; 20:363-364.
4. Gugenheim J, Stanley R, Woods G, Tullos H. Little League survey: the Houston study. *Am J Sports Med* 1976; 4:189.
5. Hang V, Lippert F, Spolek G, et al. Biomechanical study of the pitching elbow. *Int Orthop* 1979; 3:217-223.
6. Pintore E, Maffulli N. Osteochondritis dissecans of the lateral humeral condyle in a table tennis player. *Med Sci Sports Exerc* 1991; 23:889-891.
7. Bennett J, Tullos H. Ligamentous and articular injuries in the athlete. In Morrey BF (ed). *The Elbow and Its Disorders.* Philadelphia: Saunders; 1985:502-522.
8. Nestor B, O'Driscoll S, Morrey B. Ligamentous reconstruction for posterolateral rotatory instability of the elbow. *J Bone Joint Surg [Am]* 1992; 74:1235-1241.
9. O'Driscoll S, Bell D, Morrey B. Posterolateral rotatory instability of the elbow. *J Bone Joint Surg [Am]* 1991; 73:440-446.
10. Fritz R, Steinbach L. Magnetic resonance imaging of the musculoskeletal system, part 3: the elbow. *Clin Orthop Relat Res* 1996; 324:321-339.
11. Herzog R. Efficacy of magnetic resonance imaging of the elbow. *Med Sci Sports Exerc* 1994; 26:1193-1202.
12. Ho C. Sports and occupational injuries of the elbow: MR imaging findings. *AJR Am J Roentgenol* 1995; 164:1465-1471.
13. Kvitne R, Jobe F. Ligamentous and posterior compartment injuries. In Jobe FW (ed). *Operative Techniques in Upper Extremity Sports Injuries.* St. Louis: Mosby-Year Book; 1996:411-430.
14. Fleisig G, Andrews J, Dillman C, Escamilla R. Kinetics of baseball pitching with implications about injury mechanisms. *Am J Sports Med* 1995; 23:233-239.
15. Joyce M, Jelsma R, Andrews J. Throwing injuries to the elbow. *Sports Med Arthrosc Rev* 1995; 3:224-236.
16. Conway J, Jobe F, Glousman R, Pink M. Medial instability of the elbow in throwing athletes: treatment by repair or reconstruction of the ulnar collateral ligament. *J Bone Joint Surg [Am]* 1992; 74:67-83.
17. Timmerman LA, Schwartz ML, Andrews JR. Preoperative evaluation of the ulnar collateral ligament by magnetic resonance imaging and computed tomography arthrography: evaluation in 25 baseball players with surgical confirmation. *Am J Sports Med* 1994; 22:26-32.
18. Timmerman LA, Andrews JR. Undersurface tear of the ulnar collateral ligament in baseball players: a newly recognized lesion. *Am J Sports Med* 1994; 22:33-36.
19. Schwartz ML, al-Zahrani S, Morwessel RM, Andrews JR. Ulnar collateral ligament injury in the throwing athlete: evaluation with saline-enhanced MR arthrography. *Radiology* 1995; 197:297-299.
20. Safran M. Elbow injuries in athletes. *Clin Orthop Relat Res* 1995; 310:257-277.
21. Bollen S. Soft tissue injury in extreme rock climbers. *Br J Sports Med* 1988; 22:145-147.
22. Seiler J, Parker L, Chamberland P, et al. The distal biceps tendon: two potential mechanisms involved in its rupture: arterial supply and mechanical impingement. *J Shoulder Elbow Surg* 1995; 4:149-156.
23. Bourne M, Morrey B. Partial rupture of the distal biceps tendon. *Clin Orthop Relat Res* 1991; 271:143-148.
24. Nielsen K. Partial rupture of the distal biceps brachii tendon. *Acta Orthop Scand* 1987; 58:287-288.
25. Coonrad R. Tendinopathies at the elbow. *Instr Course Lect* 1991; 40:25-42.
26. Morrey B. Tendon injuries about the elbow. In Morrey BF (ed). *The Elbow and Its Disorders.* Philadelphia: Saunders; 1985:452-463.
27. Tarsney F. Rupture and avulsion of the triceps. *Clin Orthop Relat Res* 1972; 83:177-183.

28. Farrar E III, Lippert F III. Avulsion of the triceps tendon. *Clin Orthop Relat Res* 1981; 161:242.
29. Gilcreest E. Rupture of muscles and tendons. *JAMA* 1925; 84:1819.
30. Montgomery A. Two cases of muscle injury. *Surg Clin Chir* 1920; 4:871.
31. Bennett B. Triceps tendon rupture: case report and method of repair. *J Bone Joint Surg [Am]* 1962; 44:741-744.
32. Coel M, Yamada CY, Ko J. MR imaging of patients with lateral epicondylitis of the elbow (tennis elbow): importance of increased signal of the anconeous muscle. *AJR Am J Roentgenol* 1993; 161:1019-1021.
33. Rosenberg ZS, Beltran J, Cheung YY, et al. The elbow: MR features of nerve disorders. *Radiology* 1988; 23:365-369.
34. Polak J, Jolesz F, Adams D. Magnetic resonance imaging examination of skeletal muscle. Prolongation of T1 and T2 subsequent to denervation. *Invest Radiol* 1991; 23:365-369.
35. McPherson S, Meals R. Cubital tunnel syndrome. *Orthop Clin North Am* 1992; 23:111-123.
36. O'Driscoll S, Horii E, Carmichael S, Morrey B. The cubital tunnel and ulnar neuropathy. *J Bone Joint Surg [Br]* 1991; 73:613-617.

Elbow Protocols

ELBOW MRI: NON-ARTHROGRAM

Sequence No.	1	2	3	4	5	6
Sequence Type	T1	Fast spin echo with fat suppression	T1	Fast spin echo with fat suppression	T2* 20-degree flip angle	Fast spin echo with fat suppression
Orientation	Axial	Axial	Coronal	Coronal	Sagittal	Sagittal
Field of View (cm)	12-14	12-14	12-14	12-14	12-14	12-14
Slice Thickness (mm)	4	4	4	4	4	4
Contrast	No	No	No	No	No	No

ELBOW MRI: ARTHROGRAM

Sequence No.	1	2	3	4	5	6
Sequence Type	T1 with fat suppression	Fast spin echo with fat suppression	T1 with fat suppression	Fast spin echo with fat suppression	Gradient echo	Fast spin echo with fat suppression
Orientation	Axial	Axial	Coronal	Coronal	Sagittal	Sagittal
Field of View (cm)	12-14	12-14	12-14	12-14	12-14	12-14
Slice Thickness (mm)	4	4	4	4	4	4
Contrast	Intra-articular done in fluoroscopy					

Same dilution as shoulder arthrogram.

SAMPLE STANDARD REPORT

Clinical Indications

Protocol

This examination was performed using the routine protocol with multiple sequences and planes of imaging.

Discussion

1. **Joint effusion:** None; no loose bodies shown

2. **Bursitis:** No olecranon or bicipitoradial bursitis evident

3. **Osseous structures:** Normal, without osteochondritis dissecans, fractures, or other abnormalities

4. **Tendons:** Normal configuration and signal of all tendons; no medial or lateral epicondylitis

5. **Collateral ligaments:** Medial and lateral collateral ligaments are intact

6. **Nerves:** Ulnar nerve shows a normal position, size, and signal; no abnormalities of the other nerves around the elbow shown

7. **Other abnormalities:** None

Opinion

Normal MRI of the (right/left) elbow.

Wrist and Hand

12

How to Image the Wrist and Hand

See the wrist and hand protocols at the end of the chapter.

- *Coils and patient position:* Some type of surface coil is an absolute requirement for proper wrist imaging. Many different coils may be used, including dedicated wrist coils. Generally, the smaller the coil, the better the images of the wrist. If the patient is not too large, the wrist may be imaged with the patient supine and the arm alongside the body. For a larger patient, it may be impossible to image in this position; we usually have larger patients prone with the arm over the head and the elbow flexed. This position can become rapidly tiring and painful. The technologist must be aware of how to position and pad the patient properly at pressure points to ensure the patient's comfort and prevent motion during the study. Padding under the shoulder and elbow is particularly useful. The best way to under-

stand what is uncomfortable about an examination is to have it done to yourself.

- *Image orientation (Box 12-1):* We image the wrist in three anatomic orthogonal planes, based on an axial scout view obtained through the proximal carpal row; this allows for acquiring true anatomic coronal, axial, and sagittal images. Many radiologists do not obtain sagittal images in the wrist, and this may be considered an optional sequence. We prefer to have sagittal images because they provide an additional look at the osseous structures and their alignment, which may not be evaluated as well in the other imaging planes.

- *Pulse sequences and regions of interest:* Pulse sequences are a combination of T1 and some type of T2 images. Gradient echo images are particularly excellent for ligament evaluation. Three-dimensional volume acquisition using gradient echo images allows for very thin (1-2 mm) slices, which are necessary for identifying the ligaments well.

BOX 12-1

Wrist Structures to Evaluate in Different Planes

Coronal
- Osseous structures
- Scapholunate ligament
- Lunotriquetral ligament
- Triangular fibrocartilage
- Dorsal and volar radioulnar ligaments
- Extrinsic ligaments of the carpus
- Ulnar collateral ligament of thumb

Axial
- Tendons
- Median nerve
- Ulnar nerve
- Carpal tunnel
- Guyon's canal (ulnar tunnel)
- Distal radioulnar joint

Sagittal
- Carpal alignment
- Pisotriquetral synovial cyst

BOX 12-2

Intrinsic Carpal Ligaments

Scapholunate and Lunotriquetral, Most Important
- Maintain alignment among carpal bones
- Triangular, horseshoe, or bandlike shapes on proximal aspects of bone, attaching to bone or cartilage
- Low signal with areas of intermediate signal traversing (normal)
- Scapholunate abnormalities
  - Stretched or torn
  - MRI—90% accurate
    Discontinuity, absence, irregularity, thinning with high signal on T2 traversing ligament defect
    Increased intercarpal space, sometimes
    Elongation (stretching) of undisrupted ligament
- Scapholunate ligament abnormalities may lead to
  - Rotatory subluxation of scaphoid
  - Dorsal intercalated segmental instability
  - Scapholunate advanced collapse wrist
- Lunotriquetral ligament tears may lead to
  - Volar intercalated segmental instability
- Associated with triangular fibrocartilage complex tears

Two-dimensional gradient echo images that have a section thickness less than 3 mm also work well and can take less time to acquire. Protocols should be optimized for clinical indications, such as "routine" (pain), mass/infection, gamekeeper's thumb, and trauma (screening for fractures only). We do dedicated imaging of only the wrist, unless there is a clinical reason given for imaging any portion of the hand as well. The field of view for a wrist examination is approximately ±10 cm (depending on patient size), and this allows the distal radius and ulna, carpal bones, and bases of the metacarpal bones to be included. An MRI examination of the hand includes the wrist, metacarpals, and most (or all) of the fingers, using the same pulse sequences and planes of imaging as for the wrist, but the field of view is enlarged to ±14 cm to include the additional anatomy. We also perform dedicated examinations of the fingers, in which case a 6- to 8-cm field of view is used. It is important to know the clinical indications to optimize the field of view. The coronal plane of imaging shows the small ligaments of the wrist best, and it is essential to have thin slices in this plane. For evaluation of ligaments, the slice thickness should be 1 to 2 mm. A slice thickness of 3 mm can be used in the other imaging planes and for evaluation of masses, fractures, and other abnormalities aside from ligaments.

- *Contrast:* Intravenous contrast administration is used to evaluate a mass to differentiate a cystic from a solid lesion as well as to evaluate for infection to appreciate abscess formation better. Because of concern of partial tears of intrinsic ligaments and triangular fibrocartilage complex (TFCC), MR arthrography can be performed with contrast injection in the radiocarpal joint space (intrinsic ligaments) or distal radioulnar joint space.

Normal and Abnormal

LIGAMENTS

The ligaments of the wrist are divided into intrinsic and extrinsic ligaments. The intrinsic carpal ligaments connect carpal bones to one another and limit their motion. The extrinsic ligaments connect the bones of the forearm to the bones of the wrist, allowing stability of the wrist with the distal forearm.

Intrinsic Ligaments (Box 12-2)

Normal Scapholunate and Lunotriquetral Ligaments. The scapholunate ligament and the lunotriquetral ligament are the two intrinsic carpal ligaments of greatest clinical significance; disruption of these ligaments may cause instability and pain. Both of these ligaments can be evaluated best on gradient echo coronal images using thin sections. These ligaments are horseshoe-shaped, bandlike, or triangle-shaped structures on the proximal aspects of the carpal bones to which they attach (Fig. 12-1).[1,2]

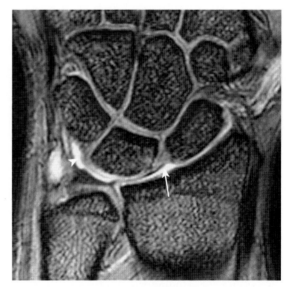

Figure 12-1 Normal intrinsic carpal ligaments. Gradient echo coronal image of the wrist. The scapholunate (*arrow*) and lunotriquetral (*arrowhead*) ligaments are located on the proximal aspects of the carpal bones to which they attach, best depicted on coronal images.

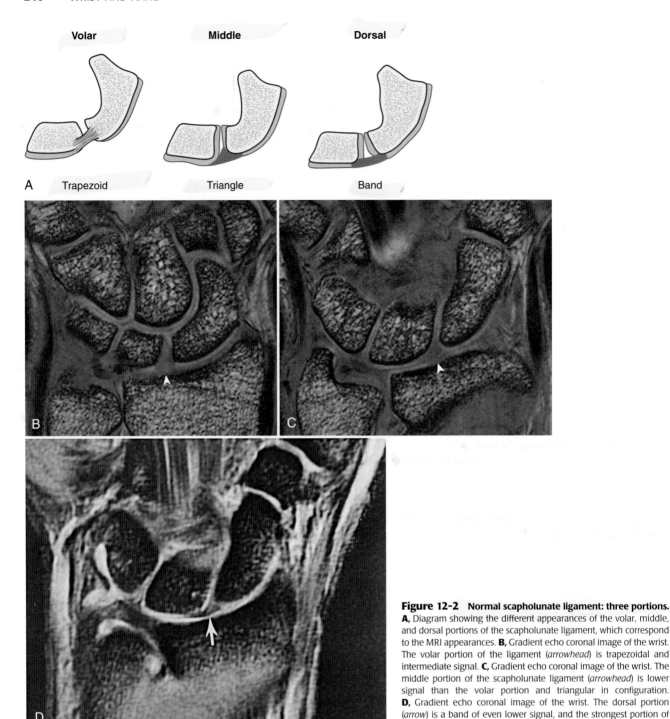

Figure 12-2 **Normal scapholunate ligament: three portions.**
A, Diagram showing the different appearances of the volar, middle, and dorsal portions of the scapholunate ligament, which correspond to the MRI appearances. **B,** Gradient echo coronal image of the wrist. The volar portion of the ligament (*arrowhead*) is trapezoidal and intermediate signal. **C,** Gradient echo coronal image of the wrist. The middle portion of the scapholunate ligament (*arrowhead*) is lower signal than the volar portion and triangular in configuration. **D,** Gradient echo coronal image of the wrist. The dorsal portion (*arrow*) is a band of even lower signal, and the strongest portion of the ligament.

The scapholunate ligament has volar, middle, and dorsal portions (Fig. 12-2). Studies have shown that only the volar and, especially, the dorsal portions are important for wrist stability. The volar portion is looser so that it can accommodate the various articulating curvatures of the scaphoid and lunate.[3] Perforations (or communicating defects) in the middle portion are common and do not seem to relate to symptoms when they are an isolated finding.[4]

The volar portion of the scapholunate ligament is trapezoidal in configuration, with intermediate signal intensity on gradient echo images. The middle portion of the scapholunate ligament is triangular in shape, with lower signal intensity than the volar component, and both portions are routinely heterogeneous in signal intensity. The dorsal portion, the most important for carpal stability, is a low signal intensity, homogeneous band. Generally, the volar portion of the scapholunate ligament attaches to cortical bone, whereas the middle and dorsal portions attach to hyaline cartilage or a combination of cartilage and cortical bone. The reason for the higher signal intensity of the volar

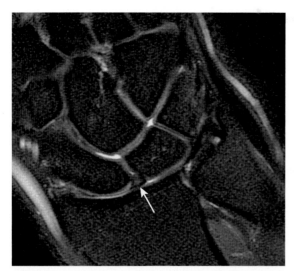

Figure 12-3 **Scapholunate ligament: normal variation.** Coronal fat-suppressed T2W image of the wrist. Intermediate signal traversing the intercarpal ligaments is a normal finding (*arrowhead*) because it does not become as high signal as fluid.

and middle portions of the scapholunate ligament compared with the dorsal portion is related to the lower density of collagen fibers and the higher proportion of loose connective tissue and vascular tissue in these regions.[5]

The lunotriquetral ligament is smaller and more taut than the scapholunate ligament, but has a similar shape and frequently displays a heterogeneous low signal intensity on coronal gradient echo images. The lunotriquetral ligament may attach to hyaline articular cartilage or cortical bone. Its stronger and thicker volar component blends with the triangular fibrocartilage (TFC).

Intermediate signal intensity may partially or completely traverse the substance of the lunotriquetral ligament and scapholunate ligament in asymptomatic individuals (Fig. 12-3). It should be considered an abnormal finding (torn ligament) only if this signal intensity is as high in signal as that of fluid on whatever type of T2 sequence is being used.

Similarly, high signal intensity between articular cartilage and the ligament should indicate an avulsed ligament only if the signal intensity is as bright as fluid.

Abnormal Scapholunate and Lunotriquetral Ligaments.

Scapholunate instability is the most common carpal instability. Clinically, patients complain of pain and weakness on the dorsal radial aspect of the wrist. Abnormalities on MRI that indicate a scapholunate ligament abnormality are listed:

1. Discontinuity of the ligament, with or without an increased space between the scaphoid and lunate bones
2. Complete absence of the scapholunate ligament
3. Distorted morphology with fraying, thinning, and irregularity
4. Elongated ligament with an increased intercarpal space (Fig. 12-4)

The accuracy of MRI has been reported as 90% compared with arthrography and 95% compared with surgery (arthroscopy and arthrotomy).[6]

Scapholunate instability occurs when the scapholunate ligament is completely torn or stretched, allowing the scaphoid and lunate bones to dissociate. The scaphoid tilts in a volar direction (rotatory subluxation), whereas the lunate tilts in a dorsal direction (dorsal intercalated segmental instability). The relationship of the osseous structures can be detected on sagittal MRIs (Fig. 12-5). Rotatory subluxation is the most common instability pattern in the wrist. The dorsal intercalated segmental instability pattern of carpal instability also can occur with an unstable fracture of the scaphoid, even though the scapholunate ligament is intact.[7,8] Partial tears more commonly affect the weaker volar ligamentous attachment.[9]

Scapholunate ligament disruption and chronic rotatory instability of the scaphoid also may lead to the capitate migrating proximally and may cause scapholunate advanced collapse (SLAC) wrist. The SLAC wrist consists of scapholunate ligament disruption, degenerative changes between the scaphoid and the distal radius, and proximal migration of the capitate between the scaphoid and lunate bones (Fig. 12-6).

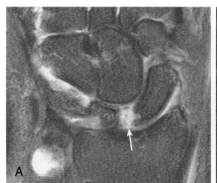
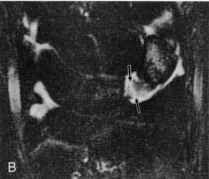
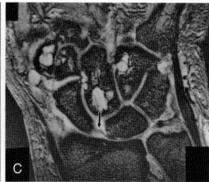

Figure 12-4 **Scapholunate ligament abnormality. A,** Coronal fat-suppressed T2W image shows fluid signal between the scaphoid and lunate (*arrow*). Scapholunate distance is wide. **B,** Fast T2 with fat saturation coronal image of the wrist (different patient than in **A**). There is distortion of the morphology of the scapholunate ligament, which is frayed and with a vertical high signal tear through it (*arrows*). **C,** Gradient echo coronal image of the wrist (different patient than in **A** and **B**). The space between the scaphoid and lunate bones is increased, and the ligament (*arrow*) is stretched, although it remains intact. This was the result of inflammation associated with rheumatoid arthritis. Multiple bone erosions, subchondral cysts, and a triangular fibrocartilage tear also are present.

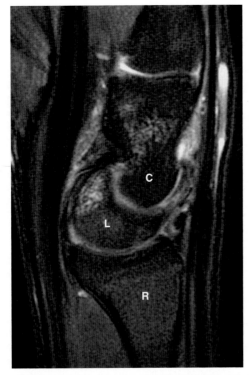

Figure 12-5 Dorsal intercalated segmental instability. Sagittal fat-suppressed T2W image of the wrist. The lunate (L) is tipped in a dorsal direction relative to the capitate (C) and radius (R) because of rotatory subluxation of the scaphoid that occurred from disruption of the scapholunate ligament.

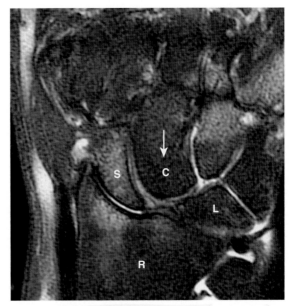

Figure 12-6 Scapholunate advanced collapse wrist. Coronal fat-suppressed T2W image of the wrist. The scapholunate ligament is absent, and the space between the scaphoid (S) and lunate (L) is increased. The capitate (C) is migrating proximally between the two bones (*arrow*). There is loss of cartilage and a decreased space between the scaphoid and radius from degenerative joint disease.

Disruption of the lunotriquetral ligament is not as easy to diagnose as disruption of the scapholunate ligament because of its smaller size. Similar abnormalities to those seen in an abnormal scapholunate ligament are present in an abnormal lunotriquetral ligament (Fig. 12-7). Tears of the lunotriquetral ligament are the second most common cause of carpal instability and result in the lunate tilting in a volar direction (volar intercalated segmental instability) secondary to the disruption of the triquetral attachment. There is a strong association between tears of the TFC and lunotriquetral liga-

ment tears. The alignment of the carpal bones on sagittal images depends on wrist position. The lunate tends to volar flex and dorsiflex relative to the radius when the wrist is placed in radial and ulnar deviation.[7] Proper positioning of the hand and wrist in the magnet is important to prevent this pitfall. Normally, the distal radius, lunate, and capitate all align colinearly, or nearly so, just as they do on a lateral wrist radiograph.

Extrinsic Ligaments

Volar and Dorsal Ligaments. The extrinsic carpal ligaments can be seen best on gradient echo coronal images; they are seen in cross section on sagittal images (Fig. 12-8). These

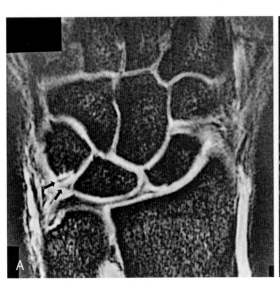

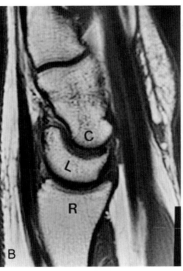

Figure 12-7 Lunotriquetral tear and consequent volar intercalated segmental instability. A, Gradient echo coronal image of the wrist. There is high signal through a disruption of the lunotriquetral ligament with fragments of the ligament (*arrow*) seen on either side of the tear. **B,** T1 sagittal image of the wrist. The lunate (L) is tipped in a volar direction relative to the capitate (C) and radius (R) because of the lunotriquetral ligament tear, resulting in carpal instability (volar intercalated segmental instability).

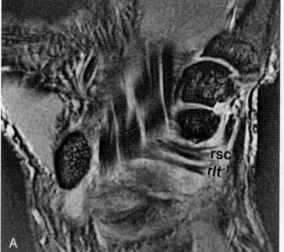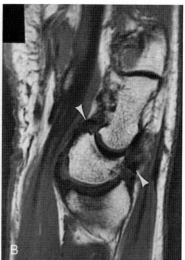

Figure 12-8 Extrinsic ligaments. **A,** Gradient echo coronal image of the wrist. Portions of the two major volar carpal extrinsic ligaments are shown coursing obliquely as striated low signal structures. rlt, radiolunotriquetral ligaments; rsc, radioscaphocapitate. **B,** T1 sagittal image of the wrist. Volar and dorsal extrinsic ligaments are seen as round, low signal structures (*arrowheads*) in cross section in this plane of imaging.

ligaments course between the carpal bones and the radius on the volar and the dorsal sides of the wrist. The extrinsic ligaments run obliquely and are best imaged on oblique sagittal images. Because imaging usually is not done in this plane, it generally requires several adjacent coronal images to see an entire ligament. The volar ligaments are stronger and thicker than the dorsal ligaments and are major stabilizers of wrist motion. Extrinsic ligaments are thickenings of the joint capsule and are intracapsular and extrasynovial. Extrinsic ligaments appear as striated fascicular structures with alternating bands of low and intermediate signal intensity on coronal MRIs.

The most important volar ligaments are the radioscaphocapitate and radiolunotriquetral ligaments. The radioscaphocapitate ligament originates on the volar surface of the radial styloid process and courses obliquely across the waist of the scaphoid without attaching to it (it acts as a seatbelt to maintain the position of the scaphoid), to insert on the

center of the capitate. The radiolunotriquetral ligament is the largest ligament of the wrist. It arises adjacent to (on the ulnar side of) the radioscaphocapitate ligament on the radial styloid. It runs obliquely to attach to the volar surfaces of the lunate and triquetrum.

The dorsal extrinsic ligaments of the wrist run obliquely between the distal radius and to each of the carpal bones of the proximal carpal row (radioscaphoid, radiolunate, and radiotriquetral ligaments).[10-12] There are other small extrinsic carpal ligaments that are not discussed here.

The good news about all of these extrinsic ligaments is that no one knows with certainty what importance they have clinically. The MRI appearance of normal extrinsic ligaments has been extensively described, but the ability of MRI to detect abnormalities is unknown. The only value in radiologists knowing about them is so that they do not cause confusion during interpretation of MRIs of the wrist. We spend little to no time analyzing these ligaments.

BOX 12-3

Triangular Fibrocartilage Complex

Components
- Triangular fibrocartilage
- Radioulnar ligaments (dorsal and volar)
- Extensor carpi ulnaris tendon sheath
- Ulnar collateral ligament
- Meniscus homologue

Function
- Absorbs axial loading forces (20% pass through ulnar side of wrist)
- Stabilizes ulnar side of wrist and distal radioulnar joint

Abnormalities
- Triangular fibrocartilage
  - Partial-thickness or full-thickness tears, detachment, degeneration
  - High signal through surface on T2 = tear
- Radioulnar ligaments
  - High signal through these structures indicates a tear
  - Tear leads to instability of distal radioulnar joint
- Extensor carpi ulnaris sheath
  - Tenosynovitis commonly affects this tendon
  - High signal surrounding tendon on axial T2 images
  - Disruption of the sheath leads to medial subluxation of extensor carpi ulnaris from its groove in ulna

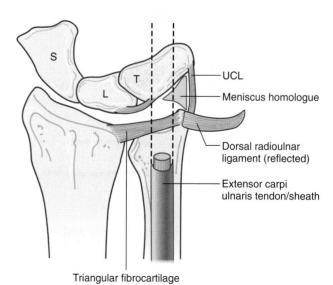

Figure 12-9 **Triangular fibrocartilage complex.** Diagram of the anatomic components of the triangular fibrocartilage complex from a dorsal perspective. L, lunate; S, scaphoid; T, triquetrum; UCL, ulnar collateral ligament.

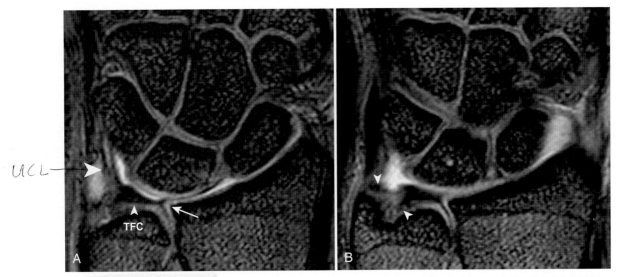

Figure 12-10 Normal triangular fibrocartilage. **A,** Coronal gradient echo image of the wrist. The triangular fibrocartilage (*small arrowhead*; TFC) is a biconcave structure attaching to the intermediate signal cartilage on the radius (*white arrow*). This image also shows the ulnar collateral ligament well (*large arrowhead*). **B,** Gradient echo coronal image of the wrist. The ulnar attachment of the triangular fibrocartilage consists of two thin bands of tissue (*arrowheads*).

TRIANGULAR FIBROCARTILAGE COMPLEX
(Box 12-3)

The TFCC is the primary stabilizer of the distal radioulnar joint and is composed of several soft tissue structures on the ulnar side of the wrist: the TFC, volar and dorsal radioulnar ligaments, meniscus homologue, ulnar collateral ligament, and the sheath of the extensor carpi ulnaris tendon (Fig. 12-9).

The functions of the structures that compose the TFCC include cushioning forces across the ulnar side of the wrist during axial loading and stabilizing the ulnar side of the wrist and the distal radioulnar joint. With neutral ulnar variance, about 80% of axial loading forces pass through the radial side of the wrist. The ulna absorbs about 20% of the axial loading forces through the TFCC.[7,13]

Triangular Fibrocartilage

Normal Triangular Fibrocartilage. The TFC is a fibrocartilaginous biconcave disk with an asymmetric bow-tie shape, similar to the temporomandibular joint disk (Fig. 12-10). The TFC is positioned in the ulnocarpal space with attachments on the medial side to the ulnar styloid process by two thin bands of TFC tissue. At its radial attachment, there is hyaline cartilage interposed between the TFC and the radius that must not be confused with a detached or torn TFC. The TFC attaches directly to the cartilage, which is the articular surface of the distal radioulnar joint. The thickness of the TFC is inversely proportional to the degree of ulnar variance. In other words, the TFC is thinner in patients with positive ulnar variance, which may predispose it to tear, and thicker in patients with negative ulnar variance. The TFC is depicted best on coronal MRIs. It may be diffusely low signal intensity regardless of pulse sequence, or have intermediate signal intensity in its substance from asymptomatic myxoid degeneration.

Abnormal Triangular Fibrocartilage. Any structure of the TFCC can be abnormal, but the TFC is the main component to show abnormalities. Clinically, patients complain of ulnar-sided wrist pain and tenderness. An audible click with pain may be elicited by rotation of the forearm. On MRI, the TFC can be evaluated similarly to the meniscus in the knee. High signal intensity within the substance of the TFC has no clinical significance, whereas high signal intensity extending through either the proximal or the distal surface of the TFC indicates a tear (Fig. 12-11).[6,14-17] TFC tears may be partial or full thickness, extending partially or completely through the substance of the TFC. Partial tears are noted more frequently at the proximal articulating surface with the distal radioulnar joint.[18] Fluid in the distal radioulnar joint was previously believed to be a secondary sign of a TFC tear, but a small amount of fluid may be present in this joint in most individuals.

The location of a tear has therapeutic implications because of the vascular supply of the TFC.[19] The peripheral 20% of the TFC on the ulnar margin is well vascularized, and tears may heal with nonoperative therapy if properly immobilized or with primary repair. The remainder of the TFC is essentially avascular, and perforations or tears in the central and radial portions of the TFC usually are débrided. Many individuals have high signal intensity within the substance of the TFC and perforations, but have no symptoms. The intrasubstance signal is probably from myxoid degeneration. The asymptomatic perforations are probably degenerative in nature because most traumatic tears are symptomatic. As with all imaging, the presence of abnormal findings does not ensure that symptoms are a consequence of the abnormalities, and correlation of the MRI and clinical findings is mandatory in planning proper management of patients. The TFC may be traumatically detached from its ulnar attachment and may become interposed between the radius and ulna, preventing proper reduction of the distal radioulnar joint (Fig. 12-12).

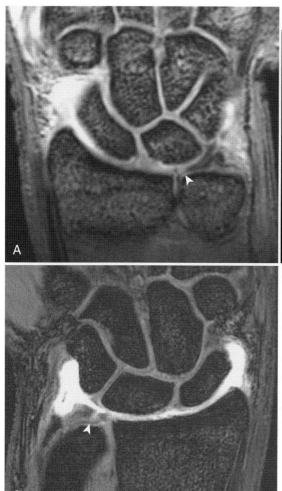

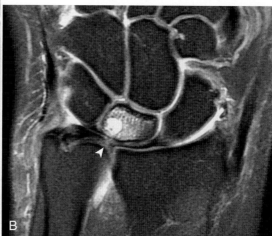

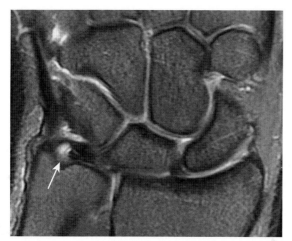

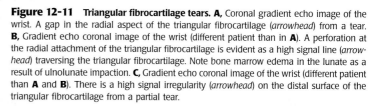

Figure 12-11 **Triangular fibrocartilage tears. A,** Coronal gradient echo image of the wrist. A gap in the radial aspect of the triangular fibrocartilage (*arrowhead*) from a tear. **B,** Gradient echo coronal image of the wrist (different patient than in **A**). A perforation at the radial attachment of the triangular fibrocartilage is evident as a high signal line (*arrowhead*) traversing the triangular fibrocartilage. Note bone marrow edema in the lunate as a result of ulnolunate impaction. **C,** Gradient echo coronal image of the wrist (different patient than **A** and **B**). There is a high signal irregularity (*arrowhead*) on the distal surface of the triangular fibrocartilage from a partial tear.

Figure 12-12 **Triangular fibrocartilage detachment.** Coronal fat-suppressed T2W image of the wrist. The ulnar attachment of the triangular fibrocartilage has been traumatically detached with discontinuity and a gap of the triangular fibrocartilage (*arrow*) through the two thin bands that attach it to the ulnar styloid process.

Traumatic tears of the TFC often are associated with injuries of adjacent structures, such as the extensor carpi ulnaris tendon sheath and lunotriquetral ligament, which can be shown readily by MRI. MRI is very accurate for diagnosing TFC tears; compared with arthrography and surgery, it has an accuracy rate of 95%. Tears in the central and radial portions are best shown, whereas tears near the ulnar attachment are less accurately diagnosed because synovitis or synovial proliferation in the prestyloid recess may mimic a tear.

Radioulnar Ligaments

Normal Radioulnar Ligaments. The volar and dorsal radioulnar ligaments are broad, striated bands that originate on the volar and dorsal cortex of the sigmoid notch of the distal radius. The ligaments pass on the volar and dorsal surfaces of the TFC and blend with it. The radioulnar ligaments attach to the ulnar styloid process medially, and to the distal

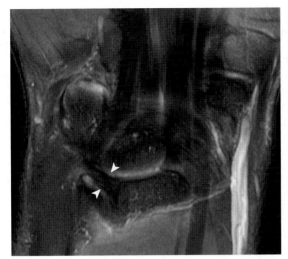

Figure 12-13 **Normal radioulnar ligament.** Coronal fat-suppressed T2W image of the wrist. The volar radioulnar ligament is seen as a low signal structure (*arrowheads*) attaching to the bones of the radius and ulna, with straight proximal and distal margins. These all are features distinguishing it from the adjacent triangular fibrocartilage proper. The dorsal radioulnar ligament has an identical appearance to the volar ligament.

radius laterally. The dorsal and volar radioulnar ligaments can be distinguished from the TFC proper because they tend to have flat superior and inferior margins, rather than being biconcave, and they attach directly to bone, rather than to cartilage on the radius (Fig. 12-13). These structures are low signal intensity on all pulse sequences and are best depicted on coronal images.[7]

Abnormal Radioulnar Ligaments. Disruption of the volar or dorsal radioulnar ligaments is associated with instability of the distal radioulnar joint.[20] Disrupted ligaments can be seen on MRI, and subluxation or dislocation of the distal radioulnar joint can be shown easily on axial MRIs (Fig. 12-14). Distal radioulnar joint instability is diagnosed when the ulna does not articulate properly with the sigmoid notch of the distal radius and is displaced in either a dorsal or volar direction from this notch.

Meniscus Homologue

The meniscus homologue can be thought of as a thickening of the ulnar side of the joint capsule that is inconsistently present. It is located just distal to the prestyloid recess and attaches to the triquetrum. If present, it is shown on coronal MRIs as a low signal intensity, triangle-shaped structure (Fig. 12-15).[13] The prestyloid recess is a triangle-shaped space bordered by the meniscus homologue distally, the TFCC attachments to the ulnar styloid process proximally, and the central TFC disk radially. The prestyloid recess normally contains fluid.

Extensor Carpi Ulnaris Sheath

Normal Extensor Carpi Ulnaris. The extensor carpi ulnaris tendon and its sheath, which is a component of the TFCC, can be seen on coronal MRIs, but is best depicted in the axial plane, as is the case with many other tendons (Fig. 12-16). The tendon sheath is not evident on MRI, unless there is

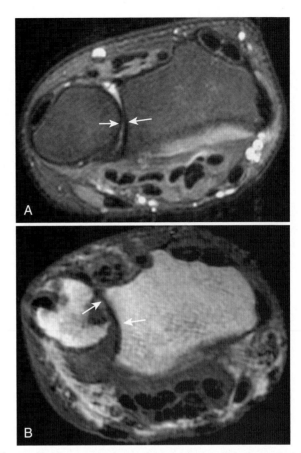

Figure 12-14 **Distal radioulnar joint: normal and abnormal. A,** Axial fat-suppressed T2W image of the wrist. The normal concentric relationship of the radius and ulna is shown (*arrows*) in the distal radioulnar joint of a patient with intact radioulnar ligaments. **B,** Axial T1W image of the wrist (different patient than in **A**). Disruption of the dorsal radioulnar ligament resulted in dorsal subluxation of the ulna relative to the radius with loss of the concentric relationship of the two bones in the distal radioulnar joint (*arrows*).

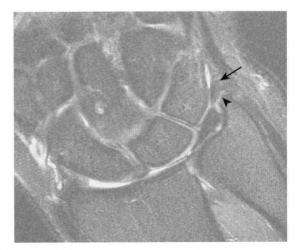

Figure 12-15 **Meniscus homologue and prestyloid recess.** Coronal fat-suppressed T2W image of the wrist. The meniscus homologue is a triangular, low signal structure (*arrow*) on the ulnar side of the wrist. It is the distal boundary of the prestyloid recess (*arrowhead*), which is a space also bounded by the triangular fibrocartilage proximally and radially.

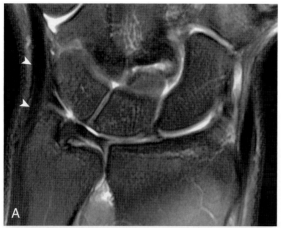

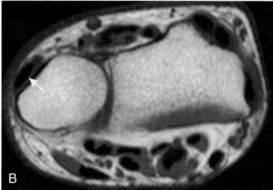

Figure 12-16 Normal extensor carpi ulnaris tendon. **A,** Coronal fat-suppressed T2W image of the wrist. The extensor carpi ulnaris tendon is seen on the ulnar and dorsal side of the wrist (*arrowheads*). **B,** T1 axial image of the wrist. The normal position of the extensor carpi ulnaris is evident in the groove on the dorsum of the ulna (*arrow*).

fluid in it. The extensor carpi ulnaris tendon is located in the groove on the dorsum of the ulna in neutral and pronation positioning of the wrist, whereas subluxation can be seen if imaged in supination.[21]

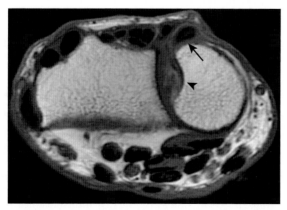

Figure 12-17 Dislocated extensor carpi ulnaris tendon. Axial T1W image of the wrist. The extensor carpi ulnaris tendon (*arrow*) is dislocated in an ulnar direction from its normal position in the groove (*arrowhead*) on the dorsum of the ulna, indicating disruption of the extensor carpi ulnaris tendon sheath, which is a component of the triangular fibrocartilage complex.

Abnormal Extensor Carpi Ulnaris Sheath. Traumatic disruption of the extensor carpi ulnaris tendon sheath can result in subluxation or dislocation of the extensor carpi ulnaris tendon at the level of the distal ulna, out of its normal groove, in a medial direction. Associated tenosynovitis is common. Subluxation and tenosynovitis are best shown on axial images (Fig. 12-17).[22]

Ulnar Collateral Ligament (Wrist)

The ulnar collateral ligament of the wrist is an additional support structure making up the TFCC that may be seen on coronal MRIs (see Fig. 12-10A). It represents a thickening of the wrist joint capsule and provides little mechanical strength. The ulnar collateral ligament extends from the ulnar styloid process to the triquetrum. A similar structure exists on the lateral side, the radial collateral ligament, which extends from the radial styloid process to the scaphoid.

ULNAR COLLATERAL LIGAMENT OF THE THUMB

Normal Ulnar Collateral Ligament of the Thumb

The normal ulnar collateral ligament of the thumb is a taut structure that attaches to the base of the proximal phalanx of the thumb and to the distal end of the first metacarpal. It stabilizes the ulnar aspect of the first metacarpophalangeal joint. On MRI, the ligament is a low signal intensity band that spans the first metacarpophalangeal joint, located deep to a similar, vertically oriented low signal intensity band, which is the adductor aponeurosis (Fig. 12-18).[23] High-resolution imaging with a small field of view oriented to anteroposterior of the view of the thumb (coronal to the thumb) is necessary to see this structure properly.

Gamekeeper's Thumb

An abduction injury to the first metacarpophalangeal joint may cause an avulsion fracture at the site of attachment of the ulnar collateral ligament to the base of the proximal phalanx of the thumb (one third of cases), or it may injure only the ulnar collateral ligament without radiographic evidence of an osseous abnormality (two thirds of cases). MRI of a tear of the ulnar collateral ligament simply shows the thin, low signal intensity ligament avulsed from the base of the thumb or discontinuity of the ligament with hemorrhage and edema surrounding the torn ends of the ligament (see Fig. 12-18). The ligament remains deep to the linear adductor aponeurosis. The edema and hemorrhage are high signal intensity on T2W images. Gradient echo images are excellent for showing the ligament well.

When the ulnar collateral ligament is retracted proximally and displaced superficial to the adductor aponeurosis, it is referred to as a *Stener lesion*. Stener lesions occur in about one third of all gamekeeper's thumbs. The interposition of the adductor aponeurosis between the torn ligament and the bone prevents healing, which may lead to chronic laxity, loss of grip, and degenerative joint disease. Treatment of a Stener lesion in the first 3 weeks after injury has a better outcome than more delayed treatment and may warrant MRI for diagnosis because physical examination is inaccurate for this lesion.

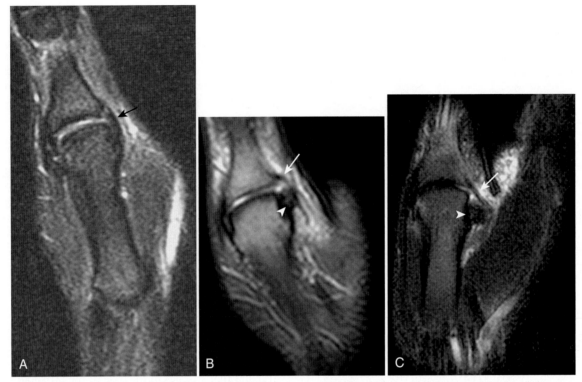

Figure 12-18 Ulnar collateral ligament of the thumb: normal and abnormal. **A,** Coronal fat-suppressed T2W image of the thumb. Normal ulnar collateral ligament (*arrow*) is spanning the first metacarpophalangeal joint as a continuous, low signal band. **B,** Coronal fat-suppressed T2W image of the thumb (different patient than in **A**). The ulnar collateral ligament (*arrowhead*) has been avulsed from its attachment to the base of the proximal phalanx of the thumb (gamekeeper's or skier's thumb), but remains deep to the adductor aponeurosis (*arrow*). **C,** Coronal fat-suppressed T2W image of the thumb (different patient than in **A** and **B**) with a Stener lesion. The ulnar collateral ligament (*arrowhead*) is detached from the base of the proximal phalanx, thickened, intermediate signal, and retracted proximally so that it gives the "yoyo on a string" appearance. The string of the yoyo is the adductor aponeurosis (*arrow*).

A Stener lesion has been described as having the appearance of a yoyo on a string on MRI.[24] The yoyo is created by the balled-up and retracted ulnar collateral ligament, and the string of the yoyo is the adductor aponeurosis (see Fig. 12-18C).

TENDONS

Normal Anatomy

Tendons in the wrist are best depicted in the axial plane. Most of the flexor tendons (nine tendons) pass through the carpal tunnel on the volar aspect of the wrist. It is unnecessary to know the names of individual flexor tendons.

The extensor tendons are located on the dorsum of the wrist and are important to know. The extensor tendons are stabilized on the dorsum of the wrist by an extensor retinaculum. Fascial septations form six dorsal compartments that contain the extensor tendons (Fig. 12-19).

The first dorsal compartment, on the radial side of the wrist, contains the abductor pollicis longus and extensor pollicis brevis tendons. The second dorsal compartment contains the extensor carpi radialis longus and brevis tendons, and is separated from the extensor pollicis longus tendon in the third dorsal compartment by Lister's tubercle, a bony protuberance on the dorsum of the radius. The fourth compartment holds the extensor digitorum and extensor indicis tendons. The extensor digiti minimi tendon lies in the fifth dorsal compartment. The extensor carpi ulnaris

tendon is located in the sixth compartment in the notch of the ulna.

It is hard enough to remember the names of these tendons, much less whether they are a longus or a brevis. A trick that helps us to remember if a tendon is a longus or a brevis is to recall that the tendon on the ulnar aspect of Lister's tubercle is the extensor pollicis longus (and it has a very longus way to go to get to the thumb). As one progresses from the extensor pollicis longus in a radial direction, the tendons alternate as to longus and brevis: extensor pollicis *longus*, extensor carpi radialis *brevis*, extensor carpi radialis *longus*, extensor pollicis *brevis*, and abductor pollicis *longus*. So, longus and brevis become easy as you get into the rhythm, and it is only the names of the tendons you are left to struggle with.

The tendons of the wrist are oval-to-round, low signal intensity structures. The extensor carpi ulnaris tendon, in particular, normally may have some high signal intensity within it for reasons that are not understood.[25] The magic angle phenomenon is a likely culprit, but it is unclear why high signal in this tendon is common in patients without symptoms. Unless the tendon has fluid around it (tenosynovitis) or is abnormally enlarged or thinned, we do not call it abnormal based on small amounts of intrasubstance high signal intensity. Small amounts of fluid in tendon sheaths are considered normal, and fluid is considered abnormal only if it completely surrounds the tendon. Striations and heterogeneous signal may be noted in the abductor pollicis

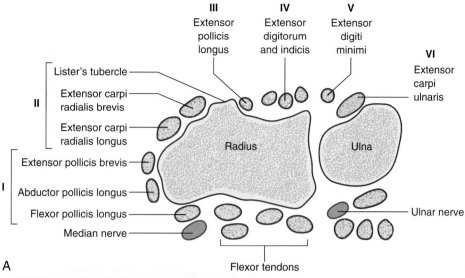

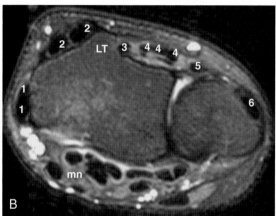

Figure 12-19 **Normal tendons of the wrist. A,** Diagram of the wrist in the axial plane at the level of the distal radioulnar joint. This shows the six dorsal compartments that contain the tendons, which are labeled. The flexor tendons and median nerve are present volarly. **B,** T2W fat-suppressed axial image of the wrist through the distal radioulnar joint. The dorsal tendons are labeled with numbers that correlate with the dorsal compartments shown in the diagram in **A**. LT, Lister's tubercle; mn, median nerve.

longus tendon simulating longitudinal tears. The appearance is due to fat interposed between tendinous fascicles and should not be misinterpreted as a pathologic condition (Fig. 12-20).[26]

Tendon Pathology

Abnormalities of the tendons in the wrist and hand are common and range from tenosynovitis to degeneration and

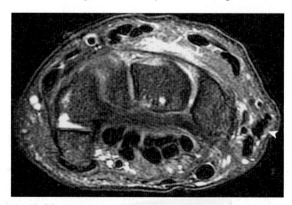

Figure 12-20 **Abductor pollicis longus striations.** Axial fat-suppressed T2W image through the proximal carpal row shows the normal appearance of the abductor pollicis (*arrowhead*). It can resemble a longitudinal split of the tendon, but the striated appearance is a result of fat interdigitating in the tendon.

tears. Chronic repetitive trauma from overuse and inflammatory arthritis are common causes for tendon problems in the wrist. Complete tears can be accurately assessed on MRI. The gap size in a torn and retracted tendon is an important factor in treatment planning. A gap measuring greater than 30 mm necessitates tendon graft rather than primary repair.[27]

de Quervain's Syndrome (Box 12-4). Entrapment and tenosynovitis of the abductor pollicis longus and extensor pollicis brevis tendons in the first dorsal compartment is known as de Quervain's syndrome.[7,22,28] The diagnosis usually is made

BOX 12-4
de Quervain's Syndrome

- Entrapment/irritation of tendons, first dorsal compartment
  - Abductor pollicis longus
  - Extensor pollicis brevis
- Associated with overuse (manual laborers) and pregnancy
- MRI appearance
  - Tendons may have normal size and signal, be thickened, or have intratendinous signal
  - Abnormal signal around tendons is common: low signal on T1; either low or high (fibrosis or tenosynovitis) on T2

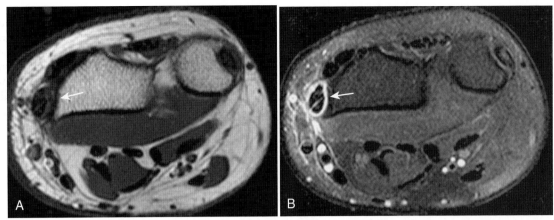

Figure 12-21   de Quervain's tenosynovitis. **A,** T1 axial image of the wrist. Painful mass over the radial styloid process proved to be tenosynovitis of the extensor pollicis brevis and abductor pollicis longus tendons (*arrow*). **B,** T2 axial image of the wrist. The tendons of the first dorsal compartment appear enlarged with fluid in the tendon sheath (*arrow*). The subcutaneous fat surrounding the tendons remains normal in this patient.

clinically, but sometimes the findings are not obvious and cannot be distinguished from the findings of a scaphoid fracture, flexor carpi radialis tenosynovitis, or degenerative arthritis of the first carpometacarpal joint. de Quervain's syndrome may be idiopathic, but also is associated with pregnancy or repetitive trauma in manual laborers.

MRI findings in de Quervain's syndrome may have a variable appearance (Fig. 12-21). There may be obliteration of subcutaneous fat surrounding the tendons, with the tendons surrounded by intermediate signal intensity tissue on all pulse sequences, or there may be tenosynovitis with high signal fluid surrounding them on T2W images. The tendons

may be normal in caliber or thickened, or there may be high signal within the tendons from partial tears or degeneration. Injection of steroids into the tendon sheath cures this disease in most patients, but surgical decompression occasionally is required.

Intersection Syndrome. The first extensor compartment tendons cross over the second extensor compartment tendons approximately 4 to 8 cm proximal to Lister's tubercle. Intersection syndrome is a result of peritendinosis of the second extensor compartment that develops secondary to overuse. This entity can be overlooked clinically, so MRI

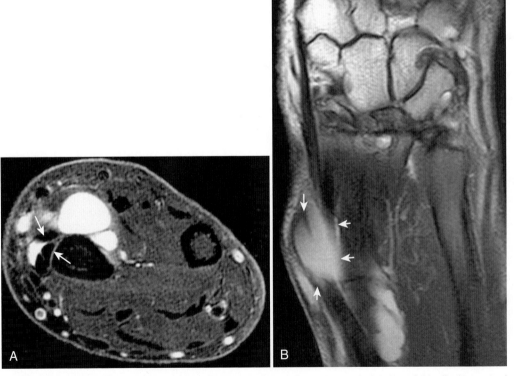

Figure 12-22   Intersection syndrome. **A,** Axial fat-suppressed T2W image located proximal to the wrist joint shows fluid collections as tendons from the first and second compartments cross (*arrows*). **B,** Coronal fat-suppressed T2W image adjacent to tendons (inhomogeneous fat suppression) shows tenosynovitis at the location of the tendon crossing (*arrows*).

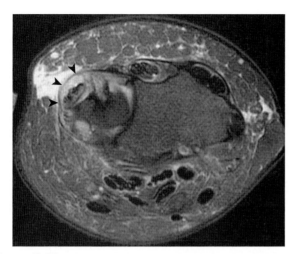

Figure 12-23 Extensor carpi ulnaris tenosynovitis and partial tears. Axial fat-suppressed T2W image of the wrist. There is extensive high signal from tenosynovitis in the soft tissues surrounding the extensor carpi ulnaris (*arrowheads*). The extensor carpi ulnaris is slightly enlarged with more than the usual high signal within it, indicating partial tears.

plays a useful role in its diagnosis. Involvement of the first and second extensor compartment tendons and tendon sheaths with abnormal signal beginning at the crossover and extending proximally is diagnostic (Fig. 12-22).[29]

Extensor Carpi Ulnaris. The extensor carpi ulnaris tendon commonly is involved with tenosynovitis or partial tears.[7,22] This involvement may occur secondary to repetitive subluxation or dislocation, which occurs when the extensor carpi

ulnaris tendon sheath has been disrupted from an injury to the TFCC. We diagnose tenosynovitis or partial tendon tears of the extensor carpi ulnaris tendon only when there is fluid surrounding the entire tendon, or the tendon is abnormally thick or thin (Fig. 12-23). High signal intensity within this particular tendon is not enough to call an abnormality because it is present in many asymptomatic individuals. Subluxation or dislocation of the extensor carpi ulnaris is diagnosed when the extensor carpi ulnaris is partially or completely dislodged from its groove on the dorsal aspect of the ulna and is displaced medially (ulnar direction). This is best evaluated on axial images.

Bowstringing. The flexor digitorum tendons in the fingers normally are closely apposed to the adjacent osseous structures because they are held in position by a system of pulley ligaments. When there is rupture of the pulley system ligaments, the tendons are free to displace from the bones of the digit, creating a "bowstring" appearance. This diagnosis, along with the quality of the displaced tendon, can be made easily by MRI when the tendons are separated from the bone to a greater extent than normal or when compared with the adjacent normal digits (Fig. 12-24). Abnormal separation between the tendon and phalanges may not be present, however, unless the finger is slightly flexed in the surface coil.

Other Tendons. Tenosynovitis and partial and complete tears also may affect other tendons of the wrist. Tenosynovitis of the flexor digitorum tendons in the carpal tunnel is a common cause of carpal tunnel syndrome. MRI cannot distinguish infected fluid from noninfected fluid, and in the

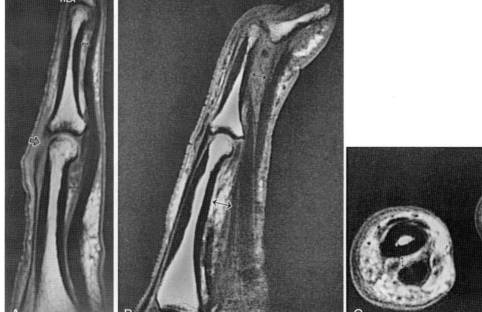
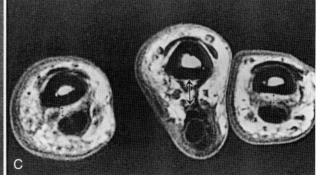

Figure 12-24 Tendon abnormalities of the fingers. **A,** T1 sagittal image of the finger. Tear of the extensor tendon (*open arrow*), which is discontinuous, intermediate signal, and thickened. This also shows the relationship of the normal flexor tendons to the phalanges (*double-headed arrows*). **B,** T1 sagittal image of the finger (different patient than in **A**). Bowstringing of the flexor tendons manifests as significant displacement (compare with **A**) of the tendons in a volar direction from the osseous phalanges (*double-headed arrows*). Scarring surrounds the tendons with partial obliteration of the volar subcutaneous fat. In addition, there is a mallet finger (flexion of the distal interphalangeal joint) from rupture of the distal extensor tendon. **C,** T1 axial image of the fingers (same patient as in **B**). The large distance between the bone and the flexor tendons is shown (*double-headed arrow*) in the middle finger from a bowstringing injury. The normal distance between bone and flexor tendons (*small double-headed arrows*) can be seen in the normal digits on either side of the injured finger.

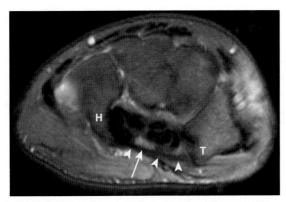

Figure 12-25   Carpal tunnel: normal anatomy. Axial T2W image of the wrist at the distal carpal tunnel at the level of the hook of the hamate (H), tubercle of the trapezium (T), and flexor retinaculum (*arrowheads*). The median nerve (*arrow*) is fasciculated and intermediate to high signal.

<table>
<tr><td>

BOX 12-5

Carpal Tunnel Syndrome

MRI Features
- Swollen median nerve (larger at level of pisiform than at distal radio-ulnar joint)
- Flattened median nerve (evaluate at level of hamate hook)
- Increased signal of nerve on T2
- Flexor retinaculum (bowing ratio >15%)

Postoperative Appearance After Carpal Tunnel Release
- Flexor retinaculum
  - Absent *or*
  - Incised free ends displaced volarly
- Flexor tendons volarly displaced

</td></tr>
</table>

flexor compartment clinical history is imperative for making a proper diagnosis when fluid is noted in the flexor compartment. A distal flexor tenosynovitis can rapidly ascend into the flexor compartment affecting the median nerve in the carpal tunnel and the other flexor tendons.

CARPAL TUNNEL

The carpal tunnel is a fibro-osseous space formed by the concave volar aspects of the carpal bones on the dorsal surface, and by the flexor retinaculum on the volar surface. The tunnel contains the flexor tendons and the median nerve. The flexor retinaculum is a dense, fibrous band that attaches to the scaphoid and tubercle of the trapezium on the radial aspect of the tunnel and to the pisiform and hook of the hamate on the ulnar side of the tunnel. The retinaculum normally shows some slight palmar bowing.[30] There is normally very little fat within the carpal tunnel, but when present, it should be found only in the dorsal aspect. The median nerve lies within the volar and radial aspect of the carpal tunnel and can be easily differentiated from the lower signal intensity tendons that surround it. It is helpful to evaluate the structures passing through the carpal tunnel at three standard locations on axial MRIs (Fig. 12-25):

1. Level of the distal radioulnar joint just before the median nerve enters the tunnel
2. Level of the pisiform bone in the proximal tunnel
3. Level of the hook of the hamate in the distal tunnel, where it is most constricted

NERVES

Median Nerve

The median nerve lies in the volar and radial aspect of the carpal tunnel, just deep to the retinaculum, although the position may vary with wrist position. The nerve has higher signal intensity and is more oval in shape than the adjacent flexor tendons in the carpal tunnel (see Fig. 12-25). The size of the median nerve is maintained or slightly decreases as it progresses distally through the tunnel. The tunnel becomes progressively smaller from proximal to distal, and the nerve may have a flattened appearance at the level of the hook of the hamate, where the tunnel is most constricted, and the nerve is in close apposition to adjacent flexor tendons.[31]

Carpal Tunnel Syndrome (Box 12-5). Carpal tunnel syndrome is the most common compressive neuropathy that

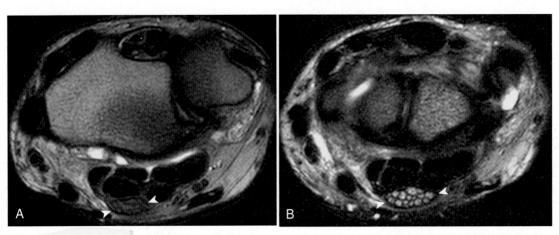

Figure 12-26   Carpal tunnel syndrome. A, Axial T2W image of the wrist at the distal radioulnar joint. The median nerve (*arrowheads*) is identified before entering the carpal tunnel. **B,** Axial T2W image of the wrist at the proximal carpal row. The median nerve (*arrowheads*) is enlarged and high signal. The flexor retinaculum is bowed volarly.

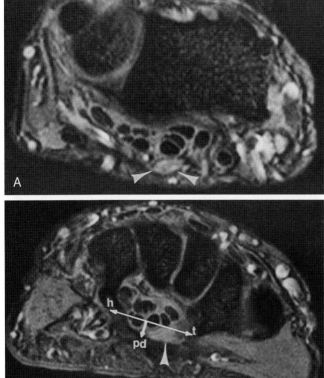
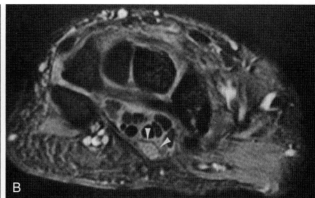

Figure 12-27   Carpal tunnel syndrome. A, Gradient echo axial image of the wrist at the distal radioulnar joint. The median nerve (*arrowheads*) has a normal appearance at this level. **B,** Gradient echo axial image of the wrist at the pisiform. The median nerve (*arrowheads*) is enlarged and has an angled or faceted appearance from pressure where it abuts the adjacent flexor tendons. **C,** Gradient echo axial image of the wrist at the distal carpal tunnel. The median nerve (*arrowhead*) is significantly larger than on more proximal images. There is an abnormal bowing ratio. The bowing ratio is calculated by drawing a line from the hook of the hamate (h) to the tubercle of the trapezium (t) and dividing that distance into the amount of palmar displacement (pd), which is the distance from line $h{\leftrightarrow}t$ to the flexor retinaculum.

affects the upper extremity, and results from the median nerve being compressed in the carpal tunnel. Symptoms generally make this an easy clinical diagnosis, so imaging is unnecessary. Patients have pain and paresthesias in the thumb, index finger, third finger, and radial half of the fourth finger, which usually worsen at night.

There are many causes of carpal tunnel syndrome. Anything that increases the volume of the contents of the tunnel or narrows the tunnel can create nerve entrapment. The most common cause of this syndrome is tenosynovitis of the flexor tendons from overuse of the hands (typists).

MRI generally is not used to diagnose carpal tunnel syndrome because nerve conduction studies and clinical history suffice in most cases. MRI may be useful to define the underlying cause of carpal tunnel syndrome if it is evident, when nerve conduction studies are equivocal, or after surgery if patients have recurrent or persistent symptoms.

MR findings of carpal tunnel syndrome are seen best on axial images. There are four major signs of carpal tunnel syndrome (Figs. 12-26 and 12-27), as follows:[30,31]

1. Focal or segmental swelling (pseudoneuroma) of the median nerve, best determined by subjectively comparing the size of the nerve at the level of the distal radius with its size at the pisiform. Normally, the nerve should stay the same size or decrease distally. If the nerve is larger on progressively more distal images, it is swollen.

2. Flattening or angulation of the nerve. This is best evaluated at the distal carpal tunnel at the level of the hook of the hamate. If the nerve is compressed against adja-

cent tendons and bones, the surface becomes faceted or angled.

3. Bowing of the flexor retinaculum caused by increased volume of the carpal tunnel contents. This is called the *bowing ratio*. The bowing ratio is calculated by drawing a line from the trapezium to the hook of the hamate on an axial image (length = TH). The distance from this line to the flexor retinaculum (palmar displacement = PD) is divided by the length TH. The ratio is up to 15% in normal subjects and ranges from 14% to 26% in patients with carpal tunnel syndrome.

4. Increased signal intensity of the median nerve on T2 images may occur from obstruction of venous return from the nerve with resultant edema.

Perhaps more important than diagnosing carpal tunnel syndrome is evaluating the cause of persistent or recurrent carpal tunnel syndrome in patients who have been treated for it surgically without success. Postoperative failures may have several causes, the most common of which is incomplete release of the flexor retinaculum.[32] MRI findings suggestive of an anatomic basis for recurrent symptoms include identification of an intact portion of the flexor retinaculum, the development of low signal intensity fibrotic scarring around the median nerve, and proximal swelling of the nerve (Fig. 12-28). MRI also may show a persistent or recurrent mass lesion within the carpal tunnel or the development of a median nerve neuroma. The normal postoperative appearance of the carpal tunnel after complete incision of the retinaculum is as follows: the retinaculum is invisible, the free ends of the retinaculum are displaced in a volar direction, and the contents of the carpal tunnel are displaced in a volar

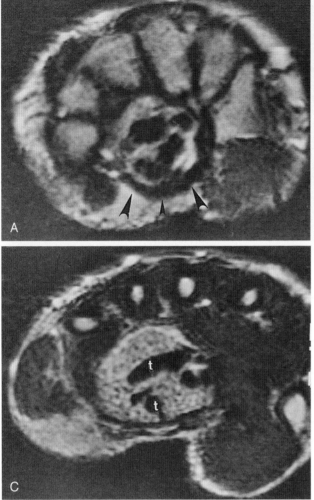

Figure 12-28   Causes of failed carpal tunnel release. A, Proton density axial image of the wrist. Incomplete release of the flexor retinaculum, which is thickened and bowed (*arrowheads*). **B,** T1 axial image of the wrist (different patient than in **A**). The median nerve (*curved white arrow*) is huge, and its volar surface is surrounded by scar (*black arrows*) from previous surgery. **C,** Proton density axial image of the wrist (different patient than **A** and **B**). Recurrent carpal tunnel syndrome occurred, caused by the development of rice bodies in the tendon sheaths surrounding the flexor tendons (t). The rice bodies give the stippled appearance in the carpal tunnel surrounding the tendons and create a mass effect on the nerve.

direction relative to the tunnel (Fig. 12-29). MRI is useful for identifying a persistent artery or vein within the carpal tunnel. This is an important observation to avoid injury to the vessel at surgery (Fig. 12-30).

Fibrolipomatous Hamartoma

Fibrolipomatous hamartoma of a nerve is a benign lesion that arises in and causes profound enlargement of a nerve.[33]

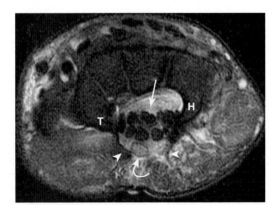

Figure 12-29   Normal postoperative appearance of the carpal tunnel. Axial T2W image of the wrist. The flexor retinaculum is partially missing, the free ends of the retinaculum are displaced volarly (*arrowheads*), and the contents of the tunnel (flexor tendons—*straight arrow*, median nerve—*curved arrow*) are displaced volarly. H, hook of hamate; T, trapezium.

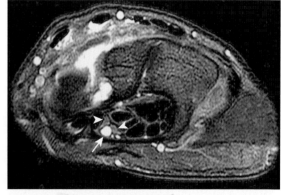

Figure 12-30   Persistent median artery. Axial T2W image of the wrist. The median nerve (*arrowheads*) is split by a vessel (*arrow*) within the carpal tunnel.

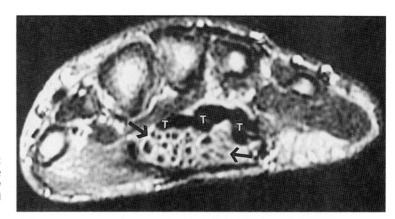

Figure 12-31 **Fibrolipomatous hamartoma.** Spin echo–T2 axial image of the wrist. The stippled area (*arrows*) volar to the flexor tendons (T) represents a gigantic median nerve. The low signal stippled appearance is from enlarged nerve fascicles and fatty tissue infiltrates around the fascicles.

The median nerve in the wrist is the most common nerve in the body to be affected. The lesion may be asymptomatic, but nerve compression may develop. Two thirds of patients with macrodactyly (macrodystrophia lipomatosa) have fibrolipomatous hamartoma. There is infiltration of the nerve by fibrous and fatty tissue.

This lesion has a distinctive MRI appearance (Fig. 12-31). It is seen as a mass along the course of the median nerve, composed of tubular low signal intensity structures, probably corresponding to nerve fascicles surrounded by epineural and perineural fibrosis, within a background of high signal intensity fat.

Ulnar Nerve

The ulnar nerve, artery, and vein pass through Guyon's canal on the ulnar side of the wrist (Fig. 12-32). The canal is formed by the flexor retinaculum and hypothenar musculature, the volar aspect is formed by a layer of fascia, and the pisiform and hook of the hamate form the osseous margins of the canal.

Ulnar Tunnel Syndrome. The ulnar nerve may become compressed along Guyon's canal. Causes for this compression include ganglion cysts (Fig. 12-33) or other masses, fracture of the hamate, or repetitive trauma to this region related to occupational or certain sports activities (biking, tennis, golf). The course, size, and signal intensity of the nerve and any adjacent masses can be assessed on axial MRIs.[34]

OSSEOUS STRUCTURES

Normal Relationships

Certain osseous anatomy of the wrist needs to be emphasized so that abnormalities are easier to understand. The relationship of the distal articular surface of the radius with the convex head of the ulna is important (Fig. 12-34). These structures are normally at the same level on coronal MRIs, and this is referred to as *neutral ulnar variance.*

If the ulna is proximal to the radial articular surface by greater than 2 mm, it is called *negative ulnar variance* (or *ulnar minus variance*). If the ulna is situated distal to the radius, it is positive ulnar (or ulnar plus) variance. Any alteration from the normal neutral ulnar variance changes the stresses on the wrist and can result in pathology. Specifically, ulnar plus variance is associated with the ulnolunate impaction syndrome and TFC tears, whereas ulnar minus variance is associated with osteonecrosis of the lunate (Box 12-6). Because of the curved surface of the ulna, care should be taken not to diagnose negative ulnar variance unless the ulna is shorter than the radius on all coronal images.

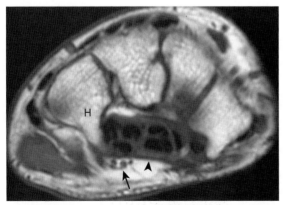

Figure 12-32 **Guyon's canal.** Axial image of the wrist. The ulnar tunnel (Guyon's canal) is formed by the flexor retinaculum (*arrowhead*), hypothenar musculature, and pisiform and hook of the hamate bones. The ulnar nerve, artery, and vein pass through the tunnel (*arrow*). H, hamate.

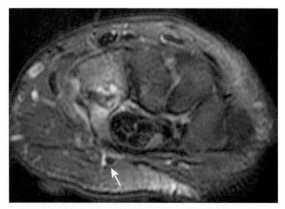

Figure 12-33 **Ulnar tunnel syndrome.** Gradient echo axial image of the wrist. There is a ganglion cyst (*arrow*) in the ulnar tunnel adjacent to the hook of the hamate, causing a compressive neuropathy of the ulnar nerve.

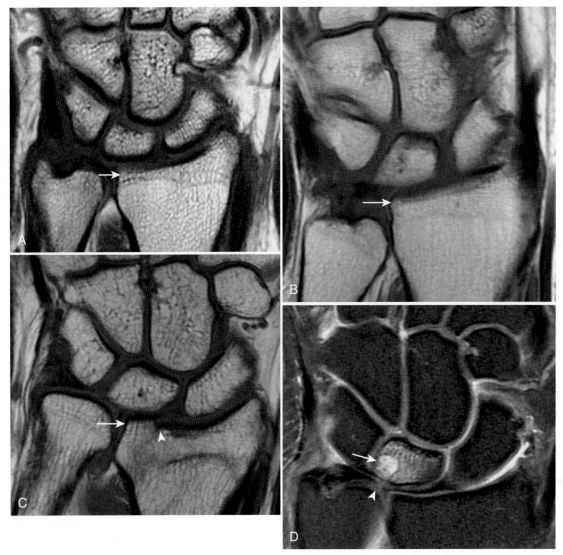

Figure 12-34 **Ulnar variance. A,** Coronal T1W image of the wrist. Neutral ulnar variance exists when the distal radius and head of the ulna are at the same level (*arrow*), or the ulna is within 2 mm proximal to the radius. **B,** Coronal T1W image of the wrist. Ulnar minus variance occurs when the head of the ulna is located proximal to the distal radius by greater than 2 mm (*arrow*). **C,** Coronal T1W image of the wrist. Ulnar plus variance results if the head of the ulna projects distal to the radius (*arrow*). Old impacted radial head fracture deformity is present (*arrowhead*). **D,** Coronal T2W image shows positive ulnar variance resulting in triangular fibrocartilage tear (*arrowhead*) and impaction on ulna (*arrow*).

Osseous Abnormalities

Os Styloideum. There are many accessory ossicles in the wrist, but the os styloideum is one that may be associated with pain and be confused with tumor or fracture. It is a common bony protuberance on the dorsal aspect of the wrist that is located at the base of the second and third metacarpals. This variant occasionally can cause pain owing to degenerative changes that develop between it and the underlying bones (Fig. 12-35), or because of an overlying bursitis or ganglion cyst as it projects from the surface of the wrist and is predisposed to injury. Presence of an os styloideum is easily seen with conventional radiographs, and MRI generally is not required to make this specific diagnosis. MRI shows a small piece of bone that articulates with the underlying capitate and trapezoid on axial or sagittal images. Bursitis and degenerative changes can be shown.

Triquetral Impaction

Occasionally, after an ulnar styloid fracture malunion, the styloid can impact the triquetrum leading to ulnar-sided wrist pain. T2W MRIs show bone marrow edema or cystic change within the triquetrum and ulnar styloid.[35,36]

Carpal Instability (Box 12-7). Carpal instability also is discussed in the sections on scapholunate and lunotriquetral ligament ruptures (see Figs. 12-5 to 12-7). Scapholunate ligament disruption may lead to scapholunate dissociation, which is the most common carpal instability syndrome. This condition results in rotatory subluxation of the scaphoid and dorsal tipping of the lunate (dorsal intercalated segmental instability). The ruptured scapholunate ligament can be diagnosed on coronal MRIs, and dorsal intercalated segmental instability can be diagnosed on sagittal images. This also may cause SLAC wrist. A tear of the lunotriquetral ligament

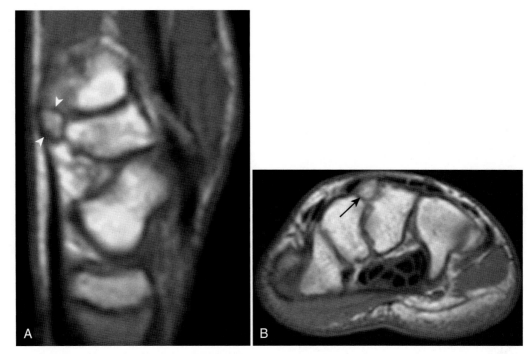

Figure 12-35 Os styloideum. **A,** Sagittal T1W image of the wrist. An os styloideum (*arrowheads*) is present on the dorsum of the wrist. **B,** Axial T1W image of the wrist. The os styloideum (*arrow*) is noted at the base of the second and third metacarpals.

can be diagnosed on coronal MRIs, and any associated instability between the lunate and triquetrum can be detected on sagittal MRIs with volar tilting of the lunate (volar intercalated segmental instability).

Ulnolunate Impaction. The ulnolunate impaction syndrome is a pain syndrome that occurs because of chronic abutment of the distal ulna against the proximal lunate. There is a strong association between ulnar plus variance and ulnolunate impaction syndrome. Ulnar plus variance leads to altered and increased forces transmitted across the ulnar side of the wrist. Ulnar plus variance may be a congenital variant, or may develop as the result of an impacted distal radial fracture. The chronic repetitive impaction of the two bones against one another initially results in degenerative changes of the cartilage covering both bones. The intervening triangular fibrocartilage often is torn. Ultimately, degenerative changes affect the bones, especially the proximal surface of the lunate.[36]

MRI can show the bone changes in the lunate when radiographs are normal. The triangular fibrocartilage tears also are easily identified. MRI shows cartilage destruction, and underlying bone marrow edema, subchondral cyst formation, or sclerosis in the proximal lunate or head of the ulna (Fig. 12-36).

Occult Fractures. Persistent pain in the wrist after trauma may be the result of bone or soft tissue injuries. MRI is the best imaging technique for identifying abnormalities affecting the osseous and soft tissue structures. If a radiographically occult fracture is the only clinical concern, a limited trauma screening MRI examination can be done. MRI offers an exquisitely sensitive and specific method of diagnosing radiographically occult traumatic bone lesions.

The scaphoid is the most commonly fractured carpal bone. Delayed fracture union and osteonecrosis of the proximal fracture fragment are complications that may be prevented by early detection of the fracture and appropriate

---

BOX 12-6

Associations With Ulnar Variance

Positive Ulnar Variance

- Triangular fibrocartilage tears
- Ulnolunate impaction syndrome
  - Cartilage degeneration of lunate and ulna
  - Triangular fibrocartilage tears
  - Proximal lunate marrow edema or subchondral cyst

Negative Ulnar Variance

- Osteonecrosis of the lunate (Kienböck's disease)

BOX 12-7

Carpal Instability

Scapholunate Ligament Disruption May Lead to

- Increased scapholunate interval
- Rotatory subluxation of scaphoid
- Dorsal tipping of lunate (dorsal intercalated segmental instability)
- Scapholunate advanced collapse wrist
  - Increased scapholunate interval
  - Degenerative changes between scaphoid and radius
  - Proximal migration of capitate between scaphoid and lunate

Lunotriquetral Ligament Disruption May Lead to

- Volar tipping of lunate (volar intercalated segmental instability)

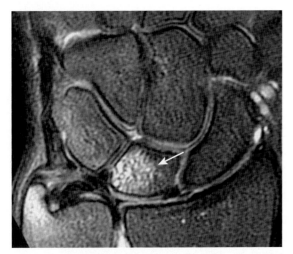

Figure 12-36   **Ulnolunate impaction.** Coronal T2W fat-suppressed image of the wrist. There is ulnar plus variance, a triangular fibrocartilage tear, and marrow edema in the lunate (*arrow*).

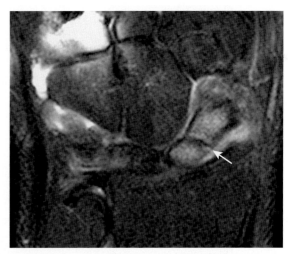

Figure 12-37   **Occult carpal fractures.** Coronal T2W image with fat suppression of the wrist. A radiographically occult scaphoid fracture is seen in this patient 3 months after the injury. The fracture line is linear low signal (*arrow*), and there is diffuse, surrounding edema throughout the bone.

treatment. About 16% of scaphoid fractures are not evident on the initial radiographs, and MRI is an excellent method for detecting these lesions (Fig. 12-37).[37-40] Many other bones in the carpus also may fracture and not be evident on radiographs. These radiographically occult fractures can be seen as marrow edema from bone contusions (Fig. 12-38) or true linear fracture lines. The appearance of contusions with marrow edema but no fracture line does not indicate a less significant injury because at follow-up a true fracture line may be evident on radiographs.[37]

Physeal Injuries. Trauma to the physis (growth plate) of the distal radius and ulna may occur in young competitive gymnasts. This injury may result in the formation of a fibrous or osseous bridge across the physis or slowing of growth in a portion of the physis, which can cause a growth disturbance. The metaphysis may have associated contusions and radiographically occult stress fractures.

MRI can show the fractures, contusions, physeal injury, or focal bridge formation. The osseous lesions are identical to those described earlier. The cartilage of the physis is thickened initially, with persistent cartilaginous foci found later within the metaphysis. Physeal bridges are focal areas of either bone or low signal intensity fibrous material that extend vertically from the metaphysis to the epiphysis, traversing the cartilaginous physis. Gradient echo or STIR sequences are excellent for showing these abnormalities.[41,42]

Osteonecrosis (Box 12-8). The two most common sites for osteonecrosis in the wrist are the proximal pole of the scaphoid after a scaphoid fracture and the lunate bone. Rarely, the proximal portion of the capitate may undergo osteonecrosis after being fractured.

The proximal pole of the scaphoid is at high risk for osteonecrosis because of its tenuous blood supply; this also can lead to delayed union or nonunion of the fracture. Assessment of the viability of the proximal fragment is important for management and for surgical planning in patients who do not heal properly.

Normal fatty marrow signal intensity on T1W images indicates viability of the fragment. Low signal intensity on T1W and T2W images indicates necrosis (Fig. 12-39). If there is low signal intensity on T1W images and high signal intensity on T2W images, the significance is less clear; the signal intensity could be the result of bone marrow edema, changes of healing, or ischemic changes.[43,44]

Kienböck's osteonecrosis of the lunate may occur as the result of repetitive trauma, acute fracture, or ulnar minus variance. Men usually are affected and describe wrist pain that worsens with activity. Most patients with this disease are involved in manual labor. The blood supply to the lunate is tenuous with much of it being supplied by end arteries. It is

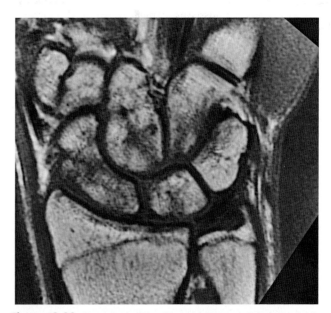

Figure 12-38   **Bone contusions.** T1 coronal image of the wrist. Patchy abnormal intermediate signal is present in the scaphoid, capitate, hamate, triquetrum, and lunate from multiple bone contusions without discrete fracture lines seen.

BOX 12-8
Osteonecrosis in the Wrist

Scaphoid
- Proximal pole at risk after fracture
- MRI
  - Low signal on T1 and T2 = osteonecrosis
  - Low signal on T1, high on T2 = questionable significance—possible ischemia, marrow edema, or healing
  - High signal on T1, intermediate on T2 (fat) = normal

Lunate (Kienböck's disease)
- Associated with repetitive trauma, fracture, ulnar minus
- MRI
  - Low signal on T1 and T2 of entire bone = osteonecrosis
  - If only a portion of the lunate is involved with low signal on T1 and T2, or there is low signal on T1 and high signal on T2, consider:
    Early stage of osteonecrosis
    Intraosseous ganglion
    Marrow edema/subchondral cyst from ulnolunate impaction (look for ulnar plus)

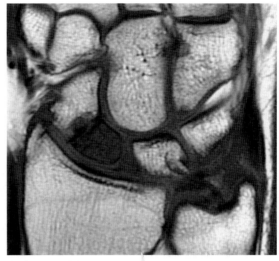

Figure 12-39 **Osteonecrosis of the scaphoid.** Coronal T1W image of the wrist. Osteonecrosis manifests as diffuse low signal in the proximal pole of the scaphoid without collapse.

subjected to strong compressive forces because of its central position in the wrist. The forces on the lunate are even greater in patients with negative ulnar variance.

MRI can show several patterns of abnormality based on the stage of the disease at the time of imaging. If there is low signal intensity on T1W and T2W images that involve the entire lunate, the findings are diagnostic for osteonecrosis (Fig. 12-40). If only a portion of the lunate is involved, or if there is increased signal intensity on T2W images, the diagnosis is less definite because other pathologies may cause a similar appearance (Fig. 12-41). High signal intensity on T2W images from osteonecrosis indicates an earlier stage of the disease process and a better outcome.[7,45,46]

Other lesions in the lunate that may simulate Kienböck's disease include intraosseous ganglion cyst and marrow edema or subchondral cyst formation that can occur from ulnolunate impaction. Both of these entities are focal and

have high signal intensity on T2W images. The diagnosis of Kienböck's disease is more definite when the entire bone is involved, or when there is low signal intensity on T1W and T2W images, but must be considered in the differential diagnosis for focal lesions that are high signal intensity on T2W images as well. Ulnolunate impaction syndrome should not be difficult to distinguish because ulnar plus variance is necessary for this entity to occur, whereas osteonecrosis of the lunate tends to occur with ulnar minus variance.

Congenital Osseous Lesions. Besides the os styloideum, there may be other congenital abnormalities of significance. Among these is congenital carpal coalition, the most common of which occurs between the lunate and triquetral bones. Lunotriquetral coalition may be osseous, fibrous, or cartilaginous. Fibrocartilaginous coalitions often have associated marrow edema or cystic changes adjacent

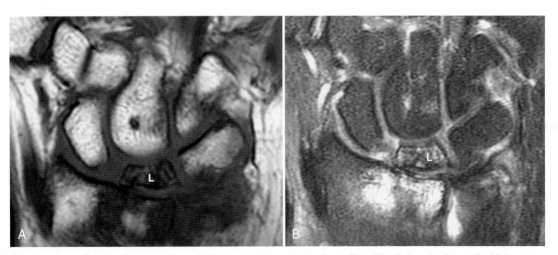

Figure 12-40 **Osteonecrosis of the lunate. A,** Coronal T1W image of the wrist. The lunate (L) is diffusely low signal from Kienböck's osteonecrosis. **B,** Fast T2W image with fat saturation. Signal in the lunate (L) remains nearly completely low signal.

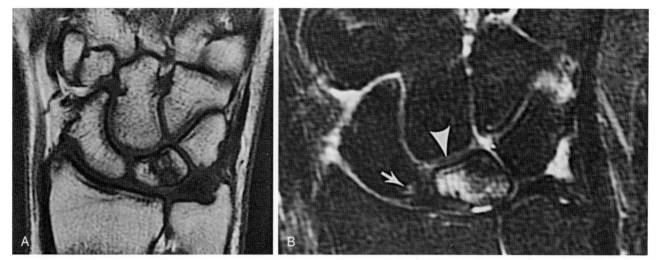

Figure 12-41 **Osteonecrosis of the lunate, partial involvement. A,** Coronal T1W image of the wrist. There is focal low signal in the lunate with normal fatty marrow on either side of the abnormality. This makes osteonecrosis less certain than if the entire lunate were involved. **B,** Coronal fast T2W with fat saturation image of the wrist (different patient than **A**). There is focal high signal in the radial side of the lunate (*arrowhead*) and a small area of high signal in the proximal pole of the scaphoid (*arrow*). Partial involvement of the lunate makes osteonecrosis a less definite diagnosis. This was proven to be osteonecrosis in the scaphoid and the lunate resulting from steroid use.

to the coalition, which mimic degenerative joint disease (Fig. 12-42).

Type II lunate has an extra facet that articulates with the proximal hamate. A type I lunate articulates only with the capitate. The articulation between the hamate and lunate that occurs with a type II lunate may lead to cartilage loss of the hamate, and MRI may show these changes as marrow edema or subchondral cysts in the proximal pole of the hamate (see Fig. 12-42). These changes are seen as a focal area of signal abnormality in the proximal hamate that is low signal on T1W and high signal on T2W images. Chondral abnormalities of the hamate are found at surgery much more commonly than are seen on MRI.

TUMORS

Bone and soft tissue tumors and tumor-like lesions of the hand and wrist are common and have various causes. Only lesions that are very common or occur almost exclusively in the wrist and hand are discussed here.

Osseous Lesions

Benign lesions of bone are far more common in the hand and wrist than malignant lesions. The most common of these lesions are enchondromas, intraosseous ganglion cysts, and epidermoid inclusion cysts.

Enchondromas. Enchondromas are cartilaginous rests within bone that have lobulated margins and often erode the endosteal surface of the cortical bone. They are located in the proximal and middle phalanges of the fingers and in the metacarpal bones. They often have calcifications seen by conventional radiography, but these may be difficult to identify by MRI. Enchondromas are low signal intensity on T1W images and become high signal intensity on T2W images. The characteristic location and lobulated configuration should allow the diagnosis to be made by MRI, where they usually are detected as incidental findings.

Intraosseous Ganglion Cysts. Intraosseous ganglion cysts are common in the carpal bones, particularly in the radial aspect of the lunate. They consist of a dense fibrous wall and a mucoid fluid inside the wall. The cysts generally are located in the subchondral region of bone and may be confined to the bone or result from extension of a soft tissue ganglion cyst into the adjacent bone. These may be painful lesions. A small ganglion cyst arising in the scapholunate ligament commonly erodes the radial aspect of the lunate bone, resulting in a common site for an intraosseous ganglion (Fig. 12-43).[47,48]

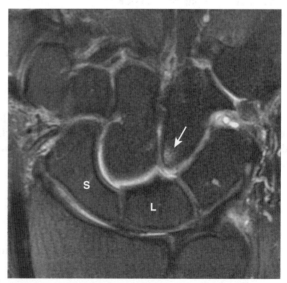

Figure 12-42 **Carpal coalition and type II lunate.** Coronal T1W image of the wrist. The space between the lunate (L) and the scaphoid (S) is narrowed. There also happens to be abnormal signal in the proximal hamate (*arrow*) because of the type II lunate, which has a facet that articulates with the hamate.

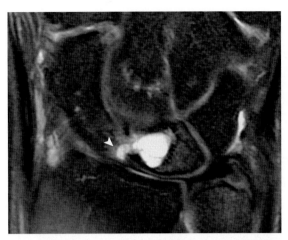

Figure 12-43 **Intraosseous ganglion cyst associated with scapholunate ligament degeneration.** Coronal T2W image of the wrist. An intraosseous ganglion cyst in the radial aspect of the lunate (*arrow*) is in continuity with a ganglion cyst in the scapholunate ligament (*arrowhead*).

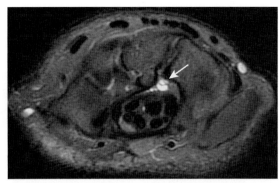

Figure 12-44 **Occult ganglion cyst of the scapholunate ligament.** Axial T2W image of the wrist. There is a small high signal mass with a septation in it representing a ganglion cyst (*arrowhead*). Incidentally noted is an intraosseous ganglion in the lunate (*arrow*).

MRI can show intraosseous ganglion cysts when radiographs are normal, and radionuclide bone scans are nonspecific. MRI can show whether the lesion is confined to bone or the result of erosion from an adjacent soft tissue ganglion cyst. These lesions are small, rounded, well-circumscribed foci with low signal intensity on T1W images and high signal intensity on T2W images.

Soft Tissue Lesions

The most common soft tissue masses in the hand and wrist are ganglion cysts, giant cell tumors of the tendon sheath, nerve sheath tumors, soft tissue chondromas, glomus tumors, and anomalous muscles.

Ganglion Cysts. The most common cause of a mass involving the wrist is a ganglion cyst.[49] These are fibrous-walled masses that contain thick mucoid fluid that resembles petroleum jelly. Ganglion cysts may be found attached by a pedicle to a tendon sheath, joint capsule, ligament, or within a fascial plane. These lesions may or may not be symptomatic. They usually occur in women in their 30s. Their cause is uncertain, but probably relates to chronic irritation at the site of formation. Ganglion cysts may erode the adjacent osseous structures. It is important to examine the scapholunate ligament carefully for small, occult ganglion cysts that are clinically not palpable but are a common source of dorsal wrist pain (Fig. 12-44).

MRI shows ganglion cysts as low signal intensity masses on T1W images, although occasionally they are higher signal intensity because of a high protein concentration. On T2W images, the lesions generally are diffusely high signal intensity. A common feature that is characteristic for ganglion cysts is the presence of thin septations within the mass that are seen as low signal intensity lines on T2W images (Fig. 12-45).[50,51]

Gadolinium may be given to differentiate a ganglion cyst from a solid mass. Enhancement is evident in the very thin fibrous wall and in the thin septations. The remainder of the lesion should show no enhancement.

Giant Cell Tumors of the Tendon Sheath. Giant cell tumors of the tendon sheath represent the second most common soft tissue mass of the hand and wrist. This tumor is an extra-articular, localized form of pigmented villonodular synovitis, a hyperplastic synovial process of unknown cause. Tumors most commonly involve the volar aspect of the fingers.

The mass shows low signal intensity on T1W and T2W images, which significantly limits the differential diagnostic possibilities (Fig. 12-46). Amyloid deposits and gouty tophi also may manifest as soft tissue masses with the same signal characteristics, but there are generally other features on the MRIs or clinical history that help to differentiate these entities. Gout usually has multiple lesions and joint involvement, and amyloid is generally a systemic process from an underlying known disease.

Glomus Tumors. Glomus tumors are benign tumors that arise from a neuromyoarterial glomus, which are present in the deepest layer of the dermis throughout the body. Glomus bodies are highly concentrated in the fingertips, especially beneath the fingernails. The lesions usually are found dorsal to the distal phalanges of the digits, but occasionally can be present on the volar surface. The glomus functions to regulate body temperature. These lesions can cause severe aching pain, point tenderness, and sensitivity to cold. Pressure erosion of the adjacent bone may occur from a glomus tumor.

Glomus tumors are small, well-defined soft tissue masses that show low signal intensity on T1W images and are hyperintense on T2W images (Fig. 12-47). Intravenous contrast administration shows these lesions to have strong enhancement. A thin capsule may be seen as low signal intensity surrounding the lesion on all pulse sequences and after contrast material is given. Axial and sagittal images are best for showing glomus tumors, and bone erosion often is evident when none is seen by conventional radiography. MRI is valuable for evaluation of glomus tumors to establish the diagnosis, to show if multiple lesions are present, and to direct surgery to the proper location because the lesions are generally extremely small and may be difficult to find.[52]

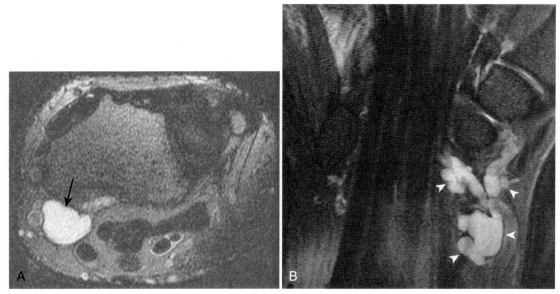

Figure 12-45 **Ganglion cyst. A,** Axial T2W image of the wrist. The ganglion cyst is a high signal mass (*arrow*) on the volar aspect of the wrist. **B,** Coronal T2W image of the wrist. The high signal ganglion cyst is more completely evaluated (*arrowheads*).

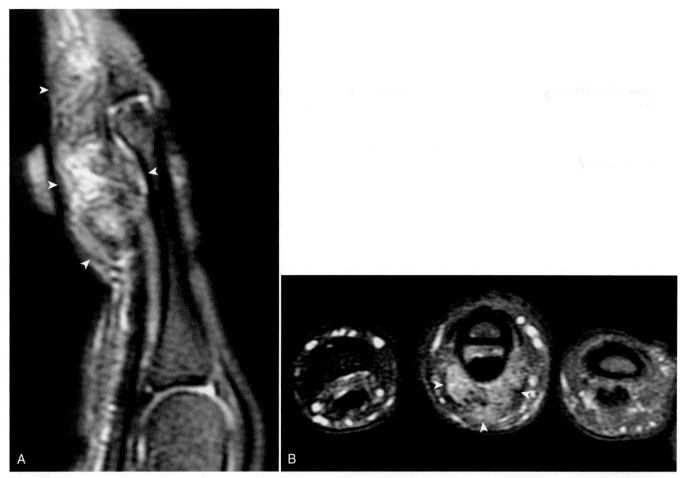

Figure 12-46 **Giant cell tumor of the tendon sheath. A,** Sagittal T2W image of the finger. There is a lobulated, intermediate to low signal mass volar to the flexor tendon of the index finger (*arrowheads*). **B,** Axial T2W image of the finger shows intermediate to low signal mass around the flexor tendon (*arrowheads*). Signal characteristics are typical of giant cell tumor of the tendon sheath.

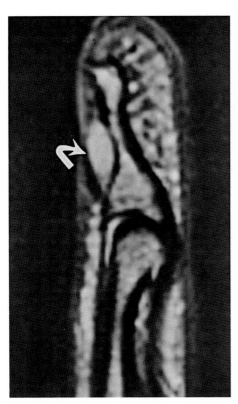

Figure 12-47 Glomus tumor. Fast T2W sagittal image of the finger. There is a small high signal mass (*curved arrow*) on the dorsum of the distal phalanx, causing bone erosion.

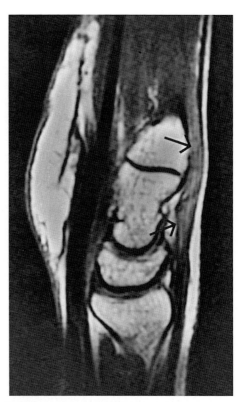

Figure 12-48 Anomalous muscle. Sagittal T1W image of the wrist. A dorsal soft tissue mass (*arrows*) with signal typical of muscle is the extensor digitorum brevis manus.

Anomalous Muscles. Anomalous muscles are common in the hand and wrist. They may manifest as a soft tissue mass, or may cause compression of the median or ulnar nerve, depending on the location of the anomalous muscle. A common anomalous muscle is the extensor digitorum manus brevis, found on the dorsum of the wrist and hand along the ulnar side of the extensor indicis tendon.[53] Clinically, this anomalous muscle may be easily confused with a ganglion cyst.

MRI documents the presence of muscle in predictable locations (Fig. 12-48). The signal intensity follows that of other skeletal muscle on all pulse sequences, which serves to differentiate it from a mass of other origin.

ARTHRITIS

Inflammatory, degenerative, and metabolic arthritides commonly affect the hand and wrist. The tomographic nature and superb contrast resolution of MRI allows erosions, subchondral cysts, synovitis, tenosynovitis, and other manifestations of arthritis to be shown in exquisite detail when other imaging techniques show no or minimal abnormalities. Chapter 6 is devoted to the findings in arthritis and the role of MRI in these diseases.

Synovial Cysts

Synovial cysts may occur in the wrist. These may be a manifestation of rheumatoid arthritis, but a synovial cyst arising from the pisotriquetral joint is so common and unrelated to an inflammatory arthritis that it warrants attention here.

Small amounts of fluid in the pisotriquetral synovial recess normally may be seen, but when it becomes large in amount, it may be a possible source of pain. These probably occur in patients who have pisotriquetral degenerative joint disease. A ball-valve mechanism may exist that allows synovial fluid to enter the cyst, but not exit it. The fluid is absorbed, and what remains behind in the synovial cyst is very thick, mucoid material similar to that found in ganglion cysts. An enlarged pisotriquetral synovial cyst is anatomically similar to a popliteal (Baker's) cyst in the knee, and may become symptomatic and usually enlarges as a response to abnormalities in the adjacent joint. We have aspirated and injected several enlarged pisotriquetral cysts with anesthetic and steroid, and patients experienced pain relief. If the injections do not relieve symptoms, surgical removal of the pisiform bone may be performed for pain relief.

The MRI appearance of the pisotriquetral synovial cyst is that of a rounded or elongated mass on the volar aspect of the wrist, just proximal to the pisiform, which is low signal intensity on T1W images and high signal intensity on T2W images (Fig. 12-49). When it measures 1 cm or more in diameter, we mention it as a synovial cyst that may be a source of pain.

INFECTION

Septic arthritis, abscesses, cellulitis, and osteomyelitis may occur in the hand and wrist. These processes are more common in other anatomic locations and are discussed in

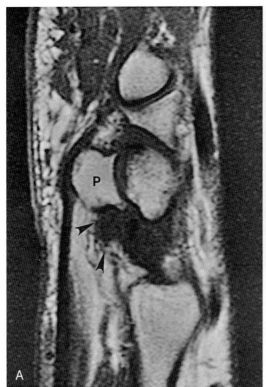

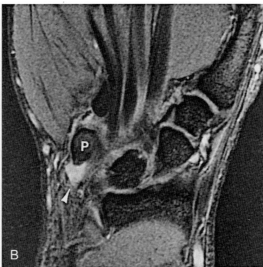

Figure 12-49   Pisotriquetral synovial cyst. **A,** Sagittal T1W image of the wrist. A low signal mass (*arrowheads*) just proximal to the pisiform (P) is a synovial cyst from the pisotriquetral joint. Note the mild degenerative changes in the joint with osteophytes. **B,** Gradient echo coronal image of the wrist. The synovial cyst becomes high signal (*arrowhead*) and is located just proximal to the pisiform (P).

detail elsewhere. The MRI findings of infection in the hand and wrist are no different than in other anatomic sites. One feature of this anatomic region to keep in mind is that infection spreads rapidly along compartments and tendon sheaths (Fig. 12-50). Any suspicion of infection needs to be aggressively worked up and treated because of the devastating consequences in the hand. Fluid in a tendon sheath (tenosynovitis) may be sterile or infected, and one should always remember to consider a purulent tenosynovitis in the differential diagnosis for tenosynovitis.

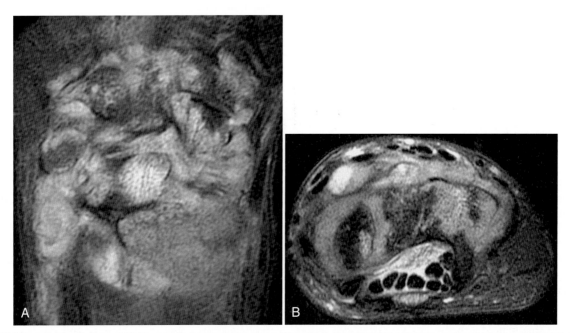

Figure 12-50   Infection. **A,** Coronal T2W image with fat suppression shows diffuse thickening of synovia with bone erosion and bone marrow edema. **B,** Axial T2W image shows lesions, bone marrow edema, and synovitis. There also is increased signal around the flexor tendons in this patient with atypical mycobacteria infection.

REFERENCES

1. Smith DK. Scapholunate interosseous ligament of the wrist: MR appearances in asymptomatic volunteers and arthrographically normal wrists. *Radiology* 1994; 192:217-221.

2. Smith DK, Snearly WN. Lunotriquetral interosseous ligament of the wrist: MR appearances in asymptomatic volunteers and arthrographically normal wrists. *Radiology* 1994; 191:199-202.

3. Berger RA. The gross and histologic anatomy of the scapholunate interosseous ligament. *J Hand Surg [Am]* 1996; 21:170-178.

4. Wright TW, Del Charco M, Wheeler D. Incidence of ligament lesions and associated degenerative changes in the elderly wrist. *J Hand Surg [Am]* 1994; 19:313-318.

5. Totterman SMS, Miller RJ. Scapholunate ligament: normal MR appearance on three-dimensional gradient-recalled-echo images. *Radiology* 1996; 200:237-241.

6. Zlatkin MB, Chao PC, Osterman AL, et al. Chronic wrist pain: evaluation with high-resolution MR imaging. *Radiology* 1989; 173:723-729.

7. Anderson MW, Kaplan PA, Dussault RG, Degnan GG. Magnetic resonance imaging of the wrist. *Curr Probl Diagn Radiol* 1998; 27:191-226.

8. Timins ME, Jahnke JP, Krah SF, et al. MR imaging of the major carpal stabilizing ligaments: normal anatomy and clinical examples. *RadioGraphics* 1995; 25:575-587.

9. Zlatkin MB, Rosner J. MR imaging of ligaments and triangular fibrocartilage complex of the wrist. *Magn Reson Imaging Clin N Am* 2004; 12:301-331.

10. Smith DK. Dorsal carpal ligaments of the wrist: normal appearance on multiplanar reconstructions of three-dimensional Fourier transform MR imaging. *AJR Am J Roentgenol* 1993; 161:119-125.

11. Smith DK. Volar carpal ligaments of the wrist: normal appearance on multiplanar reconstructions of three-dimensional Fourier transform MR imaging. *AJR Am J Roentgenol* 1993; 161:353-357.

12. Brown RR, Fliszar E, Cotten A, et al. Extrinsic and intrinsic ligaments of the wrist: normal and pathologic anatomy at MR arthrography with three-compartment enhancement. *RadioGraphics* 1998; 18:667-674.

13. Totterman SMS, Miller RJ. Triangular fibrocartilage complex: normal appearance on coronal three-dimensional gradient-recalled-echo MR images. *Radiology* 1995; 195:521-527.

14. Schweitzer ME, Brahme SK, Hodler J, et al. Chronic wrist pain: spin echo and short tau inversion recovery MR imaging and conventional and MR arthrography. *Radiology* 1992; 182:205-211.

15. Oneson SR, Timins ME, Scales LM, et al. MR imaging diagnosis of triangular fibrocartilage pathology with arthroscopic correlation. *AJR Am J Roentgenol* 1997; 168:1513-1518.

16. Golimbu CN, Firooznia H, Melone CP Jr, et al. Tears of the triangular fibrocartilage of the wrist: MR imaging. *Radiology* 1989; 173:731-733.

17. Totterman SMS, Miller RJ, McCance SE, Meyers SP. Lesions of the triangular fibrocartilage complex: MR findings with a three-dimensional gradient-recalled-echo sequence. *Radiology* 1996; 199:227-232.

18. Ruegger C, Schmid MR, Pfirrmann CWA, et al. Peripheral tear of the triangular fibrocartilage: depiction with MR arthrography of the distal radioulnar joint. *AJR Am J Roentgenol* 2007; 188:187-192.

19. Palmer AK. Triangular fibrocartilage complex lesions: a classification. *J Hand Surg [Am]* 1989; 14:594-606.

20. Staron RB, Feldman F, Haramati N, et al. Abnormal geometry of the distal radioulnar joint: MR findings. *Skeletal Radiol* 1994; 23:369-372.

21. Pfirrmann CW, Theumann NH, Chung CB, et al. What happens to the triangular fibrocartilage complex during pronation and supination of the forearm? Analysis of its morphology and diagnostic assessment with MRI arthrography. *Skeletal Radiol* 2001; 301:677-685.

22. Klug JD. MR diagnosis of tenosynovitis about the wrist. *Magn Reson Imaging Clin N Am* 1995; 3:305-312.

23. Spaeth HJ, Abrams RA, Bock GW, et al. Gamekeeper thumb: differentiation of nondisplaced and displaced tears of the ulnar collateral ligament with MR imaging—work in progress. *Radiology* 1993; 188:553-556.

24. Hinke DH, Erickson SJ, Chamoy L, Timins ME. Ulnar collateral ligament of the thumb: MR findings in cadavers, volunteers, and patients with ligamentous injury (gamekeeper's thumb). *AJR Am J Roentgenol* 1994; 163:1431-1434.

25. Rubens DJ, Blebea JS, Totterman SMS, Hooper MM. Rheumatoid arthritis: evaluation of wrist extensor tendons with clinical examination versus MR imaging—a preliminary report. *Radiology* 1993; 187:831-838.

26. Timins ME, O'Connell SE, Erickson SJ, et al. MR imaging of the wrist: normal findings that may simulate disease. *RadioGraphics* 1996; 16:987-995.

27. Drape JL, Tardif-Chestenet de Gory S, Silbermann-Hoffman O, et al. Closed ruptures of the flexor digitorum tendons: MRI evaluation. *Skeletal Radiol* 1998; 27:617-624.

28. Glajchen N, Schweitzer M. MRI features in de Quervain's tenosynovitis of the wrist. *Skeletal Radiol* 1996; 25:63-65.

29. Costa CR, Morrison WB, Carrino JA. MRI features of intersection syndrome of the forearm. *AJR Am J Roentgenol* 2003; 181:1241-1249.

30. Mesgarzadeh M, Schneck CE, Bonakdarpour A. Carpal tunnel: MR imaging, I: normal anatomy. *Radiology* 1989; 171:743-748.

31. Ikeda K, Haughton VM, Ho K-C, et al. Correlative MR-anatomic study of the median nerve. *AJR Am J Roentgenol* 1996; 167:1233-1236.

32. Murphy RX, Chernofsky MA, Osborne MA, Wolson AH. Magnetic resonance imaging in the evaluation of persistent carpal tunnel syndrome. *J Hand Surg [Am]* 1993; 18:113-120.

33. Cavallaro MC, Taylor JAM, Gorman JD, et al. Imaging findings in a patient with fibrolipomatous hamartoma of the median nerve. *AJR Am J Roentgenol* 1993; 161:837-838.

34. Binkovitz LA, Berquist TH, McLeod RA. Masses of the hand and wrist: detection and characterization with MR imaging. *AJR Am J Roentgenol* 1990; 154:323-326.

35. Cerezal L, del Pinal F, Abascal F, et al. Imaging findings in ulnar-sided wrist impaction syndromes. *RadioGraphics* 2002; 22:105-121.

36. Escobedo EM, Bergman AG, Hunter JC. MR imaging of ulnar impaction. *Skeletal Radiol* 1995; 24:85-90.

37. Breitenseher MJ, Metz VM, Gilula LA, et al. Radiographically occult scaphoid fractures: value of MR imaging in detection. *Radiology* 1997; 203:245-250.

38. Hunter JC, Escobedo EM, Wilson AH, et al. MR imaging of clinically suspected scaphoid fractures. *AJR Am J Roentgenol* 1997; 168:1287-1293.

39. Gaebler C, Kukla C, Breitenseher M, et al. Magnetic resonance imaging of occult scaphoid fractures. *J Trauma* 1996; 41:73-76.

40. Dorsay T, Major NM. Cost-effectiveness of immediate MR imaging as screening for radiographically occult scaphoid fractures versus traditional follow-up. *AJR Am J Roentgenol* 2001; 177:1257-1263.

41. Shih C, Chang C-Y, Penn I-W, et al. Chronically stressed wrists in adolescent gymnasts: MR imaging appearance. *Radiology* 1995; 195:855-859.

42. Chang C-Y, Shih C, Penn I-W, et al. Wrist injuries in adolescent gymnasts of a Chinese opera school: radiographic survey. *Radiology* 1995; 195:861-864.

43. Trumble TE. Avascular necrosis after scaphoid fracture: a correlation of magnetic resonance imaging and histology. *J Hand Surg [Am]* 1990; 15:557-564.

44. Desser TS, McCarthy S, Trumble T. Scaphoid fractures and Kienböck's disease of the lunate: MR imaging with histopathologic correlation. *Magn Reson Imaging* 1990; 8:357-361.

45. Golimbu CN, Firooznia H, Rafii M. Avascular necrosis of carpal bones. *Magn Reson Imaging Clin N Am* 1995; 3:281-303.

46. Trumble TE, Irving J. Histologic and magnetic resonance imaging correlations in Kienböck's disease. *J Hand Surg [Am]* 1990; 15:879-884.

47. Pope TL, Fechner RE, Keats TE. Intra-osseous ganglion. *Skeletal Radiol* 1989; 18:185-187.

48. Magee TH, Rowedder AM, Degnan GG. Intraosseous ganglia of the wrist. *Radiology* 1995; 195:517-520.

49. Bogumill GP, Sullivan EJ, Baker GI. Tumors of the hand. *Clin Orthop Relat Res* 1975; 108:214-222.

50. Vo P, Wright T, Hayden F, et al. Evaluating dorsal wrist pain: MRI diagnosis of occult dorsal wrist ganglion. *J Hand Surg [Am]* 1995; 10:667-670.

51. Kransdorf MJ, Murphey MD. MR imaging of musculoskeletal tumors of the hand and wrist. *Magn Reson Imaging Clin N Am* 1995; 3:327-344.

52. Drape J, Idy-Peretti J, Goettmann S, et al. Subungual glomus tumors: evaluation with MR imaging. *Radiology* 1995; 195:507-515.

53. Anderson MW, Benedetti P, Walter J, Steinberg DR. MR appearance of the extensor digitorum manus brevis muscle: a pseudotumor of the hand. *AJR Am J Roentgenol* 1995; 164:1477-1479.

Wrist and Hand Protocols

This is one set of suggested protocols; there are many variations that would work equally well.

WRIST: ROUTINE

Sequence No.	1	2	3	4	5	6
Sequence Type	T1	T2*	Turbo T2	T2*	T1	T1
Orientation	Coronal	Coronal	Coronal	Axial	Axial	Sagittal
Field of View (cm)	8-10	8-10	8-10	8-10	8-10	8-10
Slice Thickness (mm)	3	1 or 2	3	3	3	3
Contrast	No	No	No	No	No	No

WRIST: MASS OR INFECTION

Sequence No.	1	2	3	4	5	6
Sequence Type	T1	STIR	T1	STIR	T1 fat saturation	T1 fat saturation
Orientation	Coronal	Coronal	Axial	Sagittal	Coronal	Axial
Field of View (cm)	8-10	8-10	8-10	8-10	8-10	8-10
Slice Thickness (mm)	3	3	3	3	3	3
Contrast	No	No	No	No	Yes	Yes

WRIST: TRAUMA SCREENING

Sequence No.	1	2	3	4	5	6
Sequence Type	T1	Turbo T2				
Orientation	Coronal	Coronal				
Field of View (cm)	8-10	8-10				
Slice Thickness (mm)	3	3				
Contrast	No	No				

THUMB: GAMEKEEPER'S THUMB SCREENING

Sequence No.	1	2	3	4	5	6
Sequence Type	T1	T2*				
Orientation	Coronal	Coronal				
Field of View (cm)	6-8	6-8				
Slice Thickness (mm)	3	2				
Contrast	No	No				

SAMPLE REPORT STANDARD

Clinical Indications

Protocol

The routine protocol with multiple sequences and planes of imaging was used.

Discussion

1. Joint effusion: None

2. Osseous structures: No evidence of fracture or osteonecrosis; no erosions or other evidence of arthritis

3. Interosseous scapholunate and lunotriquetral ligaments: No evidence of tear

4. Triangular fibrocartilage: No tear

5. Flexor and extensor tendons: Normal position, signal, and configuration

6. Carpal tunnel: Normal; the position, morphology, and signal of the median nerve are normal

7. Guyon's canal: Normal; the ulnar nerve has a normal morphology and signal

8. Other abnormalities: None

Opinion

Normal MRI of the (right/left) wrist.

Spine

13

How to Image the Spine

See spine protocols at the end of the chapter.
- *Coils and patient position:* Phased array spine coils should be used for all spine imaging. Patients are supine in the magnet.
- *Image orientation (Box 13-1):* Sagittal and axial images are acquired in the cervical, thoracic, and lumbar regions. In the axial imaging plane, we obtain stacked cuts that cover an entire block of the spine. Acquiring images angled only through the disks (without obtaining stacked images) is considered inadequate because

portions of the spinal canal are not imaged in the axial plane, and sequestered disk fragments and spondylolysis defects are often missed.[1] Sagittal images alone are sometimes inadequate to detect a disk fragment that has migrated from the parent disk. Because sequestered disks are a cause of failed back surgery and persistent symptoms, it is important to identify them on MRI by obtaining stacked axial images in addition to sagittal images through the canal. In the unoperated lumbar spine, we obtain stacked axial images from the middle of the L3 vertebral body to the middle of the S1 vertebral body. In the postoperative spine, stacked axial images (matched images before and after contrast administra-

BOX 13-1

Spinal Structures to Evaluate in Different Planes

Sagittal
- Cord
- Disk signal, height
- Disk contour (±)
- Vertebral bodies
- Spinous processes
- Nerve roots
- Neural foramina
- Central canal
- Ligaments (anterior and posterior longitudinal, interspinous, supraspinous)
- Epidural space

Axial
- Nerve roots
- Cord
- Disk contour
- Vertebral bodies
- Neural foramina
- Central canal
- Lateral recesses
- Ligaments (ligamentum flavum)
- Epidural space
- Facet joints

Table 13-1 DISK AGING AND DEGENERATION

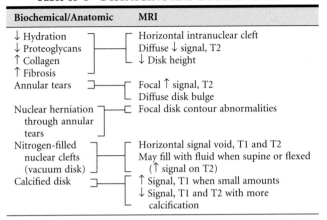

Biochemical/Anatomic	MRI
↓ Hydration ↓ Proteoglycans ↑ Collagen ↑ Fibrosis	Horizontal intranuclear cleft Diffuse ↓ signal, T2 ↓ Disk height
Annular tears	Focal ↑ signal, T2 Diffuse disk bulge
Nuclear herniation through annular tears	Focal disk contour abnormalities
Nitrogen-filled nuclear clefts (vacuum disk)	Horizontal signal void, T1 and T2 May fill with fluid when supine or flexed (↑ signal on T2)
Calcified disk	↑ Signal, T1 when small amounts ↓ Signal, T1 and T2 with more calcification

tion) are obtained by centering at the level of the previous surgery. Axial images are often better than sagittal for detecting lesions in the neural foramina. Generally, we consider axial and sagittal planes of imaging to be complementary and do not recommend doing without either. Coronal images may be useful to better define the anatomy in patients with scoliosis.

- *Pulse sequences and regions of interest:* The pulse sequences are determined by the clinical indications for the examination, based on the following major categories:
  1. Degenerative disease (including radicular symptoms)
  2. Trauma
  3. Cord compression/bone metastases
  4. Infection (disk or epidural/intradural lesion)

T1W and fast T2W images are the standard for sagittal imaging in any segment of the spine. Gradient echo sagittal sequences are used when looking for blood in the cord after trauma to take advantage of the blooming effect. A fast STIR sagittal sequence also is useful in trauma patients when looking for ligamentous injury with changes of hemorrhage and edema. Gradient echo axial images are used to detect disk disease in the cervical spine, whereas fast T2W axial images are used in the thoracic and lumbar spine for the same indications. TIW and some type of T2W images are selected in the sagittal and axial planes for most indications. Details are given in the tables of the spine protocols. Slice thickness generally is 3 or 4 mm. Axial gradient echo images through the cervical disks are 2 mm thick. The fields of view are as small as possible; larger ones are required for sagittal than for the axial imaging planes. In the cervical, thoracic, and lumbar spine, the sagittal fields of view are usually 14 cm, 16 cm, and 16 cm; recommended fields of view for the axial images are 11 cm, 12 cm, and 14 cm. Phase and frequency encoding gradients should be reversed for imaging the spine in the sagittal plane so that chemical shift artifacts at the diskovertebral inter-

faces do not obscure pathology in the vertebral body end plates or disks.

- *Contrast:* Contrast medium is always used for postoperative spine imaging, suspected infection, or intradural or nontraumatic cord lesions. If any abnormality is identified in the epidural space when evaluating for osseous metastases or cord compression, gadolinium is given to better show these lesions.

Normal and Abnormal

DEGENERATIVE CHANGES

The most prevalent abnormalities of the spine are degenerative changes of the joints and osseous structures. In the spine, the major joints consist of the paired, freely movable (diarthrodial) synovial facet joints running along the dorsal aspect of the spine and the minimally movable (amphiarthrodial) cartilaginous articulations formed by the intervertebral disks. Primary stability of the spine below C2 is provided by this three-joint complex, composed of the intervertebral disk and paired facet joints at each vertebral level. Anatomic and biochemical changes occur in these joints as the result of aging, but such changes may or may not cause symptoms.

The major focus of spine imaging over the years has been on the mechanical effect that osseous, disk, and joint structures have on adjacent nerves. Although it is important to detect this mechanical effect with imaging, most symptoms of back pain are not related to compression or stretching of an exiting or descending nerve. Pain may arise from the facet joints or disks, regardless of what these structures do to an adjacent spinal nerve root. It has been well established that asymptomatic individuals of all ages have disk abnormalities on imaging studies.[2] The source of a patient's neck or back pain must be defined carefully by integrating the findings of clinical examination and MRI, often with the aid of diagnostic injections of anesthetic to different spinal structures for confirmation.

Disk Aging and Degeneration (Table 13-1)

Features of normal and abnormal disks discussed here apply to disks at any level in the spine because they appear the same whether in the cervical, thoracic, or lumbar regions.

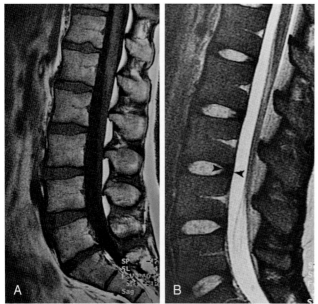

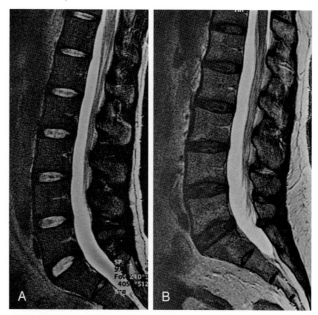

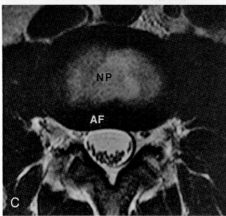

Figure 13-1 Normal disks. **A,** T1 sagittal image of the lumbar spine. Disks are intermediate signal intensity, lower signal than bone marrow, on T1W images. **B,** Fast T2 sagittal image of the lumbar spine. The nucleus is diffusely high signal, whereas the annulus fibrosus is low signal (between *arrowheads,* at L3-4). **C,** Fast T2 axial image, L3-4 disk. The nucleus pulposus (NP) is high signal, whereas the annulus fibrosus (AF) around the periphery of the disk is low signal.

Figure 13-2 Disk degeneration and aging. **A,** Fast T2 sagittal image of the lumbar spine. Horizontal low signal fibrous intranuclear clefts at each level divide the disks into upper and lower halves as an early manifestation of degeneration. **B,** Fast T2 sagittal image of the lumbar spine (different patient than in **A**). Diffuse low signal intensity throughout the disks is a more advanced change of degeneration and aging.

Normal Disk. Intervertebral disks consist of a central gelatinous nucleus pulposus composed of water and proteoglycans. The nucleus pulposus is surrounded by the annulus fibrosus. The inner portion of the annulus is composed of fibrocartilage, whereas the outer fibers are made of concentrically oriented lamellae of collagen fibers. The annulus is anchored to the adjacent vertebral bodies by Sharpey's fibers.

On MRI, the ideal normal disk is low signal intensity on T1W images, slightly lower signal than adjacent normal red marrow and very similar to muscle (Fig. 13-1). T2W images show diffuse high signal intensity throughout the disk except for the outer fibers of the annulus, which are homogeneously low signal intensity (see Fig. 13-1). Distinction between the nucleus pulposus and the inner annulus fibrosus is impossible by MRI.

Normal disks typically do not extend beyond the margins of the adjacent vertebral bodies; however, diffuse extension beyond the margins by 1 to 2 mm may occur in some histologically normal disks.[3] The posterior margins of disks tend to be mildly concave in the upper lumbar spine, straight at the L4-5 level, and slightly convex at the lumbosacral junction.

Abnormal Nucleus. With aging and degeneration, the intervertebral disks lose hydration, lose proteoglycans, and gain collagen as they become more fibrous. A horizontally oriented fibrous intranuclear cleft develops in the nucleus.

MRI shows the intranuclear cleft as a horizontal, low signal intensity line that divides the disk into upper and lower halves on T2W sagittal images (Fig. 13-2). Eventually, there is diffuse decreased signal intensity on T2W images from the increased collagen content in the nucleus (see Fig. 13-2). The disk progressively loses height with increasing degrees of degeneration.

Abnormal Annulus (Box 13-2). Aging and biochemical changes in the disks as described earlier are associated with

---

BOX 13-2

Radial Tears of the Annulus

- Also called *high intensity zones*
- Often painful
- Linear fissures through all or part of thickness of annulus
- Run perpendicular to long axis
- Usually in posterior annulus of lower lumbar disks
- Nerve ingrowth from surface of disk causes pain
- Globular or horizontal lines of increased signal in disk substance, T2 and postcontrast T1

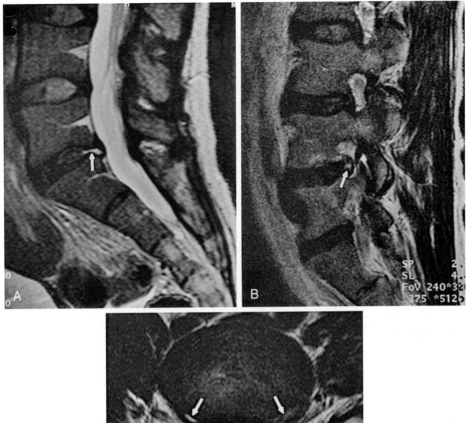

Figure 13-3 Annular tears. **A,** Fast T2 sagittal image of the lumbar spine. There is a focal line of increased signal in the posterior midline of the L5-S1 annulus (*arrow*), representing a radial tear/fissure or high intensity zone. The disk is protruding posteriorly slightly. **B,** Fast T2 sagittal image of the lumbar spine (different patient than in **A**). A focal high intensity zone (*arrow*) from a radial tear of the L4-5 annulus is seen in the region of the left neural foramen. **C,** Fast T2 axial image of L4-5 (same patient as in **B**). Short, linear segments of high signal (*arrows*) are present in the posterolateral L4-5 disk from annular tears in the foraminal regions. The disks are protruding at the sites of the tears, resulting in mild bilateral foraminal narrowing.

the development of multiple, focal annular tears. Three types of annular tears have been described, but only one type is of practical interest and that is the radial type of tear.[4]

Radial tears (or fissures) involve either part or the entire thickness of the annulus from the nucleus to the outer annular fibers. Radial tears run perpendicular to the long axis of the annulus and occur more commonly in the posterior half of the disk, usually at L4-5 and L5-S1. The radial annular tear is considered by many to be responsible for pain. It may be a pain source because vascularized granulation tissue grows into the tear and causes painful stimulation of nerve endings that also extend into the defect from the surface of the disk; this would result in diskogenic pain.[5] It also may be a pain source because of the instability of the disk that accompanies these fissures and the chemical and mechanical irritation to the nociceptive fibers that normally exist in the annulus. Radial fissures

that cause diskogenic pain can be treated by minimally invasive intradiskal therapy (thermal or chemical) or by spinal fusion.

MRI of annular tears shows focal areas of high signal intensity on T2W images or on contrast-enhanced T1W images.[6] Radial tears (Fig. 13-3) may be seen on T2W sagittal images within the posterior annulus as globular or horizontal lines of high signal intensity. On axial images, radial tears may be seen as focal areas of high signal intensity that parallel the outer disk margin for a short distance. Radial tears or fissures on MRI also are referred to as *high intensity zones.*[6]

Abnormalities in Disk Morphology (Box 13-3). The terminology for disk abnormalities is confusing and inconsistent in the literature. Many physicians have referred to any and all disk abnormalities that extend beyond the margin of the vertebral body or disk as a *herniated disk* or *herniated nucleus*

BOX 13-3

Disk Contour Abnormalities: Terminology

Herniated Disk

- All-encompassing, nonspecific term to indicate disk extends in some abnormal manner beyond margin of vertebral body

Disk Bulge

- Diffuse extension of disk by >2 mm beyond vertebral margin

Disk Protrusion

- Focal, small extension of disk beyond vertebral margin
- Anteroposterior < mediolateral diameter
- No cranial or caudal extension
- Usually asymptomatic
- Low signal T1 and T2

Disk Extrusion

- Greater extension of focal disk material than a protrusion
- Frequently symptomatic
- Anteroposterior ≥ mediolateral diameter
- May migrate craniocaudally, but maintains attachment to parent disk
- Decreased signal on T1, decreased or increased on T2

Sequestered Disk

- Loss of continuity between extruded disk material and parent disk
- Usually symptomatic
- Fragment migrates
  - Cranial or caudal (equally)
  - Anterior or posterior to posterior longitudinal ligament
  - Epidural, intrathecal, paraspinous
- Contraindication to limited disk procedures
- Common cause of failed back surgery, if unrecognized
- Decreased signal on T1, decreased or increased on T2 or contrast T1

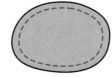

A. Diffuse Disk Bulge

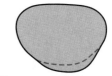

B. Broad-based Protrusion
(or focal disk bulge)

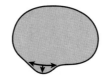

C. Focal Disk Protusion
AP< Mediolateral dimension

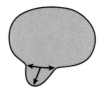

D. Disk Extrusion
AP≥ Mediolateral dimension

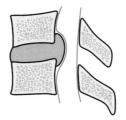

E. Disk Extrusion
Disk migrates above and/or below parent disk, maintaining continuity with it

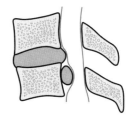

F. Sequestered Disk
Separate from parent disk

Figure 13-4 **Disk morphology.** Diagram showing abnormalities in morphology of the disks. The *dashed lines* in *A* and *B* indicate the vertebral bodies, whereas the *solid lines* represent the disks. AP, anteroposterior.

pulposus. The problem with this approach is that most of the abnormalities are of no consequence to the patient and are not associated with symptoms; this explains the high incidence of so-called disk herniations reported in an asymptomatic population.[2] Analogies to this situation would be to call benign bone islands *sclerotic foci of undetermined etiology* or calcified granulomas in the lungs on a chest x-ray *changes of infection.* These latter statements are true but of no help to the referring clinician or patient. They do not put the abnormality seen on the imaging study in proper perspective and may be misleading.

Most surgeons dealing with spine disorders are starting to use a more standardized nomenclature that helps to distinguish what are likely to be clinically relevant lesions from lesions that probably are not. We use the same terminology as our surgeons to describe abnormalities in disk morphology: *diffuse disk bulge, broad-based protrusion, focal disk protrusion, disk extrusion,* and *sequestered disk* (Fig. 13-4). *Focal disk abnormalities* occur when material from the nucleus extends either partially or completely through radial tears in the annulus. Focal disk abnormalities generally occur in a degenerated disk. The term *herniated disk* can be used to encompass all of the other, more specific terms outlined here, but in our opinion, it should never be the diagnosis in a report of a spine MRI examination.

When it has been determined that there is a diffuse or focal abnormality in disk contour, we generally try to quantify the abnormality as mild, moderate, or severe in extent. There are no agreed-on definitions for what constitutes these different categories. Our method of quantifying the severity of disk disease is *mild* if the anterior epidural fat is not obliterated, *moderate* if the epidural fat is obliterated and the thecal sac is being displaced, and *severe* if the cord is being effaced or nerve roots displaced.

This is not rocket science. The greatest difficulty is consistency and agreeing to the terms. All we are really evaluating when it comes to abnormalities in disk morphology is whether or not something is sticking out from the normal margin of a disk (like a wart from the skin surface), and by how far (how big the wart is).

Disk Bulge. A *diffusely bulging disk* extends symmetrically and circumferentially by more than 2 mm beyond the margins of the adjacent vertebral bodies. This diagnosis is based on axial and sagittal images by comparing the size of the disk with the size of the adjacent vertebral bodies and determining if the central canal and neural foramina are narrowed by the disk (Fig. 13-5). Identifying disk material protruding beyond the vertebral body margins on sagittal images does not clearly define if it is a diffuse or focal disk abnormality. The annulus can be considered lax, and a decrease in disk height and disk signal usually is present on MRI. There are tears in the annulus when there is disk bulging, although they may not be evident on MRI. A long segment of disk tissue that projects beyond the margin of the vertebral body but that does not involve the entire circum-

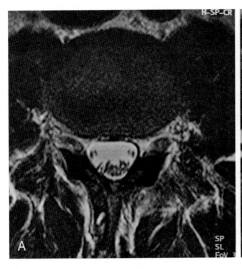

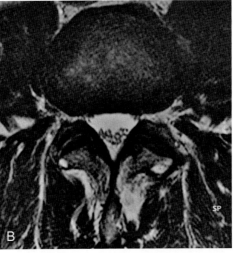

Figure 13-5 Diffuse disk bulge. A, Fast T2 axial image through a vertebral body. This shows the size of the vertebral body, which must be compared with the size of the adjacent disk (in **B**). **B,** Fast T2 axial image through the adjacent disk. The oval configuration of the disk is slightly larger than the vertebral body in **A,** indicating mild diffuse disk bulging. Also, the neural foramina and the thecal sac are slightly narrowed compared with **A,** owing to the bulging disk.

ference of the disk can be called either a *focal bulge* or a *broad-based protrusion* (Fig. 13-6).

Disk Protrusion. A *disk protrusion* is a focal, asymmetric extension of disk tissue beyond the vertebral body margin, usually into the spinal canal or neural foramen, that often does not cause symptoms. The base (the mediolateral dimension along the posterior margin of the disk) is broader than any other dimension (Fig. 13-7).[7]

Some of the outer annular fibers remain intact, and some people refer to this as a *contained disk*. The protruded disk does not extend in a cranial or caudal direction from the parent disk. MRI shows most disk protrusions and their parent disks to have low signal intensity on T1W and T2W images.

Disk Extrusion. An *extruded disk* is a more pronounced version of a protrusion and often is responsible for symptoms (Fig. 13-8). There is disruption of the outer fibers of the annulus, and the disk abnormality usually is greater in its anteroposterior dimension than it is at its base (mediolateral dimension). The extruded disk may migrate up or down behind the adjacent vertebral bodies but maintains continuity with the parent disk. These also may be referred to as *noncontained disks.* MRI shows the described contour abnormalities, and because of a significant inflammatory reaction that may occur in response to the extruded disk material, there may be high signal intensity on T2W and contrast-enhanced T1W images in or surrounding the disk. The typical appearance is the same signal intensity as the parent disk on all pulse sequences.

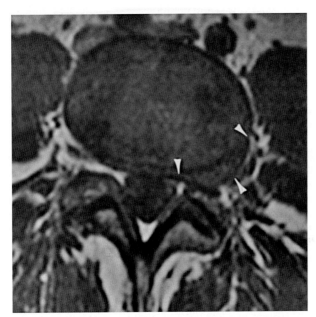

Figure 13-6   Focal disk bulge/broad-based protrusion. Tl axial image of L4-5. There is extension of disk beyond the margin of the vertebral body (between *arrowheads*) that is relatively long, referred to as either a *broad-based protrusion* or a *focal disk bulge.*

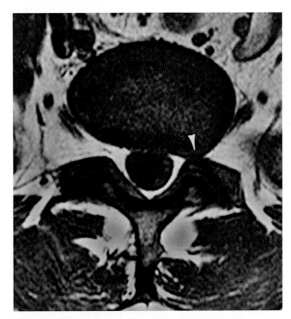

Figure 13-7   Disk protrusion. T1 axial image of L4-5. A short segment of disk protrudes into the left neural foramen (*arrowhead*), narrowing it. The base of the disk abnormality is greater than its anteroposterior dimension, typical of a focal disk protrusion.

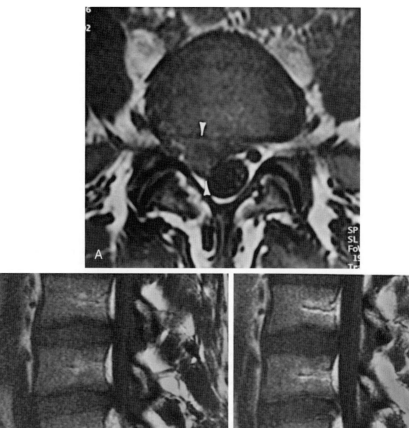

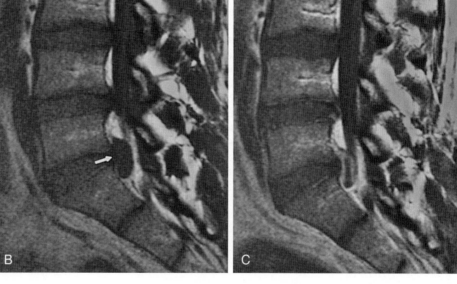

Figure 13-8 Disk extrusion. **A,** T1 axial image of L5-S1. A large piece of disk extends into the spinal canal in the right paracentral region. Its base is shorter than its anteroposterior dimension (between *arrowheads*), making this a disk extrusion. The descending S1 nerve is not identified because of displacement by the disk. **B,** T1 sagittal image of L5-S1. The disk extends superior and inferior to the level of the parent disk (*arrow*), which is an additional criterion for calling this a disk extrusion. **C,** T1 sagittal image with contrast enhancement of L5-S1. There is a peripheral rim of high signal surrounding the disk extrusion from enhancement of inflammatory reactive tissue.

Lumbar disk extrusions that cause radiculopathy but that are managed nonoperatively have been shown to do well about 90% of the time.[8] Spontaneous reduction in size of disk extrusions and protrusions that were managed conservatively has been well documented with imaging (Fig. 13-9).[9-12] The regression in disk size may not be the reason for reduction in pain. Much of the pain from extruded disks is probably from the inflammatory response to them rather than from compression of neural elements from the mass effect.

Caution is advised when using the terms *extrusion* and *extruded*. Some clinicians use the terms synonymously, whereas others apply the term *extruded* to indicate a free fragment or sequestration. This differentiation can make a huge difference. We have seen surgeons search needlessly (and without success) for a suspected sequestration because the term *extruded* was used in describing the disk bulge. Conversely, we have seen sequestrations left behind at surgery because they were called *extruded disks,* and the

surgeon thought this term was referring simply to the extrusion. Because it can be confusing and can result in patient mismanagement, some of us have abandoned the terms *extrusion* and *extruded* and replaced them with *protrusion* and *sequestration*. Others in our group have adopted the nomenclature initially mentioned, which is recommended by several spine societies.[13]

Sequestered Disk. When extruded disk material loses its attachment to the parent disk, it is called a *sequestered fragment* (Fig. 13-10). These fragments may migrate in a cranial or caudal direction with equal frequency and generally remain within about 5 mm of the parent disk. They may be located between the posterior longitudinal ligament and the osseous spine or extend through the posterior ligament into the epidural space. They almost always remain in the anterior epidural space, but occasionally the fragment may migrate into the posterior epidural space. Rarely, seques-

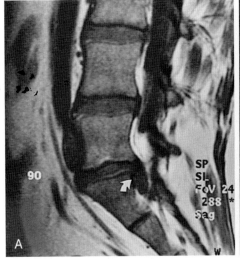

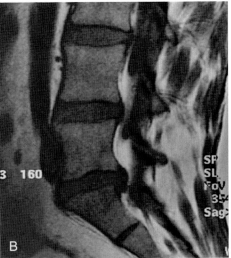

Figure 13-9 Spontaneous regression of disk extrusion. **A,** T1 sagittal image of L5-S1. A large disk extrusion extends behind the S1 vertebral body (*arrow*). **B,** T1 sagittal image of L5-S1. This image was obtained almost 1 year after the image in **A**. The patient had no surgery or other interventional therapy for the extruded disk. The disk extrusion is markedly reduced in size and now has the appearance of a disk protrusion.

tered fragments may enter the dural sac or migrate into the paraspinous soft tissues. It is extremely important to recognize these fragments because they may be overlooked at surgery. Some clinicians believe missed sequestrations are the leading cause of failed disk surgery. Sequestrations are a contraindication to chymopapain, percutaneous diskectomy, and other limited disk procedures. The fragment of disk material that migrates from the parent disk often shows peripheral or diffuse high signal intensity on T2W and contrast-enhanced T1W images, caused by the inflammatory reaction within or surrounding it. Otherwise, a low signal intensity mass resembling the signal of the parent disk is seen.

Location of Focal Disk Abnormalities (Box 13-4). A focal disk abnormality should be defined as to size, contour, location, and relationship to nerves or other important structures. The location of a focal disk abnormality needs to be conveyed accurately so that the surgical approach can be planned properly or so that it can be determined whether symptoms correlate to the anatomic abnormality seen on MRI. Focal disk abnormalities that remain at the level of the parent disk should be described as being *central, left* or *right paracentral, left* or *right foraminal,* or *left* or *right extraforaminal* (also called *lateral* or *far lateral*) (Fig. 13-11).

More than 90% of focal lumbar disk abnormalities affect the spinal canal (central and paracentral regions), whereas

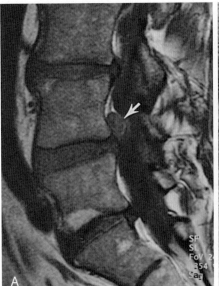

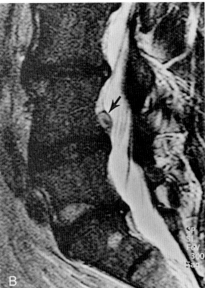

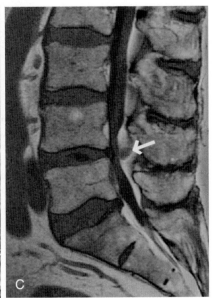

Figure 13-10 Sequestered disk. **A,** T1 sagittal image of the lumbar spine. There is a fragment of disk (*arrow*) posterior to the L4 vertebral body. There is a discrete line separating it from the L4-5 disk. Because this fragment has no attachment to a disk, it is a sequestered disk fragment. It may have originated from the L3-4 disk, which is narrowed and degenerated. **B,** Fast T2 sagittal image of the lumbar spine. The sequestered fragment (*arrow*) is much higher signal than any of the lumbar disks because of inflammatory reaction in and around the fragment. **C,** T1 sagittal image of the lumbar spine (different patient than in **A** and **B**). There is a large fragment of disk (*arrow*) in the posterior epidural space at the L4-5 level that is compressing the thecal sac. This was a sequestered fragment at surgery. MRI done 2 weeks earlier showed a disk extrusion at L4-5, but no abnormality posteriorly. MRI was repeated because of acute onset of severe back pain and radicular symptoms. Incidentally noted is Baastrup's disease involving the spinous processes (see text).

approximately 4% occur in the neural foramen, and another 4% occur in the extraforaminal regions. Individuals with symptoms of an L5 nerve abnormality almost always have a disk abnormality in the canal at the L4-5 level in the central or paracentral regions. An extraforaminal (lateral) disk at L5-S1 could cause the same symptoms as a posterior L4-5 disk, however, because it would be impinging on the L5 nerve that already exited.

About 90% of all focal disk abnormalities in the lumbar spine occur at L4-5 or L5-S1. Most focal degenerative disk abnormalities occur at C5-6 and C6-7 in the cervical spine, and very few focal disk abnormalities occur scattered throughout the thoracic spine. It is helpful to describe which nerve is affected by a disk abnormality; cervical nerves exit above the level of their respective disk level until C8, and then the nerves exit below. For example, a right paracentral C4-5 disk extrusion would impinge on the descending C6 nerve; similarly positioned right paracentral disk extrusions at T4-5 and L4-5 would nail the right descending T5 and L5 nerves. Intraforaminal extrusions at C4-5 would affect the exiting C5 nerve, whereas at T4-5 and L4-5 the exiting T4 and L4 nerves would be impinged on.

Significance of Disk Contour Abnormalities (Box 13-5). MRI is extremely sensitive in detecting abnormalities in the configuration of disks.[14-17] The problem is that many of these abnormalities do not cause symptoms, or at least not on the basis of nerve compression at that site.

Disk abnormalities are frequent in asymptomatic patients. Twenty percent of patients younger than 60 years old and 36% of patients older than 60 have one or more focal disk abnormalities of the lumbar spine, but no symptoms.[2] If the distinction is made between disk protrusions and extrusions, however, the findings are much more encouraging. Only 1% of asymptomatic patients have evidence of a disk extrusion by MRI.[7] Extrusions are much more likely to be significant and cause symptoms.

Mechanical compression of a nerve by a focal disk abnormality may cause symptoms of dysesthesias and muscle

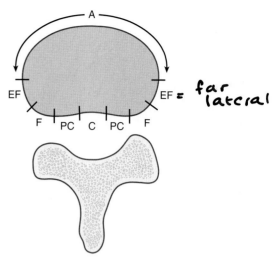

Figure 13-11 **Location of disk abnormalities.** Diagram depicting how to describe the location of disk abnormalities. Focal disk contour abnormalities may be central (C); left or right paracentral (PC); left or right foraminal (F); left or right extraforaminal (EF), which also may be called *far lateral disk abnormalities;* or anterior (A). Of focal disk contour abnormalities, 90% affect the central and paracentral regions.

weakness, but not pain symptoms. One theory for back pain is that the body reacts to displaced nucleus pulposus material with a foreign body–type inflammatory reaction. High levels of phospholipase A_2 enzyme have been found in degenerated disk material; this is also the active enzyme in snake venom

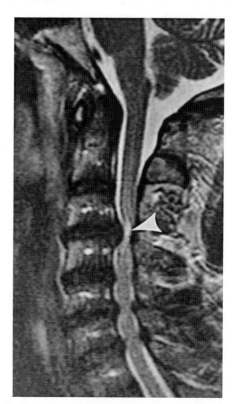

Figure 13-12 **Disk-related myelopathy.** Fast T2 sagittal image of the cervical spine. The C3-4 disk is protruding into the spinal canal, and there is compression of the cord with high signal within it (*arrowhead*). The cord abnormality is the result of cord ischemia with myelomalacia. The disks are protruding to a lesser extent at lower levels, causing multilevel canal stenosis.

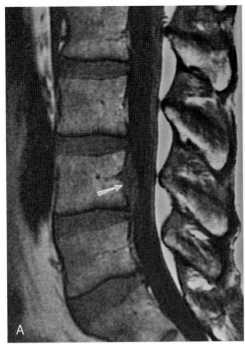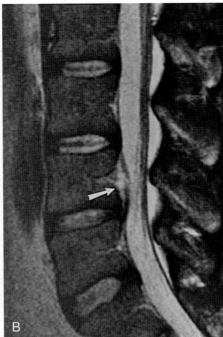

Figure 13-13 Spontaneous epidural hematoma. **A,** T1 sagittal image of the lumbar spine. There is an intermediate signal mass with a convex posterior margin posterior to L3 (*arrow*) that causes narrowing of the thecal sac. **B,** Fast T2 sagittal image of the lumbar spine. The mass becomes high signal (*arrow*). This is compatible with a spontaneous epidural hematoma. It also could be an extruded disk, but the symptoms resolved rapidly, and there is no narrowing of the disks to indicate that a large amount of disk material has been extruded.

and in the pannus of rheumatoid arthritis that generates inflammatory mediators, such as prostaglandins, leukotrienes, and platelet-activating factor. It is believed that a severe inflammatory reaction to displaced nuclear material may irritate surrounding nerves and produce pain and radicular symptoms, even in the absence of extension of disk into the spinal canal.[5,18-20]

Disk-Related Compressive Myelopathy and Epidural Hematoma. High signal intensity areas on T2W images can be seen within the spinal cord at the point of spinal stenosis secondary to a disk bulge or extrusion (Fig. 13-12). This high signal intensity may be from focal myelomalacia owing to ischemia to the cord. These cord lesions may or may not disappear after decompressive surgery.[21]

Small spontaneous epidural hematomas sometimes may occur in association with disk herniations from tearing of the fragile epidural vessels. This condition may be impossible to distinguish from a sequestered or extruded disk located posterior to the vertebral body (Fig. 13-13).

Epidural hematomas can be quite large and cause significant acute symptoms similar to those of an acute disk protrusion. They typically resolve rapidly, thus surgery is not performed. In many cases, surgery fails to detect an abnormality because at surgery the blood products are removed by the suction device (blood looks like blood at surgery), and no or only a little abnormal disk material is found. Epidural hematomas have a characteristic appearance on MRI (Fig. 13-14). They are typically large, are retrovertebral, often have some high signal on T1 sequences (blood products), and decrease in size with serial imaging.[22] We often mention that an epidural hematoma should be considered when we see what looks like a large sequestration because the treatment for each is different. With nonoperative treatment, an epidural hematoma resolves.

Disk Mimickers (Box 13-6). Abnormalities and normal variants may mimic a sequestered disk on MRI; synovial cysts from the facet joints, conjoined nerve roots, arachnoid diverticula, perineural cysts, and nerve sheath tumors arising from the nerve roots may cause confusion. We also have seen bullet fragments and cement from vertebroplasties (Fig. 13-15) within the spinal canal resembling the appearance of a sequestered disk; radiologists need to keep their minds open to the possibilities.

The signal intensity of dilated nerve root sleeves (Tarlov cysts or arachnoid diverticula), which is identical to cerebrospinal fluid (CSF), should allow differentiation from a disk fragment. A conjoined nerve is two nerve roots exiting the thecal sac at the same location; the roots can be seen within the mass on T2W images, and the lateral recess on the side of the conjoined nerve root is enlarged, indicating that this is a long-standing process.[23]

Vacuum Disks and Vertebral Bodies. Aside from abnormalities in disk contour, another manifestation of disk degeneration occurs from desiccation of the disk with the formation of cracks or clefts in the nuclear material, which may fill with nitrogen that comes out of solution from adja-

---

BOX 13-6

Mimickers of Extruded and Sequestered Disks

- Synovial cyst
- Conjoined nerve root
- Arachnoid diverticulum
- Perineural (Tarlov) cyst
- Nerve sheath tumors
- Small epidural hematoma

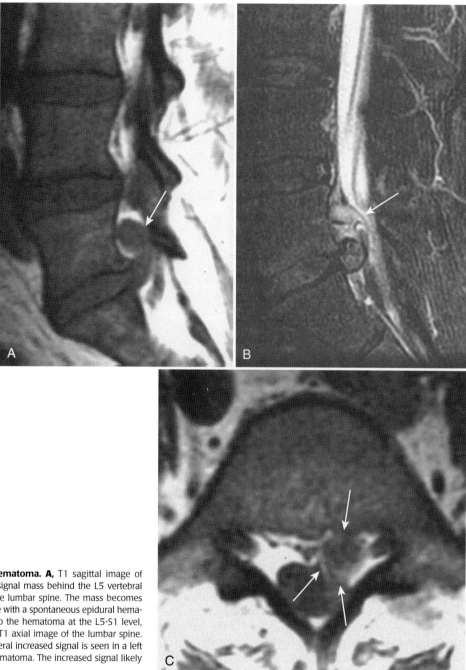

Figure 13-14   Spontaneous epidural hematoma. A, T1 sagittal image of the lumbar spine. There is an intermediate signal mass behind the L5 vertebral body (*arrow*). **B,** Fast T2 sagittal image of the lumbar spine. The mass becomes intermediate signal (*arrow*). This is compatible with a spontaneous epidural hematoma. Note the disk protrusion just caudal to the hematoma at the L5-S1 level, which has different signal characteristics. **C,** T1 axial image of the lumbar spine. A low signal mass (*arrows*) with some peripheral increased signal is seen in a left paracentral location, which is the epidural hematoma. The increased signal likely represents blood products.

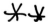

cent extracellular fluid. When this finding is present, it essentially excludes the possibility of superimposed infection or tumor involving the disk.[24] MRI shows the vacuum disk as a horizontally oriented, linear signal void on all pulse sequences (Fig. 13-16).

Cracks in the vertebral body end plates can allow nitrogen from the adjacent vacuum disk to seep into the vertebral body, forming an intraosseous vacuum cleft. This appearance has long been thought to be the result of osteonecrosis; in many cases it is simply a manifestation of degenerative disk disease and osteoporotic fractures combining to create this appearance.[25-27] The intraosseous vacuum has an appear-

ance similar to the vacuum disk, with linear signal void on all MRI pulse sequences if it is filled with gas, or intermediate signal on T1W and high signal on T2W images if it is filled with fluid (see later).

The presence of a vacuum cleft within a disk or vertebral body tends to occur with extension of the spine. The contents of the clefts may change when the patient is in a supine or flexed position. Within 1 hour of being placed supine in an MRI unit, the nitrogen-filled clefts may be replaced with fluid that is high signal intensity on T2W images (Fig. 13-17; see Fig. 13-16). These must not be confused with infection or other pathology.

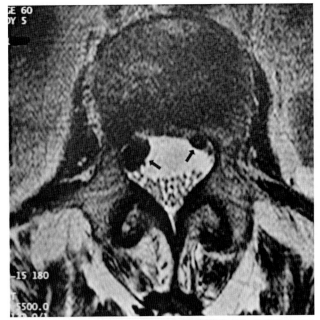

Figure 13-15   Disk mimickers. Fast T2 axial image of the lumbar spine. There are rounded low signal masses in both lateral recesses (*arrows*) in this patient with worsening radiculopathy. The signal is much lower than would be expected from sequestered disk fragments. This condition is caused by extruded cement from a vertebroplasty and is one of several entities that can mimic disk herniations.

Calcified Disks. Intervertebral disks are nourished via a vascular supply to the outermost fibers of the annulus fibrosus, but the bulk of the disk receives nourishment by diffusion through the adjacent end plates, which requires motion and stresses to occur. Calcification of the disks may occur from degenerative changes and aging, limited motion of the spine (ankylosing spondylitis, diffuse idiopathic skeletal hyperostosis, surgical fusion, old trauma, or infection), calcium pyrophosphate dihydrate crystal deposition disease, ochronosis, or hemochromatosis, among others.

MRI may show small amounts of calcium in the disks that are not evident by plain film or computed tomography (CT), which are high signal intensity on T1W images (Fig. 13-18).[28] The appearance on T2W images varies. As more calcium is deposited in the disks, they show low signal intensity on T1W and T2W images (see Fig. 13-17).

Osseous Degenerative Changes (Box 13-7)

Vertebral Bodies. The vertebral bodies respond to degenerative changes in the adjacent intervertebral disks in two major ways: (1) formation of osteophytes and (2) marrow changes paralleling the end plates. Osteophytes are the excrescences of bone that occur on the upper or lower margins of vertebral bodies. They occur as disks degenerate and bulge, placing traction stresses on Sharpey's fibers, which attach the disks to the vertebral bodies. Osteophytes usually are located anteriorly in the lumbar and thoracic spine, but are commonly anterior or posterior in the cervical spine.

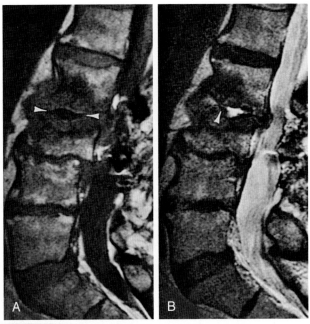

Figure 13-16   Vacuum disk. A, T1 sagittal image of the lumbar spine. There is horizontal, very low signal in the L2-3 disk (*arrowheads*) compatible with nitrogen in a vacuum disk from degeneration. The adjacent vertebral bodies have large areas of low signal marrow adjacent to the degenerated disk. **B,** Fast T2 sagittal image of the lumbar spine. This sequence was obtained later than the T1 sequence. High signal fluid is now filling most of the cleft in the disk. Low signal nitrogen is still present anteriorly (*arrowhead*) in the nondependent portion of the disk. The marrow changes remain low signal, indicating diskogenic sclerosis (type 3 marrow signal changes). This appearance could be confused with disk infection if the signal is not analyzed carefully.

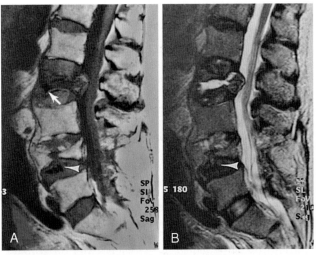

Figure 13-17   Vacuum vertebral body and calcified disk. A, T1 sagittal image of the lumbar spine. The L2 vertebral body is fractured with retropulsion into the spinal canal. The center of the vertebral body has intermediate signal except anteriorly, where very low signal (*arrow*) caused by nitrogen in a vacuum vertebra is seen. There also is linear low signal in the L4-5 disk (*arrowhead*) from a calcified disk. The low signal is too thick and irregular to be from vacuum disk. **B,** Fast T2 sagittal image of the lumbar spine. Most of the defect in the L2 vertebra has become high signal. Only a small area of low signal is present anteriorly from the small amount of nitrogen that remains. The low signal at L4-5 (*arrowhead*) persists from disk calcification.

Modic I: fluid
II: fat
III: sclerosis

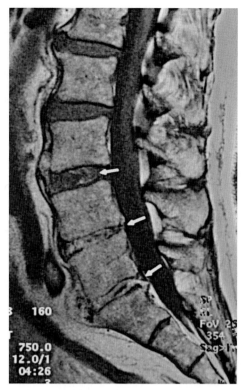

Figure 13-18 **Calcified disks.** T1 sagittal image of the lumbar spine. The lower three lumbar disks have large areas of heterogeneous high signal (*arrows*). This occurs when calcium is present in certain quantities.

* Ca++ can be high or low signal .....

In the cervical spine, disk abnormalities so commonly are accompanied by osteophytes that we refer to the combination of osteophytes and disk as *disko-osteophytic material*. Diffuse disko-osteophytic bulging or focal disko-osteophytic protrusions are common in the cervical spine. MRI of most osteophytes shows low signal intensity cortical margins with fatty marrow centers that follow the signal of fat on all pulse sequences. In the cervical spine, osteophytes may be more diffusely sclerotic (mainly cortical rather than medullary bone) and sometimes difficult to distinguish from disk material. Cervical disks are high signal intensity on gradient echo axial images, but the low signal outer fibers of the annulus and of the posterior longitudinal ligament may be difficult to distinguish from the cortical bone of osteophytes. It is sometimes difficult to determine if there is only a disk protruding into the canal, or if there is an osteophyte as well. On gradient echo axial sequences through the cervical spine, osteophytes are very low signal intensity. There may be blooming artifact from the sclerotic portions of the osteophytes that results in inaccurate overestimation of the size of osteophytes and their effect on the neural foramina or central canal. T1W images may be helpful in more accurately estimating stenosis and in determining what is osteophyte versus disk.

The marrow in vertebral bodies adjacent to degenerated disks may change in response to the disk disease. Parallel bands of abnormal signal in the end plates have been divided into two types by Modic and colleagues,[29] and a third type by other authors; these typically are called *Modic type 1, 2, or 3 changes*. These marrow changes may be focal or diffuse

along the end plate but tend to be linear and always parallel to the end plates.

Type 1 changes are the earliest marrow changes encountered. These consist of inflammatory and granulomatous tissue in the marrow that is low signal intensity on T1W images and becomes high signal intensity on T2W sequences (Fig. 13-19). This appearance may raise the question of spondylodiskitis, but disk infection has intradiskal high signal intensity on T2W images, whereas it would be unusual to have high signal intensity in an uninfected, degenerated disk adjacent to these osseous changes, making the distinction straightforward. Intact cortical end plates, lack of paraspinous inflammatory change, and preservation of the intranuclear cleft also allow the diagnosis of infection to be excluded with confidence.

Type 2 changes consist of signal intensity typical of fat on all pulse sequences, caused by focal fatty marrow conversion (see Fig. 13-19). These findings are common on spine MRI. Type 3 end plate changes result from sclerosis and have low signal intensity on all pulse sequences (see Fig. 13-16).

Facet Joints. The facet joints are formed by the inferior articular process of the vertebra above articulating with the superior articular process of the lower vertebra. The articular surfaces are covered with hyaline cartilage. The osseous structures are enveloped in a joint capsule lined by synovium; these are true synovial joints. The anterior aspects of the facet joints and the laminae are covered by the ligamentum flavum.

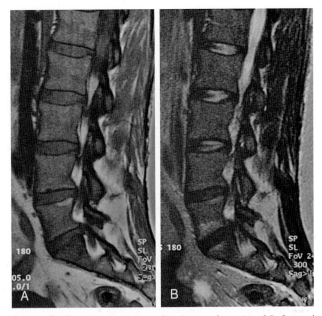

Figure 13-19 Osseous degenerative changes (type 1 and 2 changes). **A,** T1 sagittal image of the lumbar spine. Linear high signal fat parallels the inferior end plate of L4 and superior end plate of L5 from type 2 marrow signal changes associated with adjacent degenerative disk disease. **B,** Fast T2 sagittal image of the lumbar spine. High signal fat in the L4 and L5 end plates is still evident because fat is not suppressed on fast T2 sequences. There also is linear high signal paralleling the inferior end plate of L5 and superior end plate of S1 that was not evident on the T1 sequence, compatible with type 1 marrow signal changes from the degenerative disk disease.

These joints frequently undergo degenerative changes, especially in the middle and lower cervical spine and the lower lumbar spine and lumbosacral junction. Degenerative changes of the facet joints manifest as cartilage fibrillation with joint space narrowing, subchondral sclerosis, subchondral cysts, and osteophyte formation that result in overgrowth or hypertrophy of the osseous portions of the joints. Changes in the marrow of pedicles adjacent to facet degenerative joint disease may occur, similar to that seen in vertebral body end plates adjacent to degenerative disk disease, as a result of increased stresses. Synovial cysts may develop from degenerated spinal facet joints and project either anteriorly (through the ligamentum flavum) or posteriorly from the joints. Loss of cartilage from degenerative changes in the facet joints in concert with loss of disk height from degenerative disk disease leads to inward buckling of the ligamentum flavum, which causes narrowing of the neural foramina or central canal.

Symptoms from degenerative changes of the facet joints may result from compression of adjacent neural structures (spinal stenosis) by overgrowth of the bone, inward buckling of the ligamentum flavum, protrusion of synovial cysts into the spinal canal, or the joints themselves being painful. Degenerated facet joints not only can cause local pain at the facet joints but also frequently are responsible for referred pain patterns to the shoulders or interscapular regions from cervical disease or to the buttocks, thighs, and hips from lumbar facet syndromes.[30,31] As always, the presence of abnormalities on MRI examination does not indicate which,

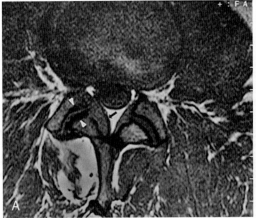

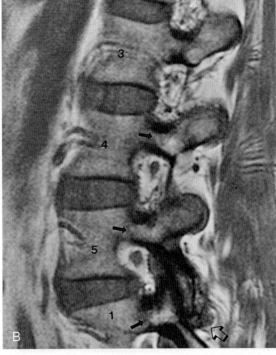

Figure 13-20 Degenerative facet joint disease. **A,** T1 axial image of the lumbar spine. The right facet joint shows mild hypertrophic changes of the bones from osteophyte formation, subchondral sclerosis (*arrowheads*), and ligamentum flavum thickening (*arrow*), all of which are different in appearance than on the normal left side. **B,** T1 sagittal image of the lumbar spine. Severe degenerative disease of the L5-S1 facet is seen (*open arrow*) with hypertrophic changes, a large inferior recess, and inward buckling of the ligamentum flavum into the neural foramen. Marrow signal intensity changes are evident in the pedicles, which are associated with adjacent degenerative facet joint disease. High signal fat (type 2 changes) is seen in the pedicles of L4, L5, and S1 (*arrows*). The L3 pedicle has normal signal that matches the signal in the adjacent vertebral body.

if any, of these joints is responsible for pain in a given patient. Additional work-up with injection of anesthetic into facet joints is the only way to document if a facet joint is responsible for some or all of the symptoms.

MRI of degenerative facet joint disease (Fig. 13-20) is typical of degenerative changes in any joint (subchondral sclerosis is low signal intensity on all pulse sequences; cysts are low signal intensity on T1W and high signal intensity on T2W images). There often are increased amounts of fluid in the joints, seen as high signal on T2W images. The osteophytes and hypertrophic osseous changes create a rounded and enlarged (Portobello mushroom) appearance of the articular processes of the facets on axial images that may affect the appearance of the adjacent spinal canal, lateral recesses, or neural foramina. Signal intensity changes (Modic changes) in the pedicles adjacent to facet joint degeneration may be seen (see Fig. 13-20) and sometimes are easier to identify than the degenerative changes themselves. These can be Modic type 1, 2, or 3 signal changes but are most commonly type 2 (fat signal).

Synovial cysts are rounded masses of varying size and sometimes variable signal intensity (Fig. 13-21). They are generally low signal intensity on T1W images, but because of hemorrhage into the cyst or high protein content, they occasionally may be relatively high signal intensity on T1W images. T2W images generally show high signal intensity or mixed signal intensity relating to the presence of calcifications (in ≤30%) and vacuum phenomenon. Contrast-enhanced images show peripheral enhancement with an appearance similar to a sequestered disk. Most sequestered disk fragments are not located posteriorly in the spinal canal or are not diffusely high signal intensity on T2W images, whereas a synovial cyst is. A synovial cyst always lies immediately adjacent to the facet joint, but a communication is not shown on MRI. A synovial cyst can be differentiated from a sequestered disk fragment with certainty by injecting contrast material into the facet joint and showing filling of the cyst under fluoroscopy.

Posterior Spinous Processes. Degenerative changes of the spinous processes and intervening interspinous soft tissues (kissing spine or Baastrup's disease) may occur as the result of hyperlordosis in the cervical or lumbar spine or from associated degenerative disk or facet joint disease, which places increased stresses on these posterior structures.[32] Close apposition of adjacent spinous processes causes laxity of the overlying supraspinous ligament and damage to the intervening interspinous ligaments. The interspinous ligament becomes fibrillated and torn, producing spaces in the ligament that may lead to formation of bursae or, eventually, true synovial joints between spinous processes. Breakdown of the interspinous ligaments causes excessive motion and leads to instability with direct contact between spinous processes that may result in eburnation of the bone, a faceted appearance, osteophytes, or degenerative enthesophytes. These changes sometimes cause pain symptoms.

The main appearance to be aware of on MRI is the high signal intensity bursal fluid collections between spinous processes on T2W images (Fig. 13-22). Also, the lack of space between adjacent spinous processes, flattening of the superior or inferior surfaces (faceted appearance), and low signal intensity eburnation (sclerosis) on all pulse sequences are

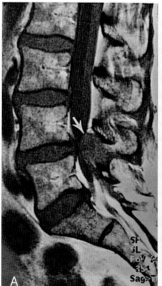
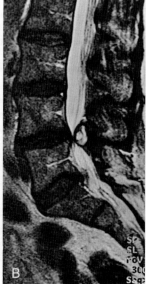
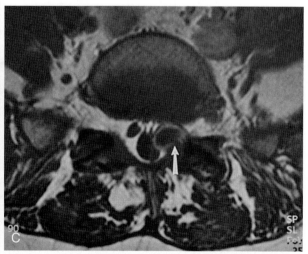

Figure 13-21 **Synovial cyst from degenerative facet joint disease. A,** T1 sagittal image of the lumbar spine. There is an intermediate signal mass (*arrow*) in the posterior epidural space compressing the thecal sac at the L4-5 level. **B,** Fast T2 sagittal image of the lumbar spine. The mass becomes mainly high signal with a low signal rim. **C,** T1 contrast-enhanced axial image of the lumbar spine. There is peripheral rim enhancement of the left-sided mass (*arrow*). It is immediately adjacent to the degenerated left facet joint, but a communication cannot be seen. The thecal sac and nerve are displaced.

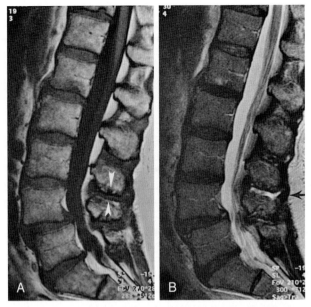

Figure 13-22 Baastrup's disease (kissing spine). **A,** T1 sagittal image of the lumbar spine. The spinous processes of L3 and L4 are closer together than at the other levels. There is sclerosis in the bones (*arrowheads*) where they abut one another, and the bones are angled and faceted from chronic wear against each other. **B,** Fast T2 sagittal image of the lumbar spine. There is high signal between the L3 and L4 spinous processes from breakdown of the interspinous ligament and formation of a bursa (*arrow*).

identified. Sometimes, degenerative cysts are noted in the spinous processes where they chronically abut; these cysts have low signal intensity on T1W images that becomes hyperintense on T2W images.

SPINAL STENOSIS (Box 13-8)

Spinal stenosis is narrowing of the central spinal canal, neural foramen, lateral recess, or any combination of these anatomic regions, by soft tissue or osseous structures that impinge on neural elements and may result in symptoms. The standard classification for spinal stenosis is based on cause and includes congenital (eg, short pedicle syndrome,

---

BOX 13-8

Spinal Stenosis

Sites of Involvement
- Central canal
- Neural foramina
- Lateral recesses

Causes
- Degenerative
  - Disk contour abnormalities (bulges, herniations)
  - Vertebral body osteophytes
  - Degenerative spondylolisthesis
  - Facet joint degeneration, osteophytes, synovial cysts
  - Ligamentum flavum buckling
- Congenital short pedicles
  - Usually requires superimposed degeneration to be symptomatic
- Any mass arising from bone, disk, or within canal
  - Osseous tumor, fracture fragments
  - Spondylolysis, spondylolisthesis
  - Ossification of posterior longitudinal ligament
  - Epidural lipomatosis, hematoma, abscess, tumor, scarring

Complications
- Pain symptoms
- Cord myelomalacia from ischemia
- Nerve root edema

---

achondroplasia) or acquired (usually degenerative) causes. Even if there are congenital abnormalities of the spine that narrow the canal, patients rarely have symptoms of spinal stenosis, unless they have superimposed degenerative changes (acquired stenosis). Among some miscellaneous causes of spinal stenosis are spondylolysis (pars defect) with spondylolisthesis (anterior or posterior subluxation), ossification of the posterior longitudinal ligament, epidural lipomatosis, or osseous abnormalities such as fracture or Paget's disease, among many others.

Symptoms from multilevel spinal stenosis are often nonspecific and include back pain, intermittent neurogenic claudication, extremity radiculopathy, pain with hyperextension relieved by flexion, and pain on standing relieved by lying down. The presence of imaging findings of spinal stenosis does not indicate that a patient has symptoms from the stenosis. Just as arteriosclerotic calcification of the coronary arteries on a chest CT scan does not confirm that the patient's

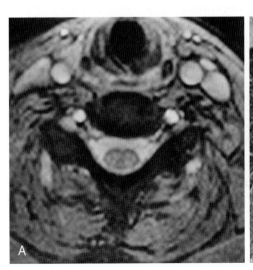

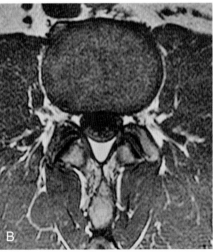

Figure 13-23 Normal central spinal canal. A, T2* axial image of the cervical spine. The central canal is normal, with the high signal thecal sac having a rounded, plump oval configuration. **B,** T1 axial image of the lumbar spine. The central canal is normal at this level, with the low signal thecal sac again having the appearance of a rounded, plump oval.

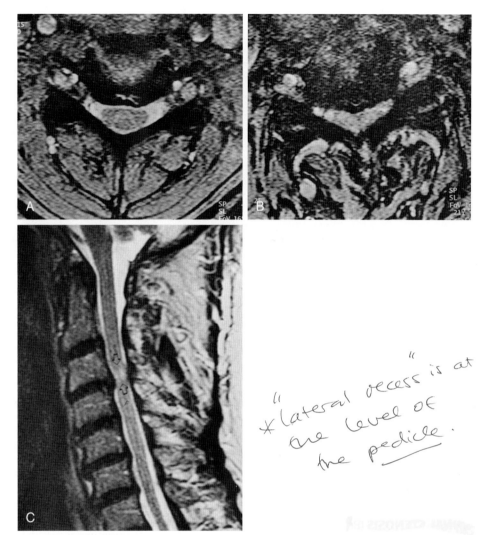

Figure 13-24 Central canal stenosis: cervical (acquired). **A,** T2* axial image of the cervical spine. There is diffuse disko-osteophytic bulging into the central canal, causing the thecal sac to lose its rounded appearance. This is mild in extent because there is still cerebrospinal fluid present between the osteophyte and the cord. The neural foramina are normal and unaffected by the degenerative process. **B,** T2* axial image of the cervical spine (same patient as in **A** but different level). The central canal is markedly narrowed with essentially no cerebrospinal fluid seen, and the cord is flattened by the diffuse disko-osteophytic bulge. Both neural foramina are narrowed from osteophytes, worse on the right than on the left side. **C,** Fast T2 sagittal image of the cervical spine (different patient than in **A** and **B**). There is focal high signal in the cord (*open arrows*) at the level of the bulging disk and osteophytes from myelomalacia.

"lateral recess is at the level of the pedicle."

chest pain is from angina, abnormalities of the spine on imaging do not indicate the patient must have symptoms relating to the abnormalities. Clinical examination and other tests must be correlated with MRI studies in the spine (and elsewhere) to avoid errors in managing patients.

Spinal stenosis may occur at one or more levels in the spine and almost always is the result of several degenerative processes occurring in concert. When disks degenerate and lose height, and the articular cartilage in the facet joints is lost, there may be motion of one vertebral segment relative to the adjacent one; this motion causes degenerative spondylolisthesis, which results in spinal stenosis. As the spine loses height from these same degenerative changes, the ligamentum flavum buckles inward toward the canal and neural foramina, also resulting in spinal stenosis. Other degenerative changes that lead to spinal stenosis include diffuse or focal abnormalities in disk contour, vertebral body osteophytes, facet joint osteophytes (hypertrophy), and facet joint synovial cysts.

Central Canal Stenosis

Central canal stenosis usually is the result of facet joint osteophytes and inward buckling of the ligamentum flavum

posteriorly, with disk bulging anteriorly in the canal. Vertebral body osteophytes (especially in the cervical spine) also may contribute to central canal stenosis, as can postoperative scarring. We do not use measurements to determine if there is central stenosis, but use the shape of the canal and thecal sac instead. Normally, the central canal and thecal sac are round or nearly round (a plump oval) structures on axial images (Fig. 13-23); if they become flattened ovals or triangular in shape, it indicates central stenosis (Figs. 13-24 to 13-26). We quantitate the degree of stenosis as mild, moderate, or severe as part of our dictated report, but there are no universally agreed-on objective definitions for these terms. Severe central stenosis can cause edema in the affected nerve roots, or, in the cervical spine, there may be abnormalities of the cord, probably myelomalacia from ischemia at the site of stenosis, which is high signal intensity on T2W images (see Fig. 13-24).

Lateral Recess Stenosis. Lateral recess stenosis usually is caused by hypertrophic degenerative changes of the facet joints, or less commonly by a disk fragment or postoperative fibrosis. Lateral recesses are located on the medial aspects of pedicles. Nerve roots lie in these recesses after leaving the thecal sac, but before entering the exiting neural foramina.

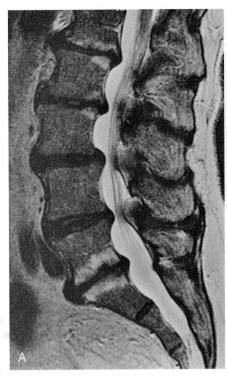

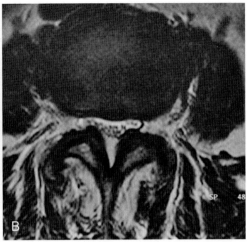

Figure 13-25   Central canal stenosis: lumbar (acquired). **A,** Fast T2 sagittal image of the lumbar spine. Disks and ligamentum flavum protrude into the spinal canal, causing multilevel canal stenosis with narrowing of the thecal sac at the disk levels. **B,** Fast T2 axial image of the lumbar spine. The central canal is markedly narrowed and has a triangular shape, rather than the normal plump oval. The central stenosis is from a diffusely bulging disk in concert with bilateral facet degenerative joint disease.

There is a neural foramen bordering the upper and the lower margins of a lateral recess. Measurements are not used to determine if this recess is stenotic. If there is deformity in the shape of the recess, and the descending nerve is displaced or compressed, there is lateral recess stenosis (Fig. 13-27). This space is best evaluated in the axial plane of imaging.

Neural Foramen Stenosis

Neural foramen stenosis occurs as a result of degenerative osteophytes of the facet joints or of the uncovertebral joints in the cervical spine; inward buckling of the ligamentum flavum (which forms the posterior aspect of the foramina); a foraminal disk protrusion, extrusion, or sequestered fragment; a diffuse disk bulge; or postoperative fibrosis. Narrowing of the neural foramina can be evaluated on sagittal and

axial images. On sagittal images, the normal neural foramen has the appearance of a vertical oval. If disk material extends into the foramen, the oval narrows inferiorly, creating a keyhole shape (Fig. 13-28). Axial images may be more accurate for diagnosis because they show more of the extent of each foramen (Figs. 13-29 and 13-30).

Something that really impinges on our nerves is the concept we repeatedly hear from our residents that the nerve must be unaffected by a disk abnormality if they see the nerve surrounded by fat in the superior aspect of the neural foramen on sagittal images. They see a big disk abnormality in the lower neural foramen and say, "but the nerve got out." This thinking is inaccurate and not based on anatomic fact.

What we see in the superior portion of the neural foramen is the large dorsal root ganglion and ventral root cut in cross section. As the nerve progresses laterally and inferiorly in the

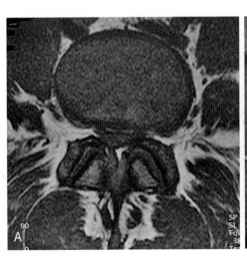

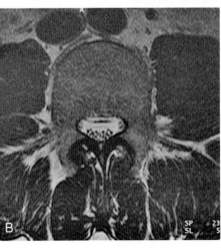

Figure 13-26   Central canal stenosis: lumbar (congenital with superimposed acquired). **A,** T1 axial image of the lumbar spine. There are mild hypertrophic changes of the left facet joint from degenerative disease and a very mild diffuse disk bulge. The central canal is severely narrowed, with a flattened thecal sac and triangular shape of the canal. **B,** Fast T2 axial image of the lumbar spine (same patient as in **A**). An image obtained through the pedicles shows that the pedicles are congenitally short, and the central canal is small at this level (a flattened oval rather than a plump oval), even without the presence of superimposed degenerative changes.

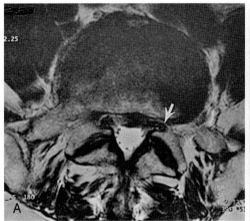 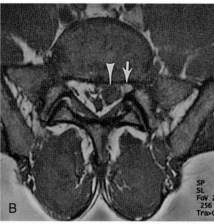

Figure 13-27 Lateral recess stenosis. **A,** Fast T2 axial image of the lumbar spine. Both lateral recesses are narrowed as the result of osteophytes from facet degenerative joint disease. The left side is more severe than the right (*arrow*), and the nerve that runs in the lateral recess is compressed between osteophyte and the vertebral body. **B,** T1 axial image of the lumbar spine (different patient than in **A**). There is a large, extruded disk fragment (*arrowhead*) narrowing the left lateral recess (*arrow*) and compressing the nerve in it.

neural foramen, it divides into approximately 15 fascicles, which compose the short segment spinal nerve. The fascicles, which cannot be seen well on MRI, regroup to form the dorsal and ventral rami. The dorsal and ventral nerve roots, the spinal nerve, and the dorsal and ventral rami run obliquely through the neural foramen in a superior-to-inferior and medial-to-lateral direction; this can be appreciated on coronal MR images through the neural foramen (Fig. 13-31). Disk or other material that narrows the mid or inferior portion of the neural foramen may compress or irritate the spinal nerve or dorsal and ventral rami, whereas the dorsal root ganglion looks pristine and unaffected, sur-

rounded by fat in the superior portion of the foramen. In addition, any mass projecting lateral to the foramen may impinge on the nerve that exited through the foramen at one level above and cause nerve symptoms. The point is that anything narrowing *any* portion of the neural foramen may affect a nerve because there is nerve passing through all levels of the foramen and just outside the foramen—we just happen to see the nerve best in the superior and medial aspect of the foramen because we are looking at the large dorsal root ganglion. NOTE

POSTOPERATIVE CHANGES

Uncomplicated Postoperative MRI (Box 13-9)

Many changes occur in the osseous and soft tissues of the spine after surgery. It is important to know their MRI appearance so as not to confuse normal postoperative changes with pathology that requires treatment. Osseous abnormalities include removal of portions of the spine (lamina, facets) or additions of bone graft or hardware to the spine. Dura and CSF sometimes may protrude through

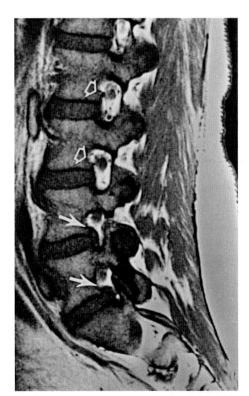

Figure 13-28 Foraminal stenosis. Normal neural foramina on sagittal images should have a vertical oval appearance (*open arrows*). Stenosis from disk abnormalities creates narrowing of the lower portion of the foramen so that it has a keyhole appearance (*solid arrows*). The dorsal root ganglion is evident in the superior portion of the lumbar foramina.

BOX 13-9

Postoperative Changes: Uncomplicated

Vertebral Marrow
- Unchanged from before surgery; no enhancement (unless Modic 1 changes are present)

Nerve Roots
- May enhance for 6 months

Disks
- Contrast enhancement of posterior annulus, and increased signal on T2 for years

Epidural
- Scarring/fibrosis common
- Contrast enhancement of fibrosis for years
- Fibrosis is often nodular, resembling persistent or recurrent disk extrusion
  - Peripheral enhancement may mimic disk extrusion in first 6 months
  - Diffuse enhancement is typical after 6 months, allowing differentiation from disk (peripheral enhancement only)

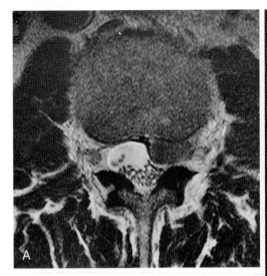

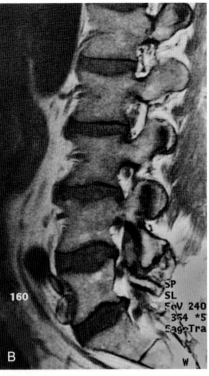

Figure 13-29 Foraminal stenosis: lumbar. **A,** Fast T2 axial image of the lumbar spine. There is a large L3-4 intra-foraminal disk extrusion that essentially obliterates the left neural foramen. **B,** T1 sagittal image of the lumbar spine. The disk extrusion seen on axial images was not evident on any of the sagittal images. It is essential to use axial and sagittal images to evaluate the neural foramina and extraforaminal regions because they are sometimes complementary to one another.

a lamina defect and result in a postoperative meningocele (Fig. 13-32). Distinguishing a meningocele from a pseudo-meningocele (a defect in the dura with leak of spinal fluid) generally is impossible on MRI. Marrow in the vertebral bodies adjacent to an operated disk generally remains normal after surgery (or maintains the same disk-related Modic marrow abnormalities that were present before surgery) and does not enhance with contrast material (although Modic 1 changes do enhance).

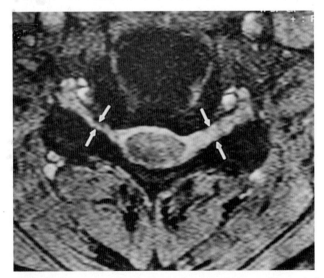

Figure 13-30 Foraminal stenosis: cervical. T2* axial image of the cervical spine. There is moderate narrowing of the right neural foramen compared with the normal left foramen (*arrows*). The stenosis of the right foramen is from osteophytes arising from the uncovertebral joint.

Epidural scarring after osseous decompression or disk surgery is extremely common and occurs to a variable extent in different individuals. Fibrosis is shown to best advantage after injection of intravenous gadolinium. The degree of contrast enhancement is greatest during the first year after surgery, but contrast enhancement may persist for years. The fibrosis or scarring in the anterior epidural space where surgery was performed is often an irregular epidural mass that mimics a persistent or recurrent disk (Fig. 13-33).[33-35] The mass effect from scarring at the operated disk level may take months to resolve and may never resolve completely. During the first 6 months after surgery, there may be peripheral contrast enhancement of the mass of granulation tissue and fibrosis, making it impossible to distinguish scarring from disk in the early postoperative period. Enhancement of intrathecal nerve roots after contrast administration is common during the first 6 months after surgery, but should not persist after that (Fig. 13-34).[33-35]

Postoperative changes in disks often are seen after intravenous gadolinium is given and may persist for years (Fig. 13-35). Most patients have enhancement of the posterior annulus at the operative site as a result of curettage, whereas only a few have enhancement within the center of the disk. These disk changes have the appearance of high signal intensity on T2W and contrast-enhanced T1W images. This appearance should not be confused with a disk infection because the adjacent vertebral bodies should maintain a normal appearance postoperatively.

Failed Back Surgery

Patients may have persistent, recurrent, or new and different symptoms after surgery of the spine. The reasons for these

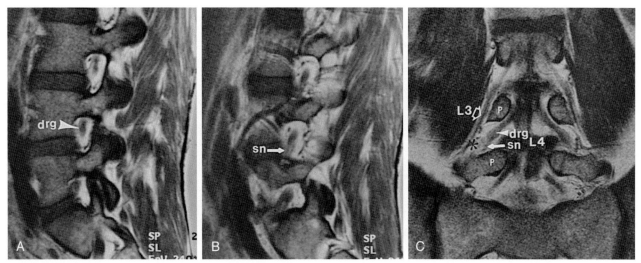

Figure 13-31   **Neural foramen anatomy: how the nerve really gets out. A,** T1 sagittal image of the lumbar spine. The oval neural foramina are seen with the dorsal root ganglia (drg; *arrowhead*) cut in cross section in the superior foramina. **B,** T1 sagittal image of the lumbar spine. This is one cut more lateral than that in **A**. The lateral aspect of the neural foramen is imaged, and the striated fascicles of the spinal nerve (sn; *arrow*) are evident in the inferior aspect of the foramen at the level of the disk. If the dorsal root ganglion is surrounded by fat, but there is a disk protruding into the inferior foramen, the nerve did not "get out"—the dorsal root ganglion got out, but the spinal nerve or dorsal and ventral rami did not. There *is* nerve traversing the lower foramen at the level of the disk. **C,** T1 coronal image of the lumbar spine. The neural foramen is shown between the pedicles (p). The nerve runs through it obliquely from superomedial to infero-lateral. The dorsal root ganglion (drg; *arrowhead*) is located in the superomedial foramen, whereas the spinal nerve (sn; *arrow*) is located in the inferior and lateral portion of the foramen. The L3 nerve (*open arrow*) is seen coming from above, and it is obvious why a far lateral disk in the location marked by the *asterisk* (*) could affect the L3 or L4 nerves.

problems are many and varied. The most common reasons are recurrent or persistent disk extrusions, postoperative scarring, nerve root damage (neuritis), and inadequate surgery (missed free fragments, inadequate decompression of spinal stenosis, wrong level treated, or what was treated was not the pain source). Spondylodiskitis and epidural abscess, epidural hematoma (Fig. 13-36), failure of fusion of bone graft material, arachnoiditis, and a defect in the dural sac that creates a pseudomeningocele all may occur as complications of spinal surgery.

Distinguishing postoperative scarring (epidural fibrosis) from extruded disk material is one of the most important

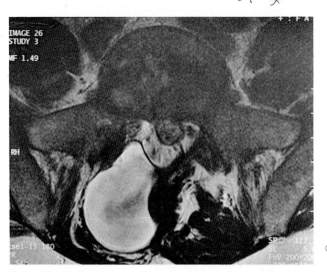

Figure 13-32   **Postoperative changes: meningocele.** Fast T2 axial image of L5. There are postoperative changes of a right laminectomy, through which a large, high signal mass protrudes into the posterior soft tissues.

tasks for radiologists in evaluating postoperative MRI studies. All postoperative spine MRI studies are done with contrast enhancement to distinguish between these two common causes of symptoms in postoperative patients.[36] Scar tissue that is more than 6 months old enhances diffusely and early after the intravenous administration of gadolinium (high signal intensity on T1W images) (see Fig. 13-33). Disk material does not enhance until late, if at all, and usually enhances only peripherally (Fig. 13-37). These rules do not work as well during the first 6 months after surgery, when asymptomatic fibrosis may show peripheral rather than diffuse contrast enhancement that is indistinguishable from an extruded disk. MRI has more value in differentiating scar from disk material after the first 6 months postoperatively. Extruded disk material may be an indication for another operation, whereas there is no benefit from reoperating on a patient with epidural fibrosis.

Other signs that may help distinguish epidural fibrosis from a disk abnormality are that epidural fibrosis often has irregular margins; it may not be contiguous with the adjacent disk; and, instead of producing a mass effect on the dural sac, it may cause retraction. Recurrent disk herniations, conversely, usually are contiguous with the disk, have sharp margins, and cause mass effect on the dural sac.

INFLAMMATORY CHANGES

Spondylodiskitis (Box 13-10)

Infection of the spine generally occurs from hematogenous spread of *Staphylococcus aureus* from a distant site. In adults, the marrow in the region of a vertebral body end plate

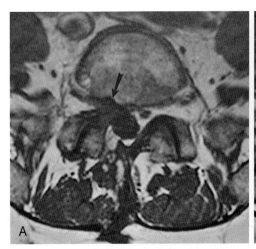

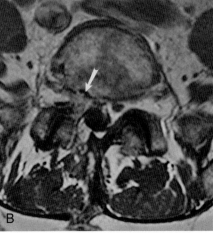

Scar

Figure 13-33 Postoperative changes: scarring/fibrosis (versus disk). **A,** T1 axial image of L5. There is an intermediate signal mass (*arrow*) in the right paracentral region of this patient with a right laminectomy. The descending right L5 nerve is not seen. This could be a disk fragment or scarring. **B,** T1 contrast-enhanced axial image (same level as in **A**). There is diffuse enhancement of the right paracentral mass, indicating this is from scarring/fibrosis, rather than from a disk fragment.

usually is affected first (osteomyelitis or spondylitis), and the infection rapidly spreads to the adjacent disk (diskitis) and to the closest adjacent vertebral body. When the bone and the disk are infected, it is referred to as *spondylodiskitis.* In contrast to adults, children have disks with significant vascularity, so the initial infection may occur in the disk and then spread secondarily to the adjacent bone.

The MRI appearance depends on the extent of disease and the body's response to it at the time of imaging. Patients usually do not present for imaging until the infection has spread across a disk and involves at least two adjacent vertebral bodies. The MRI findings consist of a triad of findings:

1. Low signal intensity on T1W images in vertebral body marrow
2. Contrast enhancement of marrow on T1W images, and possibly of the disk if an abscess has not formed
3. High signal intensity of the disk on T2W images (Fig. 13-38)[37]

High signal intensity in marrow on T2W images is sometimes present, but if reactive changes or sclerosis in the bone exist, the marrow may be low signal intensity on T2W images. Associated abnormalities that may be detected with spondylodiskitis include decreased disk height; destruction of the low signal intensity cortical end plate; and subligamentous, epidural, or paraspinous inflammatory phlegmon

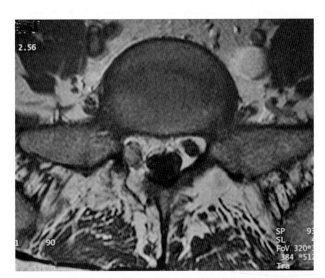

Figure 13-34 Postoperative changes: nerve root enhancement. T1 contrast-enhanced axial image of L5. The right lamina is surgically absent. The right descending L5 nerve is enlarged and high signal compared with the normal left nerve. This is expected during the first 6 months after surgery.

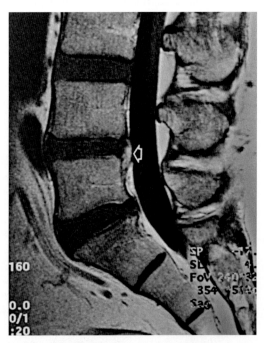

Figure 13-35 Postoperative changes: disk enhancement. T1 contrast-enhanced sagittal image of the lumbar spine. The posterior annulus of the L4-5 disk shows focal enhancement (*open arrow*) from previous surgery with curettage. This finding may last indefinitely after surgery.

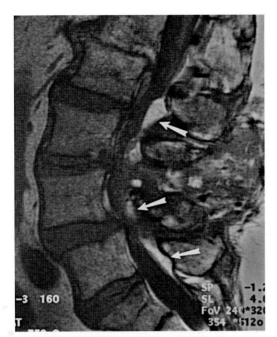

Figure 13-36 Postoperative complications: epidural hematoma. T1 sagittal image of the lumbar spine. There was posterior decompression surgery at the L4 level. While still hospitalized, the patient developed pain and weakness. MRI shows a heterogeneous hematoma posteriorly at the level of the L4 spinous process. In addition, there are irregular high and intermediate signal masses in the posterior epidural space (*arrows*), representing a subacute hematoma that is compressing the dural sac and cauda equina.

Granulomatous infections, such as tuberculosis or fungal infections, may be more clinically indolent than pyogenic infections. Bone destruction is almost always evident at the time of imaging, rather than just marrow edema. The disks may be spared, or nearly so, as the infection spreads beneath the anterior or posterior longitudinal ligaments of the spine to adjacent vertebrae.[38] The posterior elements often are involved, and epidural and paraspinous abscesses are common and large at the time of presentation.

Epidural Abscess

Direct extension of infection from spondylodiskitis can cause an epidural abscess, as described earlier. Other times, there is hematogenous seeding of the epidural space from infection at a remote site, or direct implantation of bacteria from instrumentation may occur (Fig. 13-39). Spondylodiskitis is present in 80% of patients with an epidural abscess at the time of imaging.[39] Two stages may be evident: the phlegmon (diffuse soft tissue inflammation), which progresses to an abscess (focal fluid collection), with MRI features as described earlier.

Arachnoiditis

Arachnoiditis is an inflammatory process that may occur after surgery from agents being injected into the subarachnoid space, such as anesthetics, contrast material, or

or abscess. MRI of soft tissue inflammatory or hyperemic phlegmonous response shows soft tissue swelling or a mass in the epidural or paraspinous regions that is high signal on T2W images or enhances diffusely with contrast material on T1W images. If an abscess has formed, the soft tissue mass is low signal intensity on T1W images, high signal intensity on T2W images, and shows peripheral rim enhancement on contrast-enhanced T1W images. Contrast administration is mandatory for complete evaluation of a spine with a suspected infection.

Figure 13-37 Postoperative complications: recurrent disk (versus scarring). A, T1 axial image of L5-S1 disk. A right laminectomy has been performed. The patient has recurrent symptoms, and MRI shows intermediate signal in the right paracentral region that could be either scarring or a recurrent disk extrusion. The descending S1 nerve root is not identified. **B,** T1 contrast-enhanced axial image of L5-S1. There is a thin peripheral rim of enhancement (*arrowheads*) around the mass, typical of a disk, rather than scarring, which would have diffuse enhancement.

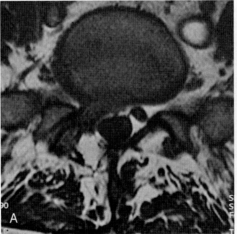

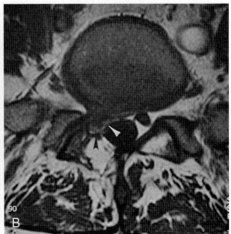

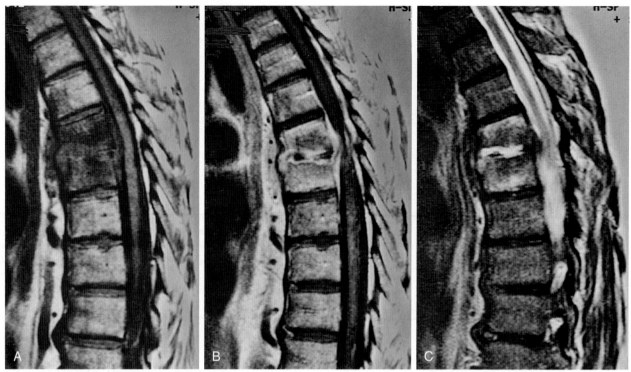

Figure 13-38 **Spondylodiskitis. A,** T1 sagittal image of thoracic spine. There is abnormal low signal in two adjacent vertebral bodies. The end plates show destruction. Soft tissue masses extend anterior and posterior to the vertebral bodies. The posterior mass is displacing the cord. **B,** T1 contrast-enhanced sagittal image of the thoracic spine. The marrow shows contrast enhancement, as does the mass in the anterior epidural space and the mass anterior to the spine. The diffuse enhancement of the soft tissue masses indicates that these are phlegmonous masses rather than abscesses. The disk shows rim enhancement only, which means there is an abscess in the disk. **C,** T2 sagittal image of the thoracic spine. The vertebral bodies show heterogeneous high signal. The soft tissue phlegmon is difficult to see compared with the contrast-enhanced images. The pus in the disk is diffusely high signal.

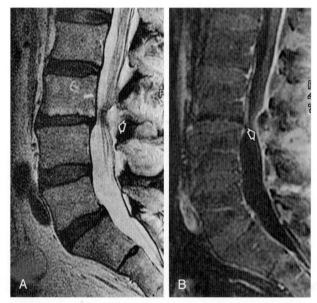

Figure 13-39 **Epidural abscess. A,** Fast T2 sagittal image of the lumbar spine. Fever and neurologic symptoms occurred in this patient after instrumentation for placement of an epidural catheter. There is a high signal mass (*arrow*) displacing the dura and cauda equina anteriorly. **B,** T1 sagittal image with fat suppression and contrast enhancement of the lumbar spine. There is peripheral rim enhancement (*arrow*) of the mass, which indicates it is cystic (abscess).

steroids; from infection; or from intrathecal hemorrhage. An inflammatory response occurs, and adhesions form; fibrous inflammatory masses also occasionally may be evident. On MRI, the findings are best shown on T2W images (Figs. 13-40 to 13-42). The nerve roots may be clumped instead of evenly distributed through the thecal sac. Nerves may adhere to the dura so that there is the appearance of an empty thecal sac without nerve roots present. On sagittal images, the nerves of the cauda equina may have an irregular, angled, or wavy appearance, rather than the normal gentle curve as they descend. Contrast administration serves no useful purpose for making this diagnosis.[40]

Ankylosing Spondylitis

Many different arthritides may affect the spine, but ankylosing spondylitis involves the spine by definition. Occasionally, young patients with back pain are sent for MRI, and we are able to diagnose ankylosing spondylitis first by MRI. Although we do not believe MRI is routinely necessary to diagnose early ankylosing spondylitis, there are occasions where the sequence of events creates such a situation, and it is necessary to know the MRI changes in the spine.

The classic changes of ankylosing spondylitis involve the sacroiliac joints and spine, usually clinically manifesting in patients in their late teens or early 20s. The earliest changes are sacroiliitis with microerosions of the cartilage and subchondral bone and associated marrow edema. The changes in the sacroiliac joints on spine MRI consist of high signal

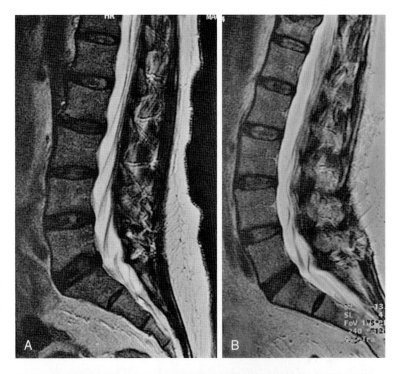

Figure 13-40 Arachnoiditis: normal and abnormal nerves, sagittal plane. **A,** Fast T2 sagittal image of the lumbar spine. This is an example of the normal appearance of the cauda equina nerves descending in the dural sac with a gentle curve. Compare with arachnoiditis in **B**. **B,** Fast T2 sagittal image of the lumbar spine (different patient than in **A**). The nerves of the cauda equina have a wavy, angled, and irregular appearance typical of arachnoiditis in the sagittal plane.

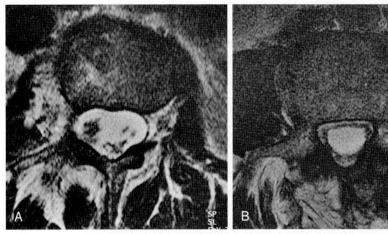

Figure 13-41 Arachnoiditis: axial plane. **A,** Fast T2 axial image of the lumbar spine. The nerve roots are clumped and show an uneven distribution in the thecal sac from arachnoiditis. **B,** Fast T2 axial image of the lumbar spine (different patient than in **A**). The nerves adhere to the dura, creating the empty thecal sac appearance of arachnoiditis.

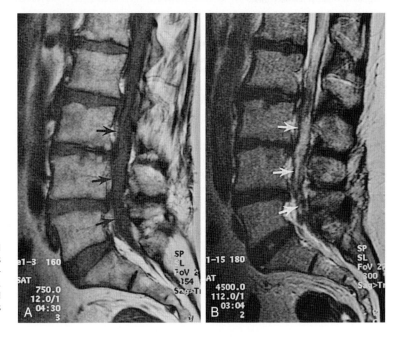

Figure 13-42 Arachnoiditis: fibrous mass. **A,** T1 sagittal image of the lumbar spine. The thecal sac has heterogeneous intermediate signal, rather than the normal low signal of cerebrospinal fluid (*arrows*). **B,** Fast T2 sagittal image of the lumbar spine. There is persistent heterogeneous intermediate signal in the dural sac (*arrows*). These are changes of a fibrous inflammatory mass from arachnoiditis.

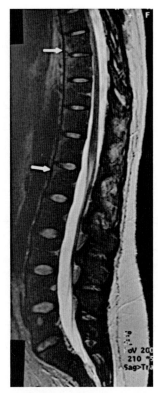

Figure 13-43 *Ankylosing spondylitis: early changes.* Fast T2 sagittal image of the thoracolumbar spine. MRI shows abnormal high signal in the anterior vertebral bodies of several lower thoracic and upper lumbar vertebral bodies (between *arrows*) from marrow edema. The vertebrae also are squared.

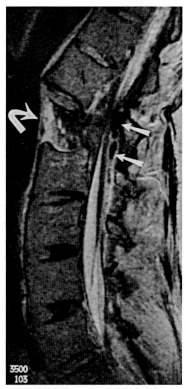

Figure 13-44 *Ankylosing spondylitis: fracture.* Fast T2 sagittal image of the thoracolumbar junction. There is a fracture through the disk (*curved arrow*) with marked displacement of fragments. Low signal in the posterior spinal canal from an epidural hematoma (*arrows*) is present. Changes of ankylosing spondylitis are evident in the vertebral bodies inferior to the fracture; the squared bodies are fused anteriorly with high signal evident in the disks from ossification and calcification.

intensity on T2W images that parallel the joints, involving the iliac side of the joint to a greater extent than the sacral side. This appearance can be very similar to insufficiency fractures, but these diseases usually affect patients of different ages and gender, and usually no osteoporosis is seen in young patients with ankylosing spondylitis. Infection of the sacroiliac joint could have an identical appearance, but this is usually a unilateral process, whereas ankylosing spondylitis affects the sacroiliac joints bilaterally.

The earliest changes of ankylosing spondylitis in the spine occur from marrow edema at the anterior corners of the vertebral bodies at the thoracolumbar junction. This edema is caused by inflammatory changes beneath the attachments of the anterior longitudinal ligament to the spine and where Sharpey's fibers from the disk annulus attach to the vertebral body. The MRI appearance is low signal intensity on T1W images (or no abnormality evident at all) and high signal intensity on T2W images (Fig. 13-43). The sequence of events would lead to squaring of the vertebral bodies from the erosion of bone and sclerosis of the corners of the vertebral bodies ("shiny corner" sign on conventional radiographs) as the bone attempts to heal from the inflammatory process. The sclerotic bone would be low signal intensity on T1W and T2W images.

Because of the stiffness and rigidity of the spine in patients with more advanced ankylosing spondylitis, fractures may occur, often through the disks. These may be difficult to

identify on conventional radiographs, but MRI may be useful in showing the fracture and any associated epidural hematomas, which are particularly common in patients with this disease (Fig. 13-44).

TRAUMATIC CHANGES

Spondylolysis and Spondylolisthesis (Box 13-11)

Spondylolysis is an osseous defect (fracture) of the pars interarticularis of the spine. These usually occur in the lower

---

BOX 13-11

Spondylolysis

Direct Evidence
- Defect in pars interarticularis
  - Difficult diagnosis by MRI
  - Sclerotic (low signal) intact pars may mimic lysis

Indirect Evidence
- Neural foramen
  - Obliquely oriented figure-of-eight configuration
- Modic marrow changes in adjacent pedicles
- Decreased posterior vertebral body height
- Widened canal compared with L1 level by >25% (even when no spondylolisthesis is present)

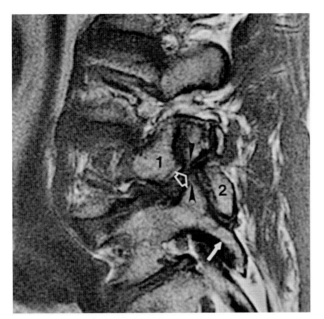

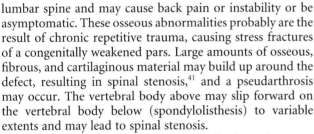

Figure 13-45 **Spondylolysis: sagittal plane.** T1 sagittal image of the lumbar spine. The normal pars interarticularis at L5 is shown for reference (*solid white arrow*). The pars at L4 is in two separate fragments (1, 2), and a large spondylolytic defect in the pars is shown (*open arrow*). The gap created by the L4 pars defect is filled by inferior and superior articular processes that are resting on each other (*arrowheads*), so that the foot of the "Scottie dog" above is resting on the ear of the one below.

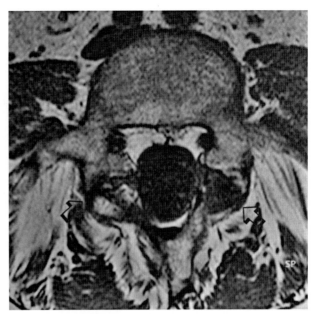

Figure 13-46 **Spondylolysis: axial plane.** T1 axial image of the lumbar spine. Oblique, irregular defects (*open arrows*) are evident bilaterally in the posterior ring of L4 from spondylolysis. A cut through the mid–vertebral body at the inferior aspect of the pedicles should have a solid ring of bone, without any defects from facet joints, spondylolysis, or other entities. The anteroposterior diameter of the canal is elongated from displacement of bone as the result of the lysis.

lumbar spine and may cause back pain or instability or be asymptomatic. These osseous abnormalities probably are the result of chronic repetitive trauma, causing stress fractures of a congenitally weakened pars. Large amounts of osseous, fibrous, and cartilaginous material may build up around the defect, resulting in spinal stenosis,[41] and a pseudarthrosis may occur. The vertebral body above may slip forward on the vertebral body below (spondylolisthesis) to variable extents and may lead to spinal stenosis.

Findings of spondylolysis may be difficult to detect on MRI (Fig. 13-45). Direct visualization of the defect in the pars is possible, but it is not as easily seen as it is on radiographs or CT. On sagittal MR images, the break in the pars may be seen as a focus of low signal intensity. An intact pars sometimes has sclerosis with low signal intensity on all pulse sequences, which appears to be a spondylolytic defect on MRI when none is present. It is helpful to identify a pars defect directly on axial images, where a cut through the mid–vertebral body (at the inferior aspect of the pedicles) shows disruption of the pars where normally there is an intact bony ring made of the pedicles and laminae (Fig. 13-46). This disruption of the pars has an appearance similar to a cut through the facet joints (with the pars defects mimicking the facet joints), but the facet joints should not be present at this location.

Because of the difficulty in making the diagnosis of spondylolysis on MRI, especially when no spondylolisthesis is present, several secondary signs have been described that may help (Fig. 13-47).[42] The neural foramen at the affected level becomes horizontal in orientation and may have a lobulated, oblique, figure-of-eight appearance. The pedicles and articular processes adjacent to the pars defect may have

reactive marrow changes (Modic changes) from abnormal stresses, usually with fatty marrow that has signal intensity that follows fat on all pulse sequences. Wedging, with a decreased height of the posterior vertebral body at the level of the spondylolysis, can be seen as a secondary finding. Widening of the anteroposterior diameter of the canal at the affected level can occur even when there is no anterior spondylolisthesis because the posterior elements displace slightly posteriorly. This widened spinal canal can be shown as abnormal if it measures 25% greater or more in anteroposterior diameter compared with the diameter of the canal at the L1 level. If CT or conventional radiographs of the spine are available, they should be immediately reviewed because the diagnosis of spondylolysis can be made much more easily and confidently with these modalities than with MRI.

Intraosseous Disk Herniations

Disk material not only projects into the spinal canal, but also may directly herniate into the adjacent vertebral bodies through the end plates, in which case it is known as a Schmorl's or cartilaginous node. These may occur because bone is weakened by osteoporosis, tumor, metabolic diseases, or congenital weak points in the end plates. Although usually asymptomatic, Schmorl's nodes may occur from trauma with axial loading forces and may be acutely painful in this latter situation. Multiple thoracic Schmorl's nodes can occur in very active teens from axial stresses and result in irregularity of several end plates, loss of disk height, and narrowing of the height of the affected anterior vertebral bodies from fractures, with a resultant kyphosis (Scheuermann's disease) (Fig. 13-48).

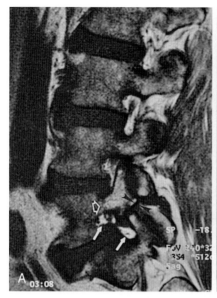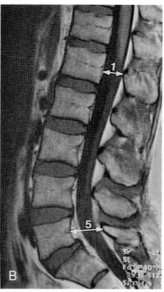

Figure 13-47 **Spondylolysis: secondary signs. A,** T1 sagittal image of the lumbar spine. A spondylolytic defect is seen between the *arrowheads* at L5. Secondary evidence includes the lobulated, oblique figure-of-eight L5-S1 neural foramen (*solid arrows*) and the high signal fat from reactive type 2 marrow changes in the pedicle and superior articular process of L5 (*open arrow*). **B,** T1 sagittal image of the lumbar spine. There is wedging of the posterior L5 vertebral body. The spinal canal at L5 (5; *arrows*) is more than 25% wider compared with the anteroposterior diameter of the canal at L1 (1; *arrows*).

An inflammatory, foreign body–type response to intraosseous disk herniation may occur, with vascularization around the disk material and surrounding marrow edema, which may cause severe pain (Fig. 13-49).[43] Vascularized Schmorl's nodes on MRI tend to have large, dome-shaped regions of marrow edema surrounding them; marrow edema is low signal on T1W and high signal on T2W and contrast-enhanced T1W images. A rim of contrast enhancement around the periphery of the Schmorl's node is seen in addition to the surrounding marrow edema. These can have an aggressive look, similar to a tumor, and careful evaluation is necessary to make the proper diagnosis.

Major Trauma (Box 13-12)

MRI for evaluation of traumatic changes in the spine usually is performed to look for soft tissue injury; however, certain fractures in the spine also are well depicted with MRI. Generally, ligament rupture, traumatic disk extrusions, cord injury, epidural hematomas, and paraspinous hematomas are shown better with MRI than with other imaging techniques. There are some logistical difficulties in performing MRI examinations in critically injured spinal trauma patients, and these must be weighed against the potential benefits of the examination.

We use MRI (after conventional films and CT) in patients who have sustained major spinal trauma for several different indications, as follows: radiographs suggesting ligamentous injury, some thoracolumbar burst fractures to look for intact ligaments, cervical facet dislocations to look for a disk extrusion or epidural hematoma before performing a closed reduction, incomplete neurologic deficits to assess the cord and ligaments to help determine what type of surgery will be done and the patient's prognosis, neurologic deficits in the face of no radiographic traumatic abnormalities (eg, central cord syndrome) or if the neurologic deficit does not match the level of a radiographic traumatic abnormality, and in obtunded trauma patients with no radiographic abnormalities to determine the need to keep them in a cervical collar. Generally, there is no purpose in doing MRI in patients with a complete neurologic deficit because the treatment and outcome are unlikely to be affected.[44]

Osseous. Osseous spinal injuries are well identified by radiographs and CT. Any fracture through cortical bone would

Figure 13-48 **Scheuermann's disease.** T1 sagittal image of the lumbar spine. The end plates are irregular at multiple levels in the lower thoracic and throughout the lumbar spine from intraosseous disk herniations. There also is loss of the normal lumbar lordosis and loss of disk and vertebral body height.

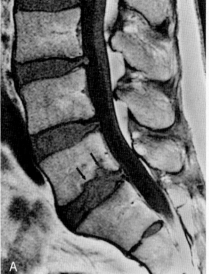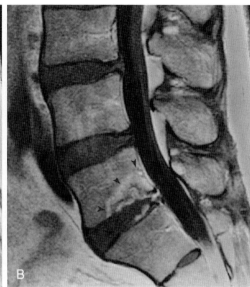

Figure 13-49 **Vascularized (painful) Schmorl's nodes. A,** T1 sagittal image of the lumbar spine. The inferior end plate of L5 is irregular from intraosseous disk herniation (*arrows*). **B,** T1 contrast-enhanced sagittal image of the lumbar spine. An enhancing rim is present in the marrow surrounding the Schmorl's node (*arrowheads*), and there is peripheral enhancement around the herniated intraosseous disk itself. This patient had disk surgery in the remote past, which accounts for the enhancing posterior periphery of the L5-S1 disk.

be difficult to identify on MRI compared with CT; many posterior element fractures definitely would be missed on MRI, and MRI should not be done as a replacement examination for detecting spinal fractures. Fractures of the vertebral bodies may be evident on MRI, however, when they are

not identifiable on CT or radiographs because of the marrow edema and hemorrhage in the trabecular bone, for which MRI is very sensitive (Fig. 13-50). Vertebral body fractures appear as amorphous regions of high signal intensity on T2W images and may be intermediate signal intensity on T1W images, if evident at all on this sequence; linear fracture lines are usually not evident.

Ligaments. The anterior and posterior longitudinal ligaments of the spine, the ligamentum flavum, the interspinous

---

BOX 13-12

Major Spinal Trauma

Osseous
- Posterior element (cortical) fractures, easily missed on MRI
- Vertebral body (marrow) fractures, easily detected

Ligaments
- Increased signal on T2 from hemorrhage/edema directs attention to sites of acute ligament injury
- Ligament partial tears: Thickening and intrasubstance increased signal
- Complete tears: Discontinuity of ligament

Disks
- Traumatic extrusions

Epidural Fluid
- Hematoma
- Pseudomeningocele

Vascular
- Vertebral artery occlusion

Cord
- Early
  - Transection
  - Hemorrhage
  - Hemorrhage surrounded by edema
  - Edema (contusion)
- Delayed
  - Myelomalacia
  - Intramedullary cysts
  - Syrinx
  - Infarction

Nerves
- Avulsion, contusion

Paraspinous Soft Tissues
- Hematoma, muscle strains

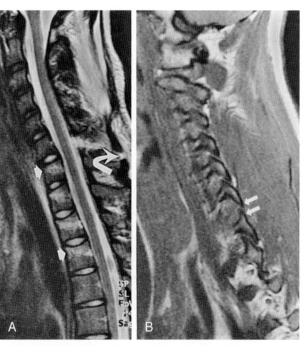

Figure 13-50 **Major trauma: osseous. A,** Fast T2 sagittal image of the cervical spine. There is marrow edema from fractures of C7 through T3 (between *solid white arrows*); radiographs and CT were normal. The supraspinous ligament is discontinuous from a tear (*curved arrow*) at C6-7. **B,** T1 sagittal image of the cervical spine (different patient than in **A**). Perched facets (*arrows*) are easy to see in the lower cervical spine because of the tomographic nature of MRI.

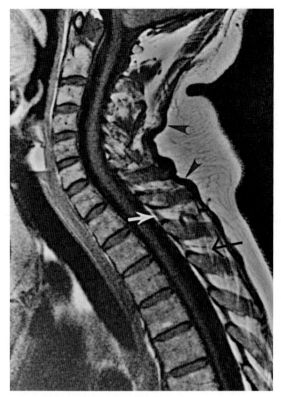

Figure 13-51 **Spinous ligaments: normal.** T1 sagittal image of the cervical spine. The supraspinous ligament is shown (*arrowheads*). The ligamentum flavum is a vertical, low signal structure anterior to the spinous processes (*white arrow*). The interspinous ligaments are difficult to see, and the presence of fat between spinous processes is the best indication of normal (*black arrow*). The normal anterior and posterior longitudinal ligaments are not seen on this sequence because they blend with adjacent cortical bone and other low signal structures.

ligaments, and the supraspinous and nuchal ligaments must be carefully evaluated in trauma patients. These supporting ligaments of the spine are made of collagen and generally appear as taut, low signal intensity bands on all pulse sequences on MRI (Fig. 13-51).[45] An exception to this MRI appearance involves the normal interspinous ligaments, which run vertically between adjacent spinous processes and may have a striated or patchy appearance with areas of intermediate signal intensity interspersed with large areas of high signal intensity fat on T1W images. Another exception involves the supraspinous and nuchal ligaments, which are not always taut and normally have areas that are wavy and may have high signal intensity within them from the magic angle phenomenon on short TE pulse sequences.

Ligaments may be partially or completely torn. Some type of T2W sequence, especially with fat suppression (eg, STIR), is necessary for showing high signal intensity edema and hemorrhage in and around an injured ligament (Fig. 13-52). Discontinuity of the ligament indicates a complete rupture, but partial tears with ligamentous thickening and intrasubstance high signal intensity also can be seen. Obliteration of the fat between spinous processes on T1W images, with high signal intensity on T2W images, indicates interspinous ligament sprain. The high signal intensity areas of edema and hemorrhage are extremely useful for directing one's attention to the sites of ligamentous injury, which otherwise may be subtle on MRI. For this reason, MRI should be performed as soon as possible after the trauma, before the edema resolves (preferably within 3 days).

Traumatic Disks. Acute traumatic disk extrusions are important in specific situations. An 11% incidence of

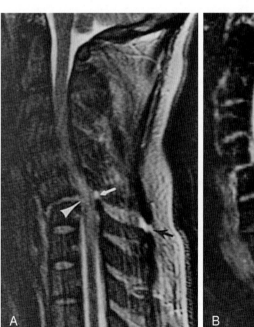 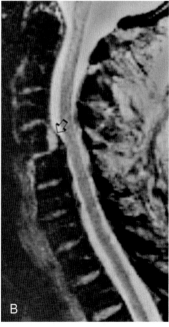

Figure 13-52 **Major trauma: ligaments. A,** STIR sagittal image of the cervical spine. The supraspinous ligament is torn (*black arrow*), as is the ligamentum flavum (*white arrow*) and posterior longitudinal ligament at the C6-7 level (*arrowhead*). There is high signal in the cord from contusion at the same level. **B,** T2* sagittal image of the cervical spine (different patient than in **A**). There is subluxation of C4 on C5. The linear, low signal posterior longitudinal ligament (*open arrow*) is displaced from the adjacent vertebral body by blood or disk material, but remains intact, which has a significant impact on management.

increased neurologic compromise as a result of unrecognized disk extrusions was reported in patients who had reduction of cervical facet dislocations under anesthesia.[46] If a traumatic disk extrusion is shown by MRI, careful consideration should be given to open reduction of the dislocated facets, or at least in not performing the reduction under general anesthesia, to prevent progressive neurologic deficits. Acute disk herniations also may be associated with traumatic cord abnormalities before reducing or manipulating the spine (Fig. 13-53).

T2W images of traumatic disk extrusions may show them as either low or high signal intensity, depending on whether or not there is hemorrhage involving the disk. Disks at the injured level have signal intensity identical to adjacent intact disks on T2W images if there is no hemorrhage; there is higher signal intensity than the normal disk in the presence of hemorrhage, and the disk height often is decreased.

Epidural Fluid Collections. Trauma may result in an epidural hematoma (Fig. 13-54) or a pseudomeningocele. Pseudomeningoceles occur from a rent in the dura (as from avulsion of a nerve root) with leakage of CSF into the epidural space and beyond.

Vascular Abnormalities. The vertebral arteries of patients with cervical trauma have been reported as abnormal from occlusion in 24% of patients.[47] MRI shows vertebral artery asymmetry, with lack of the normal, low signal intensity from flow void in the vertebral artery on the abnormal side (Fig. 13-55). Asymmetry of signal intensity also may occur in asymptomatic, nontraumatized patients because of asymmetry in size and of flow in the arteries. This may be evaluated best on axial images, but also on sagittal cervical spine

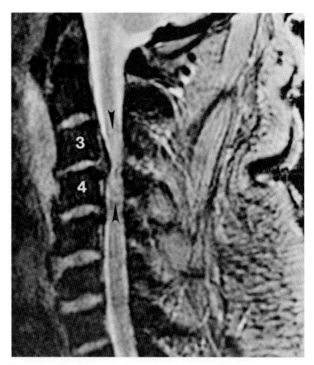

Figure 13-53 **Major trauma: disks.** T2* sagittal image of the cervical spine. There is a traumatic disk herniation at C3-4. The posterior longitudinal ligament remains intact, draped over the displaced disk material. There is abnormal signal in the cord (*arrowheads*), centered at the level of the abnormal disk from hemorrhage/edema.

MRI. Treatment for this entity is controversial for patients with a concomitant spinal cord injury because it is undesirable to give anticoagulants to these patients, and because the frequency of vertebrobasilar ischemia in trauma patients is low.

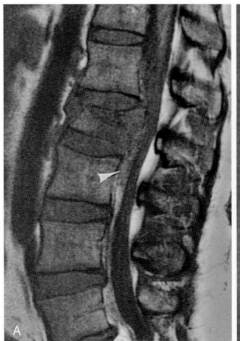
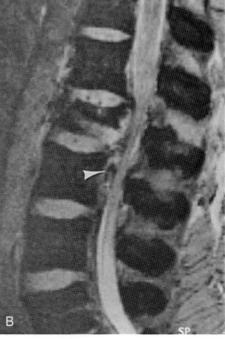

Figure 13-54 **Major trauma: epidural hematoma. A,** T1 sagittal image of the lumbar spine. A burst fracture of L2 protrudes into the spinal canal. Intermediate signal in the anterior epidural space (*arrowhead*) is from blood. **B,** T2* sagittal image of the lumbar spine. There is very low signal and blooming in the epidural hematoma (*arrowhead*) from blood. The canal is narrowed secondary to the retropulsed fracture and the epidural hematoma.

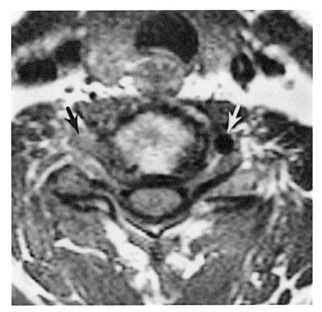

Figure 13-55 Major trauma: vascular. T1 axial image of the cervical spine. There is asymmetry in the appearance of the vertebral arteries bilaterally. The left side is normal (*white arrow*) with low signal from flow void. The right side has abnormal increased signal in the vertebral artery (*black arrow*) because of decreased flow from occlusion.

Cord Injuries. Three abnormal patterns may occur in the cord as a result of trauma:

1. Contusion (edema)
2. Hemorrhage
3. A combination of central hemorrhage with peripheral, surrounding edema (Fig. 13-56)[48]

Cord transection may occur, with hemorrhage in the gap between the segments. The cord may be either enlarged or normal in size.

The appearance of hemorrhage in the cord is a function of the chronicity of the lesion.[49] The signal characteristics listed in Table 13-2 are based on conventional spin echo techniques, but gradient echo sequences also may be valuable in showing blood because it shows blooming. The mnemonic we use to help remember the progression of MRI changes from hemorrhage is discussed in detail in Chapter 3 (**It Be IdDy BidDy BaBy Doo Doo** mnemonic; see Table 13-2).

Cord edema without hemorrhage or fractures is a common manifestation of the central cord syndrome, which occurs with a hyperextension injury, usually in older individuals with degenerative changes in the cervical spine that cause spinal stenosis. The osteophytes and bulging disks impinge against the cord during the injury, resulting in central cord edema. Patients have symptoms of weakness or paralysis of the upper limbs and sparing of the lower extremities. Edema manifests on MRI as being isointense to the cord on T1W images and high signal intensity on T2W images (Fig. 13-57).[46]

There is a better prognosis with contusion of the cord than with hemorrhage; recuperation of neurologic function is unlikely with cord hemorrhage. Other possible sequelae of trauma to the cord include myelomalacia, intramedullary cysts, syrinx, and infarction.

Other Soft Tissues. Muscles, nerves, and prevertebral and other paraspinous soft tissues may show evidence of injury on MRI after trauma. The paraspinous muscles may be strained and show high signal intensity on T2W images from

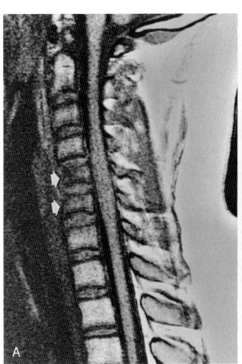

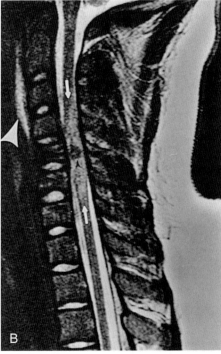

Figure 13-56 Major trauma: cord injury. **A,** T1 sagittal image of the cervical spine. Vague decreased signal in the C5 and C6 vertebral bodies (*arrows*) is from fractures (not evident on radiography or CT). The cord has normal signal, but is increased in caliber posterior to the abnormal vertebral bodies. The patient had a significant neurologic deficit. **B,** Fast T2 sagittal image of the cervical spine. There is a focal area of low signal (*black arrowhead*) in the cord from hemorrhage. There is diffuse increased signal from edema (*arrows*) surrounding the hemorrhage. There is a small, high signal prevertebral hematoma (*white arrowhead*).

Table 13-2 CORD HEMORRHAGE*

Age	Blood Products	T1 Signal	T2 Signal	Mnemonic
Hyperacute (0-1 day)	Oxyhemoglobin/serum	Isointense to cord	Bright	It Be (**IB**)
Acute (1-3 days)	Deoxyhemoglobin	Isointense to cord	Dark	IdDy (**ID**)
Early subacute (4-7 days)	Intracellular methemoglobin	Bright	Dark	BiDdy (**BD**)
Late subacute (>7 days)	Extracellular methemoglobin	Bright	Bright	BaBy (**BB**)
Chronic (>2 wk)	Hemosiderin	Dark	Dark	Doo Doo (**DD**)

*Hemorrhage into soft tissues other than the cord and brain goes through the same sequence of changes, but often slower and in a less predictable fashion because of the lower oxygen tension.

edema, or hemorrhage into muscle may have variable signal depending on the age of the injury (Fig. 13-58). Nerves may be injured, either avulsed or contused, and leakage of CSF may be seen with nerve avulsions (Fig. 13-59). A contused nerve has high signal intensity, usually with enlargement, on T2W images in the injured segment.

OSSEOUS SPINE TUMORS (Box 13-13)

Benign Bone Tumors

The most common benign osseous tumors of the spine are hemangiomas, osteoid osteoma, osteoblastoma, giant cell tumor, osteochondroma, and aneurysmal bone cyst. Before the age of 30 years, tumors of the spine are uncommon and generally benign.

Hemangiomas in the vertebral bodies are so common that they are discussed separately. Otherwise, a few simple rules,

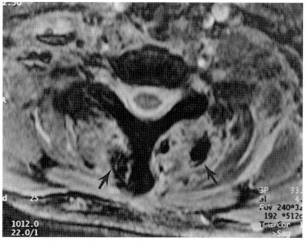

Figure 13-58 Major trauma: muscle strain. T2* axial image of the cervical spine. This patient had severe neck pain, but negative radiographs and CT. MRI shows muscle strains in the paraspinous muscles with areas of high signal and focal areas of low signal with blooming (*arrows*) from hemorrhage in torn muscle.

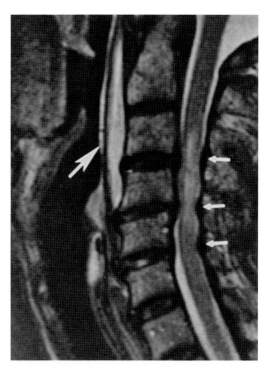

Figure 13-57 Major trauma: central cord syndrome. Fast T2 sagittal image of the cervical spine. The central spinal canal is stenotic from bulging disks and ligamentum flavum (*small arrows*) at several levels. There is increased signal in the cord at the level of the stenosis from contusion. There are no fractures or traumatic disk herniations. There also is prevertebral soft tissue hemorrhage/edema (*large arrow*).

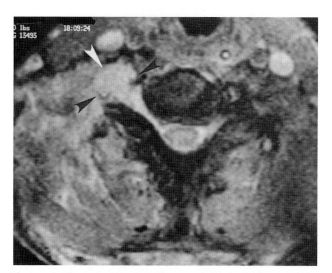

Figure 13-59 Major trauma: nerve root avulsion. T2* axial image of the cervical spine. The right neural foramen is high signal and appears empty compared with the normal left side. There is a bulbous collection (*arrowheads*) of high signal just outside of the neural foramen, compatible with a pseudomeningocele associated with nerve root avulsion and leak of spinal fluid.

BOX 13-13

Osseous Spine Tumors: Decreasing Order of Frequency

Benign
- Hemangiomas (increased signal T1 and T2)
- Osteoid osteoma (posterior elements)
- Osteoblastoma (posterior elements)
- Giant cell tumor (sacrum)
- Osteochondroma (protrude from bone)
- Aneurysmal bone cyst (posterior elements)

Malignant
- Metastases (multiple)
- Myeloma (multiple)
- Lymphoma (multiple)
- Chordoma (sacrum)
- Sarcomas
  - Ewing's sarcoma, osteosarcoma, chondrosarcoma

Most tumors discovered before age 30 years are benign.
Most tumors discovered after age 30 years are malignant.

such as the location of spine lesions, help to narrow the differential diagnosis on MRI. Osteoid osteomas, osteoblastomas, and aneurysmal bone cysts are most likely to occur in the posterior spinal elements. In addition, aneurysmal bone cysts are expansile and usually have fluid-fluid levels within them, whereas osteoid osteomas are small and usually have a target appearance because of the calcified central nidus and large surrounding areas of edema in the marrow and soft tissue structures adjacent to the lesion (Fig. 13-60). Giant cell tumors of the spine are rare and nonspecific in appear-

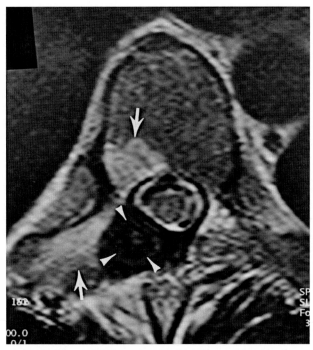

Figure 13-60 **Benign bone tumors: osteoid osteoma.** Fast T2 axial image of T10. A target lesion (*arrowheads* indicate the inner circle of the lesion) in the right lamina represents the osteoid osteoma, which is surrounded by high signal edema in the posterior vertebral body, pedicle, transverse process, and soft tissues (*arrows*). There is mild central canal narrowing from the lesion. The low signal in the cerebrospinal fluid that surrounds the cord is simply flow artifact from the normal motion of the fluid.

ance, but when they occur in the spine, they most frequently involve the sacrum.

Intraosseous Hemangiomas. Spinal hemangiomas are common and frequently multiple. The vertebral bodies are more commonly affected than the posterior elements.

Most ordinary hemangiomas have a classic appearance and are asymptomatic (Fig. 13-61). On T1W images, they are round lesions of high signal intensity, caused by the large fat component of typical hemangiomas; on T2W images, they also are high signal intensity (higher than fat) because of the slow-flowing blood in the lesions. Thick, low signal intensity, vertical trabecular struts may be seen within the lesions. The high signal intensity of hemangiomas on T2W sequences distinguishes them from focal areas of marrow conversion, which consist almost entirely of fat and have a lower signal intensity than hemangiomas on T2W images. Fast T2W sequences without fat saturation show fat as high signal intensity, which may make it difficult to distinguish hemangiomas from focal areas of marrow fat conversion.

A small percentage of hemangiomas have a completely different appearance than the above-described fatty lesions; these are referred to as *aggressive* or *atypical hemangiomas*.[50] These have diffuse low signal intensity on T1W images, enhance with contrast material, and are high signal on T2W images. Aggressive hemangiomas are composed predominantly of vessels, rather than fat. These lesions tend to be symptomatic because of fracture and collapse of the vertebral body, or extension of the hemangioma into the epidural space, with mass effect that may result in neurologic symp-

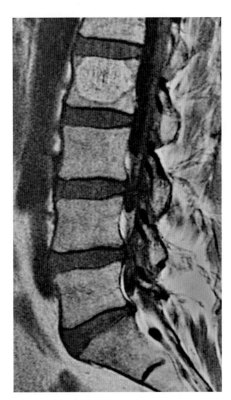

Figure 13-61 **Benign bone tumors: hemangioma.** T1 sagittal image of the lumbar spine. There is a large, round, high signal fat lesion in the L2 vertebral body with thick, low signal vertical struts in its center, typical of a hemangioma.

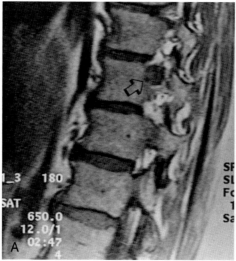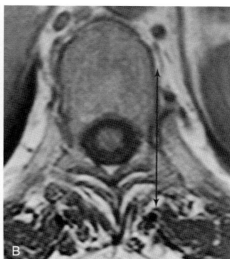

Figure 13-62 Malignant bone tumors: a pitfall. **A,** T1 sagittal image of the thoracic spine. A focal, low signal round lesion in the posterosuperior vertebral body and pedicle (*open arrow*) resembles a metastatic lesion. **B,** T1 axial image of the thoracic spine. The sagittal slice obtained through the costovertebral joint (*double-headed arrow*) shows the focal "lesion" in the sagittal plane (**A**), but it is due simply to volume averaging.

toms and pain. These have an appearance similar to that of metastatic disease or other aggressive lesions of bone.

Malignant Bone Tumors

The most common malignant osseous lesions to affect the spine usually occur after age 30 years and include metastases, multiple myeloma, lymphoma, chordoma, and sarcomas (Ewing's sarcoma, osteosarcoma, and chondrosarcoma, in decreasing order of frequency). Ewing's sarcoma and osteosarcoma occur at a younger age than any of the other malignant lesions, usually during the second decade.

Metastases and Multiple Myeloma. Metastases and multiple myeloma are common and are discussed in detail in Chapter 2. The spine is the site of most bone metastases and myeloma because of its high red marrow content; the thoracolumbar spine in particular is affected. In the spine, MRI is extremely useful not only to show the presence and location of lesions, but also to depict any epidural spread and its effect on the cord or nerves. Gadolinium frequently is used to better show epidural extension of tumor arising from bone.

Metastases are usually focal and multiple, but may cause diffuse homogeneous marrow disease, or occasionally be a solitary focal lesion. Lytic metastases are generally low signal intensity on T1W images and become bright on T2W images, especially if untreated. Most sclerotic metastases have low signal on T1W and T2W sequences. Myeloma has the following patterns on MRI with increasing severity of disease: normal marrow appearance, focal lesions (the "mini brain" appearance is characteristic if present,[51] but otherwise they look like metastases), variegated pattern, and diffuse pattern.

There is a pitfall to be aware of in the thoracic spine that may mimic a metastasis or myeloma. Sagittal T1W images through the costovertebral joint may give the appearance of a focal low signal lesion in the posterosuperior vertebral body, extending into the pedicle (Fig. 13-62). The location on the lateral margin of the vertebral body, and in its posterosuperior aspect, makes the true nature of this finding obvious. This appearance may be seen at multiple levels, mimicking multiple lesions.

Acute osteoporotic compression fractures in the spine may have features similar to metastatic disease, and it is a common problem to try to differentiate the two on spine MRI examinations of elderly individuals. This is discussed in Chapter 2, but also is briefly reviewed here. A fractured vertebral body is statistically more likely to be from metastatic disease than from an acute osteoporotic fracture with surrounding hemorrhage and edema if it meets the following criteria:

1. The pedicles and posterior elements have abnormal signal intensity.
2. There is an associated soft tissue mass.
3. There are multiple lesions in other bones, especially round, focal lesions.
4. The entire vertebral body has abnormal signal intensity, without any areas of fatty marrow.
5. The posterior vertebral body wall has a convex rather than an angled appearance.

and

6. No linear fracture line is present.

Follow-up MRI (in 6 to 8 weeks) or biopsy is generally necessary to make a definitive distinction between acute osteoporotic fractures and pathologic fractures from metastases.

Chordomas. Chordomas and other primary bone tumors that may arise in the spine are rare. Chordomas arise from notochordal remnants, and most spinal chordomas are located in the sacrum or coccyx (the differential diagnosis includes metastases, plasmacytoma, or giant cell tumor). Rarely, chordomas are present in vertebral bodies elsewhere in the spine. More than one adjacent vertebral segment commonly may be involved by this tumor. The MRI appearance is nonspecific, showing a mass that is heterogeneous, low signal intensity on T1W images and hyperintense on T2W images, and that may involve more than one adjacent level (Fig. 13-63).

Primary Bone Tumors. Bone sarcomas that arise in the spine have features identical to their appearance in any other bone.

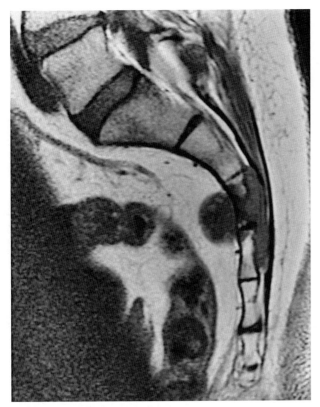

Figure 13-63 **Malignant bone tumors: chordoma.** T1 sagittal image of the sacrum. There is destruction of the S3 and S4 vertebral bodies with extension of tumor into the spinal canal and presacral space. The sacral location and involvement of adjacent segments is typical of a chordoma.

SPINAL CANAL CONTENTS

Most abnormalities affecting the spine were described in earlier sections. The osseous structures and joints are the sites of origin for the bulk of spine abnormalities. Many abnormalities of the structures within the spinal canal are secondary to abnormalities of the adjacent bones and joints of the spine.

As musculoskeletal radiologists, our goals in evaluating the spinal canal contents are (1) not to miss anything of importance, and (2) to make the diagnosis or to have a reasonable list of differential diagnostic possibilities for the abnormal findings, without crowding too much of our brain with erudite details of spinal canal pathology. Abnormalities involving the contents of the canal are covered accordingly in this chapter, and additional information can be obtained from other texts devoted to these topics.

The classic division of spinal structures into intramedullary, intradural extramedullary, and extradural is not used here. These terms are ingrained in the literature from work initially done with myelography, but we find it easier with MRI to discuss the precise location of a lesion because that is virtually always possible to ascertain with MRI. For instance, why use the vague term *extradural*, which includes everything from the dural sac to the Atlantic Ocean? We do not refer to an osteoid osteoma in the shaft of a femur as being an intracortical, extramedullary, subperiosteal lesion; it is simply a cortical lesion, a medullary lesion, or a subperiosteal lesion. The same simplicity should apply to the spine;

we use the terms *cord, intradural space,* and *epidural space* to define the location of lesions within the spinal canal.

Epidural Space (Box 13-14)

The epidural space extends from the foramen magnum to the sacral hiatus in the craniocaudal direction; it lies external to the thecal sac and deep to the osseous structures and ligaments of the spine within the spinal canal. It is composed mainly of fat and blood vessels. MRI shows the normal epidural space with signal characteristics that follow fat on all pulse sequences.

Lesions that occur in the epidural space include epidural lipomatosis, epidural hematoma, epidural abscess, and certain kinds of cysts. Many lesions from the adjacent bones, disks, and ligaments may secondarily encroach on the epidural space.[52] Masses within the epidural space often are surrounded by a rim of epidural fat, which helps to place the lesions within this anatomic compartment.

BOX 13-14

Epidural Abnormalities

Abscess
- Usually associated with spondylodiskitis

Hematoma
- Trauma, surgery, anticoagulation, or spontaneous
  - Spontaneous, probably secondary to disk disruption

Lipomatosis
- Increased fat in thoracic/lumbar spine may cause stenosis symptoms

Cysts
- Synovial cysts
  - Facet joint degeneration
- Arachnoid cysts (includes sacral meningoceles)
  - Defect in dura allows arachnoid and CSF herniation
  - May compress nerves or displace cord
  - May erode bone
  - Often have static flow, increased signal on T2 relative to CSF
- Arachnoid diverticula
  - Dilation of nerve root sleeves
  - Common, multiple, may erode bone
  - Occur above sacral level
  - Asymptomatic or mimic disk extrusion
  - Signal follows CSF, no enhancement differentiates from nerve sheath tumors
- Perineural (Tarlov cysts)
  - Dorsal nerve root fibers involved with cyst
  - Affect sacral nerve roots usually
  - Asymptomatic, or may cause nerve compression symptoms
  - May erode bone, cysts present in central canal or neural foramina or both
  - Signal follows CSF, or higher than CSF on T2 (static flow)
- Pseudomeningoceles
  - Traumatic, nerve root avulsion often associated
  - Rent in dura and arachnoid with CSF collection in epidural space and beyond
- Lateral thoracic meningoceles
  - Associated with neurofibromatosis, other manifestations usually present (dural ectasia)

Miscellaneous
- Any bone or disk abnormality extending into epidural space
- Ossification, posterior longitudinal ligament

CSF, cerebrospinal fluid.

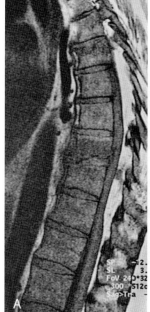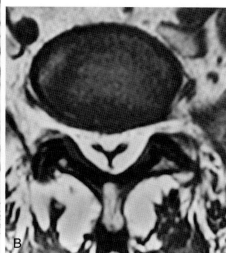

Figure 13-64 **Epidural space: epidural lipomatosis. A,** T1 sagittal image of the thoracic spine. There is a large amount of high signal fat in the posterior epidural space of the thoracic spine. It causes compression of the dural sac anteriorly. The sac widens distally, where the fat becomes thinner. **B,** T1 axial image of the lumbar spine (different patient than in **A**). High signal fat is filling the central canal, and the dural sac is compressed into a small triangular structure.

Epidural Abscess. Epidural abscess was discussed earlier in the section on infection. It is a localized fluid collection with rim enhancement that usually is associated with adjacent spondylodiskitis (see Figs. 13-38 and 13-39).

Epidural Hematoma. Focal collections of blood in the epidural space occur from acute trauma (see Fig. 13-54), as a complication of surgery (see Fig. 13-36), from anticoagulation, or spontaneously (see Figs. 13-13 and 13-14). The appearance of a hematoma on MRI depends on its age; this was described earlier in the trauma section.

Spontaneous epidural hematomas are believed to occur from tearing of fragile epidural veins at the time of an acute disk disruption. Annular tears or focal disk herniations usually are present at the level of a spontaneous epidural hematoma; symptoms are those of an acute disk herniation, but resolve more rapidly. Spontaneous epidural hematomas are largest in the anteroposterior diameter at the mid–vertebral body level (adjacent to the basivertebral venous plexus) and taper as they extend to the adjacent disk level.[22] Spontaneous epidural hematomas are often quite small and may be difficult to distinguish from a sequestered disk or extrusion, depending on their signal intensity at the time of imaging.

Epidural Lipomatosis. Deposition of excessive quantities of fat in the epidural space usually affects patients who are taking corticosteroids or who have endogenous hyperadrenocorticism, but also may occur in obese individuals or for no apparent reason. This entity is often an incidental finding on MRI and causes no symptoms. Only the thoracic or lumbar spine or both are involved (Fig. 13-64). Symptoms of spinal stenosis may exist. MRI shows large amounts of epidural fat that follow the signal intensity of fat on all pulse sequences and a decreased thecal sac size caused by compression by the fat.

Epidural Cysts. Several different cystic structures may be found in the epidural space. Synovial cysts that arise from degenerative facet joint disease may impinge on the epidural space (see Fig. 13-21). They may be located deep to the ligamentum flavum, or break through the ligament so that they are directly within the epidural space and may compress nerves. The MRI appearance was discussed earlier in the section on degenerative changes.

Arachnoid cysts occur when the arachnoid protrudes into the epidural space through a congenital or traumatic defect in the dura and is filled with CSF. The mass effect may cause neurologic symptoms by compressing adjacent soft tissue structures in the canal (cord and nerves). There may be pressure erosions of adjacent osseous structures (posterior vertebral bodies or inner aspects of pedicles). MRI shows an epidural mass that is low signal intensity on T1W and high signal intensity on T2W images (Fig. 13-65).

Sacral meningoceles are arachnoid cysts that occur in a specific location. They protrude through a developmental dural defect and may erode the sacrum (intraosseous or intrasacral meningoceles); these may or may not be symptomatic. Cyst size does not seem to relate to the presence of symptoms, but cysts that communicate with the subarachnoid space are usually asymptomatic, whereas cysts that do not communicate are symptomatic. Compression of nerves by the cystic mass may cause symptoms. These cysts are similar in signal intensity to CSF, but often have slightly higher signal intensity on T2W images, caused by static flow (Fig. 13-66).

Arachnoid diverticula are common cysts, formed by dilation of nerve root sleeves (Fig. 13-67). These are commonly multiple, bulbous dilations of the dura and arachnoid that are filled with CSF and can clinically mimic disk extrusions or compression by other masses. These diverticula may erode bone. Arachnoid diverticula typically affect nerve root sleeves above the sacral level. There is no contrast enhance-

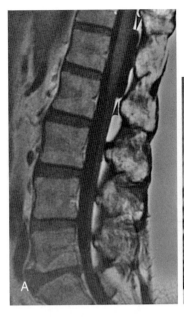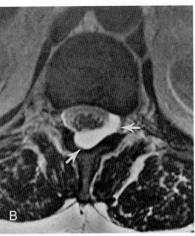

Figure 13-65 Epidural space: arachnoid cyst. **A,** T1 sagittal image of the lumbar spine. A low signal mass (*arrowheads*) replaces the posterior epidural fat posterior to L1. **B,** Spin echo–T2 axial image of L1. The high signal cystic mass in the posterior epidural space (*arrows*) compresses the dural sac.

ment, which differentiates them from tumor, and the signal intensity follows that of the fluid in the subarachnoid space on all pulse sequences, allowing differentiation from most disk herniations.

Perineural cysts, or Tarlov cysts, occur in the sacral region and have nerve fibers within the wall of the cyst or coursing through the cyst (Fig. 13-68). They may cause nerve compression or bone erosion, but usually are asymptomatic.

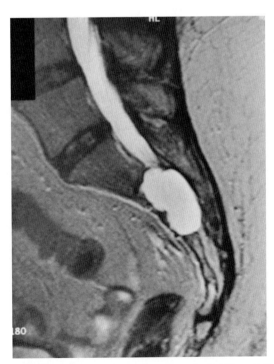

Figure 13-66 Epidural space: sacral meningocele. Fast T2 sagittal image of the lumbar spine. There is a large, high signal, cystic mass in the sacral canal that is eroding the bone of the sacrum from pressure. A sacral meningocele has higher signal than the cerebrospinal fluid because of the relatively slower flow within it.

They have no direct connection to the thecal sac, but are continuous with the dura and arachnoid of the posterior nerve roots in the sacral region. The signal intensity follows that of CSF, or, because of an increased protein content or absence of flow, they often have higher signal intensity on T2W images than CSF.

Other cystic lesions that may occur in the epidural space are lateral thoracic meningoceles (which typically occur in neurofibromatosis, but other spinal abnormalities, such as dural ectasia, are present to help make the diagnosis) and traumatic pseudomeningoceles (which tend to extend out of the epidural space through neural foramina and are large). Scalloping of posterior vertebral bodies may occur from the different epidural cysts described earlier and from dural ectasia seen in neurofibromatosis, Marfan syndrome, and Ehlers-Danlos syndrome, and from erosion by any soft tissue tumor mass and in patients with acromegaly and achondroplasia.

Miscellaneous. Many different abnormalities can secondarily affect the epidural space from the adjacent ligaments, bones, and joints. Most of these entities have been discussed elsewhere (eg, disk herniations, osteophytes, bone tumors). These lesions are directly visible on MRI, so it is clear from where they arose. Ossification of the posterior longitudinal ligament of the spine usually affects the cervical spine, resulting in thickening of the posterior longitudinal ligament, which impinges on the epidural space and may cause symptoms relating to spinal stenosis (Fig. 13-69). This entity is very common in patients with diffuse idiopathic skeletal hyperostosis and should be looked for closely in this disorder.

Intradural Space (Box 13-15)

The intradural space is the CSF-filled subarachnoid space between the dura and the spinal cord; nerve roots are included in this space. Benign intradural lesions include nerve sheath tumors, meningiomas, paragangliomas, and

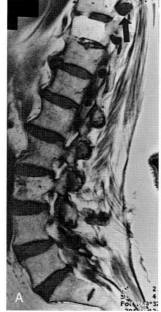
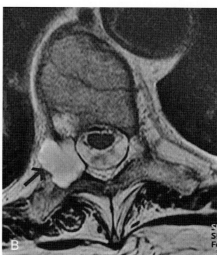

Figure 13-67 Epidural space: arachnoid diverticulum. A, T1 sagittal image of the thoracolumbar spine. There is a rounded, low signal mass in the right neural foramen at T8-9 (*arrow*). Smaller, but similar-appearing low signal masses are evident in several neural foramina below T9. Hemangiomas are in T10 and L3 (focal fat within the vertebral bodies). **B,** Fast T2 axial image through T8-9 neural foramina. The high signal arachnoid diverticulum is evident in the right foramen (*arrow*), separate from the dural sac. There is pressure erosion of the anterior aspect of the transverse process and the posterior vertebral body.

assorted cysts. Nerve sheath tumors and spinal meningiomas compose about 90% of all intradural benign and malignant tumors. Metastases are the most common malignant abnormality to affect this space. A common artifact in the intradural space on MRI occurs from turbulent flow of the CSF, which must not be mistaken for a true mass in this region. It appears as elongated, oblong regions of low signal within the spinal fluid on all pulse sequences, best seen on T2W images (Fig. 13-70).

Nerve Sheath Tumors. Pathologic and MRI features of nerve sheath tumors were discussed in detail in Chapter 4 and are not repeated here. Nerve sheath tumors consist of

neurofibromas and schwannomas (neurilemomas). Most nerve sheath tumors (75%) arise within the dura, but a few are located intradurally and in the epidural space ("dumbbell" lesions), and a few more are located completely outside the dura (either epidural or paraspinous) (Fig. 13-71). They may be solitary or multiple.

Meningioma. Most spinal meningiomas are benign and occur in the thoracic spine or, less commonly, the cervical spine, usually in women. They have a broad attachment to the dura, and on MRI show signal intensity similar to the cord on all pulse sequences and diffuse homogeneous enhancement with contrast material (Fig. 13-72).

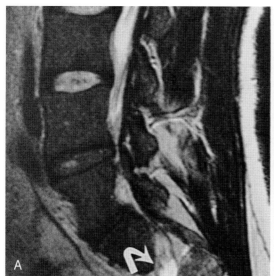
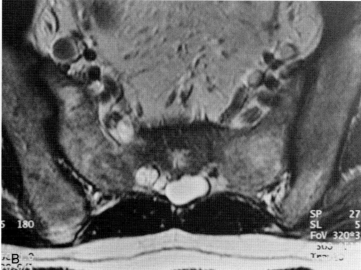

Figure 13-68 Epidural space: perineural (Tarlov cyst). A, Fast T2 sagittal image of the lumbar spine. A high signal cyst surrounds the right S2 nerve in the neural foramen (*curved arrow*). **B,** Fast T2 axial image of S2. The perineural cyst is evident in the right sacral foramen and in the central canal as high signal intensity.

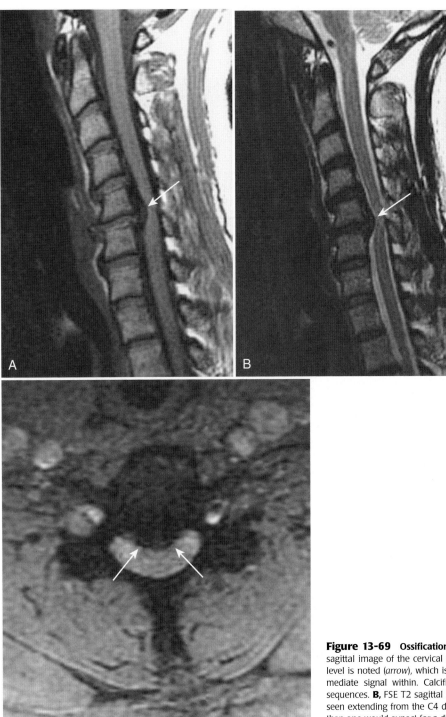

Figure 13-69 **Ossification of the posterior longitudinal ligament. A,** T1 sagittal image of the cervical spine. A mass impression on the cord at the C5-6 level is noted (*arrow*), which is predominantly low in signal, but has some intermediate signal within. Calcification is sometimes increased in signal on T1 sequences. **B,** FSE T2 sagittal image of the cervical spine. This process (*arrow*) is seen extending from the C4 disk level to the C6 vertebral body, a longer extent than one would expect for a disk or osteophyte. **C,** T2* axial image of the cervical spine. This image through the C6 body shows a low signal mass (*arrows*) impressing the cord. This is ossification of the posterior longitudinal ligament.

Some meningiomas may show areas of dense calcification, which have low signal intensity on all pulse sequences.

Other Tumors. Paragangliomas are rare lesions that may occur in several locations in the body. Pheochromocytomas of the adrenal glands are the most common paraganglioma. In the spine, paragangliomas occur in the filum terminale and the cauda equina. MRI shows a mass that is isointense to cord on T1W images and becomes slightly hyperintense to cord on T2W images (Fig. 13-73). Paragangliomas are vascular and show marked contrast enhancement; they may have a heterogeneous appearance from hemorrhage. Ependymomas often arise from the filum terminale or conus medullaris and should be considered along with paragangliomas and the much more common nerve sheath tumors

Intradural Abnormalities

- Nerve sheath tumors*
  - Neurofibroma or schwannoma
  - Most are intradural; dumbbell lesions are intradural and extradural
- Meningiomas*
  - Usually women
  - Thoracic > cervical
- Ependymomas†
- Paragangliomas†
- Cysts
  - Epidermoid (lumbar usually)
  - Dermoid (lumbar usually, signal resembles fat)
  - Arachnoid (posterior thoracic, usually)
- Metastases
  - Multiple nodules or sheetlike pattern involving leptomeninges in conus/cauda equina region
  - Contrast enhancement essential to make diagnosis
- Lipomas

*Nerve sheath tumors and meningiomas constitute 90% of intradural lesions.
†Conus/filum terminale/cauda equina region (include nerve sheath tumor and metastasis in differential for this area).

or metastases in the differential diagnosis for masses in this anatomic region.

Lipomas. Fatty masses that have signal characteristics typical of fat on all pulse sequences occur in several locations and forms in the spine, including an intradural location (Fig. 13-74). Intradural lipomas most commonly are found on the dorsal surface of the cord. This is a congenital abnormality associated with occult spinal dysraphism. Much more common than an intradural lipoma are lipomas associated with myelomeningoceles (lipomyelomeningoceles) and tethered cords. Another lipomatous lesion is the filum terminale fibrolipoma, or "fatty filum." The fatty filum is a common MRI finding of no clinical significance. It consists of a filum that has a normal size and shape, but is infiltrated

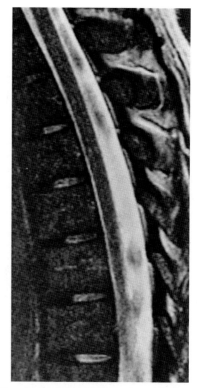

Figure 13-70 **Intradural space: pitfall.** Fast T2 sagittal image of the thoracic spine. There are multiple low signal, oblong regions in the cerebrospinal fluid posterior to the thoracic cord secondary to turbulent cerebrospinal fluid flow. These are not true masses, and they would remain low signal on T1 sequences also.

with fat and follows the signal of fat on all pulse sequences (Fig. 13-75).

Intradural Cystic Lesions. Intradural cystic lesions include epidermoid, dermoid, and arachnoid cysts. Epidermoid cysts are either congenital, in which case they occur in the

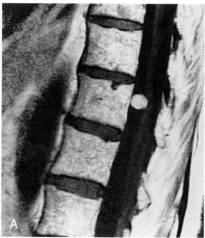
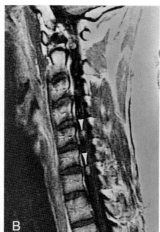
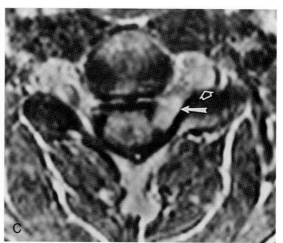

Figure 13-71 **Intradural space: nerve sheath tumors. A,** T1 contrast-enhanced sagittal image of the lumbar spine. There is a round, enhancing mass posterior to an upper lumbar vertebral body within the dural sac. This was found to be a schwannoma at surgery. **B,** T1 contrast-enhanced sagittal image of the cervical spine (different patient than in **A**). Two enhancing lesions are present in the anterior dural sac (*arrowheads*), surrounded by cerebrospinal fluid. These were neurofibromas. **C,** T1 contrast-enhanced axial image of the cervical spine (same patient as in **B**). A neurofibroma is present in the intradural space (*solid arrow*) and extends into the epidural space in the neural foramen (*open arrow*). This is a dumbbell neurofibroma that is intradural and extradural.

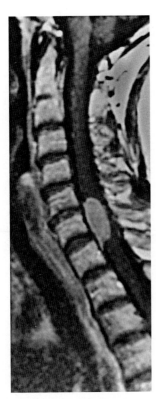

Figure 13-72   Intradural space: meningioma. T1 contrast-enhanced sagittal image of the cervical spine. There is an enhancing mass in the anterior intradural space with a broad-based attachment to the anterior dura. This is a typical appearance for a meningioma.

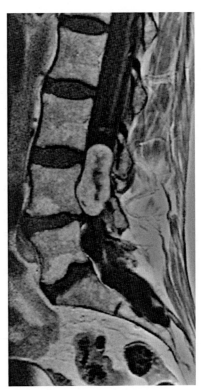

Figure 13-73   Intradural space: paraganglioma. T1 contrast-enhanced sagittal image of the lumbar spine. There is a large mass involving the cauda equina that fills the dural sac and erodes the posterior L4 vertebral body, indicating it is a long-standing lesion. The center of the mass is low signal from necrosis or hemorrhage. This was a paraganglioma at surgery; the differential diagnosis should include ependymoma, metastasis, and nerve sheath tumor.

cauda equina or conus, or acquired from lumbar punctures, in which case they occur in the lower lumbar region. MRI features vary and are nonspecific, but generally show a mass of low signal intensity on T1W and high signal intensity on T2W images (higher than spinal fluid).

Dermoid cysts are congenital tumors that arise from epithelial inclusions in the neural groove during development. They may be located either intradurally or within the cord in equal numbers. They usually are found in the lumbar spine, and signal characteristics on MRI are similar to fat.

Arachnoid cysts are rare lesions that usually arise in the posterior aspect of the thoracic spine. Their cause is uncertain. Adhesions in the subarachnoid space from previous trauma and bleeding may be a cause of these cysts. They communicate with the subarachnoid space and have the signal characteristics of CSF on MRI examinations, so they may be difficult or impossible to see except for the mass effect they have on the cord by displacing it.

Metastases. Metastases to the subarachnoid space usually involve the lumbosacral spine. They are multiple and are deposited in the arachnoid and pia mater. The conus and cauda equina may be diffusely involved, with a sheetlike infiltrative pattern or with multiple nodules. The leptomeninges (the arachnoid that lines the dural sac and the pia that covers the cord and nerve roots) may be involved by metastases from primary tumors arising in the central nervous system or from any other primary

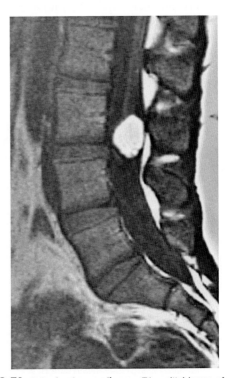

Figure 13-74   Intradural space: lipoma. T1 sagittal image of the lumbar spine. There is a high signal mass in the dural sac from an intradural lipoma. The patient presented with atrophy in a lower extremity resulting from nerve compression.

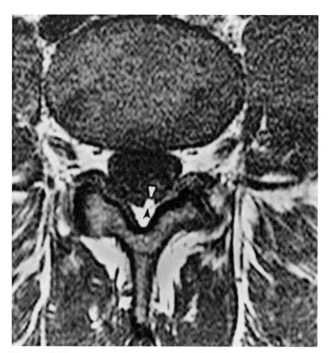

Figure 13-75 **Intradural space: fatty filum terminale.** T1 axial image of the lumbar spine. When fat infiltrates a normal-sized filum terminale, it is of no consequence and is known as a lipoma of the filum, or simply as a fatty filum (*arrowheads*).

carcinoma, lymphoma, or leukemia. MRI may not show these lesions unless an intravenous contrast agent is used. There may be thickened nerve roots or multiple small intradural nodules that are high signal intensity from contrast enhancement on T1W images. Contrast enhancement of the leptomeninges also can be seen in inflammatory causes of meningitis.

Spinal Cord Lesions
(Box 13-16 and Table 13-3)

Lesions arising within the cord are varied and numerous, but their MRI appearance is as limited as abnormalities of tendons. Just about all that can happen with abnormalities in the cord is that there is signal intensity different from the normal cord (usually, high signal intensity on T2W or contrast-enhanced T1W images), and the caliber of the cord may increase, decrease, or remain normal. Lesions most commonly found in the spinal cord generally are caused by **d**emyelinating diseases, **c**ysts, **i**nfarction, or **t**umor—hence our mnemonic DCIT: **d**amn **c**ord **i**s **t**rouble. This is not an exhaustive list of all abnormalities that can affect the cord, but it covers most abnormalities and the most common entities.

Demyelination Abnormalities. Demyelination abnormalities include myelomalacia, multiple sclerosis, transverse myelitis (usually from infection or post vaccination), compressive myelopathy (as from a disk extrusion or spinal stenosis), and radiation myelopathy. These lesions usually are difficult to identify on T1W unenhanced images, have high signal intensity on T2W images, and may have diffuse or patchy increased signal or no enhancement on T1W enhanced images. The margins of these lesions may not be as distinct as compared with a syrinx. The cord caliber is usually normal, but may be enlarged or atrophic. Plaques from multiple sclerosis usually are located in the posterior and lateral regions of the cord, and post-traumatic myelomalacia occurs at the site of previous spinal trauma; other demyelinating lesions have no predilection for a specific site. Myelomalacia is discussed further in the section on cysts of the cord (see next) because post-traumatic myelomalacia may lead to cyst or syrinx formation, and it may be difficult or impossible to differentiate among these entities by MRI.

Table 13-3   SPINAL CORD LESIONS: MRI FEATURES

	Cord Contour	T2 Signal	Contrast-Enhanced T1 Signal
Demyelination	↑, normal, ↓	↑ (or sometimes normal with cord atrophy)	↑ (diffuse or patchy), or none
Cysts	↑ usually	↑	None
Infarction	↑, normal, ↓	↑ H pattern in gray matter	↑ (patchy or diffuse), or none
Tumors	↑ usually	↑	↑ (patchy or diffuse), or none

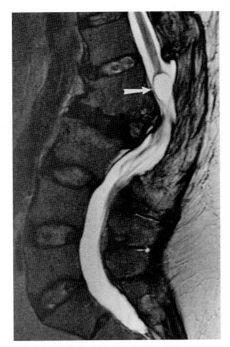

Figure 13-76 Cord: progressive post-traumatic myelomalacic myelopathy. Fast T2 sagittal image of the thoracolumbar spine. There is an old healed fracture in the upper lumbar spine with a secondary acute angle kyphosis. A rounded, high signal, cystic cord lesion (*arrow*) is present posterior to the fracture site. This is compatible with an area of previous myelomalacia in the cord that developed cysts, which coalesced into a rounded cyst, known as progressive post-traumatic myelomalacic myelopathy. This is likely to progress proximally into a typical elongated syrinx.

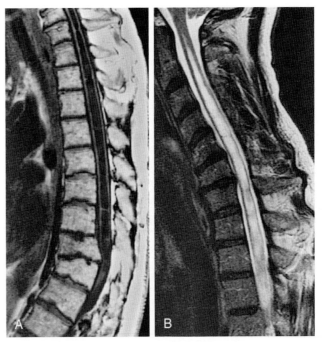

Figure 13-77 Cord: syrinx. **A,** T1 sagittal image of the thoracic spine. Old fracture of the lower thoracic spine is evident with retropulsion into the spinal canal. There is very low signal throughout the thoracic cord proximal to the site of previous injury, compatible with a syrinx. **B,** Fast T2 sagittal, cervicothoracic spine (same patient as in **A**). The abnormality within the cord follows the signal of cerebrospinal fluid, is elongated, and progresses proximally from the site of trauma, typical of a syrinx. The cord is markedly atrophic, but the overall contour of the cord is increased in size because of the syrinx.

Cysts. Hematomyelia and hydrosyringomyelia cause cysts in the cord that are unrelated to underlying neoplasm. Hematomyelia was described earlier in the trauma section, and the appearance of blood varies with its age. After trauma, myelomalacia may develop at the site of trauma. Eventually, small cysts may form in the area of myelomalacia and coalesce into an apparent rounded, post-traumatic intramedullary cyst, which is known as progressive post-traumatic myelomalacic myelopathy (Fig. 13-76). The cavities that form in the areas of myelomalacia may progress to a typical elongated syrinx.

A syrinx may be the sequela of trauma, occurring several months to many years after the traumatic event, and it occurs at the site of the trauma. Post-traumatic syringomyelia probably occurs from bleeding, which leads to arachnoid adhesions, tethering of the cord to the dura (usually dorsally, where blood pools with the patient supine), and consequent turbulent flow of CSF, which initiates cord cavitation. Syringomyelia also occurs in association with several congenital abnormalities, in particular the Chiari malformation.

A syrinx has sharply demarcated margins from the cord and usually has signal intensity that is isointense to CSF on all pulse sequences (Fig. 13-77). The cystic lesions do not show contrast enhancement. The cord caliber often appears increased, but actually is reduced from atrophy, and the intramedullary cyst or syrinx causes focal expansion of the cord contour. Myelomalacia and a post-traumatic cyst or syrinx can look very similar on MRI (Fig. 13-78). Proton

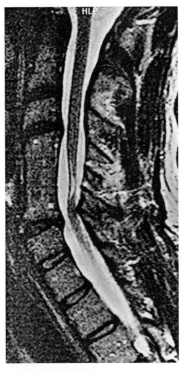

Figure 13-78 Cord: myelomalacia. Fast T2 sagittal image of the cervical spine. There was previous trauma to the spine with fusion of the mid–cervical vertebral bodies. The cord posterior to the site of the trauma and fusion is atrophied and has linear high signal within it. The atrophy allows the diagnosis of myelomalacia to be made, but the high signal within the cord could otherwise be from a syrinx and from malacia.

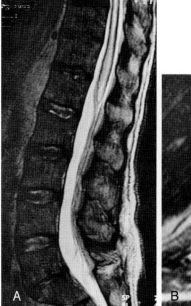

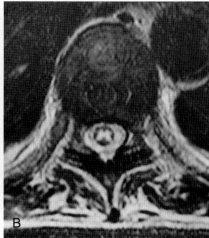

Figure 13-79   Cord: infarction. **A,** Fast T2 sagittal image of the lumbar spine. There is increased signal throughout the distal cord in this diabetic patient with severe atherosclerotic disease. **B,** Fast T2 axial image of the thoracic spine (same patient as in **A**). The high signal in the center of the cord has an H shape, which is typical of a cord infarction.

density images may be useful in the differentiation because myelomalacia has intermediate to high signal intensity on this sequence, whereas a syrinx has low signal intensity. Generally, however, a syrinx follows the signal intensity of CSF, whereas myelomalacia is slightly different in appearance even on standard T1W and T2W images. Differentiating between myelomalacia and syringomyelia on standard spine MRI examinations is usually impossible. Cord atrophy without signal abnormalities is another manifestation of myelomalacia that would clearly not be confused with a syrinx.

Infarction. Arteriosclerotic disease, arteriovenous malformations, aortic dissection, and disk extrusions or other masses all may cause cord infarction. The MRI appearance is high signal intensity on T2W images and shows contrast enhancement as diffuse or patchy or not at all. The high signal may occur in an H pattern in the central cord because the gray matter is affected preferentially as a result of the blood supply to the cord (Fig. 13-79). The cord is enlarged initially, but later may be atrophic. Arteriovenous malformations may be seen on MRI as punctate or serpen-

Figure 13-80   Cord: ependymoma. Fast T2 sagittal image of the cervical spine. There is a cystic mass in the cervical cord with focal increase in caliber of the cord. The findings are good for a glioma, but nonspecific as to which type. This happened to be an ependymoma, although these are typically more common in the conus and without a cystic component.

BOX 13-17

Tethered Cord

Clinical

- Occurs in children or adults
- Pain, dysesthesias, spasticity, loss of bowel and bladder control

Possible Associations

- Scoliosis
- Dysraphic spine
- Thickened filum terminale
- Lipoma
- Diastematomyelia
- Myelomeningocele

MRI Findings

- Conus distal to L1-2 disk
- No sharp transition between conus and filum (conus appears elongated)
- *Pitfall:* Layering of cauda equina may mimic low-lying cord; must depend on axial images for diagnosis
- May see associated findings listed above (eg, lipoma)

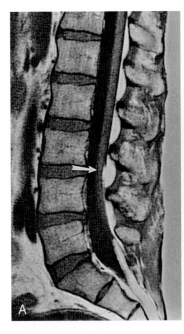
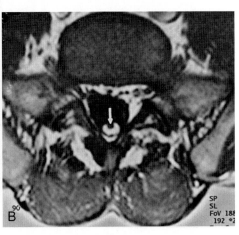

Figure 13-81 Tethered cord: associated dorsal lipoma. **A,** T1 sagittal image of the lumbar spine. The cord is abnormally low, extending at least as far as the L4 vertebra (*arrow*). **B,** T1 axial image of L5 (same patient as in **A**). There is a high signal intradural lipoma in the dorsal aspect of the lower lumbar spine, which is surrounding a thickened filum terminale (*arrow*).

tine areas of low signal intensity from flow void in vessels in or on the surface of the cord. This appearance should not be confused with the much more commonly encountered areas of signal intensity loss in the CSF from turbulent flow artifact.

Tumors. Ependymomas and astrocytomas constitute about 95% of all cord gliomas. Hemangioblastomas and metastases (especially from lung or breast primaries) are other tumors occurring in the cord. Ependymomas are more common than astrocytomas and usually affect the conus or filum.

Ependymomas often become necrotic or hemorrhagic. Astrocytomas often have associated cysts and are long lesions. Cysts also may be seen with ependymomas (Fig. 13-80), however, and occur frequently with hemangioblastomas. Metastases often have edema surrounding them that is out of proportion to the size of the lesion. Neoplasms usually cause enlargement of the caliber of the cord. Lesions are low signal intensity on T1W images and diffuse or patchy high signal intensity on T2W and T1W enhanced images, with heterogeneous areas present if there has been hemorrhage.

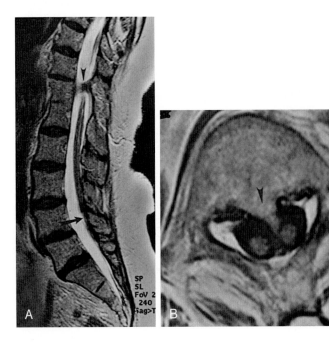

Figure 13-82 Tethered cord: associated diastematomyelia. **A,** Fast T2 sagittal image of the lumbar spine. The cord terminates at approximately the L4 level (*arrow*). There is congenital fusion of the T12-L1 vertebrae, with a spike of bone running through the spinal canal at that level (*arrowhead*). **B,** T1 axial image of T12. The bone spike (*arrowhead*) separates the spinal canal and cord into two halves.

Tethered Cord (Box 13-17)

Many congenital abnormalities affect the spine, but only a few are discussed in this chapter. Many osseous abnormalities are evaluated best using CT or conventional radiography. Lesions that appear at birth or shortly thereafter are not diagnostic dilemmas for us because they have been thoroughly worked up by the time we see them in our practice, which consists mainly of adults. Congenital lesions, such as myeloceles, meningoceles, myelomeningoceles, and lipomyelomeningoceles (among other congenital lesions), are not described here. One category of congenital spinal abnormalities that may not manifest until adulthood is that of the tethered cord.

The conus of the spinal cord ends normally at or above the L1-2 disk level; if it exists below this level, it is considered an abnormal tethered cord. An abnormally low (tethered) cord is a common feature of many congenital spinal malformations, and a thickened filum terminale usually is associated with it. Symptoms may manifest in childhood or adulthood and consist of pain, dysesthesias, spasticity, or loss of bowel and bladder control. Abnormalities that are associated with a tethered cord include, in descending order of frequency, lipoma (a tethered cord often terminates in a dorsally located lipoma) (Fig. 13-81), tight filum terminale, diastematomyelia (Fig. 13-82), and myelomeningocele.[52]

MRI of a tethered cord shows the conus located caudal to the L1-2 level and lack of a sharp transition between the conus and filum (the conus appears elongated). It is essential to evaluate the axial images when a tethered cord is suspected because the nerve roots of the cauda equina that layer posteriorly in the thecal sac may mimic a low-lying conus on sagittal MR images. There may be associated findings of scoliosis, spinal dysraphism, lipoma, diastematomyelia, or myelomeningocele also present on the imaging study.

REFERENCES

1. Singh K, Helms CA, Fiorella D, Major NM. Disc space-targeted angled axial MR images of the lumbar spine: a potential source of diagnostic error. *Skeletal Radiol* 2007; 36:1147-1153.
2. Boden S, Davis D, Dina T, et al. Abnormal magnetic resonance scans of the lumbar spine in asymptomatic subjects: a prospective investigation. *J Bone Joint Surg [Am]* 1990; 72:403-408.
3. Yu S, Haughton V, Sether LA. Anulus fibrosus in bulging intervertebral disks. *Radiology* 1988; 169:761-763.
4. Yu S, Haughton VM, Sether LA, et al. Criteria for classifying normal and degenerated intervertebral disks. *Radiology* 1989; 170:523-526.
5. McCarron R, Wimpee M, Hudkins P, et al. The inflammatory effect of nucleus pulposus: a possible element in the pathogenesis of low back pain. *Spine* 1987; 12:760-764.
6. Schellhas KP, Pollei SR, Gundry CR, Heithoff KB. Lumbar disc high-intensity zone: correlation of magnetic resonance imaging and discography. *Spine* 1996; 21:79-86.
7. Jensen M, Brant-Zawadzki M, Obuchowski N, et al. Magnetic resonance imaging of the lumbar spine in people without back pain. *N Engl J Med* 1995; 331:69-73.
8. Saal JA, Saal JS. The non-operative treatment of herniated nucleus pulposus with radiculopathy: an outcome study. *Spine* 1989; 14:431-437.
9. Bozzao A, Gallucci M, Masciocchi C. Lumbar disk herniation: MR imaging assessment of natural history in patients treated without surgery. *Radiology* 1992; 185:135-141.
10. Guinto FC, Hashim H, Stuner M. CT demonstration of disc regression after conservative therapy. *AJNR Am J Neuroradiol* 1984; 5:632-657.
11. Pardatscher K, Fiore D, Barbiero A. The natural history of lumbar disc herniations assessed by a CT follow-up study. *Neuroradiology* 1991; 33:84.
12. Teplick J, Haskin M. Spontaneous regression of herniated nucleus pulposus. *AJNR Am J Neuroradiol* 1985; 6:331-335.
13. Fardon DF, Milette PC. Nomenclature and classification of lumbar disc pathology. *Spine* 2001; 26:461-462.
14. Modic M. Degenerative disorders of the spine. In Modic M, Masaryk T, Ross J (eds). *Magnetic Resonance Imaging of the Spine.* Chicago: Year Book; 1989.
15. Modic M, Masaryk T, Boymphrey F. Lumbar herniated disc disease and canal stenosis: prospective evaluation by surface coil MR, CT, and myelography. *AJNR Am J Neuroradiol* 1986; 7:709-717.
16. Brown B, Schwartz R, Frank E, et al. Preoperative evaluation of cervical radiculopathy and myelopathy by surface coil MR imaging. *AJR Am J Roentgenol* 1988; 151:1205-1212.
17. Modic M, Masaryk T, Mulopulos G, et al. Cervical radiculopathy: prospective evaluation with surface coil MR imaging, CT with metrizamide, and metrizamide myelography. *Radiology* 1986; 161:753-759.
18. Vanharanta H, Scahs B, Ohnnmeiss D, et al. Pain provocation and disc deterioration by age: a CT/discography study in a low back pain population. *Spine* 1989; 14:420-423.
19. Franson R, Saal JA, Saal JS. Human disc phospholipase A2 is inflammatory. *Spine* 1992; 17:129-132.
20. Olmarker K, Rydenik B, Nordborg C. Autologous nucleus pulposus induces neurophysiologic and histologic changes in porcine cauda equina nerve roots. *Spine* 1993; 18:1425-1432.
21. Takahashi M, Jameshita Y, Sakamoto Y, Kojima R. Chronic cervical cord compression: clinical significance of increased signal intensity on MR images. *Radiology* 1989; 173:219-224.
22. Dorsay TA, Helms CA. MR imaging of epidural hematoma in the lumbar spine. *Skeletal Radiol* 2003; 31:677-685.
23. Helms CA, Dorwart RH, Gray M. The CT appearance of conjoined nerve roots and differentiation from a herniated nucleus pulposus. *Radiology* 1982; 144:803-807.
24. Schweitzer ME, El-Noueam KI. Vacuum disc: frequency of high signal intensity on T2-weighted MR images. *Skeletal Radiol* 1998; 27:83-86.
25. Malghem J, Maldague B, Labaisse M-A, et al. Intravertebral vacuum cleft: changes in content after supine positioning. *Radiology* 1993; 187:483-487.
26. Dupuy DE, Palmer WE, Rosenthal DI. Vertebral fluid collection associated with vertebral collapse. *AJR Am J Roentgenol* 1996; 167:1535-1538.
27. Lafforgue P, Chagnaud C, Daumen-Legré V, et al. The intravertebral vacuum phenomenon ("vertebral osteonecrosis"): migration of intradiscal gas in a fractured vertebral body? *Spine* 1997; 22:1885-1891.
28. Major NM, Helms CA, Genant HK. Calcification demonstrated as high signal intensity on T1-weighted MR images of the disks of the lumbar spine. *Radiology* 1993; 189:494-496.
29. Modic MT, Steinberg PM, Ross JS, et al. Degenerative disk disease: assessment of changes in vertebral body marrow with MR imaging. *Radiology* 1988; 166:193-199.
30. Dussault RG, Kaplan PA. Facet joint injection: diagnosis and therapy. *Appl Radiol* 1994; 23:35-39.
31. Dussault RG, Kaplan PA, Anderson MW, Whitehill R. Interventional musculoskeletal radiology of the spine. In Taveras JM, Ferrucci JT (eds): *Radiology: Diagnosis—Imaging—Intervention.* Philadelphia: Lippincott-Raven; 1998.
32. Sartoris DJ, Resnick D, Tyson R, Haghighi P. Age-related alterations in the vertebral spinous processes and intervening soft tissues: radiologic-pathologic correlation. *AJR Am J Roentgenol* 1985; 145:1025-1030.
33. Boden S, Davis D, Dina T. Contrast-enhanced MR imaging performed after successful lumbar disc surgery: prospective study. *Radiology* 1992; 182:59-64.
34. Ross J, Masaryk T, Modic M. Lumbar spine: postoperative assessment with surface coil MR imaging. *Radiology* 1987; 164:851-860.
35. Deutsch A, Howard M, Dawson E, et al. Lumbar spine following successful surgical discectomy: magnetic resonance imaging features and implications. *Spine* 1993; 18:1054-1060.
36. Ross TS, Masaryk TJ, Schrader M, et al. MR imaging of the postoperative lumbar spine: assessment with gadopentetate dimeglumine. *AJR Am J Roentgenol* 1990; 155:867-872.

37. Dagirmanjian A, Schils J, McHenry M, Modic MT. MR imaging of vertebral osteomyelitis revisited. *AJR Am J Roentgenol* 1996; 167:1539-1543.

38. Roos AE, Meerten EL, Bloem JL, Bluemm RG. MRI of tuberculous spondylitis. *AJR Am J Roentgenol* 1986; 147:79-82.

39. Numaguchi Y, Rigamonti D, Rothman MI, et al. Spinal epidural abscess: evaluation with gadolinium-enhanced MR imaging. *RadioGraphics* 1993; 13:545-559.

40. Johnson CE, Sze G. Benign lumbar arachnoiditis: MR imaging with gadopentetate dimeglumine. *AJR Am J Roentgenol* 1990; 155:873-880.

41. Major NM, Helms CA, Richardson WJ. MR imaging of fibrocartilaginous masses arising on the margins of spondylolysis defects. *AJR Am J Roentgenol* 1999; 173:673-676.

42. Ulmer JL, Mathews VP, Elster AD, et al. MR imaging of lumbar spondylolysis: the importance of ancillary observations. *AJR Am J Roentgenol* 1997; 169:233-239.

43. Stäbler A, Bellan M, Weiss M, et al. MR imaging of enhancing intraosseous disk herniation (Schmorl's nodes). *AJR Am J Roentgenol* 1997; 168:933-938.

44. Slucky AV, Potter HG. Use of magnetic resonance imaging in spinal trauma: indications, techniques, and utility. *J Am Acad Orthop Surg* 1998; 6:134-145.

45. Grenier N, Greselle J-F, Vital J-M, et al. Normal and disrupted lumbar longitudinal ligaments: correlative MR and anatomic study. *Radiology* 1989; 171:197-205.

46. El-Khoury GY, Kathol MH, Daniel WW. Imaging of acute injuries of the cervical spine: value of plain radiography, CT, and MR imaging. *AJR Am J Roentgenol* 1995; 164:43-50.

47. Millar W. Vertebral artery injury after acute cervical spine trauma: rate of occurrence as detected by MR angiography and assessment of clinical consequences. *AJR Am J Roentgenol* 1995; 164:443-447.

48. Kulkarni MV, McArdle CB, Kopanicky D, et al. Acute spinal cord injury: MR imaging at 1.5 T. *Radiology* 1987; 164:837-843.

49. Bradley WG Jr. MR appearance of hemorrhage in the brain. *Radiology* 1993; 189:15-26.

50. Friedman DP. Symptomatic vertebral hemangiomas: MR findings. *AJR Am J Roentgenol* 1996; 167:359-364.

51. Major NM, Helms CA, Richardson WJ. The "mini brain": plasmacytoma in a vertebral body on MR imaging. *AJR Am J Roentgenol* 2000; 175:261-263.

52. Raghavan N, Barkovich AJ, Edwards M, Norman D. MR imaging in the tethered spinal cord syndrome. *AJR Am J Roentgenol* 1989; 152:843-852.

Spine Protocols

This is one set of suggested protocols; there are many variations that would work equally well.

CERVICAL SPINE: DEGENERATIVE

Sequence No.	1	2	3	4	5	6
Sequence Type	T1	Fast T2	T1	T2*		
Orientation	Sagittal	Sagittal	Axial	Axial		
Field of View (cm)	14	14	11	11		
Slice Thickness (mm)	4	4	4	2		
Contrast	No	No	No	No		
			Stacked			

THORACIC SPINE: DEGENERATIVE

Sequence No.	1	2	3	4	5	6
Sequence Type	T1	Fast T2	T1	T2*		
Orientation	Sagittal	Sagittal	Axial	Axial		
Field of View (cm)	16	16	12	12		
Slice Thickness (mm)	3	3	9	4		
Contrast	No	No	No	No		
			Stacked			

LUMBAR SPINE: DEGENERATIVE

Sequence No.	1	2	3	4	5	6
Sequence Type	T1	Fast T2	T1	Fast T2		
Orientation	Sagittal	Sagittal	Axial	Axial		
Field of View (cm)	16	16	14	14		
Slice Thickness (mm)	4	4	4	4		
Contrast	No	No	No	No		
				Stacked mid L3 to mid S1		

SPINE: POSTOPERATIVE

Sequence No.	1	2	3	4	5	6
Sequence Type	T1	Fast T2	T1	T1	T1	
Orientation	Sagittal	Axial	Axial	Axial	Sagittal	
Field of View (cm)	Depends on site (same as for degenerative protocols)					
Slice Thickness (mm)						
Contrast	No	No	No	Yes	Yes	
		Stacked	Stacked	Stacked		

Note: May also routinely do a fast T2 sagittal sequence if you have time to spare on the scanner.

SPINE: TRAUMA

Sequence No.	1	2	3	4	5	6
Sequence Type	T1	Fast T2*	T2*	T2*	T1	Fast STIR
Orientation	Sagittal	Sagittal	Sagittal	Axial	Axial	Sagittal
Field of View (cm)	Depends on site (same as for degenerative spine protocols)					
Slice Thickness (mm)	4	4	4	4	4	4
Contrast	No	No	No	No	No	No
				Stacked	Stacked	

OSSEOUS SPINE METASTASES/CORD COMPRESSION

Sequence No.	1	2	3	4	5	6
Sequence Type	T1	STIR	T1	Fast T2	†	
Orientation	Sagittal	Sagittal	Axial	Axial		
Field of View (cm)	Depends on site covered (same as for degenerative spine protocols)					
Slice Thickness (mm)	4	4	8	8		
Contrast	No	No	No	No		
				Stacked	Stacked	

†If mass is seen in epidural space or cord, administer intravenous contrast agent, and repeat sagittal and axial T1 sequences through abnormal regions.

Spine Protocols (Continued)

This is one set of suggested protocols; there are many variations that would work equally well.

SPINE: INFECTION/INTRADURAL LESIONS

Sequence No.	1	2	3	4	5	6
Sequence Type	T1	Fast T2	T1	Fast T2	T1	T1
Orientation	Sagittal	Sagittal	Axial	Axial	Sagittal	Axial
Field of View (cm)	Depends on site covered (same as for degenerative spine protocols)					
Slice Thickness (mm)	4	4	4	4	4	4
Contrast	No	No	No	No	Yes	Yes
			Stacked	Stacked		Stacked

SAMPLE STANDARD REPORTS

MRI of the Cervical Spine

Clinical Indications

Protocol

The routine protocol with multiple sequences and planes of imaging was used.

Discussion

1. **Craniocervical junction:** No abnormalities identified

2. **Cervical spinal cord:** The size, signal, and configuration of the cord appear normal

3. **Osseous structures:** The bone marrow is normal; alignment is anatomic

4. **Disk spaces:** Levels C2-3, C3-4, C4-5, C5-6, C6-7, and C7-T1 have a normal appearance without evidence of degenerative changes, disk herniation, or other abnormalities; there is no evidence of spinal or foraminal stenosis

Opinion

Normal MRI of the cervical spine.

MRI of the Dorsal Spine

Clinical Indications

Protocol

The routine protocol with multiple sequences and planes of imaging was used

Discussion

1. **Dorsal spinal cord:** Normal signal and configuration

2. **Osseous structures:** The bone marrow is normal; alignment is anatomic

3. **Disk spaces:** Appear normal without evidence of degenerative changes or disk herniation; no central canal or foraminal stenosis

Opinion

Normal MRI of the dorsal spine.

MRI of the Lumbar Spine

Clinical Indications

Protocol

The routine protocol with multiple sequences and planes of imaging was used.

Discussion

1. The cord terminates at _____

2. **Lumbar spinal cord/conus:** Normal size, signal, and configuration

3. **Osseous structures:** The bone marrow appears normal; alignment is anatomic; no spondylolysis is shown

4. **Disk spaces, neural foramina, spinal canal, and facet joints:** Disk levels L1-2, L2-3, L3-4, L4-5, and L5-S1 are normal without evidence of degenerative changes, herniated disks, canal or foraminal stenosis, or facet joint arthrosis

Opinion

Normal MRI of the lumbar spine.

Scout		**Final Image**
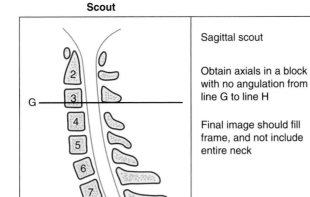	Sagittal scout Obtain axials in a block with no angulation from line G to line H Final image should fill frame, and not include entire neck	Stacked axials (no angulation) 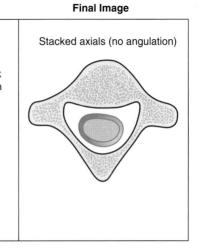

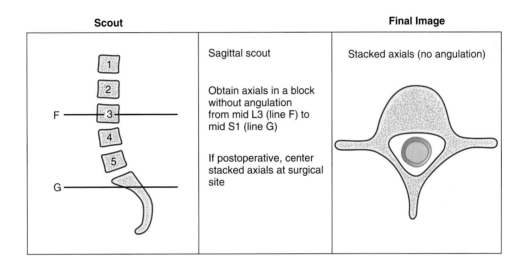

Scout		**Final Image**
	Sagittal scout Obtain axials in a block without angulation from mid L3 (line F) to mid S1 (line G) If postoperative, center stacked axials at surgical site	Stacked axials (no angulation)

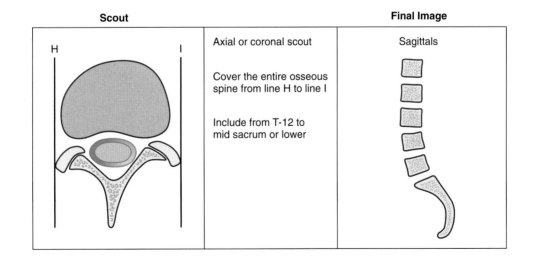

Scout		**Final Image**
	Axial or coronal scout Cover the entire osseous spine from line H to line I Include from T-12 to mid sacrum or lower	Sagittals

Hips and Pelvis

14

How to Image the Hips and Pelvis

See the hip and pelvis protocols at the end of the chapter.

- *Coils and patient position:* Generally, when evaluating the hips for entities such as avascular necrosis (AVN) or fractures, it is possible in many patients to use a torso phased array coil. For larger patients, the body coil is necessary. Both hips and the entire pelvis are imaged simultaneously for most clinical indications. The patient is placed supine in the magnet. For evaluation of smaller structures in the hip joint, such as the labrum or cartilage, a surface coil, such as a flexible wrap coil, is recommended, and then only the symptomatic hip is evaluated with thinner slice thickness and smaller interslice gap. The addition of intra-articular contrast material, such as a dilute gadolinium solution, is helpful for additional evaluation of the labrum.
- *Image orientation (Box 14-1):* The most useful information for evaluating hip pathology can be obtained in the axial and coronal planes. Sagittal images sometimes can be difficult to interpret because the fovea centralis may mimic pathology, and these images generally give no additional information. For evaluation of labral tears and femoroacetabular impingement, oblique coronal and oblique axial images are helpful.
- *Pulse sequences and regions of interest:* A large field of view (24-30 cm) is necessary when evaluating both hips and the pelvis simultaneously, as is done for AVN or trauma. Especially in the setting of trauma, the entire osseous pelvis should be evaluated. We routinely scan from the iliac crest to the lesser trochanter. To scan the pelvis in a timely fashion, a slice thickness of 6 or 7 mm with an interslice gap of about 3 mm is reasonable. When assessing joint pathology, such as labral detail, a smaller field of view is recommended (14-24 cm), with a smaller slice thickness. We have found that 3-mm slice thickness with a 10% interslice gap (0.3 mm for those who do not wish to do the math) is satisfactory. The coverage for a dedicated hip MRI examination should include the supra-acetabular location through the

Structures to Evaluate in Different Planes

Coronal

- Osseous structures
  - Acetabulum
  - Femoral head, neck
  - Greater, lesser trochanter
  - Sacrum
  - Ilium
  - Sacroiliac joints
- Muscles
  - Gluteal muscles
  - Adductors
  - Abductors
  - Hamstrings
  - Quadriceps
- Labrum
- Pulvinar

Axial

- Osseous structures
  - Acetabulum
  - Femoral head, neck
  - Greater, lesser trochanter
  - Sacrum
  - Ilium
  - Sacroiliac joints
- Muscles
  - Gluteus maximus, medius, and minimus
  - Sartorius, rectus femoris
  - Gracilis, pectineus, adductor longus, brevis, and magnus
  - Tensor fascia lata
  - Piriformis
  - Obturator internus, externus
  - Gemelli superior and inferior
  - Quadratus femoris
- Labrum
- Pulvinar

Sagittal

Not standard or necessary to perform

bottom of the lesser trochanter. A T1W sequence is necessary for showing anatomic detail. Some type of T2W image in the same planes also is recommended. T2W images show edema or fluid that may not be appreciated on T1W images. Fast spin echo T2W images with fat suppression and (fast) STIR images show fluid and edema with increased conspicuity compared with other types of T2 sequences.

- *Contrast:* Intravenous contrast administration is generally unnecessary except to differentiate a cystic from a solid mass. Intra-articular contrast administration is of great benefit, however, when assessing labral pathology. The dilution technique is the same as for the shoulder or any other joint. A 1/200 dilution of gadolinium in normal saline is injected into the joint after confirmation with a small amount of radiopaque contrast material. The high signal contrast (gadolinium) compared with the low signal labrum makes identification of tears easier. Additionally, we recommend fat suppression with T1W and T2W images after intra-articular contrast injection to make the gadolinium more conspicuous.

Normal and Abnormal

OSSEOUS STRUCTURES

Osseous and ligamentous structures and the musculotendinous components help to characterize and constrain the dynamic movements of the hip. The hip is important in the transfer of weight and energy between the appendicular and axial skeleton but is crucial in the execution of lower limb motion, such as walking, running, jumping, and kicking. Despite its importance in everyday maneuvers, the hip is less understood than other joints.

Normal Osseous Structures

The hip is a ball-and-socket joint, allowing for considerable motion with flexion and extension, internal and external rotation, and abduction and adduction. The acetabulum covers 40% of the femoral head and is formed from ilium, ischium, and pubic bones. At birth, these three bones are separated by the triradiate cartilage, a Y-shaped physeal plate. The acetabulum is tilted anteriorly, which explains the greater potential for flexion of the hip compared with extension. Because of the concave shape of the acetabulum, the hip is inherently stable. The depth of the acetabulum is increased by the dense fibrocartilaginous labrum that surrounds it. The combination of the labrum and transverse acetabular ligament makes a complete ring around the acetabulum.

The femur is the longest and strongest bone in the body. The proximal femur comprises a head, neck, and greater and lesser trochanters. The femoral head is spherical in shape, but is slightly flattened anteriorly and posteriorly. With the exception of the fovea, it is covered by articular cartilage that ends approximately at the level of the epiphyseal plate at the femoral head-neck junction. The fovea is seen as an indentation in the normal round contour of the femoral head on its medial aspect and is the site of attachment of the ligamentum teres.

The trochanters are apophyses, which add to the width of bone. The greater trochanter serves as the insertion site for the tendons of the gluteus medius and minimus, the obturator internus and externus, and the piriformis muscles. The lesser trochanter receives the iliopsoas tendon (Fig. 14-1).

The bone marrow of the pelvis and hips is generally diffuse or patchy intermediate signal (but higher signal than muscle on T1W images) because of the large amount of red marrow that persists in this region throughout life. The epiphyses and apophyses should have high signal fatty marrow on T1W images. Occasionally, a small rim of red marrow may parallel the subchondral bone of the femoral epiphysis; this is considered normal. Thick stress trabeculae in the femoral neck (calcar) can be seen as low signal lines on MRI, as can linear physeal scars at the femoral head-neck junction.

Vascular Abnormalities of Bone

Osteonecrosis (Avascular Necrosis) (Box 14-2). One of the major indications for MRI of the hip is for detection of osteonecrosis of the femoral head. The presumed mechanism of mechanical failure of the femoral head is accumulated stress fractures of necrotic trabeculae that are not repaired. MRI is capable of detecting the early stages of ischemic necrosis, which is important clinically so that therapy

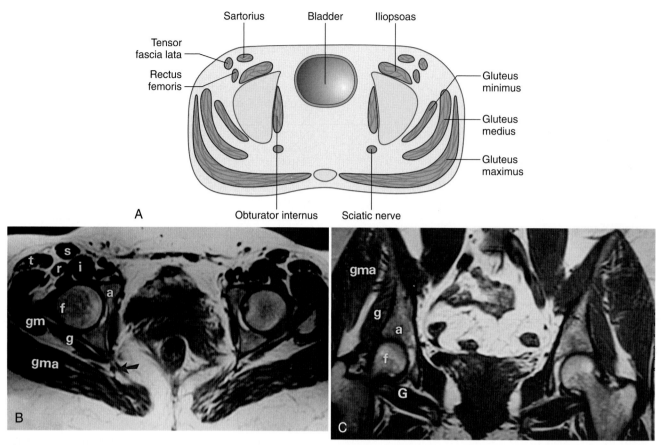

Figure 14-1   **Normal anatomy of the pelvis. A,** Sketch showing normal anatomy. **B** and **C,** Axial (**B**) and coronal (**C**) T1W images through a normal pelvis. *Arrow* points to the sciatic nerve. a, acetabulum; f, femoral head; G, gemellus; g, gluteus minimus; gm, gluteus medius; gma, gluteus maximus; I, iliopsoas; r, rectus femoris; t, tensor fascia lata; s, sartorius.

can be instituted before the onset of femoral head collapse, fragmentation, degenerative change, and hip replacement. Early diagnosis can lead to joint-sparing techniques, such as core decompression, rotational osteotomy, or free vascularized fibular graft.

Numerous causes of AVN have been cited, including trauma, steroids, hemoglobinopathies, alcoholism, pancreatitis, Gaucher's disease, and radiation. AVN is considered idiopathic when no cause can be identified. Anabolic and catabolic steroid use can result in AVN.

AVN is bilateral in 40% of hips, so both hips should be imaged simultaneously for this indication. The classification scheme for AVN observed on radiographs cannot be used for MRI. MRI is most useful when plain films are negative.[1] MRI also is more sensitive than computed tomography (CT) or radionuclide bone scintigraphy.[2] Additionally, MRI can provide information regarding articular cartilage, marrow conversion, joint fluid, and associated insufficiency fractures, which also are common in patients taking steroids.

The appearance of AVN on MRI includes a diffuse pattern of bone marrow edema early (similar in appearance to transient bone marrow edema), subsequently becoming more focal in the femoral head; a serpiginous line of low signal intensity surrounding an area of fatty marrow in the femoral head between the 10-o'clock and 2-o'clock positions on coronal images (usually anterior in the femoral head) is characteristic for AVN (Figs. 14-2 and 14-3). This is the typical geographic pattern of AVN that is seen most often. Collapse of bone and sclerosis may result in a focal area of low signal on T1W images that is variable signal on T2W images (Fig. 14-4)—in other words, not a fatty center. This

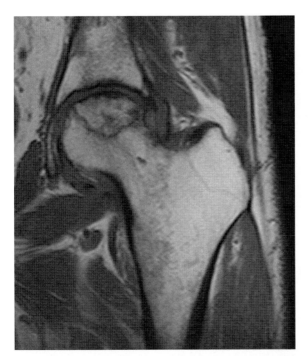

Figure 14-2 Avascular necrosis. Coronal T1W image in a 51-year-old man with left hip pain and normal bone scintigraphy. A serpiginous low signal area in the subchondral location is noted in the femoral head with fat in center.

latter appearance is uncommon and is less specific than the geographic pattern.

On spin echo T2W images, the "double-line sign" has been described as an appearance typical of ischemic necrosis. The *double line* is a line of low signal that surrounds an inner line of high signal on spin echo T2W images. The *double-line sign* represents a chemical shift artifact and is not currently seen with the updated high field MRI scanners because of the spectral presaturation fat suppression that is always applied with the T2W FSE/TSE sequences to eliminate the high signal of the fatty tissue. MRI signal abnormalities such as the double-line sign initially were thought to be helpful in staging osteonecrosis because they corresponded to histologic findings[3]; however, because the prognostic significance is unclear, staging based on signal characteristics generally is not recommended.

Important additional findings necessary to report to the clinician include the volume of the head that is involved with AVN; this is best determined with axial imaging. Additionally, findings of degenerative disease, such as joint space narrowing and osteophytes, are important to report because this helps with staging of the disease. Similarly, it is important to report collapse of the femoral head (see Fig. 14-4). The presence and amount of a joint effusion often correspond to the severity of clinical pain symptoms.

Misinterpretation of osteonecrosis may occur if one is unfamiliar with a few potential pitfalls (Box 14-3).

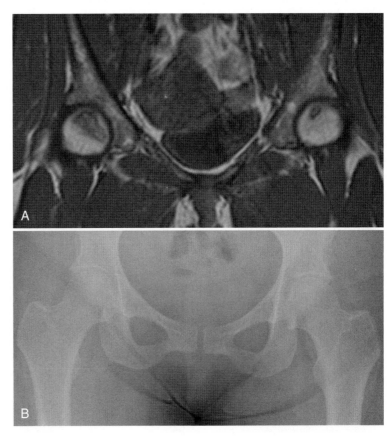

Figure 14-3 Avascular necrosis. A, Coronal T1W image showing serpiginous, low signal areas in the proximal femora compatible with avascular necrosis. **B,** Conventional radiography interpreted as normal in this patient without risk factors for avascular necrosis.

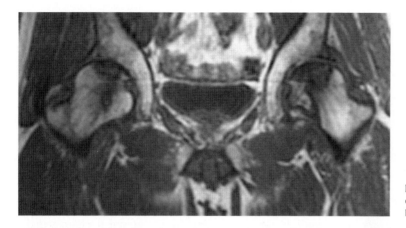

Figure 14-4 **Avascular necrosis.** Coronal T1W image shows curvilinear, serpiginous low signal intensity in the femoral heads bilaterally. The lesions are diffusely low signal.

BOX 14-3

Pitfalls for Focal Avascular Necrosis

- Hematopoietic marrow
- Synovial herniation pit
- Fovea centralis

BOX 14-4

Legg-Calvé-Perthes Disease

- Idiopathic avascular necrosis of femoral head
- Age 4-10 years
- May lead to growth arrest
- MRI findings: Diffuse low signal on T1W and T2W images ± collapse of femoral head
- MRI predictors of growth arrest
  - Physeal bridging
  - Signal change in physis/metaphysis

Occasionally, normal hematopoietic marrow can be identified in the femoral head. The signal intensity of hematopoietic marrow is higher in signal than AVN on T1W images. A synovial herniation pit, which represents a tiny defect in the bone that allows joint fluid to fill this space (analogous to a subchondral cyst, but removed from the articular surface), can erroneously be interpreted as an area of AVN (Fig. 14-5).[4] The fovea centralis, a normal anatomic finding, inadvertently may be diagnosed as a site of AVN with subchondral collapse (Fig. 14-6). Subchondral cysts from degenerative joint disease of the hip may appear similar to AVN, but the low signal margins of the cyst are smooth and regular, rather than serpiginous as with AVN. Also, abnormalities on both sides of the joint usually are present, with evidence of degenerative cysts and degenerative cartilage loss and osteophytes. Metastases occasionally may have an appearance similar to AVN that is diffusely low signal on T1W images.

Legg-Calvé-Perthes disease is an idiopathic AVN of the growing femoral epiphysis that results in a progressive deformity and outward displacement of the femoral head; it occurs in children 4 to 10 years old (Box 14-4). MRI has been reported to be useful for assessing Legg-Calvé-Perthes disease. Diffuse low signal in the femoral head on T1W and T2W images is the most common finding. Collapse of the femoral epiphysis also can occur.[5,6] Jaramillo and associates[7] showed that physeal bridging and deformity of the femoral head with abnormal low signal in the head on MRI were statistically significant predictors of growth arrest. Abnormalities of the epiphysis did not relate to growth arrest. Depiction of physeal bridging at MRI was the best predictor

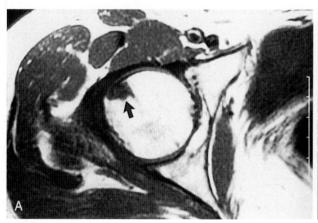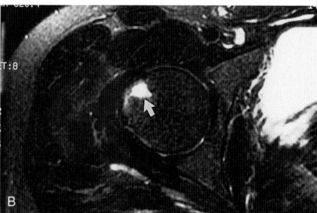

Figure 14-5 **Avascular necrosis pitfalls: synovial herniation pit.** **A,** Axial T1W image shows a wedge-shaped area of low signal at the 10-o'clock position (*arrow*). **B,** Axial fast spin echo image with fat suppression shows high signal (*arrow*) (similar to that of fluid in the bladder). This is a characteristic location for a synovial herniation pit.

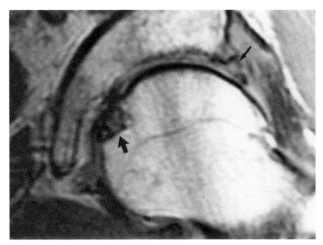

Figure 14-6 **Avascular necrosis pitfalls: fovea centralis.** Coronal T1W image shows a low signal area medial in location (*large arrow*). This represents a prominent fovea centralis (a normal structure). A superior labral tear also is incidentally noted (*small arrow*).

of growth arrest in their study. MRI allows earlier diagnosis and diagnosis of coexistent contralateral disease and monitoring of therapy (Figs. 14-7 and 14-8).

Idiopathic Transient Osteoporosis of the Hip (Transient Painful Bone Marrow Edema) (Box 14-5). Idiopathic transient osteoporosis of the hip (ITOH) also has been referred to as *transient painful bone marrow edema*. The first well-documented description was reported in three women during the last trimester of pregnancy.[8] ITOH is an uncom-

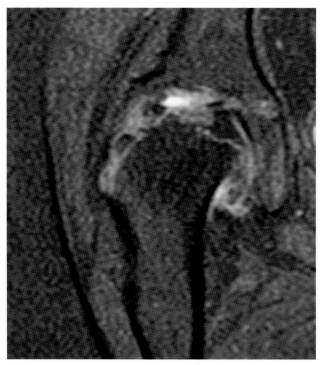

Figure 14-7 **Legg-Calvé-Perthes disease.** Coronal T1W image with fat suppression and intra-articular contrast administration shows fragmentation of the epiphysis.

mon and usually self-limited clinical entity of unknown cause that primarily affects middle-aged men (40-55 years old). Although the underlying cause is uncertain, a vascular basis almost certainly exists. When women are affected, it is usually during the third trimester of pregnancy. There are anecdotal reports of ITOH occurring in early pregnancy with resolving hip pain after spontaneous or therapeutic abortions. The male-to-female ratio is 3:1. This condition is rare in children,[9] and there are no known predisposing factors except pregnancy.[10-12] Generally, only one hip is affected at a time. Recurrence in the same hip can occur.[12] This entity is known as *regional migratory osteoporosis* when it migrates to other joints.[12]

Clinically, patients present with disabling pain without a history of trauma. Conventional radiography shows osteopenia isolated to the affected hip. It is important to make the proper diagnosis so that correct treatment can be instituted. ITOH generally resolves spontaneously in 6 to 8 months after protected weight bearing and symptomatic support.

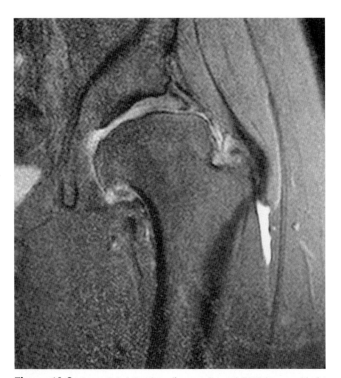

Figure 14-8 **Legg-Calvé-Perthes disease.** Coronal T2W image with fat suppression and intra-articular contrast administration shows irregularity of the left femoral head with widening of the femoral neck. Physes are closed. Note abnormal signal within the labrum.

BOX 14-5
Idiopathic Transient Osteoporosis of the Hip

- Middle-aged men
- Pregnant women
- Male-to-female ratio 3:1
- No history of trauma
- Spontaneous resolution (6-8 mo)
- MRI: Low T1 signal; high T2 signal femoral head to intertrochanteric region
- Differential diagnosis: Septic hip, avascular necrosis (early), osteoid osteoma (younger age group)

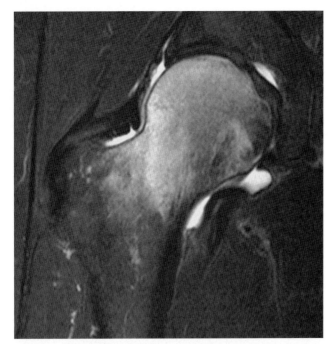

Figure 14-9 **Idiopathic transient osteoporosis of the hip.** Coronal fat-suppressed T2W image shows high signal in the femoral head and neck, representing bone marrow edema from hyperemia. Note the large joint effusion.

Insufficiency fractures of the hip may occur without protected weight bearing because of the severity of the localized osteoporosis. MRI in ITOH shows decreased signal on T1W images and increased signal on T2W images extending from the femoral head to the intertrochanteric region (Fig. 14-9). These findings have been attributed to bone marrow edema. The signal intensity in the acetabulum is normal. These characteristics have been reported within 48 hours after the onset of symptoms of ITOH.[10]

Because early AVN can have a similar appearance on imaging, and the treatments are different, it is important to differentiate ITOH from AVN. There is some controversy as to whether ITOH represents a very early, reversible stage of AVN.[10-12] VandeBerg and colleagues[13] developed criteria to increase sensitivity and specificity of irreversible changes of ITOH that would lead to a diagnosis of AVN. They suggested that the absence of a subchondral low signal intensity on T2W images or postcontrast T1W images suggests a favorable outcome (reversible disease). The presence of a low signal subchondral area measuring more than 4 mm in thickness and greater than 12.5 mm in length on T2W images or postcontrast T1W images suggests an irreversible lesion (AVN). An intra-articular osteoid osteoma of the hip can cause marrow edema in a similar distribution as ITOH, and a cortically based, small, round lesion should be carefully searched for to exclude this; however, different age groups generally are affected by these two disease processes. Infection of the proximal femur with a septic joint also should be considered in the differential diagnosis based on the MRI appearance.

Fractures (Box 14-6)

Fatigue Fractures. Stress fractures occur commonly around the hips and in the pelvis. Stress fractures are divided into

fatigue fractures and insufficiency fractures. Fatigue fractures result from increased or abnormal stress applied to normal bone. MRI is superb for evaluating this abnormality and may be positive when conventional radiography is negative.[14] Bone scintigraphy is sensitive but not specific for stress fractures or stress reactions. MRI is sensitive and specific because it can show the linear fracture or marrow edema from a stress reaction (Figs. 14-10 to 14-12). Because of the exquisite contrast and intrinsic spatial resolution of MRI, this abnormality can be diagnosed early, leading to early appropriate treatment.

Stress reactions occur typically in the femoral neck along the medial aspect (compressive surface) or the superior lateral surface (tensile surface). Additional locations of stress fractures in the pelvis include the pubic rami (superior and inferior) and sacrum. Sacral stress fractures are most often seen in athletes, especially runners. Patients often present with low back pain, and lumbar spine MRI is ordered. The sacrum should be evaluated for this abnormality. The diagnosis can be overlooked because the bone marrow edema may not be conspicuous on non–fat-suppressed T2W images (Fig. 14-13). Stress fractures image as linear low signal surrounded by bone marrow edema.

Insufficiency Fractures. Insufficiency fractures may occur in osteoporotic patients. These are fractures that occur from physiologic stresses on bone weakened by osteoporosis. In

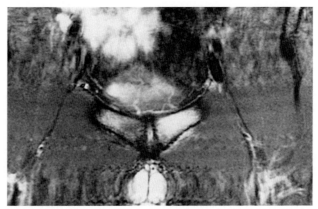

Figure 14-10 **Stress reaction: pubic symphysis.** Coronal fat-suppressed T2W image shows high signal in the pubic bones bilaterally, compatible with stress reaction.

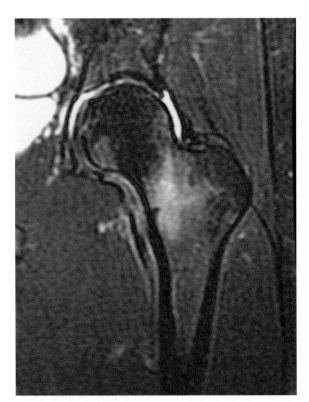

Figure 14-11 **Stress (fatigue) fracture.** Coronal T2W image in a 22-year-old woman with groin pain while training for a road race. Low signal is noted in the medial aspect of the femoral neck. Periosteal thickening is evident. Bone marrow edema around the fracture makes linear low signal easy to identify.

the clinical setting of a painful hip in an osteoporotic patient (even with no significant history of trauma, and despite the fact that the patient may be able to bear weight), a radiographically occult fracture may exist.[15] MRI is the fastest, most cost-effective, and most sensitive and specific method for making the diagnosis in this setting. A limited MRI examination consisting of coronal and axial images of the entire pelvis using T1W and fat-suppressed T2W sequences can be done to evaluate for this entity. Any marrow sequence would suffice. Sometimes the fracture is more readily appreciated on T1W images, and sometimes T2W images are better, so both are recommended for screening.

MRI shows linear low signal with surrounding bone marrow edema on T1W images (Fig. 14-14). The fracture remains low signal on T2W images, but surrounding bone marrow edema is high in signal intensity. Images of the entire pelvis with larger field of view are recommended because hip pain may be referred from abnormalities outside of the hip, such as sacral insufficiency fractures. Multiple fractures often coexist. The most common locations for insufficiency fractures around the pelvis are subcapital, intertrochanteric, sacral, supra-acetabular, pubic bones, and superior or inferior pubic rami.

A sacral insufficiency fracture has a pathognomonic appearance on MRI. T1W images show linear low signal (representing the fracture), usually paralleling the sacroiliac joint with surrounding bone marrow edema (low signal on T1W images and high signal on T2W images). Generally, the bone marrow edema is confined to the sacral ala with the fracture and does not extend across the midline, unless

the fracture is bilateral (Figs. 14-15 and 14-16). If the linear component of the fracture is not evident, the abnormality of the sacral marrow may mimic metastatic disease.

Supra-acetabular insufficiency fractures are reliably diagnosed with MRI by noting a curvilinear (eyebrow-shaped) low signal fracture line that parallels the roof of the acetabulum, accompanied by surrounding bone marrow edema

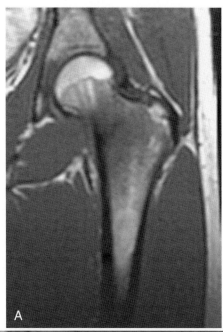

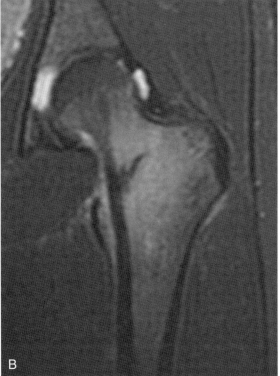

Figure 14-12 **Femoral neck (fatigue) fracture. A,** Coronal T1W image shows low signal in the femoral neck with focal linear low signal (fracture). **B,** Coronal T2W image with fat suppression shows marrow edema with low signal fracture line.

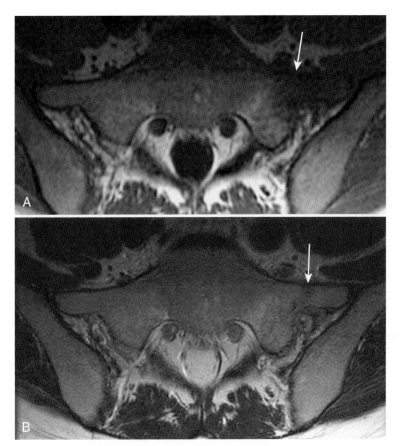

Figure 14-13 **Sacral stress fracture. A,** Axial T1W image in a 21-year-old elite tennis player shows bone marrow edema in left lateral sacrum (*arrow*). **B,** FSE T2W image shows fracture line (*arrow*).

(low signal on T1W images that becomes high signal on T2W images) (Fig. 14-17).[16] These fractures are seen in the same patient population with sacral insufficiency fractures (ie, patients with osteoporosis and especially patients who had previous pelvic radiation, which significantly weakens the bone). The characteristic curvilinear low signal fracture line should be identified, along with the geographic appearance of the bone marrow edema, so that insufficiency fractures are not confused with metastatic disease, which generally has diffuse edema and perhaps an associated soft tissue mass with destruction of the acetabulum.

Insufficiency and fatigue fractures have a predilection for the femoral neck and pubic bones (although they have been reported in the sacrum). Supra-acetabular and sacral fractures are almost exclusively of the insufficiency type in osteoporotic individuals.

Salter Fractures (Box 14-7). Traumatic epiphyseal slip can occur in skeletally immature individuals as a result of birth trauma or accidental or nonaccidental trauma. If the femoral head ossification center is not mineralized, conventional radiography may suggest developmental dysplasia of the hip (DDH) (owing to lateral displacement of the femoral shaft). A T2W sequence, particularly fast spin echo with fat suppression or (fast) STIR imaging, shows edema and hemorrhage through the physis and is diagnostic of a shear injury.

Slipped capital femoral epiphysis is predominantly an adolescent occurrence, typically observed in boys 10 to 17 years old and in girls 8 to 15 years old. Boys generally are more frequently affected than girls, and this entity is more common in blacks than whites. The incidence is especially high in overweight children. Proposed causes include adolescent growth spurt, hormonal influences, increased weight, and activity, all of which result in repetitive stresses, resulting in a Salter 1 fracture of the proximal femoral growth plate.

If conventional radiography is equivocal, MRI can be used to assess the relationship of the femoral head and neck. MRI shows a widened growth plate with abnormal high signal on the T2W image through the growth plate, with medial and posteriorly located femoral epiphysis with respect to the metaphysis. On the coronal T1W image, the growth plate appears wider than normal, as evidenced by increased width of the low signal physis (Fig. 14-18). These findings can aid the surgeon with operative planning. An additional important advantage of MRI is its ability to identify early osteonecrosis, which can be seen in 15% of children with this entity.

BOX 14-7

Slipped Capital Femoral Epiphysis

- Age 10-17 years (males), 8-15 years (females)
- Male > female
- Increased incidence in overweight children
- MRI: Widened growth plate with high T2 signal
  - Epiphyseal slip

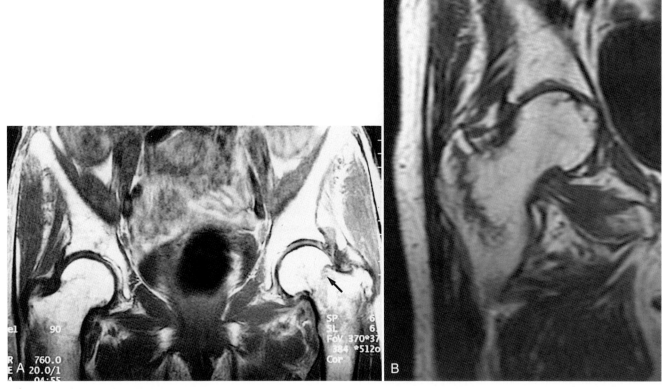

Figure 14-14 **Insufficiency fracture, femoral neck.** An elderly woman with left hip pain and normal plain films. **A,** Coronal T1W image shows linear low signal in the femoral neck (*arrow*). **B,** Coronal T1W image shows linear low signal through intertrochanteric location compatible with insufficiency fracture.

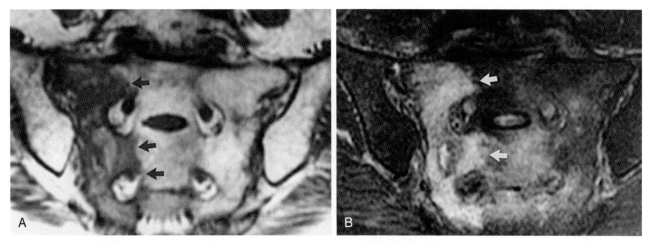

Figure 14-15 **Sacral insufficiency fracture with hip pain. A,** Axial T1W image in a 57-year-old woman with a history of breast cancer and right hip pain. Low signal is identified in a linear orientation through the right sacral ala (*arrows*). **B,** Axial FSE image with fat suppression shows high signal from a sacral insufficiency fracture in the same area (*arrows*).

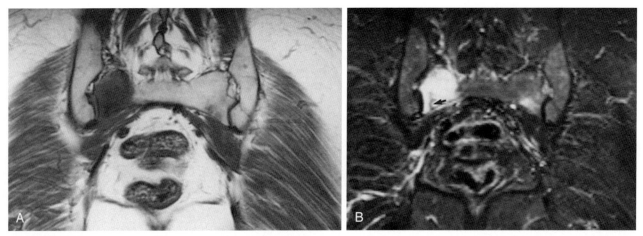

Figure 14-16 Sacral insufficiency fracture. **A,** Coronal T1W image shows linear low signal in the right sacral ala with surrounding poorly defined, low signal edema that does not cross the midline. A small left sacral insufficiency fracture is beginning. **B,** Coronal STIR image shows bone marrow edema (high signal) bilaterally with linear low signal, representing the fracture line on the right side (*arrow*).

Herniation Pits

A commonly encountered aperture in the femoral neck cortex is termed a *herniation pit*. It is seen on the anterior surface of the femoral neck. Ingrowth of fibrous and cartilaginous elements occurs through a perforation in the cortex, resulting in unilateral or bilateral, small, rounded radiolucent areas in the anterolateral aspect of the femoral neck on conventional radiography (in the upper outer quadrant of the femoral neck in the coronal plane). Generally, these lesions are unchanging and asymptomatic, although they may enlarge in individuals of all ages, perhaps related to changing mechanics, such as the pressure and abrasive effect of the overlying hip capsule and anterior muscles. Herniation pits also may be a manifestation of femoroacetabular impingement from chronic repetitive stresses. MRI generally shows a focus of low signal intensity on T1W images and high signal intensity of T2W images consistent with that of fluid (Fig. 14-19) or intermediate signal consistent with fibrous tissues in the typical location, as described earlier.

Osseous Tumors

Benign Osseous Lesions (Box 14-8). The hip is not a site unique to any particular bone tumor. An enchondroma is a benign lesion that can be found incidentally. As in other long bones, it is well defined, lobular in contour, and low to

---

BOX 14-8

Common Osseous Tumors of the Hip and Pelvis

Benign
- Enchondroma
- Chondroblastoma
- Giant cell tumor
- Geode

Malignant
- Metastatic disease
- Myeloma (plasmacytoma)
- Chondrosarcoma

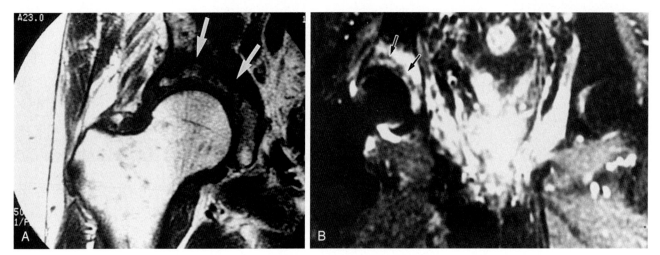

Figure 14-17 Supra-acetabular insufficiency fracture. **A,** Coronal T1W image in an 80-year-old man with prostate carcinoma and right hip pain. Curvilinear low signal is identified paralleling the roof of the acetabulum (*arrows*). Surrounding edema also is present. **B,** Coronal (fast) STIR image shows edema pattern and curvilinear signal diagnostic of supra-acetabular insufficiency fracture (*arrows*).

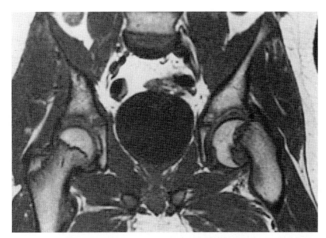

Figure 14-18 **Slipped capital femoral epiphysis.** Coronal T1W image shows marked inferior slip of femoral head from the growth plate in the left hip. Note normal relationship of right femoral head and neck.

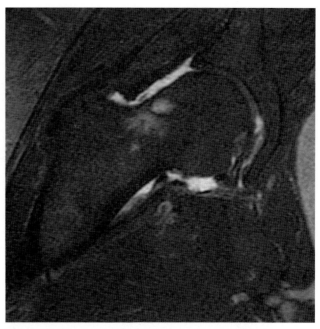

Figure 14-19 **Synovial herniation pit.** Coronal FSE T2W image with fat suppression shows high signal in a well-defined lesion in a characteristic location for synovial herniation pit.

intermediate in signal intensity on T1W images (depending on how much calcification is present) and high in signal intensity on T2W images with low signal representing calcified components (Fig. 14-20).

Another lesion that can be seen in the epiphysis, trochanters (apophysis), or flat bones of the pelvis is a giant cell tumor. The appearance on conventional radiographs is usually characteristic. MRI is helpful if conventional imaging is not diagnostic. Giant cell tumor is low signal on T1W images and intermediate on T2W images. This tumor usually does not get very bright on T2W images. MRI can show areas of cortical destruction and the extent of the soft tissue component.

In children and young adults, a chondroblastoma occasionally is encountered around the hip. As with giant cell tumor, chondroblastoma also has a predilection for the epiphysis or apophysis. MRI shows a rounded lesion with low signal on the T1W image; the T2W image also shows low to intermediate signal intensity, generally with a large area of surrounding marrow edema (low signal on T1W and high signal on T2W images). Calcified chondroid matrix may be identified as punctate areas of low signal within the lesion, but is better appreciated on CT or conventional radiography than with MRI (Fig. 14-21). Periosteal elevation

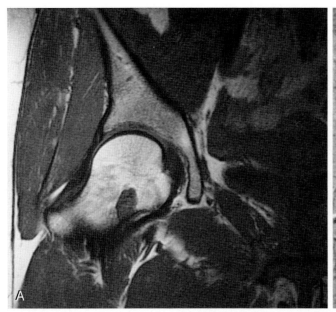
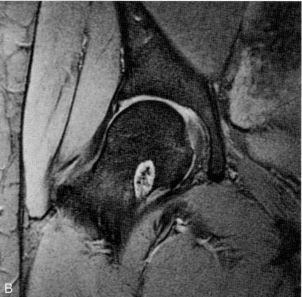

Figure 14-20 **Enchondroma. A,** Coronal T1W image shows lobular contour of low signal in the femoral neck. **B,** Coronal T2W image shows high signal chondroid with some areas of punctate low signal, which is consistent with calcification seen on conventional radiographs.

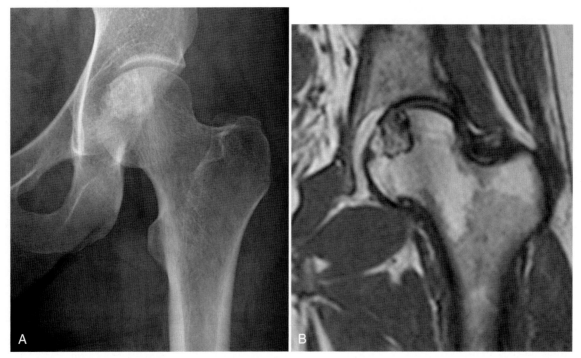

Figure 14-21 **Chondroblastoma. A,** Conventional radiograph shows epiphyseal chondroid lesion in a 32-year-old patient. **B,** Coronal T1W image shows chondroid lesion with some fatty elements. This proved to be "burned-out" chondroblastoma.

also can be seen occasionally with this lesion. It is not unusual to have a small soft tissue component with this benign lesion (Fig. 14-22).

Occasionally, a subchondral cyst in the femoral head or acetabulum can become very large, mimicking an aggressive lesion, AVN, or something more sinister than what it is. Subchondral cysts may enlarge over time. A search for associated abnormalities, such as joint space narrowing, osteophyte formation (osteoarthritis), or pannus formation (rheumatoid arthritis), can help make the diagnosis of a subchondral cyst. Subchondral cysts image as low signal

intensity on T1W images that becomes high in signal (fluidlike) on T2W images.

Malignant Osseous Lesions. No primary malignant tumor of bone is site-specific for the hip or pelvis. Chondrosarcoma occurs in this location more than other malignant tumors of bone. As mentioned in Chapter 7, it can be difficult sometimes to differentiate an enchondroma from a chondrosarcoma. A soft tissue mass, bone marrow edema, and periosteal reaction are helpful signs that indicate the more aggressive chondrosarcoma. Metastatic lesions and myeloma

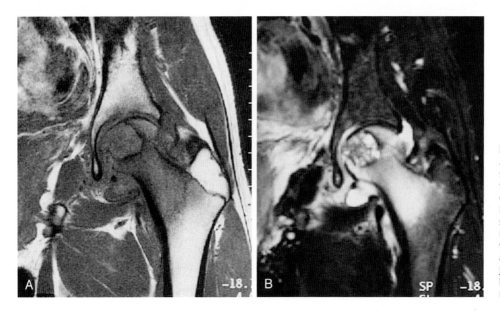

Figure 14-22 Chondroblastoma. A, Coronal T1W image shows round, low signal abnormality in the epiphysis of this child, with surrounding bone marrow edema. **B,** Coronal STIR image shows the lesion in the femoral epiphysis with some low signal areas. This appearance is typical for chondroid matrix; without the low signal foci on T2, this could just as easily be osteomyelitis with a septic joint. Bone marrow edema is noted as high signal in the femoral neck and surrounding the lesion.

(plasmacytoma) are the most common malignant processes that affect the hip and pelvis and are discussed in detail in Chapter 2.

SOFT TISSUES

Muscle and Tendon Abnormalities

Normal Capsule and Ligaments. The capsule of the joint attaches to the margin of the acetabular rim and extends distally to cover the femoral neck, inserting anteriorly along the intertrochanteric line and posteriorly halfway down the femoral neck. The greater and lesser trochanters are extracapsular structures. The capsule is lined by synovium, which is not evident on MRI when it is normal. The capsule is reinforced externally by three ligaments: the iliofemoral (the strongest), pubofemoral, and ischiofemoral. The iliofemoral ligament inserts on the intertrochanteric line and explains why almost the entire femoral neck is intracapsular. In approximately 15% of individuals, there is a hiatus between the iliofemoral and pubofemoral ligaments; this hiatus allows connection between the hip joint and the adjacent iliopsoas bursa. The capsule is more easily identified when the joint is distended (either with joint fluid or intra-articular contrast material) and images as a thin, low signal structure. Occasionally, capsular thickening can occur in the setting of recurrent joint effusions, which can lead to adhesions and fibrotic thickening of the capsule.

Normal Muscles (Box 14-9). Four muscle groups that affect hip motion can be identified. The anterior femoral muscles—including the sartorius and the rectus femoris—flex, abduct, and externally rotate the thigh. The medial group—including the gracilis, pectineus, adductor longus, adductor brevis, and adductor magnus—act as adductors, but also internally rotate and flex the hip. The lateral muscles—the tensor fascia

---

BOX 14-9

Normal Soft Tissue Structures of the Hip and Pelvis

Muscles
- Anterior (flex and abduct)
  - Sartorius
  - Rectus femoris
- Medial (adduct, internally rotate, flex)
  - Gracilis
  - Pectineus
  - Adductor longus, brevis, magnus
- Lateral (extend, abduct)
  - Tensor fascia lata
  - Gluteus maximus, medius, minimus
- External rotators
  - Piriformis
  - Obturator internus, externus
  - Gemelli superior, inferior
  - Quadratus femoris
- Posterior—hip extension, knee flexion (hamstrings)
  - Biceps femoris
  - Semimembranosus
  - Semitendinosus
- Iliopsoas—flexes hip and externally rotates thigh

BOX 14-10

Muscle Abnormalities

- Muscle strains
  - Hamstring strain, avulsion
  - Gluteus medius tendon tears (greater trochanter pain syndrome)
- MRI findings
  - Isointense to muscle on T1W image
  - High signal in the tendon T2W image
  - Disruption of tendon fibers (may have edema in adjacent bone and muscle)

---

lata and the gluteus maximus, medius, and minimus—extend and abduct the hip; the piriformis, the obturator internus and externus, the gemelli superior and inferior, and the quadratus femoris produce external rotation. The posterior femoral muscles (the hamstring muscles) include the biceps femoris, semimembranosus, and semitendinosus, which integrate hip extension and knee flexion. The iliopsoas (composed of the iliacus and the psoas major and minor) is the strongest hip flexor.

Muscle Strains (Box 14-10). Injuries to the thigh muscles and their pelvic attachments are common in trained and untrained athletes.[17] The injury pattern is discussed in great detail in Chapter 3. Patients may undergo MRI for evaluation of pain after a fall when conventional radiography is normal (shows no fracture). Muscle abnormalities may account for the symptoms, but MRI also is very valuable in assessing the underlying bone for an occult fracture. The hamstring muscles are injured most frequently, but tears in quadriceps and adductor muscles also occur (Fig. 14-23).

Gluteus Medius and Minimus Tendon Tears. Tears of the gluteus medius and minimus tendon also have been referred to as *greater trochanter pain syndrome* and *rotator cuff tears of the hip*. Patients complain of chronic dull, aching pain around the hip or groin region that is aggravated by weight bearing and resisted hip abduction. The symptoms often mimic intra-articular hip pathology. The pain is associated with tendinopathy or tears of the gluteus medius or minimus tendons and associated muscle. This entity affects middle-aged to elderly women about four times more often than men and is thought to be a result of a degenerative and progressive process (Fig. 14-24).[18-20]

MRI examinations show abnormal high signal in the gluteus medius or minimus muscles on T2W images; discontinuity of the tendons may be evident (Fig. 14-25). The signal intensity on T1W images is isointense to musculature, and it is not appreciated as abnormal. T2W images must be performed to make this diagnosis. The coronal images are the most helpful in making the diagnosis. The gluteus medius tendon attaches to the posterosuperior portion of the greater trochanter, whereas the minimus attaches to the anterosuperior trochanter.

Athletic Pubalgia. Groin pain in a competitive athlete is a common and challenging entity. It is most often described in sports involving twisting and turning movements, such as football, ice hockey, and soccer. Of the four adductor muscles, the adductor longus is chiefly implicated in groin

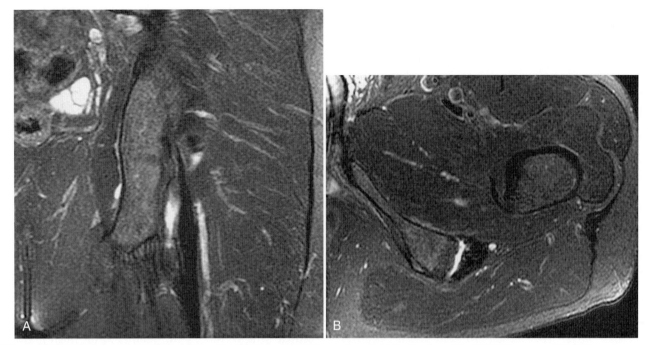

Figure 14-23 **Partial tear, hamstring. A,** Coronal fast T2W fat-suppressed image shows fluid signal in the origin of the left hamstring. The findings are consistent with a partial tear of the hamstring. **B,** Axial T2W image with fat suppression shows fluid signal at tendon-bone interface.

pain in athletes. It is usually associated with a microtear at the pubic attachment of the adductor longus (Fig. 14-26). The identification of a secondary cleft sign or bone edema at the symphysis should increase the index of suspicion that groin pain symptoms relate to an injury at the symphysis pubis.[21,22]

Hamstring Injuries. Buttock pain is a common complaint of all age groups. Often, this is due to a spouse, but a cause that is underappreciated is a hamstring injury. Patients often are presumed to have sciatic symptoms, and a lumbar spine study is ordered. The hamstrings are not imaged in this study, but are nicely seen in a study of the pelvis or even a unilateral hip. The origin of the hamstrings on the ischial tuberosity should be evaluated. The tendons include biceps

femoris, semitendinosus, and semimembranosus. These tendons may avulse or have partial tears leading to buttock pain (Fig. 14-27).

Piriformis Syndrome. The sciatic nerve exits the pelvis at the greater sciatic notch and is intimately associated with the piriformis muscle. The nerve usually is located immediately anterior to the piriformis muscle. There can be variations in the relationship between these structures: the sciatic nerve can split through the piriformis muscle; the nerve itself can split, and a portion of the split nerve can go through the piriformis muscle; or the nerve can be split, and a portion of the nerve can be superficial to the piriformis muscle. Because of this variation in location of the sciatic nerve, compression, hypertrophy, or injury to the piriformis muscle

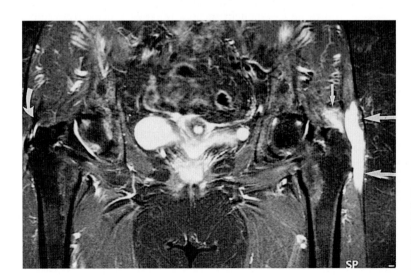

Figure 14-24 **Torn gluteus medius tendon and trochanteric bursitis.** Coronal STIR image shows abnormal high signal in the location of the gluteus medius muscle and tendon (*short arrow*). *Curved arrow* points to normal gluteal insertion on the right. Note also the high signal fluid collection adjacent to the greater trochanter, representing greater trochanteric bursitis (*large arrows*).

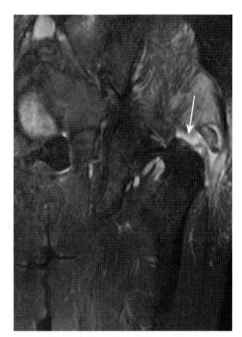

Figure 14-25 **Torn gluteus medius tendon.** Coronal T2W image with fat suppression shows increased signal in gluteal musculature. No tendon insertion is identified (*arrow*).

can cause irritation to the sciatic nerve, mimicking radicular symptoms from disk disease.

MRI may show asymmetry in the size of one piriformis muscle compared with the contralateral side. There usually is no abnormal signal or size of the piriformis muscle in patients with the piriformis syndrome, unless there has been direct trauma. In the case of trauma to the piriformis muscle, high signal may be identified on T2W images, caused by edema and hematoma.

Other Muscles and Tendons. Injuries also can occur to the other muscle groups around the hip. The findings on MRI are the same for injured tendons located anywhere. Fat-suppressed T2W or STIR images show the abnormal fluid/edema with increased conspicuity and are recommended for evaluation of these structures. Tendons may be thinned or thickened, have abnormal high signal within them on any pulse sequence, or be discontinuous or avulsed from their osseous attachments. In the setting of hip pain and evaluation for an occult fracture, muscle strain or hematoma may account for pain when no fracture is identified. Appropriate therapy can be instituted to address the pain source.

Nerves

Normal Nerves. The largest nerve adjacent to the hip joint is the sciatic nerve. It is located immediately posterior to the posterior column of the acetabulum and lateral to the ischial tuberosity. It generally arises from the ventral L4-S3 nerve roots, exits the infrapiriform portion of the greater sciatic foramen, and courses between the ischial tuberosity and the greater trochanter. It is surrounded by fat and located between the quadratus femoris muscle anteriorly and the gluteus maximus muscle posteriorly. On MRI, the sciatic nerve is easiest to identify as an intermediate signal intensity

stippled structure surrounded by fat just lateral to the hamstring origin (ischial tuberosity) on axial images (see Fig. 14-1).

Abnormal Sciatic Nerve. The sciatic nerve can be compressed by a nearby mass, or can be traumatized from a direct blow; this may result in swelling of the nerve. The location of the nerve around the hip joint makes it susceptible to traumatic injury. The appearance of the nerve is similar to any other nerve injury, in which the nerve may be enlarged focally or diffusely and has increased signal on T2W images. Chapter 4 contains a more comprehensive discussion. Another entity that can affect the sciatic nerve is fibrolipomatous hamartoma (Fig. 14-28).

Bursae (Box 14-11)

Iliopsoas Bursa. The iliopsoas bursa is the largest bursa of the hip (and of the entire body). The iliopsoas bursa can be distended and cause groin pain. It communicates with the joint in 15% of the population and can become distended when the joint is distended, when there is no significant joint effusion, or even when it does not communicate with the hip

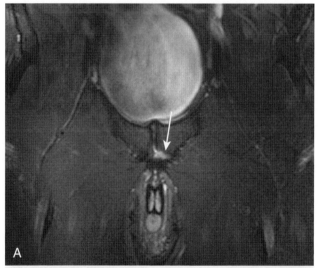

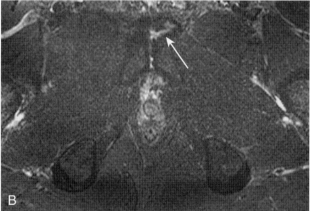

Figure 14-26 **Athletic pubalgia. A,** Coronal T2W image with fat suppression shows fluid signal in the pubic symphysis and along the insertion of the adductor tendons on the left (*arrow*) in this professional hockey player. **B,** Axial T2W image with fat suppression in the same patient shows fluid signal between the bone-tendon interface (*arrow*).

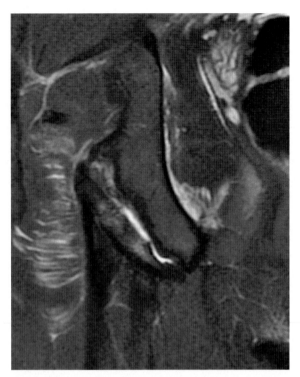

Figure 14-27 **Hamstring avulsion.** Coronal T2W image with fat suppression shows abnormal signal in the hamstring tendon origin and in the bone.

fluid, which is isointense to joint fluid (see Fig. 14-29); that is, it is low signal on T1W images and high signal intensity on T2W images. After the administration of intravenous contrast material, the bursa is more readily diagnosed because the fluid does not enhance, but the lining of the bursa does; this helps to distinguish a potentially confusing anterior groin mass from the fluid-filled bursa (Fig. 14-30). These bursae can be treated acutely with direct intrabursal steroid injections, but if they are inflamed because they are in communication with an abnormal hip joint, they cannot be treated permanently without addressing the joint problem.

Greater Trochanteric Bursitis. Trochanteric bursitis is another cause of hip pain. Patients usually localize the pain to the lateral aspect of the hip. Often this entity results from repetitive hip flexion. It can be impossible to distinguish it on clinical grounds from a torn gluteus medius or minimus

joint. It usually becomes distended in patients with rheumatoid arthritis or osteoarthritis (Fig. 14-29).[23] Distention of this bursa can help explain the patient's pain.

The iliopsoas bursa is located immediately anterior to the hip joint and adjacent to the femoral vessels, femoral nerve, and iliopsoas muscle. It is not seen unless distended with

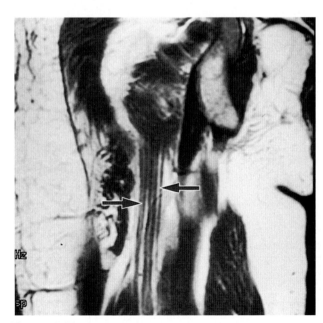

Figure 14-28 **Fibrolipomatous hamartoma of sciatic nerve.** Coronal T1W image shows multiple fascicles of sciatic nerve surrounded by fat (*arrows*) in this patient with sciatic nerve symptoms.

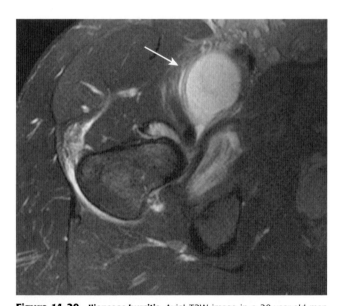

Figure 14-29 **Iliopsoas bursitis.** Axial T2W image in a 30-year-old man with rheumatoid arthritis and right hip pain. A high signal mass is noted adjacent to the iliopsoas tendon (*arrow*), consistent with an iliopsoas bursitis. The neck leading to connection with joint space is evident.

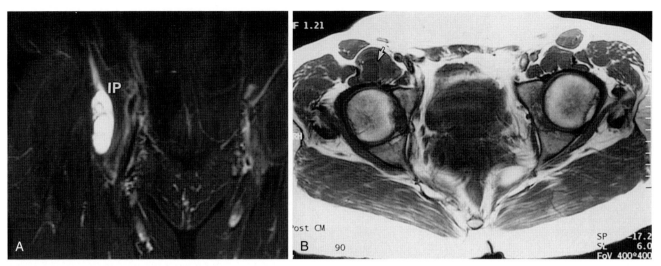

Figure 14-30   Iliopsoas bursa. **A,** Coronal STIR image shows a high signal mass adjacent to iliopsoas muscle (IP). **B,** Axial T1W image after contrast administration shows peripheral enhancement of the mass (*arrow*), confirming the fluid nature of this mass.

tendon or muscle, which occurs in a similar middle-aged and elderly population. Patients generally are treated with anti-inflammatory medications. If pain is refractory to anti-inflammatory medications, a steroid injection into the bursa can be beneficial.

The findings on MRI for trochanteric bursitis consist of no perceptible abnormality on T1W images because the fluid is isointense to surrounding musculature. T2W images show increased signal intensity, however, paralleling the greater trochanter. This does not have to be a well-defined fluid collection, but rather a focus of high signal interdigitating around the tendons of the greater trochanter (Fig. 14-31). A small amount of bursal fluid is often present bilaterally in patients who have no clinical symptoms of bursitis. If the

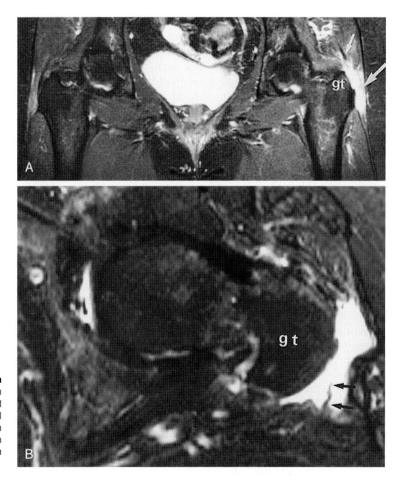

Figure 14-31 Greater trochanteric bursitis and torn gluteus medius tendon. A, Coronal STIR image shows focal high signal around the greater trochanter (gt; *large arrow*). The torn and retracted gluteus medius tendon also is seen (*small arrow*). **B,** Axial image shows the well-defined fluid collection, compatible with greater trochanteric bursitis. The gluteus medius tendon is torn (*arrows*). Greater trochanteric bursitis often is seen in association with gluteus medius tendon tears.

quantity of fluid is asymmetric, a diagnosis of bursitis can be suggested.

Soft Tissue Tumors (Box 14-12)

Benign Soft Tissue Tumors. No soft tissue tumors are particularly unique to the hip region. A lesion that occurs with some frequency is a lipoma, which can occur in the subcutaneous tissues or can be intramuscular. Lipoma is easily identified on MRI because the signal intensity of the lesion follows that of fat on all imaging sequences; it is high in signal intensity on T1W images and suppresses on fat-suppressed images. Another soft tissue mass that can occur around the pelvis is a desmoid, which is a benign fibrous tumor that is locally aggressive. Generally, the imaging features of desmoids are similar to most soft tissue tumors, low signal intensity on T1W images and increased signal intensity on T2W images. Because of the predominant fibrous component in this tumor, however, it can remain low in signal on T2W images. This is a useful sign, when present.

Malignant Soft Tissue Tumors (see Box 14-12). The most common malignant soft tissue tumor is malignant fibrohistiocytoma. This tumor is not unique to the hip and pelvis area, but should be considered in the differential diagnosis for a mass that occurs in the soft tissues that is low in signal on T1W images. T2W images may show some high signal intensity, but because of the fibrous component may have some intermediate to low signal elements.

Other soft tissue sarcomas, such as liposarcoma and synovial cell sarcoma, also can occur and are nonspecific in their imaging characteristics (low signal on T1W images and high signal on T2W images). Occasionally, synovial cell sarcoma resembles fluid-like signal on the T2W image (ie, very intense signal). Gadolinium is helpful in differentiating a cystic col-

lection from a solid mass. Liposarcomas have variable fat content and may not be high in signal on T1W images, as would be expected for a fat-containing mass.

JOINTS

Normal Ligamentum Teres

The ligamentum teres and the pulvinar (extrasynovial fibrofatty tissue) are contained within the acetabular fossa—the nonarticular medial wall of the acetabulum. The ligamentum teres runs from the acetabular fossa to the fovea centralis of the femoral head. Although the ligamentum teres does not normally contribute to hip joint stability, it does carry the artery of the ligamentum teres that supplies blood to the femoral head in children. In adults, the blood supply associated with the ligamentum teres tends to involute.

Labrum (Box 14-13)

The acetabular labrum is a rim of fibrocartilaginous tissue around the margin of the acetabulum that deepens the acetabular fossa and provides additional coverage for the femoral head. The labrum is innervated by nerves that play a role in proprioception and pain production. The normal labrum is a triangular structure on axial, sagittal, and coronal imaging that is attached to the rim of the acetabulum.[24,25] The normal labrum is low signal on all imaging sequences (Fig. 14-32). Using surface coils, the labrum can be imaged in exquisite detail.

Labral Tears. Symptoms of labral tears include persistent pain, clicking, or decreased range of motion.[24] Labral tears can result from an acute injury, chronic stress (femoroacetabular impingement), or DDH. Protocol adjustments need to be made to evaluate the labrum effectively. If a labral abnormality is the clinical question, MR arthrography with small field of view, thin slice thickness, and a smaller interslice gap is recommended, rather than imaging the entire pelvis.[26]

A surface coil is imperative for adequate signal in this region. Because of the oblique orientation of the labrum, it has been postulated that radial imaging of the labrum may be helpful in further evaluation of pathology. In a study by Yoon and associates,[27] radial imaging did not show any labral tear not seen in standard imaging planes.

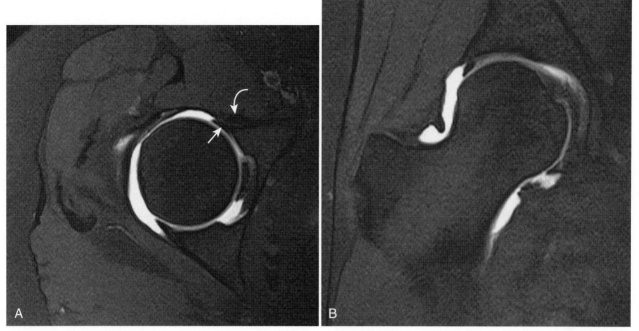

Figure 14-32   Normal labrum. A, Axial T1W image with fat suppression and intra-articular contrast administration shows a triangular, low signal structure, representing normal appearance of the labrum (*small arrow*). The low signal structure adjacent to the labrum is the iliopsoas tendon (*curved arrow*). The normal relationship between the labrum and iliopsoas tendon should be understood so that a tear in the labrum is not erroneously diagnosed. **B,** Coronal T1W image shows a triangular low signal structure representing a normal labrum.

A helpful addition to the protocol for evaluation of the labrum and coincident femoroacetabular impingement is oblique coronal and oblique axial images oriented along the plane parallel to the femoral neck. This orientation is especially helpful for identifying anterior labral tears and recognizing bone contour deformity, which can be seen in femoroacetabular impingement.

The MRI appearance of an abnormal labrum is that of linear or diffuse high signal in the labrum, deformity in contour of the labrum (loss of the normal triangular structure) (Fig. 14-33), and detachment from the acetabulum (Figs. 14-34 and 14-35). Amorphous, round high signal within the substance of the labrum is a result of degeneration of the labrum, which is not thought to be clinically significant.[25] Hip arthroscopists have used a classification system called the *Lage classification.* It is the only published arthroscopic classification system for hip labral tears. It does not correlate well with Czerny's MR arthrography classification system, however, which has been used previously by radiologists.[28] Using a clock-face description to localize tears, along with a description of the signal of the labrum, has been proposed as a helpful way to characterize the extent of labral pathology.[29] Using quadrants to describe labral tears is useful. This requires the use of two planes to characterize the location adequately. As in the shoulder, a small para-articular cyst can form as a result of a labral tear (Fig. 14-36). The presence of a para-articular cyst is a strong indicator of an associated labral tear.

One pitfall in imaging is the extension of the acetabular cartilage along the medial aspect of the labrum, which should

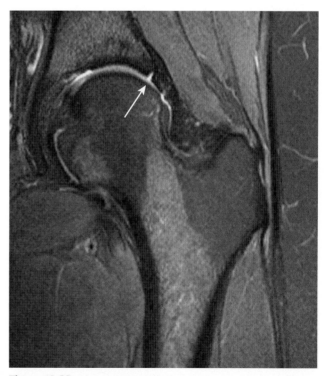

Figure 14-33   Linear labral tear. Coronal T1W image with fat suppression and intra-articular contrast administration. Linear high signal is identified through the undersurface of the labrum (*arrow*). The remaining portion of the labrum is no longer triangular in configuration.

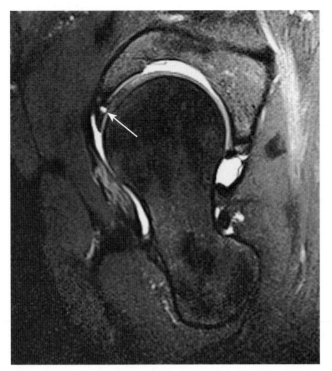

Figure 14-34 Anterosuperior labral tear. Oblique coronal T1W image with fat suppression and intra-articular contrast administration shows triangular labrum avulsed from acetabular attachment (*arrow*). Fluid is identified through labral detachment.

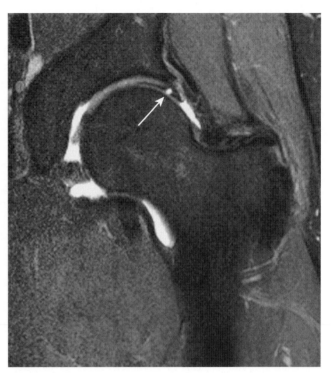

Figure 14-35 Superior acetabular labral tear. Coronal T2W image with fat suppression and intra-articular contrast administration shows fluid at labral–cartilage interface (*arrow*).

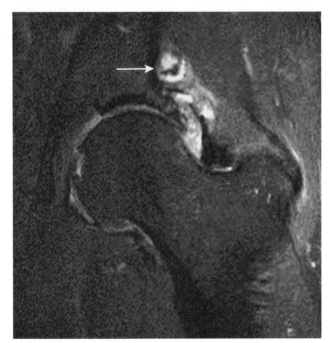

Figure 14-36 Labral tear with paralabral cyst. Coronal FSE-T2W image with fat suppression shows a fluid collection adjacent to the labrum, compatible with a paralabral cyst (*arrow*). Note presence of osteophytes in this patient with degenerative disease.

not be confused with a labral tear or detachment. Another pitfall may be the iliopsoas tendon where it crosses anterior to the labrum. It is important to understand this relationship because the high signal between these two low signal structures could mimic a tear of the labrum (see Fig. 14-32). In the United States, most labral tears generally are anterior and superior in location, whereas in Asian countries the defect is more commonly found posteriorly. A possible explanation for this disparity is the squatting position many Asians assume for relaxation. Surgery generally is indicated to repair labral defects. Previous literature would suggest the presence of an anterosuperior sublabral foramen. This has not proved to be the case subsequently.

Normal Articular Cartilage

The acetabulum is not entirely covered by articular cartilage. Surrounding the nonarticular medial aspect of the acetabulum (acetabular fossa) is the articulating portion of the acetabulum, which is covered by articular cartilage. The cartilage is thin, measuring no more than 3 mm.

Abnormal Articular Cartilage

The cartilage is best evaluated with fluid in the joint, a small field of view, and use of a surface coil to optimize signal-to-

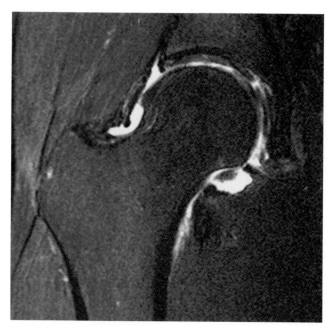

Figure 14-37 **Chondral defects.** Coronal T2W image with fat suppression and intra-articular contrast administration shows irregularity along the surface of the acetabulum and femoral head.

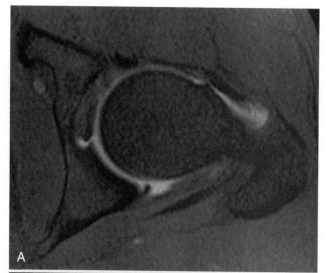

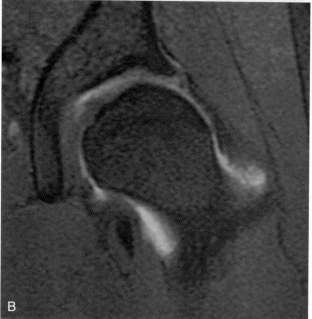

Figure 14-38 **Femoroacetabular impingement (cam). A,** Axial T1W image with fat suppression and intra-articular contrast administration shows a bony protuberance at the junction of the femoral head and neck. **B,** Coronal T1W image with fat suppression with intra-articular contrast administration shows a torn labrum as evidenced by the abnormal signal throughout the labrum.

noise ratio. Cartilage images as intermediate signal, and abnormalities are identified in 30% of patients with labral pathology and often noted in patients with femoroacetabular impingement. Defects are identified by noting fluid signal replacing the normal intermediate signal intensity of the cartilage (Fig. 14-37).

Femoroacetabular Impingement (Box 14-14)

Femoroacetabular impingement is a major cause of early osteoarthritis of the hip. It is especially identified in young (20-40 years old) and active patients. Generally, patients complain of groin pain either with hip rotational activity or immediately after activity. It is due to early pathologic contact during hip joint motion between bony prominences of the acetabulum or femoral neck or both that limits the range of motion of the hip. This pathologic contact is identified especially during flexion and internal rotation. The excursion of the femoral head as it glides around the acetabulum is limited.

Two subgroups of femoroacetabular impingement have been described, the "cam" and the "pincer" types, although some overlap may exist between the two. The cam type is more common in young athletic men and involves abutment of an abnormally shaped (nonspherical) femoral head into the acetabular rim, particularly during hip flexion. This abutment can lead to chondral and labral injury secondary to the shearing forces produced from the reduced excursion of the femoral head clearance (Fig. 14-38).[30-32] The labrum

---

BOX 14-14

Femoroacetabular Impingement

Cam

- Young, active individuals
- Abnormal offset at femoral head–neck junction (pistol grip deformity of femoral head–neck)
- Limited internal rotation and flexion of hip
- Labral fraying or tears or both
- Adjacent cartilage irregularity/defect superior and anterior
- Associated herniation pit
- Os acetabuli

Pincer

- More common in women
- Overcoverage of acetabulum
- Synovial herniation pit
- Acetabular fraying/tears
- Cartilage irregularity/defects posterior acetabulum

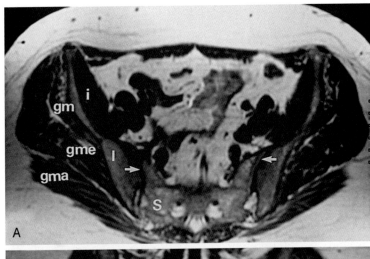
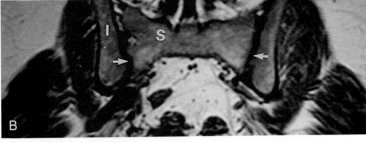

Figure 14-39 Normal sacroiliac joints. **A** and **B**, Axial (**A**) and coronal (**B**) T1W images of the sacroiliac joints. True synovial portion (*arrows*). gm, gluteus minimus; gma, gluteus maximus; gme, gluteus medius; I, ilium; i, iliacus; S, sacrum.

is abnormal in signal, deformed or detached, and the chondral surface on the acetabulum immediately adjacent to the labrum may have abnormal signal from partial-thickness or full-thickness defects. It is useful to have intra-articular fluid and oblique planes to make these assessments. Findings that have been seen in association with this entity include synovial herniation pits, flattening of the junction of the head and neck (pistol grip deformity of the femoral head), and an os acetabuli. The synovial herniation pit generally is located at the junction of the femoral head and neck. The more characteristic pistol grip deformity is shown with additional ossification at the junction of the head and neck or in a patient who had a prior slipped capitofemoral epiphysis.

The pincer type is more common in middle-aged women and involves contact between the acetabular rim and the femoral head-neck junction secondary to overcoverage of the femoral head by the acetabulum.[30] The acetabulum can reduce femoral head clearance leading to impingement. Anterior acetabular overcoverage (acetabular retroversion), protrusio acetabuli, and coxa profunda have been implicated as causes of impingement.[33] MRI shows abnormal signal or deformed or detached labrum with chondral abnormalities most often in the posterior aspect of the acetabulum.[34]

Inflammatory Arthritides

Arthritis affecting the hip joint can be from a variety of causes. Rheumatoid arthritis can affect the hip, most often symmetrically bilaterally with axial joint space narrowing. Differentiating an inflammatory arthritis from a septic joint generally is impossible when only a single joint is known to

be involved. Subchondral cyst formation, pannus, and joint effusion are common.

Sacroiliitis is a nonspecific term suggesting an inflammatory process involving the sacroiliac joints (Fig. 14-39). A variety of disease processes can affect the sacroiliac joint, including the human leukocyte antigen (HLA) B-27 spondyloarthropathies, such as ankylosing spondylitis, inflammatory bowel disease, psoriasis, and Reiter's syndrome. Other common entities that affect these joints include osteoarthritis, gout, rheumatoid arthritis, and infection. The appearance on MRI is similar for each of these entities. The joint space may show erosions that appear as foci of high signal along the joint space on T2W images. Bone marrow edema may be seen immediately adjacent to the joint within the iliac bone and sacral ala. Erosions can be seen with any of the aforementioned abnormalities. The symmetry of the appearance may help with the differential diagnosis because ankylosing spondylitis and inflammatory bowel disease are nearly always bilateral and symmetric. Psoriasis and Reiter's syndrome are bilateral and symmetric about 40% of the time.

Infection of the sacroiliac joint may show fluid that appears high signal on T2W images within the joint space, but which does not enhance after the administration of contrast material (Fig. 14-40). The inflammatory reaction (phlegmon) may enhance, but the abscess collection or associated joint fluid does not enhance The appearance of a septic joint may be impossible to differentiate by MRI from an uninfected inflammatory arthritis (seronegative spondyloarthropathy or rheumatoid arthritis). If the process is bilateral, it is highly unlikely to be from infection.

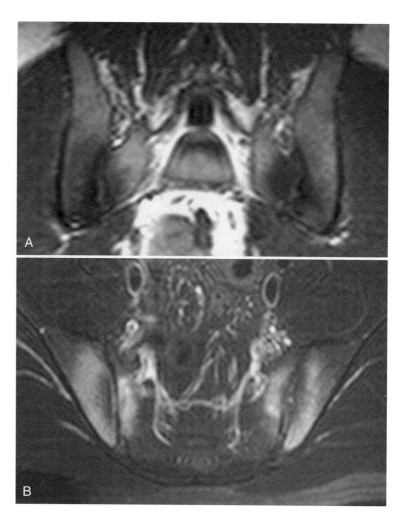

Figure 14-40 **Sacroiliitis. A,** Coronal T1W image shows low signal in the bilateral sacral and iliac bones. **B,** Axial fast T2W fat-suppressed image shows abnormal signal in the bones. The findings are consistent with sacroiliitis.

The sacroiliac joints are composed of two parts, the true joint and a strong ligamentous attachment between the two bones (see Fig. 14-39). The true joint, a synovial joint, comprises the anteroinferior half to two thirds of the joint. The articular surfaces are covered with cartilage and separated by a joint space. Hyaline cartilage exclusively lines the sacral surface, whereas a thinner mixture of hyaline and fibrocartilage lines the iliac surface. This discrepancy likely accounts for why disease processes begin along the iliac margin first. Many joint abnormalities may affect the articular cartilage, as described subsequently.

Degenerative Joint Disease

Osteoarthritis also affects the hip and is much more common than rheumatoid arthritis. The findings of joint space narrowing (superolateral and anteriorly), osteophyte formation, and subchondral cysts can be noted easily on MRI. Often, the only finding initially is a nonspecific joint effusion or marrow edema in the subchondral bone (Fig. 14-41). It can be useful to have conventional radiographs of the hip available when evaluating the MR images for suspected arthritis because they can be complementary studies.[35]

Developmental Dysplasia (Box 14-15)

DDH, formerly called *congenital dislocation of the hip*, occurs in 1% of newborns. The disorder is more common in newborn girls and newborns with a positive family history. The left hip is more commonly affected.[36] Early intervention can lead to normal hip development in 95% of patients with DDH. DDH has been classified according to the configuration of the acetabulum and labrum.[37] Type 1 is characterized by positional instability; type 2, by subluxation of femoral head and eversion of the labrum; and type 3, by frank dislocation of the femoral head posterosuperiorly.

BOX 14-15

Developmental Dysplasia of the Hip

- Occurs in 1% of newborns
- Females slightly more affected than males
- Left hip > right hip
- 95% normal development after intervention
- If undetected, early hip degeneration ensues (patients in their 30s)
- MRI useful in cases refractory to reduction attempts
  - Possible causes: Redundant labrum, excess pulvinar, transverse acetabular ligament, capsular hypertrophy, constriction of iliopsoas tendon, deformities of acetabulum or femoral head
  - Femoral head located superior to acetabulum, upturned lateral aspect of acetabular roof, shallow/steep acetabulum
- Common associated findings in adults
  - Labral tears
  - Degenerative joint disease

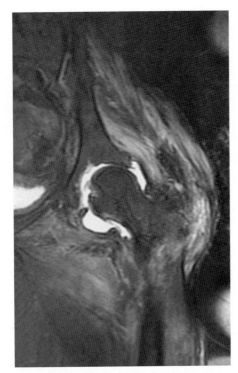

Figure 14-41 **Hip joint effusion.** Coronal T2W image with fat suppression shows a distended joint as shown by fluid signal surrounded by joint capsule.

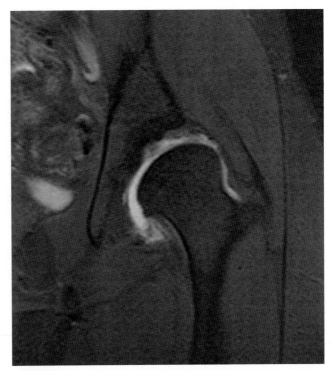

Figure 14-42 **Developmental dysplasia of the hip.** Coronal T1W image with fat suppression and intra-articular contrast administration shows shallow acetabulum, abnormal configuration and signal of the labrum, and abnormal appearance to femoral head.

DDH ideally is diagnosed at birth by physical examination; however, the diagnosis can be missed, delaying therapy. These infants present for evaluation and treatment at several months to years of age. Ultrasound still should be regarded as the principal means of investigation in newborns.[38] MRI should be considered for DDH when reduction has been attempted but is unsuccessful. Because of the ability of MRI to resolve tissue types, structures that may prevent reduction of the femoral head can be identified. These include an abnormal labrum, pulvinar, transverse acetabular ligament (connects anterior with posterior labrum), capsular hypertrophy, constriction of iliopsoas tendon, and deformities of the acetabulum or femoral head.[37] The fact that a child can be imaged in cast material is another advantage of MRI. Sedation is necessary to perform MRI on most younger patients.

Young adults, usually in their 30s, may develop severe hip pain from DDH that was never diagnosed as a child. The DDH leads to early degenerative joint disease and labral tears, both of which are a source of pain. Degenerative joint disease in the hip, whether or not it is caused by DDH, usually begins in the far anterior aspect of the hip joint. MRI shows edema in the subchondral bone of the acetabular region or femoral head early in the process; this progresses to subchondral cysts in the same locations. A careful search for the typical abnormal configuration of the osseous structures of the hip can be made on MRI and radiography when degenerative changes are seen at a young age; the degenerative changes generally are easier to identify than DDH on MRI. On MRI examination, the abnormal hip is

located superiorly to the acetabulum. Irregular shape and shallow acetabulum also can be identified (Fig. 14-42). Instead of the lateral aspect of the roof of the acetabulum turning downward, as is normal, it is directed superiorly (like a raised eyebrow). Careful inspection of the joint space should be performed to identify if the pulvinar (fat; high signal on T1W images) is trapped in the joint space, preventing reduction. A redundant labrum also can prevent reduction. This structure images as low signal on all sequences and should be evaluated as a cause of nonreducible hip.

Intra-articular "Tumors" (Synovial Processes) (Box 14-16)

Pigmented Villonodular Synovitis. Pigmented villonodular synovitis (PVNS) is an uncommon disorder characterized by synovial proliferation with hemosiderin deposition

---

BOX 14-16

Intra-articular Tumors

- Pigmented villonodular synovitis—low T1, low T2, owing to hemosiderin
- Synovial chondromatosis—low T1, high T2, following cartilage signal
- Synovial osteochondromatosis—low T1, high or low T2, depending on fatty marrow or sclerotic bodies
- Amyloid arthropathy—low T1, low to intermediate T2

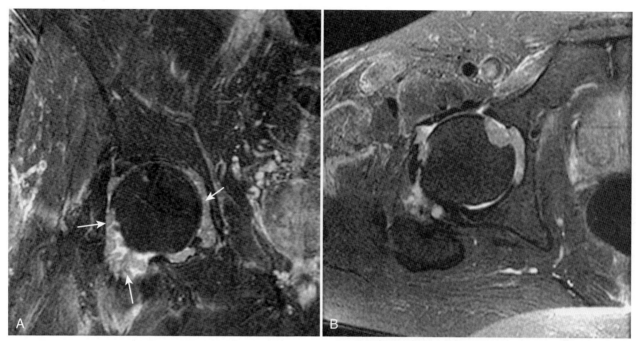

Figure 14-43 **Synovial chondromatosis. A,** Coronal T2W image with fat suppression shows multiple intra-articular loose bodies of similar size (*arrows*) and signal intensity in the hip joint. **B,** Axial T2W image with fat suppression shows masslike intermediate signal intensity compatible with a conglomerate mass of loose bodies, which can be seen in primary synovial chondromatosis.

in the involved synovial tissue. Pressure erosions of bone by the synovial masses may occur. PVNS occurs most commonly in the second through fifth decades and is usually monarticular. The hip is among the joints most commonly affected by this disease process. Synovial involvement may be localized, although a diffuse form of synovial involvement may be evident in 75% of cases. Because incomplete excision of PVNS guarantees recurrence, the entire joint must be evaluated carefully on MRI. A complete synovectomy is necessary for successful treatment.

T1W and T2W images are necessary to evaluate hemosiderin deposition, which is shown as large, globular areas of low signal intensity on all imaging sequences. Gradient echo imaging shows blooming of the hemosiderin elements, making them more prominent.[39] The presence of hemosiderin makes the diagnosis of PVNS on MRI virtually pathognomonic.

Primary Synovial Chondromatosis. Primary synovial chondromatosis is the result of metaplastic proliferation of the synovium, resulting in multiple cartilaginous or osseous loose bodies (Fig. 14-43). Secondary osteochondromatosis also is referred to as *degenerative* owing to loose body formation as a result of cartilage fragments being knocked off in the joint from degenerative disease. Primary synovial chondromatosis is not associated with degenerative changes until very late in the disease process. It is impossible to distinguish PVNS from synovial chondromatosis (nonossified) with conventional radiography. MRI makes

the differentiation between these two processes possible. As stated earlier, the hemosiderin deposits characteristic of PVNS are low in signal on all imaging sequences. Synovial chondromatosis follows the signal characteristics of cartilage, however. Cartilaginous loose bodies are low in signal on T1W and higher in signal on T2W images, following the signal of the articular cartilage.[40] Ossified loose bodies allow the diagnosis of synovial osteochondromatosis to be made on conventional radiography. On MRI, the ossified bodies may have low signal cortical margins with a fatty ("chewy nougat") center that follows the appearance of fat on all pulse sequences. Some ossified bodies are diffusely dense and sclerotic (low signal on all pulse sequences) throughout. Often, a mix of cartilaginous and ossified bodies is present.

Amyloid Arthropathy. Amyloid arthropathy is rare in terms of the hip. Typically, patients have renal failure and present with hip pain clinically similar to that of rheumatoid arthritis. Conventional radiography may show erosions within the acetabulum and femoral head or neck. MRI shows the erosions to be low in signal on T1W images and to remain low to intermediate signal on T2W images. This arthropathy often manifests as mass lesions within the joint space. The radiographic features of this entity can be confused with PVNS on conventional radiography and MRI. History and a careful search for hemosiderin (PVNS) should allow the two diagnoses to be distinguished (Fig. 14-44).

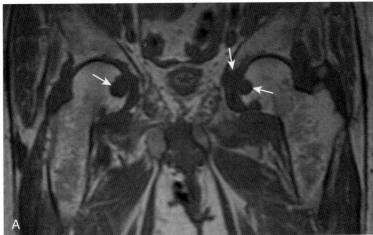

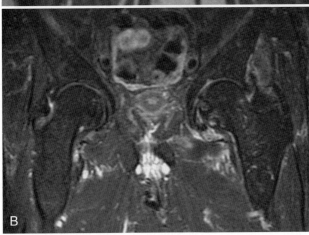

Figure 14-44 **Amyloid arthropathy. A,** Axial T1W image shows multiple low signal erosions in the femoral head and acetabulum (*arrows*). **B,** Coronal T2W image with fat suppression shows that the erosions do not become high in signal. This finding is compatible with amyloid arthropathy.

REFERENCES

1. Coleman B, Kressel H, Dalinka M, et al. Radiographically negative avascular necrosis: detection with MR imaging. *Radiology* 1988; 168:525-528.
2. Beltran J, Herman L, Burk J. Femoral head avascular necrosis: MR imaging with clinical-pathological and radionuclide correlations. *Radiology* 1988; 166:215-220.
3. Mitchell D, Rao V, Dalinka M. Femoral head avascular necrosis: correlation of MR imaging, radiographic staging, radionuclide imaging, and clinical findings. *Radiology* 1987; 162:709-715.
4. Nokes SR, Vogler JB, Spritzer CE, et al. Herniation pits of the femoral neck: appearance at MR imaging. *Radiology* 1989; 172:231-234.
5. Rush B, Bramson R, Ogden J. Legg-Calvé-Perthes disease: detection of cartilaginous and synovial changes with MR imaging. *Radiology* 1988; 167:473-476.
6. Bluemm R, Falke T, des Plantes B, Steiner R. Early Legg-Perthes disease (ischemic necrosis of the femoral head) demonstrated by magnetic resonance imaging. *Skeletal Radiol* 1985; 14:95-98.
7. Jaramillo D, Galen TA, Winalski CS, et al. Legg-Calvé-Perthes disease: MR imaging evaluation during manual positioning of the hip—comparison with conventional arthrography. *Radiology* 1999; 212:519-525.
8. Curtiss P, Kincaid W. Transitory demineralization of the hip in pregnancy: a report of three cases. *J Bone Joint Surg [Am]* 1959; 41:1327-1333.
9. Nishiyama K, Sakamaki T. Transient osteopenia of the hip joint in children. *Clin Orthop Relat Res* 1992; 275:199-203.
10. Guerra J, Steinberg M. Distinguishing transient osteoporosis from avascular necrosis of the hip. *J Bone Joint Surg [Am]* 1995; 77:616-624.
11. Yamamoto T, Kubo T, Hirasawa Y. A clinicopathologic study of transient osteoporosis of the hip. *Skeletal Radiol* 1999; 28:621-627.
12. Major NM, Helms CA. Idiopathic transient osteoporosis of the hip. *Arthritis Rheum* 1997; 40:1178-1179.
13. VandeBerg BC, Malghem JJ, Lecourt FE, et al. Idiopathic bone marrow edema lesions of the femoral head: predictive value of MR imaging findings. *Radiology* 1999; 212:527-535.
14. Stafford S, Rosenthal D, Gebhardt M, et al. MRI in stress fracture. *AJR Am J Roentgenol* 1986; 147:553-556.
15. Bogost GA, Lizerbram EK, Crues JR. MR imaging in evaluation of suspected hip fracture: frequency of unsuspected bone and soft-tissue injury. *Radiology* 1995; 197:263-267.
16. Otte MT, Helms CA, Fritz RC. MR imaging of supra-acetabular insufficiency fractures. *Skeletal Radiol* 1997; 26:279-283.
17. Ishikawa K, Kai K, Mizuta H. Avulsion of the hamstring muscles from the ischial tuberosity: a report of two cases. *Clin Orthop Relat Res* 1988; 232:153-155.
18. Chung CB, Robertson JE, Cho G, et al. Gluteus medius tendon tears and avulsive injuries in elderly women: imaging findings in six patients. *AJR Am J Roentgenol* 1999; 173:351-353.
19. Kingzett-Taylor A, Tirman PFJ, Feller J, et al. Tendinosis and tears of gluteus medius and minimus muscles as a cause of hip pain: MR imaging findings. *AJR Am J Roentgenol* 1999; 173:1123-1126.
20. Dwek J, Pfirrmann C, Stanley A, et al. MR imaging of the hip abductors: normal anatomy and commonly encountered pathology at the greater trochanter. *Magn Reson Imaging Clin N Am* 2005; 13:691-704, vii.
21. Cunningham PM, Brennan D, O'Connell M, et al. Patterns of bone and soft-tissue injury at the symphysis pubis in soccer players: observation at MRI. *AJR Am J Roentgenol* 2007; 188:W291-W296.
22. Schilders E, Bismil Q, Robinson P, et al. Adductor-related groin pain in competitive athletes: role of adductor enthesis, magnetic resonance

imaging, and entheseal pubic cleft injections. *J Bone Joint Surg [Am]* 2007; 89:2173-2178.

23. Pritchard R, Shah H, Nelson C, FitzRandolph R. MR and CT appearance of iliopsoas bursal distention secondary to diseased hips. *J Comput Assist Tomogr* 1990; 14:797-800.

24. Fitzgerald R. Acetabular labrum tears: diagnosis and treatment. *Clin Orthop Relat Res* 1995; 311:60-68.

25. Czerny C, Hoffman S, Urban M, et al. MR arthrography of the adult acetabular capsular-labral complex: correlation with surgery and anatomy. *AJR Am J Roentgenol* 1999; 173:345-349.

26. Toomayan GA, Holman WR, Major NM, et al. Sensitivity of MR arthrography in the evaluation of acetabular labral tears. *AJR Am J Roentgenol* 2006; 186:449-453.

27. Yoon LS, Palmer WE, Kassarjiana A. Evaluation of radial-sequence imaging in detecting acetabular labral tears at hip MR arthrography. *Skeletal Radiol* 2007; 36:1029-1033.

28. Lage LA, Patel JV, Viller RN. The acetabular labral tear: an arthroscopic classification. *Arthroscopy* 1996; 12:269-272.

29. Blankenbaker DG, De Smet AA, Keene JS, et al. Classification and localization of acetabular labral tears. *Skeletal Radiol* 2007; 36:391-397.

30. Ganz R, Parvizi J, Beck M, et al. Femoroacetabular impingement: a cause for osteoarthritis of the hip. *Clin Orthop Relat Res* 2003; 417:112-120.

31. Notzli HP, Wyss TF, Stoecklin CH, et al. The contour of the femoral head-neck junction as a predictor for the risk of anterior impingement. *J Bone Joint Surg [Br]* 2002; 84:556-560.

32. Kassarjian A, Yoon LS, Belzile E, et al. Triad of MR arthrographic findings in patients with cam-type femoroacetabular impingement. *Radiology* 2005; 236:588-592.

33. Sietenrock KA, Schoeniger R, Ganz R. Anterior femoroacetabular impingement due to acetabular retroversion: treatment with periacetabular osteotomy. *J Bone Joint Surg [Am]* 2003; 85:278-286.

34. Tannast M, Siebenrock KA, Anderson SE. Femoroacetabular impingement: radiographic diagnosis—what the radiologist should know. *AJR Am J Roentgenol* 2007; 188:1540-1552.

35. Sanchez R, Quinn S. MRI of inflammatory synovial processes. *Magn Reson Imaging* 1989; 7:529-540.

36. Johnson N, Wood B, Jackman K. Complex infantile and congenital hip dislocation: assessment with MR imaging. *Radiology* 1988; 168:151-156.

37. Guidera K, Einbecker M, Berman C, et al. Magnetic resonance imaging evaluation of congenital dislocation of the hips. *Clin Orthop Relat Res* 1990; 261:96-101.

38. Terjesen T, Runden T, Johnsen H. Ultrasound in the diagnosis of dislocation of the hip joints in children older than two years. *Clin Orthop Relat Res* 1991; 262:159-169.

39. Flandry F, Hughston J, McCann S, Kurtz D. Diagnostic features of diffuse pigmented villonodular synovitis of the knee. *Clin Orthop Relat Res* 1994; 298:212-220.

40. Hermann G, Abdelwahab IF, Klein M, et al. Synovial chondromatosis. *Skeletal Radiol* 1995; 24:298-300.

Hip/Pelvis Protocols

This is one set of suggested protocols; there are many variations that would work equally well.

DEDICATED HIP MRI (NOT ARTHROGRAM)

Sequence No.	1	2	3	4
Sequence Type	T1	Fast spin echo with fat saturation	T1	Fast spin echo with fat saturation
Orientation	Axial	Axial	Coronal	Coronal
Field of View (cm)	14	14	14	14
Slice Thickness (mm)	4	4	4	4
Contrast	No	No	No	No

DEDICATED HIP MRI (ARTHROGRAM)

Sequence No.	1	2	3	4
Sequence Type	T1 with fat saturation	Fast spin echo T2 with fat saturation	T1 with fat saturation	Fast spin echo T2 with fat saturation
Orientation	Coronal	Coronal	Axial	Axial
Field of View (cm)	14	14	14	14
Slice Thickness (mm)	4	4	4	4
Contrast	(Intra-articular fluoroscopic guidance)*			

*Same solution as used for shoulders (see Chapter 10). Inject ~12-15 mL.

PELVIS MRI (FRACTURES/AVASCULAR NECROSIS)

Sequence No.	1	2	3	4
Sequence Type	T1	Fast spin echo with fat saturation	T1	Fast spin echo with fat saturation
Orientation	Coronal	Coronal	Axial	Axial
Field of View (cm)	32	32	32	32
Slice Thickness (mm)	7	7	7	7
Contrast	No	No	No	No

SAMPLE STANDARD REPORTS

MR Arthrogram of the Hip

Clinical Information

Protocol

After the intra-articular injection of contrast material, the MRI examination was performed according to the routine protocol

Discussion

1. **Acetabular labrum:** Normal; no tears, detachment, or degeneration shown

2. **Hip joint:** No synovitis, osteoarthritis, loose bodies, or other abnormalities

3. **Osseous structures:** Normal; no avascular necrosis, fractures, or other abnormalities

4. **Bursae:** No trochanteric or iliopsoas bursitis

5. **Soft tissues:** Muscles, tendons, and all other extra-articular soft tissues surrounding the hip appear normal

6. **Other abnormalities:** None

Opinion

Normal MR arthrogram of the (right/left) hip.

MRI of the Pelvis and Hips

Clinical Information

Protocol

The examination was performed using the routine protocol with multiple sequences and planes of imaging

Discussion

1. **Osseous structures:** Normal; no fracture, avascular necrosis, or other lesions

2. **Hip and sacroiliac joints:** Normal, without evidence of joint effusion or other abnormalities; no gross abnormalities of the acetabular labra are shown, but an MR arthrogram would be necessary for complete evaluation of the labra, if clinically indicated

3. **Bursae:** No trochanteric or iliopsoas bursitis shown

4. **Soft tissues:** Muscles and tendons of the pelvis and of both hips show no atrophy, edema, mass, tears, or other abnormalities

5. **Other abnormalities:** None

Opinion

Normal MRI of the pelvis and hips.

Knee

15

How to Image the Knee

See the protocols for knee MRI at the end of this chapter.

MRI of the knee is the most frequently requested MRI joint study in musculoskeletal radiology. The reasons for this are simple: it works, and so referring physicians request it. MRI provides a comprehensive examination of the knee, giving surgeons information they cannot obtain clinically or noninvasively. It also provides a road map for a surgeon performing arthroscopic or open surgery. It has proved to be very accurate, with sensitivity and specificity 90% to 95% for the menisci and close to 100% for the cruciate ligaments. This chapter shows how that kind of accuracy can be obtained.

- *Coils and patient position:* There are many ways to image the knee adequately, with different centers having differing imaging protocols based solely on personal preferences. We not only give which recipes work but also, more importantly, stress what should not be used. As with all joint imaging, a dedicated surface coil must be used. Most centers have a knee coil of some sort, and one seems to work as well as another. (At a cost of $10,000-$20,000 each, they should work well!) A small field of view should be used to maximize resolution. Generally, we use 14 to 16 cm, depending on the size of the patient. Slice thickness can be 3 to 5 mm, with 4 mm being the standard in most centers. A small interslice gap (0.4 mm) is used to reduce cross talk, unless volume imaging is employed. Having slice thickness less than 4 mm does not seem to increase accuracy and leads to more images to interpret, or information overload. A matrix of 256 × 192 or 256 × 256 is standard, with neither being better than the other. We try to have the knee in about 5 degrees of external rotation so that the anterior cruciate ligament (ACL) is orthogonal to the sagittal plane of imaging. This is typically the position of the knee in the relaxed state, and no effort at externally rotating the knee needs to be made in most patients.

- *Pulse sequences:* The menisci are best evaluated using sagittal images. It is necessary to have a short TE to see meniscal tears effectively. This can be in the form of conventional spin echo T1W, proton density, or gradient echo sequences. It has been shown conclusively that fast spin echo (FSE)–proton density (PD) images are unacceptable. Although there seems to be conflicting data on this subject, with several articles touting FSE-

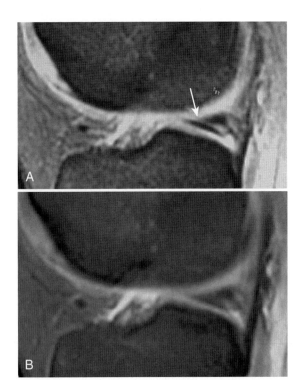

Figure 15-1 Meniscus tear not seen with fast spin echo sequence. **A,** Sagittal conventional spin echo–proton density (TR/TE 2000/20) image with fat suppression shows an oblique tear of the posterior horn of the medial meniscus (*arrow*). **B,** Sagittal fast spin echo–proton density (TR/TE 3000/16; ETL 4) image with fat suppression prospectively was called *normal*.

PD,[1,2] and others condemning it,[3,4] we strongly believe that many meniscal tears are missed using FSE-PD sequences. We compared conventional proton density sequences and FSE-PD sequences in 216 consecutive knees and found that the FSE-PD examination missed 42 tears that were seen on the conventional proton density sequences (Fig. 15-1). Our overall sensitivity for interpreting the menisci using conventional proton density sequences is 90% to 95%; using FSE-PD, our sensitivity was 80%.[5] Why is there such a difference in our results and in those of other investigators? In fact, there is not much difference. If one calculates the sensitivity for meniscal tears in the articles published on this subject, one would find that every publication has a sensitivity of around 80%. It seems all of the articles have the same results; however, the conclusions differ. It makes no sense to us to sacrifice accuracy in finding meniscus tears for the small decrease in imaging time that fast spin echo sequences give. The savings in time do not allow enough of a savings to increase patient throughput, and even if it did, it would not justify missing about 10% of the meniscal tears, which is exactly what happens with FSE-PD sequences. This may change with 3T imaging, but that remains to be seen. For evaluating the menisci, we use a 4-mm-thick sagittal spin echo–proton density sequence that has fat suppression. Fat suppression makes a more esthetic-looking image when looking at the menisci (Fig. 15-2). It increases the range of signal in the menisci and makes tears more conspicuous than without fat suppression. It has not been shown that it increases accuracy (in side-to-side comparison of hundreds of cases with and without fat suppression, we have found no examples of tears seen on one sequence and not on the other). Nevertheless, it gives the reader more confidence and makes for a pretty image, which is not all bad. We also use a 4-mm-thick sagittal FSE-T2W image with fat suppression, which is excellent for examining the cruciate ligaments, cartilage, and bones. A sagittal conventional spin echo–T2W image would suffice similarly, but does not have the same high signal-to-noise ratio or resolution as fast spin echo and takes more time. A STIR image also would suffice. A gradient echo sagittal image (volume or single slice) would do nicely for the cartilage and cruciates, but is unacceptable for examining the bones. Some centers use sagittal gradient echo to replace the T1W and the T2W image in the sagittal plane. This is a

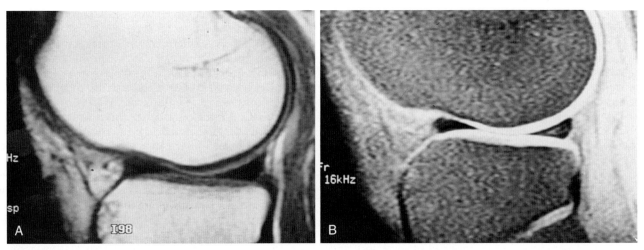

Figure 15-2 Use of fat suppression for the meniscus. **A,** Sagittal conventional spin echo–T1W image of the lateral meniscus without fat suppression shows most of the signal emanating from the marrow in the femur and tibia. **B,** The same sequence with fat suppression shows the meniscus to better advantage because of the suppression of signal from the marrow.

considerable time-saving technique. The marrow signal is examined with a marrow-sensitive sequence in the coronal or axial planes. The coronal plane is used to examine the collateral ligaments and serves as another plane to examine the cruciate ligaments if doubt exists on the sagittal plane. The coronal plane also is used to inspect the cartilage. It has not been shown to be a useful plane for the menisci. It is rare to see a meniscus tear on the coronal plane that is not seen on the sagittal images. We compiled the results of more than 200 consecutive knees in which we repeated our meniscus-sensitive sagittal sequence in the coronal plane and interpreted the coronal images separately from the sagittal images. In more than 400 menisci (two menisci/knee, >200 knees) we had only two menisci in which we saw tears that were not seen on the sagittal images. Arthroscopy was done on one meniscus, and no tear was found. We believe that a meniscus-sensitive sequence is unnecessary in the coronal plane. The coronal plane should have some sort of T2W image. If fast spin echo sequences are employed, fat suppression is recommended. It can be difficult to differentiate fat from fluid on high field strength magnets with fast spin echo. It is important to determine if fluid lies between the medial meniscus and the medial collateral ligament (MCL) to diagnose a meniscocapsular separation. A small fat pad often separates these structures and can be mistaken for fluid unless fat suppression is used. For many years, the coronal plane images were solely T1W. It took us years to realize that little, if any, information was gained using this sequence, but gradually we all moved to coronal T2W images. Only in hindsight do we see how foolish we were not to question why we were using T1W images in the coronal plane when we never saw any abnormalities. Most of us used T1W images in the coronal plane because everyone else did. (Talk about the emperor's new clothes!) The axial plane also should be imaged with some sort of T2 sequence. As in the coronal plane, nothing is gained using a T1W image, and much can be overlooked. This is the best plane to examine the patellar cartilage. The trochlear cartilage also is well seen on this sequence. Medial patellar plicae are best seen in this plane. A second (or third) look at the cruciate ligaments can be made on the axial images, and, similarly, the collateral ligaments can be reinspected. A knee protocol that works well consists of three planes of FSE-T2W images with fat suppression and a sagittal sequence that is conventional proton density with fat suppression. That's right, fat suppression on all four sequences, leaving us open to missing the dreaded lipoma of the knee. In 3 years of monitoring our accuracy using our MRI interpretations against the arthroscopy reports, we are satisfied that this is a solid imaging protocol that allows us a high accuracy for menisci, cruciate ligaments, collateral ligaments, and cartilage.

- *Contrast:* There is no place for gadolinium in routine imaging of the knee. MR arthrography has been advocated as useful in the postoperative knee to help differentiate between a repaired meniscus and a torn meniscus, but we have little experience with this.

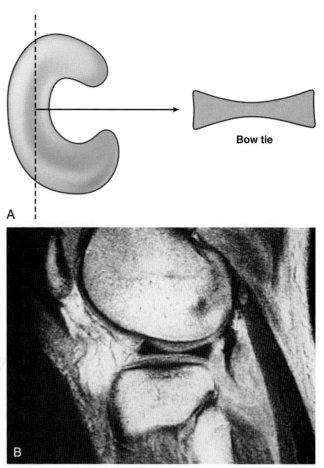

Figure 15-3 **Normal body segment of meniscus. A,** Schematic shows how a sagittal slice through the body of the meniscus gives an image of the meniscus that resembles a bow tie. **B,** Sagittal T1W image through the body of the lateral meniscus shows the normal bow tie appearance.

lateral m: A = P
Medial M: A < P

Normal and Abnormal

MENISCI

Normal

The menisci in the knee are C-shaped, fibrocartilaginous structures that are thick peripherally and thin centrally. A sagittal slice through the body segment should show the meniscus as an elongated rectangle or a bow tie, depending on how peripheral the sagittal slice is (Fig. 15-3). The medial and the lateral menisci should have two contiguous images of the body of the meniscus if 4- or 5-mm-thick slices are obtained. Three or four sagittal images should be seen through the anterior and posterior horns of the menisci (Fig. 15-4), with the posterior horn of the medial meniscus usually larger than the anterior horn. The anterior and posterior horns of the lateral meniscus are equal in size. The posterior horn of either meniscus should never be smaller than the anterior horn if it is normal.

The normal meniscus is devoid of signal on all imaging sequences, with the exception of children and young adults, who typically have some intermediate to high signal in the

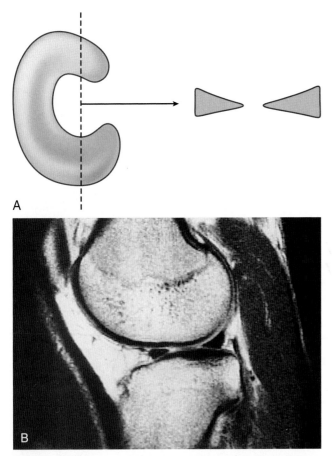

A

B

Figure 15-4 Normal anterior and posterior horns of the meniscus.
A, Schematic shows the appearance of a sagittal slice through the anterior and posterior horns of the meniscus. **B,** Sagittal T1W image through the anterior and posterior horns of the lateral meniscus.

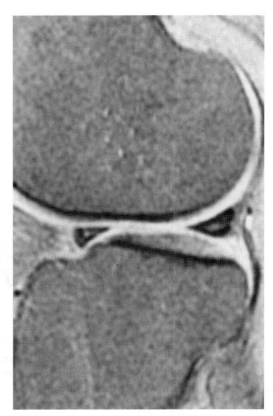

Figure 15-5 Myxoid or intrasubstance degeneration. Sagittal proton density image with fat suppression through the lateral meniscus shows some high signal in the anterior and posterior horns that does not disrupt an articular margin of the meniscus. This is myxoid degeneration.

posterior horns near the meniscal attachment to the capsule. This signal represents normal vascularity and should not be misinterpreted as meniscus degeneration. The vascularity of the meniscus is greatest near the periphery and is almost nonexistent near the free edge. Peripheral tears can be repaired, whereas more central tears cannot.

Abnormal

Several grading schemes for abnormal meniscus signal have been developed. They are not generally in widespread use because the only abnormal signal that has any real significance is that which disrupts the articular surface of a meniscus, representing a tear. Any signal that does not disrupt an articular surface, with one exception, which is covered in detail subsequently, is intrasubstance or myxoid degeneration (Fig. 15-5). Presumably, myxoid degeneration is a result of aging or wear and tear, but its cause is unknown. It is not a source of symptoms, does not always lead to meniscus tears, and is not treated clinically or surgically. Why mention it? If myxoid degeneration is prominent, it can be mentioned so that anyone else looking at the study would know we saw it, but judged the signal not to be a tear, rather than thinking

it was simply overlooked. Also, if it is especially prominent, there is a possibility that it might represent a meniscal cyst. Meniscal cysts are discussed in more detail later.

Tears

If high signal clearly disrupts an articular surface of the meniscus, it is an easy call: it is a torn meniscus. If high signal comes close to the articular surface, but does not quite reach the articular surface, it is an easy call: it is not a tear, it is intrasubstance degeneration. It is not always that clear-cut. In many cases, it is too close to call. In these situations, do the same thing radiologists do all the time—hedge. We are not being facetious. If you tell your orthopedic surgeons that when you call a tear or when you call no tear they can count on a correct diagnosis in more than 90% of the cases, they will find MRI examinations and your readings to be very helpful. You will be able to give a definitive diagnosis in about 90% of cases. You should explain that about 10% of the time you will be unable to discern definitely if the meniscus is torn or not. In those cases, the clinical examination is paramount. If the patient gets better with conservative care, it was probably not a torn meniscus. If the patient does not improve, the surgeon may decide to perform an arthroscopic procedure, in which case you would have told the surgeon where to look for a possible meniscus tear. It seems that 10% is the hedge rate for the menisci.[6-8]

Types of Meniscal Tears

- Oblique or horizontal
- Vertical
  - Flap
  - Bucket handle
- Peripheral
- Medially flipped flap tear
- Radial (parrot beak tear)
- Meniscocapsular separation

It has been shown that sensitivity for meniscal tears decreases considerably if there is an associated ACL tear.[9] There are several reasons for this. First, the meniscal tears that seem to occur when the ACL is torn are located in two places: the posterior horn of the lateral meniscus and in the periphery of the menisci (medial and lateral menisci). These are not the usual locations for meniscus tears and consequently often are overlooked. Also, several pitfalls occur in the posterior horn of the lateral meniscus that can be confused with meniscal tears, all of which are mentioned later in this chapter. Suffice it to say that when the ACL is torn, a close inspection should be done for a peripheral tear or for a tear in the posterior horn of the lateral meniscus.

Oblique or Horizontal Tears. There are many types of meniscal tears (Box 15-1). The most common is an *oblique* or *horizontal tear* (these are synonymous terms; some surgeons prefer one term over the other, and others use them interchangeably) that affects the undersurface of the posterior horn of the medial meniscus (Fig. 15-6). These commonly are degenerative in nature, rather than as a result of trauma.

Bucket-Handle Tears. Vertical longitudinal tears (Fig. 15-7) make up the common bucket-handle tear that occurs in about 10% of meniscal tears. The normal meniscus has a body width of about 9 mm, which is seen on two consecutive

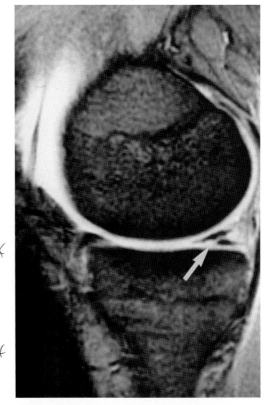

Figure 15-6 **Meniscus tear.** Sagittal image through the medial meniscus reveals an oblique tear of the posterior horn (*arrow*).

sagittal images as a single slab of meniscal tissue that has a shape similar to a bow tie. When the inner edge of the meniscus displaces, a bucket-handle tear is easily diagnosed by noting only one instead of the normal two body segments present on the outermost sagittal images through the meniscus (Fig. 15-8). This is called the *absent bow tie sign* because the body segments normally have a bow tie appearance on the sagittal images.[10] A displaced meniscal fragment should

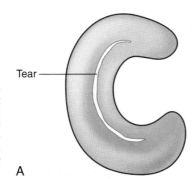

Figure 15-7 **Vertical longitudinal meniscus tear. A,** Schematic shows a meniscus with a vertical longitudinal tear. If the inner edge displaced, it would be called a *bucket-handle tear*. **B,** Sagittal image through a meniscus with a vertical tear (*arrow*).

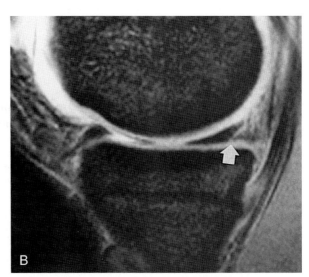

Bucket-Handle
Tear signs:
- absent bow-tie
- double PCL
- anterior flipped meniscus.

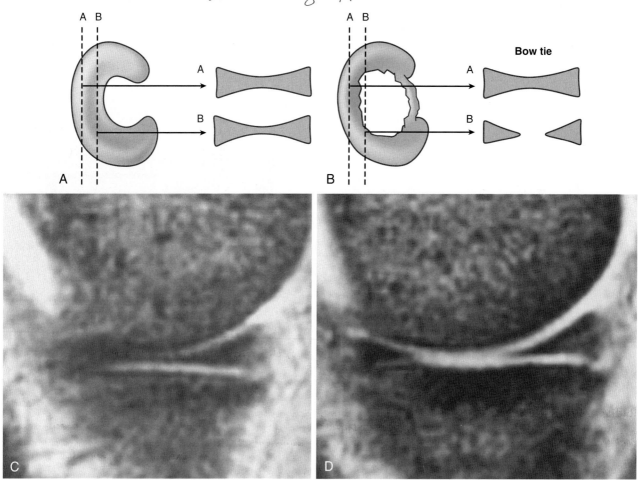

Bow tie

Figure 15-8 **Use of bow tie appearance to detect a bucket-handle tear. A,** Schematic shows how two sagittal images through the body normally produce two images of the meniscus that have a bow tie appearance. **B,** Schematic shows how, in a bucket-handle tear with the free edge of the meniscus displaced, only one sagittal image has a bow tie appearance. **C,** The first sagittal image through the medial meniscus in a patient with a bucket-handle tear shows the normal bow tie appearance. **D,** The next sagittal image in the same patient shows anterior and posterior horns, rather than another bow tie. This appearance is characteristic of a bucket-handle tear of the meniscus.

always be found, most often in the intercondylar notch (Fig. 15-9). A careful search for a fragment should be made when only one body segment is seen on the sagittal images. The displaced meniscal fragment can lie in front of the posterior cruciate ligament (PCL), which is called a *double PCL sign* (Fig. 15-10). The displaced fragment also may flip over the anterior horn of the affected meniscus, which is called an *anterior flipped meniscus sign* (Fig. 15-11). In any case, the absent bow tie sign is a very sensitive sign for a bucket-handle tear.

Although our original publication on the absent bow tie sign had a 97% sensitivity,[10] a subsequent publication of ours showed a sensitivity of around 90%.[11] Another publication[12] looked at all the MRI signs for a bucket-handle tear and reported only a 71% sensitivity for the absent bow tie sign. Nevertheless, it was the most reliable sign for detecting bucket-handle tears. Also, in the prospective reading of their 74 cases of bucket-handle tears, the investigators had only a 46% sensitivity (using the absent bow tie sign increased their

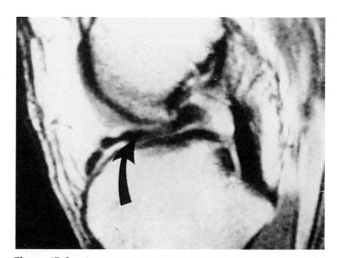

Figure 15-9 **Displaced fragment in a bucket-handle tear.** Sagittal image through the intercondylar notch in a patient with a bucket-handle tear shows the displaced fragment (*arrow*).

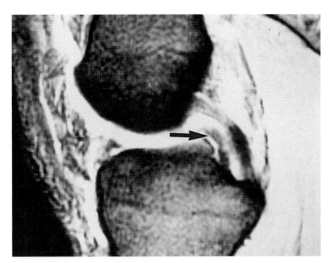

Figure 15-10 **Double posterior cruciate ligament sign.** Sagittal image through the intercondylar notch in a patient with a bucket-handle tear shows the displaced fragment anterior to the posterior cruciate ligament (*arrow*)—the double posterior cruciate ligament sign.

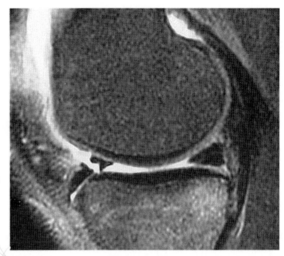

Figure 15-11 **Anterior flipped meniscus.** Sagittal image of the lateral meniscus in a patient with a bucket-handle tear shows the displaced fragment flipped onto the anterior horn—the anterior flipped meniscus sign.

sensitivity from 46% to 71%). We now rely on the absent bow tie sign only if we can identify the displaced meniscal fragment.

Radial or Free Edge Tears. The absent bow tie sign also is positive in free edge tears (also called *radial tears* or *parrot beak tears*). Free edge tears are common and are an unusual source of symptoms, unless they are large. The absent bow tie sign is useful in recognizing these tears. They are easily differentiated from bucket-handle tears because the second body segment, or bow tie, has only a small gap, rather than the large gap seen in bucket-handle tears (Fig. 15-12), and no displaced fragment is present. An investigation of about 200 knees that underwent arthroscopy by a single surgeon showed a 15% incidence of radial tears.[13] In that report we described three basic appearances of radial tears: (1) ghost,

(2) cleft, and (3) truncated triangle. A ghost meniscus is seen when a radial tear has completely traversed the meniscus (Fig. 15-13). The MRI slice is parallel to the tear, and partial volume averaging of the adjacent meniscal tissue creates an intermediate or gray signal. This is a severe type of meniscal tear and results in profound loss of the "hoop-stress" or springlike resistance of the meniscus. The meniscus usually extrudes off of the tibia (Fig. 15-14), and osteoarthritis ensues because of the lack of cushioning or protective effect of the meniscus with axial loading.

A cleft is the most reliable sign for a radial tear and is seen when the MRI slice is perpendicular to the tear (see Fig. 15-12). When the MRI slice is parallel to the same tear with a cleft, it results in a truncated triangle (Fig. 15-15). A radial tear usually, but not always, will have two of the signs,

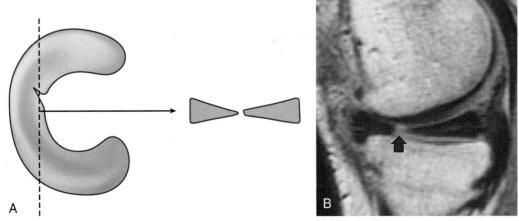

Figure 15-12 **Radial tear.** **A,** Schematic of a free edge or radial tear shows how the sagittal image has a small gap in the expected bow tie appearance. **B,** The sagittal image in a meniscus with a free edge or radial tear shows a small gap in the bow tie (*arrow*).

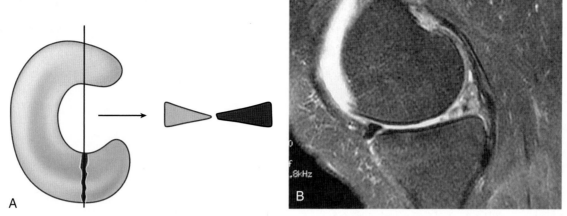

Figure 15-13 **Radial tear with a ghost meniscus. A,** Schematic shows how an image parallel to a large radial tear that involves the entire width of the meniscus posterior horn gives a ghost meniscus. **B,** Sagittal image through a large radial tear of the posterior horn with no normal posterior horn visible.

depending on the orientation of the tear to the imaging plane. At surgery, the free edge of a meniscus with a radial tear is treated with débridement and smoothing.

Medial Flipped Meniscus. A meniscus tear that can be seen with MRI but can be overlooked at arthroscopy is a flap tear of the medial meniscus with the flap of meniscus flipped into the medial gutter underneath the meniscus.[14] It can be missed at surgery if the surgeon fails to probe the medial gutter and deliver the flipped fragment. These are common tears and should be considered when the body segments look thinner than normal or have a piece of meniscus missing from the undersurface (Fig. 15-16). The medial flipped fragment can be seen on the coronal images lying just below and medial to the medial meniscus.

Description of Meniscal Tears. When a meniscal tear is identified and characterized as to which type (see Box 15-1), additional descriptors should include location (anterior horn, posterior horn, body); extent of the tear (which meniscal surface and length); and associated findings such as

meniscal cyst, discoid meniscus, or displaced fragments or flaps.

Cysts

Meniscal cysts occasionally are seen that involve a meniscus without the meniscus having a tear that extends to the articular surface. With weight bearing, the fluid in the cyst can be expressed into the adjacent soft tissues, where it is called

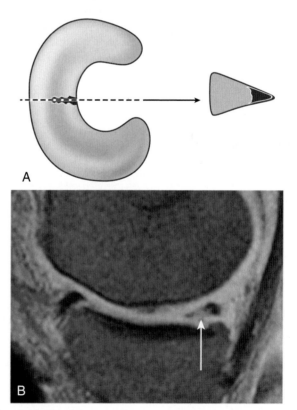

Figure 15-14 **Extruded meniscus resulting from a radial tear.** Coronal image through the posterior knee shows a cleft (*large arrow*) that has caused the meniscus to extrude off of the tibia (*small arrows*).

Figure 15-15 **Radial tear with a truncated triangle sign. A,** Schematic shows how an image parallel to a radial tear gives a truncated triangle. **B,** Sagittal image through a radial tear of the posterior horn shows a truncated triangle (*arrow*).

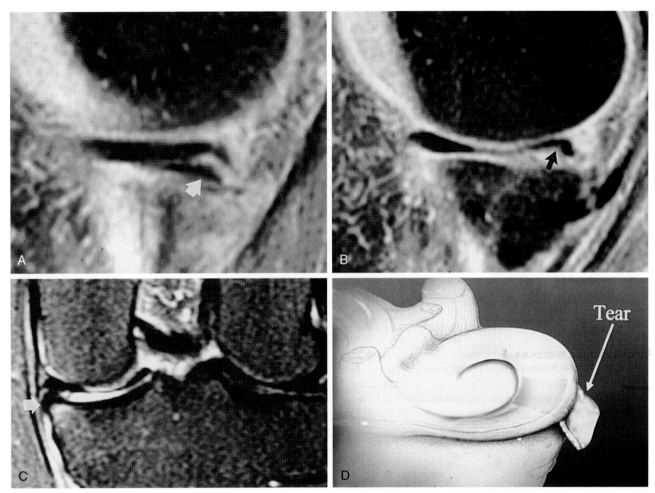

Figure 15-16   Medial flipped meniscus. A, The first sagittal image through the body of the medial meniscus in a patient with a medially displaced flap tear shows a small fragment of meniscus inferiorly displaced (*arrow*). **B,** The next adjacent sagittal image reveals a defect in the undersurface of the posterior portion of the body of the meniscus (*arrow*). This defect is the donor site for the displaced flap of meniscus seen in **A**. **C,** Coronal image shows the medially displaced flap of meniscus inferior to the body of the meniscus (*arrow*). **D,** An artist's depiction of a medially displaced flap tear.

a *parameniscal cyst* (Fig. 15-17). It is important to advise the surgeon of the presence of such a cyst because without a meniscal tear the cyst can be missed at arthroscopy. Also, many surgeons decompress a meniscal cyst that does not have a meniscal tear by an extra-articular approach, rather than via arthroscopy.[15] Most meniscal cysts do not exhibit marked high signal with T2W images, but the parameniscal component usually is very high in signal. When the cyst is confined to the meniscus, the signal resembles intrasubstance degeneration, only it is much more pronounced (Fig. 15-18). If a mass effect makes the meniscus appear swollen, it is an easy diagnosis; otherwise, it is a difficult call.

These cases are handled by suggesting a meniscal cyst versus severe intrasubstance degeneration—at least the surgeon is aware of the possibility of a meniscal cyst. A meniscal cyst often is noticed first by seeing on the most medial or lateral sagittal images through the body of the meniscus that the normal bow tie appearance has a horizontal stripe, which represents the collapsed meniscal cyst (Fig. 15-19). This often is called a *horizontal cleavage tear,* but that term is inappropriate because a true meniscal tear is not always present.

Discoid Meniscus

If more than two body segments are present on the sagittal images, a discoid meniscus should be considered (Fig. 15-20). A discoid meniscus is most likely a congenital (although some insist it is acquired) malformation of the meniscus in which the meniscus, in the most extreme form, is disk-shaped rather than C-shaped. Most discoid menisci are not completely disk-shaped, but have a wider than normal body of the meniscus. The lateral meniscus is most commonly affected, with an incidence reported of around 3%, whereas the medial meniscus is uncommonly affected. Often a discoid meniscus is enlarged and affects the anterior or posterior horns of the meniscus asymmetrically. In such a case, the anterior or posterior horn is much larger than its counterpart. Although often encountered incidentally, discoid menisci are more prone to undergo cystic degeneration with subsequent tears than a normal meniscus. Even without cystic changes or a tear, a discoid meniscus can cause symptoms and require surgery.[16]

A discoid meniscus that can cause symptoms without being torn is a Wrisberg variant of a discoid lateral meniscus.[17] This is a discoid meniscus that lacks attachments to the capsule via the normal struts or fascicles and lacks attachment to the tibia via the coronary or meniscotibial ligaments at the posterior horn of the meniscus (Fig. 15-21). This allows the posterior horn to sublux or fold into the joint with knee flexion, akin to a rug sliding or folding up on a slippery floor if it is not attached. In a Wrisberg variant of a discoid lateral meniscus, the only attachment to the posterior horn is the Wrisberg ligament—hence the name. It is important to inspect every discoid lateral meniscus closely for the normal struts or fascicles that surround the popliteus tendon and attach the meniscus to the capsule. If recognized, the surgeon can reattach the meniscus to the capsule and the tibia, rather than performing a meniscectomy. These are typically seen in children, and a meniscectomy at an early age leads to advanced osteoarthritis.

It is extremely valuable to recognize the normal bow tie appearance of the body segments in the medial and the lateral menisci as seen on sagittal images on every examination. Many of the aforementioned abnormalities can be rec-

ognized easily by noting the absence of the normal two body segments. These include the bucket-handle tear, radial tear, medially flipped flap tear, and meniscal cyst (Box 15-2). A discoid meniscus exhibits more than two body segments. Our routine search pattern on sagittal images includes a close inspection of the body segments to be certain there are two, and only two, bow ties that are not deformed in any way. Exceptions to this expectation would include a large patient (Shaquille O'Neal would undoubtedly have three or four bow ties), or very thin slices (the two bow tie rule applies only to slice thicknesses of 4 or 5 mm), and, as mentioned previously, a discoid meniscus.

Exceptions to the two bow tie rule that can mimic a bucket-handle tear (Box 15-3) can be seen in children or small adults in whom the menisci are small—only one bow tie is seen, but this is followed by only two or three images showing the anterior and posterior horns, rather than the usual three or four images; also, it occurs in both menisci. Simultaneous medial and lateral bucket-handle tears are rare. Another exception is in the postoperative knee where the free edge of the meniscus has been débrided. To recognize this situation, we have every patient fill out a form before the MRI examination that asks about prior surgery. The two bow tie rule can be broken if severe osteoarthritis is present or in older patients (>65 years old). These patients can wear down the free edge of the meniscus, leaving a very thin body segment that can be confused with a bucket-handle tear. None of these exceptions to the two bow tie rule would have a displaced meniscus as would a bucket-handle tear.

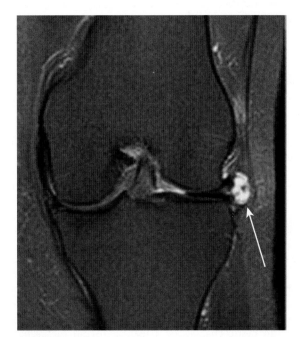

Figure 15-17 Meniscal cyst. Coronal image in a patient with a meniscal cyst of the lateral meniscus. A small parameniscal cyst (*arrow*) has resulted from the fluid in the meniscus being expressed into the adjacent soft tissues.

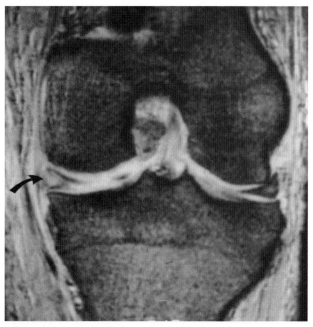

Figure 15-18 Meniscal cyst. Medial meniscal cyst is noted (*arrow*), which gives a slightly swollen appearance to the meniscus. The lateral meniscus has marked intrasubstance degeneration, which should not be mistaken for a meniscal cyst.

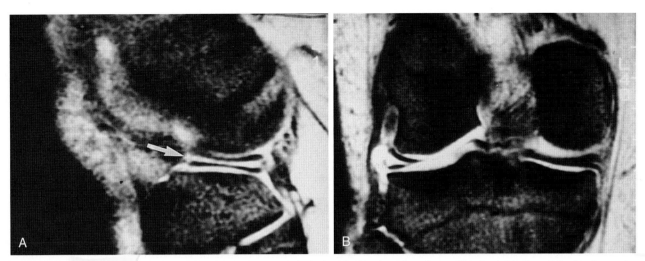

Figure 15-19   Meniscal cyst. A, Sagittal gradient echo image through the body of the lateral meniscus shows a high signal stripe (*arrow*) bisecting the meniscus. **B,** Coronal image reveals a meniscal cyst with a small parameniscal cyst attached.

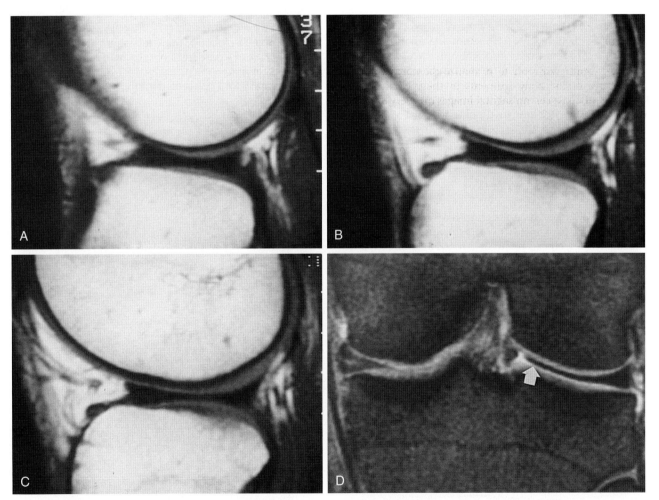

Figure 15-20   Discoid lateral meniscus. A-C, Successive sagittal images through the lateral meniscus show a bow tie appearance, indicating the body segment is present on more than two images. This appearance should suggest a discoid meniscus. **D,** Coronal image reveals that the meniscus extends almost into the intercondylar notch (*arrow*), indicative of a discoid lateral meniscus.

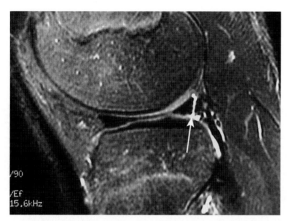

Figure 15-21 **Wrisberg variant of a discoid lateral meniscus.** Sagittal image in a young boy with a discoid lateral meniscus reveals no attachment of the meniscus to the capsule (*arrows*), which is indicative of a Wrisberg variant.

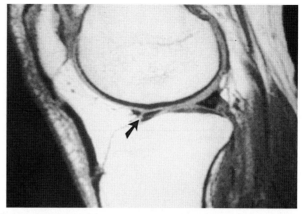

Figure 15-22 **Transverse ligament.** Sagittal image through the lateral meniscus shows a transverse ligament inserting onto the anterior horn (*arrow*), creating a pseudotear.

Pitfalls

A few pitfalls involving the menisci warrant mention.

Transverse Ligament. An easy pitfall to recognize is the insertion of the transverse ligament on the anterior horns of the menisci. The transverse ligament runs across the anterior aspect of the knee in Hoffa's fat pad from the anterior horn of the medial meniscus to the anterior horn of the lateral meniscus. Its function is unknown, and it is not present in every knee. At its insertion on the anterior horn of the lateral meniscus, it often has the appearance of a meniscus tear (Fig. 15-22). It can reliably be differentiated from a tear by following it across the knee in Hoffa's fat pad on sequential sagittal images. It uncommonly causes a similar pseudotear appearance on the medial meniscus.

Speckled Anterior Horn Lateral Meniscus. The anterior horn of the lateral meniscus occasionally has a speckled appearance, which can resemble a macerated or torn anterior horn (Fig. 15-23). This appearance is caused by fibers of the ACL inserting into the meniscus. It is reported to be seen in 60% of normal patients.[18]

Meniscofemoral Ligament Insertion. The posterior horn of the lateral meniscus has several pitfalls that mimic tears. Insertion of the meniscofemoral ligament of Humphry or Wrisberg can give the appearance of a meniscal tear (Fig. 15-24). A meniscofemoral ligament is present in about 75% of knees. It originates on the medial femoral condyle and runs obliquely across the knee in the intercondylar notch (Fig. 15-25), anterior (ligament of Humphry) or posterior (ligament of Wrisberg) to the PCL (Fig. 15-26), and inserts

into the posterior horn of the lateral meniscus. When considering a pseudotear from the insertion of one of the meniscofemoral ligaments, one needs to follow the ligament through the intercondylar notch to the PCL on sequential sagittal images. In 2% to 3% of knees, both ligaments (Humphry and Wrisberg) are present. The function of the meniscofemoral ligament has not been clearly established, and no injury to it has been described.

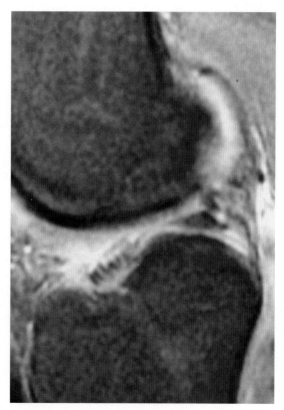

Figure 15-23 **Speckled anterior horn lateral meniscus.** Sagittal image through the lateral meniscus shows the anterior horn with a speckled appearance. This is a normal variant created by fibers of the anterior cruciate ligament inserting into the meniscus.

BOX 15-3

Pitfalls in Absent Bow Tie Sign

- Children or small adults
- Postoperative
- Severe osteoarthritis
- Older patients (>65 years old)

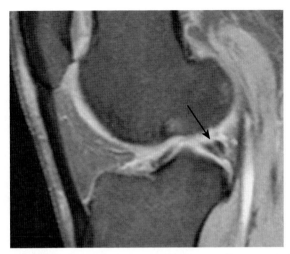

Figure 15-24 Pseudotear from meniscofemoral ligament. Sagittal image through the lateral meniscus shows the posterior horn with a pseudotear (*arrow*) caused by the insertion of one of the meniscofemoral ligaments.

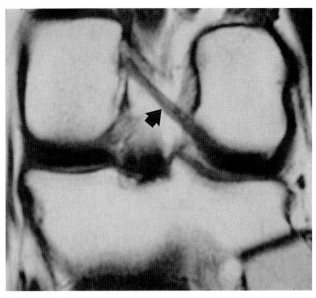

Figure 15-25 Meniscofemoral ligament. Coronal image shows a meniscofemoral ligament (*arrow*) extending obliquely across the intercondylar notch.

Pulsation From Popliteal Artery. The popliteal artery is just posterior to the posterior horn of the lateral meniscus, and pulsation artifact can extend through the meniscus, making it difficult to examine or, in some instances, giving the appearance of a torn meniscus (Fig. 15-27). This appearance is rectified easily by swapping the phase and frequency direction before scanning so that the vessel pulsation extends superior to inferior rather than anterior to posterior.

Magic Angle Phenomenon. Occasionally, the posterior horn of the lateral meniscus has an ill-defined, hazy appear-ance with diffuse intermediate signal seen on proton density or T1W images (Fig. 15-28A and B). This is due to the magic angle phenomenon.[19] The posterior horn of the lateral meniscus slopes upward at around 55 degrees, which is the angle at which high signal begins to be seen in certain collagen-containing structures if the TE is short.[20] It disap-pears on the T2W sequences or if the 55-degree angle is

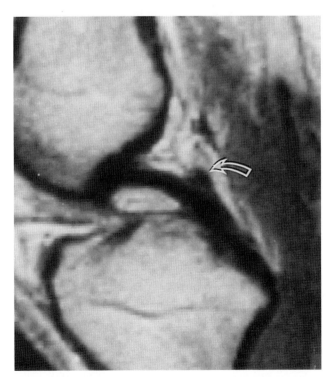

Figure 15-26 Ligament of Wrisberg. Sagittal image through the intercondylar notch shows a ligament of Wrisberg (*arrow*) just posterior to the posterior cruciate ligament.

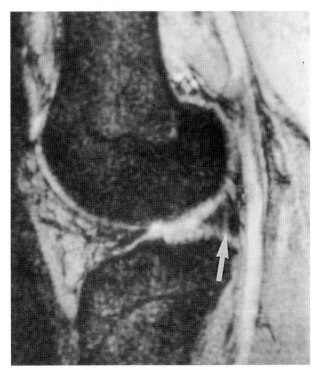

Figure 15-27 Popliteal artery pulsation artifact. Sagittal gradient echo image through the lateral meniscus has a pulsation artifact from the popliteal artery that mimics a tear of the posterior horn (*arrow*).

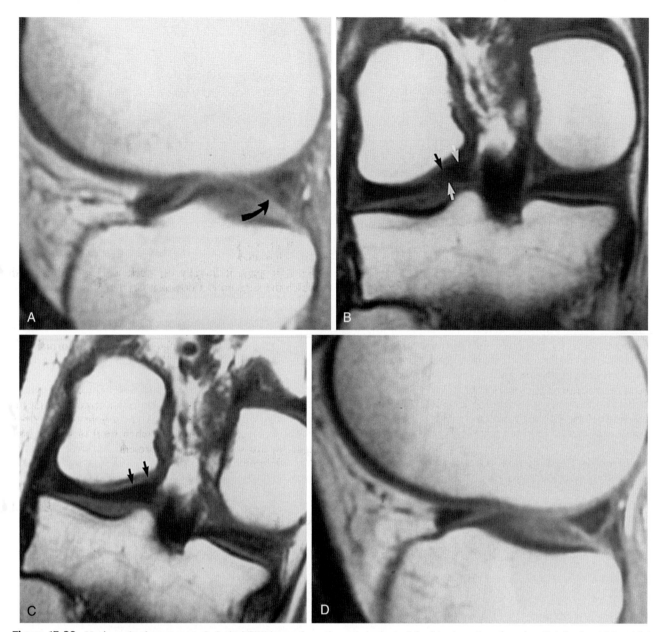

Figure 15-28 **Magic angle phenomenon. A,** Sagittal T1W image shows the posterior horn of the lateral meniscus (*arrow*) as ill-defined and intermediate signal. **B,** Coronal T1W image again shows the posterior horn to be ill-defined and intermediate in signal (*arrows*). The posterior horn slopes upward at an angle of about 55 degrees. **C,** Coronal T1W image taken with the knee abducted to flatten out the angle of the posterior horn now shows the meniscus sharply and without signal (*arrows*). **D,** Sagittal T1W image through the abducted lateral meniscus shows the posterior horn sharply and without intermediate signal. The signal and hazy appearance in **A** and **B** are from the magic angle effect.

changed (see Fig. 15-28C and D). This has not proved to be a big problem in hiding meniscus tears, so imaging with the knee abducted has not been recommended.

Popliteus Tendon Pseudotear. The popliteus tendon originates on the lateral femoral condyle and extends inferiorly between the posterior horn of the lateral meniscus and the joint capsule. It runs obliquely and extends posteriorly to join its muscle belly, which lies just posterior to the proximal tibia. Where the tendon passes between the meniscus and the capsule, it can give the appearance of a meniscus tear

(Fig. 15-29); this should be recognized as a normal structure and not confused with a tear. A vertical tear of the posterior horn of the lateral meniscus should not be confused with the popliteus tendon (Fig. 15-30). This type of tear often occurs when there is an ACL tear, and care should be taken to account for the normal popliteus tendon so that a meniscus tear is not overlooked.

Because the sensitivity for meniscal tears is known to decrease when the ACL is torn, and many of the missed tears occur in the posterior horn of the lateral meniscus, close attention should be directed to this area when an ACL tear

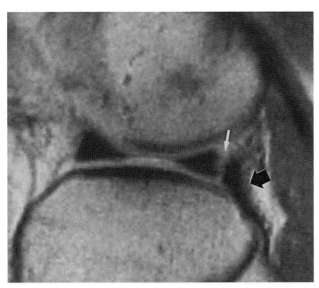

Figure 15-29 **Popliteus tendon pseudotear.** Sagittal image through the lateral meniscus shows the popliteus tendon (*black arrow*) passing close to the posterior horn of the meniscus, creating a pseudotear (*white arrow*) appearance.

is present. Knowing the pitfalls that involve the posterior horn of the lateral meniscus is imperative to a high accuracy rate (Box 15-4).

LIGAMENTS

Anterior Cruciate Ligament

The normal ACL has straight, taut fibers that run parallel to the roof of the intercondylar notch (Fig. 15-31). It typically has a striated appearance with some high signal within it, especially at its insertion on the tibia. T2W sagittal images are recommended for evaluating the ACL. If the ACL is not

BOX 15-4

Pitfalls Involving the Posterior Horn of the Lateral Meniscus

- Meniscofemoral ligament insertion
- Pulsation artifact from popliteal artery
- Magic angle phenomenon
- Popliteus tendon

clearly seen as normal or as torn on sagittal images, axial and coronal images should be used to examine the ACL further, but this is unnecessary except in rare instances. Accuracy of MRI for the ACL is extremely high, approaching 95% to 100% in almost all reported series.[21-23]

A torn ACL usually is obvious by the fact that no normal-appearing fibers of the ACL can be identified (Fig. 15-32). When it tears, it literally explodes, leaving nothing with which the surgeon can do a primary repair. A tendon graft (usually from the patella tendon or the hamstrings) is used to reconstruct the ACL when necessary. Occasionally, an ACL tear is seen in which the fibers of the torn ACL are seemingly intact, but the angle is flatter than normal (Fig. 15-33). As mentioned, the fibers should be parallel to the roof of the intercondylar notch.

A partial tear of the ACL is treated nonoperatively, and the imaging literature has very little concerning accuracy in diagnosing partial tears of the ACL. A sprain or partial tear of the ACL can be mentioned when focal or diffuse high signal or laxity of the ACL is present. There is no way of determining the validity of these findings because surgeons are equally unable to diagnose partial tears confidently. A pitfall that can lead the unwary to call an ACL tear when it is an essentially normal ligament is an ACL cyst. An ACL cyst is an entity of unknown cause in which the ACL is distended with mucinous fluid (Fig. 15-34). The normal ACL fibers are not clearly identified and appear to be disrupted; however, these patients have no instability and usually are

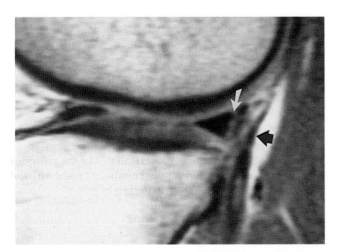

Figure 15-30 **Popliteus tendon pseudotear.** Sagittal image through the lateral meniscus shows a peripheral vertical tear of the posterior horn (*white arrow*), which erroneously was thought to be the popliteus tendon. The popliteus tendon can be seen just posterior to the meniscus (*black arrow*).

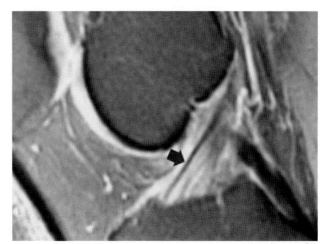

Figure 15-31 **Normal anterior cruciate ligament.** Sagittal fast spin echo–T2W image through the intercondylar notch shows a normal anterior cruciate ligament (*arrow*), with the anterior band parallel to the roof of the notch.

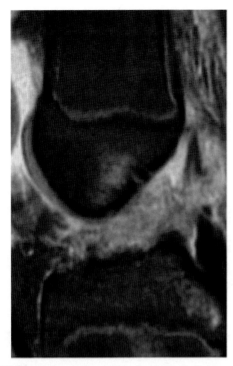

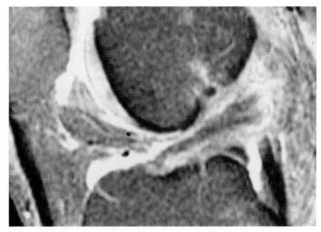

Figure 15-33 Torn anterior cruciate ligament. Sagittal image through the intercondylar notch shows the anterior cruciate ligament to be flatter than the roof of the notch. Also, its origin off the femur could not be identified. This is a torn anterior cruciate ligament.

Figure 15-32 Torn anterior cruciate ligament. Sagittal image through the intercondylar notch shows the anterior cruciate ligament to be disrupted, with no normal fibers identified.

asymptomatic. At most, they have a feeling of swelling or fullness in the knee and are unable to flex the knee fully because of the mass effect. The ACL has a drumstick appearance on sagittal images and appears cystic on coronal or axial images. We have seen this in about 1% of all our knee MRI examinations. One report in the surgery literature tells of mistaking an ACL cyst for a tumor, with subsequent resection of the normal ACL.[24]

After surgery to reconstruct the ACL, we occasionally are asked to reimage a patient because of pain or instability. The ACL graft should be present as a taut structure, usually with some increased signal on T2W sagittal images (Fig. 15-35). If the graft is disrupted or absent, it has failed. The

tibial tunnel should be parallel to the roof of the femoral intercondylar notch. If it is too steep, the graft is impinged by the femur on extension of the knee (Fig. 15-36). If it is too flat, it may be too lax and not provide the needed stability.

One of the most common reasons for pain after knee arthroscopy is the presence of arthrofibrosis (scar) in Hoffa's fat pad. This arthrofibrosis can have several appearances and may require reoperation. A round mass of scar in Hoffa's fat pad, called a *cyclops lesion,* can interfere with knee extension and often needs to be resected (Fig. 15-37). A linear scar that extends to the inferior pole of the patella can restrict patellar motion and cause pain (Fig. 15-38).[25]

Posterior Cruciate Ligament

The PCL normally is seen as a low signal structure in the intercondylar notch, gently curving between the posterior tibia and the femur (Fig. 15-39). It is infrequently torn and even less frequently surgically repaired. When it tears, it typically does not have an actual disruption of the fibers, as is seen with other ligaments, but rather it stretches and is not

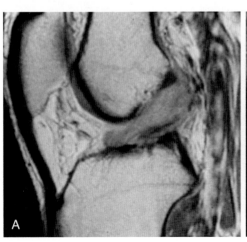

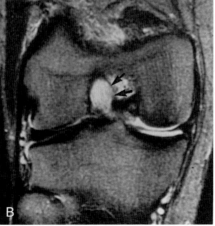

Figure 15-34 Anterior cruciate ligament cyst. **A,** Sagittal proton density image through the intercondylar notch shows the anterior cruciate ligament as a cystic, drumstick-shaped structure without clearly identifiable fibers. **B,** Coronal fast spin echo–T2W image shows the anterior cruciate ligament to have a cystic appearance (*arrows*). This is characteristic of an anterior cruciate ligament cyst.

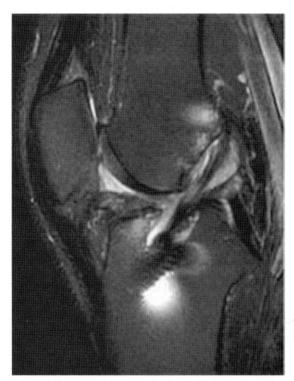

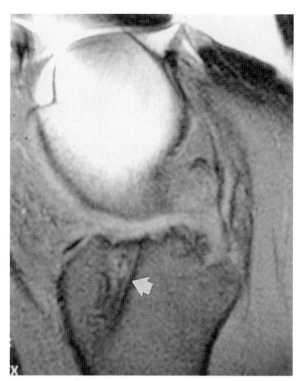

Figure 15-35 **Anterior cruciate ligament graft intact.** Sagittal T2W image through the intercondylar notch in a patient with a prior anterior cruciate ligament reconstruction shows the anterior cruciate ligament graft to be intact. It has some increased signal, which is normal in reconstructions.

Figure 15-36 **Torn anterior cruciate ligament graft.** Sagittal fast spin echo–T2W image in a patient with a prior anterior cruciate ligament reconstruction fails to show the anterior cruciate ligament graft because it is disrupted. The tibial tunnel (*arrow*) is steeper than the roof of the intercondylar notch, allowing the femur to impinge on the graft when the knee is in extension.

structurally competent, more like overstretching the elastic in one's socks. On MRI, it most commonly has a fat, gray appearance on proton density or T1W images (Fig. 15-40) and does not have high signal on T2W images (Fig. 15-41) (although PCL tears have been reported to be high signal on STIR sequences). Because this appearance is contrary to

most injured structures, it has been our experience that tears of the PCL frequently are missed. If the PCL avulses from its tibial attachment, it is easily diagnosed, but this is an uncommon presentation. Orthopedic surgeons are repairing the PCL more frequently than in the past, but in most cases a

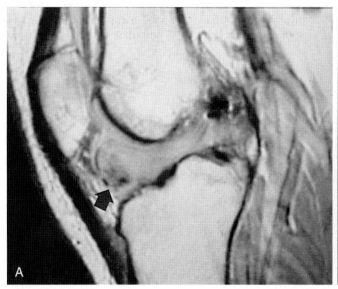

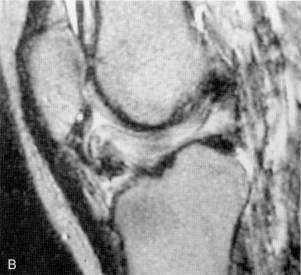

Figure 15-37 **Cyclops lesion. A,** Sagittal proton density image in a patient with a prior anterior cruciate ligament reconstruction shows scar tissue in Hoffa's fat pad (*arrow*). **B,** On a sagittal T2W image, the scar stays low in signal. It has a rounded configuration, which has been termed a *cyclops lesion*. This is arthrofibrosis secondary to the surgery.

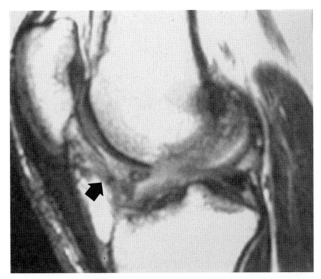

Figure 15-38   Arthrofibrosis. Sagittal proton density image in a patient with a prior anterior cruciate ligament reconstruction shows scar tissue in Hoffa's fat pad (*arrow*), which is linear in configuration and extends to the inferior pole of the patella. This form of arthrofibrosis can cause patellar pain and patellar tracking abnormalities.

torn PCL is not repaired. For most cases, it does not matter what you say about the PCL—the surgeon will not even inspect it at arthroscopy. We should be able to tell the surgeon with a high degree of accuracy if the PCL is torn or not, however.

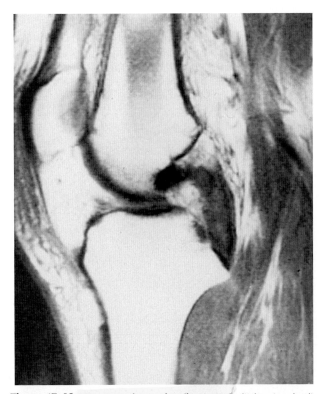

Figure 15-40   Torn posterior cruciate ligament. Sagittal proton density image through the intercondylar notch shows a torn posterior cruciate ligament that is thicker than normal and has uniform intermediate signal, rather than low signal.

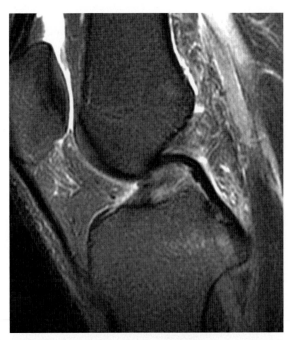

Figure 15-39   Normal posterior cruciate ligament. Sagittal T1W image through the intercondylar notch shows a normal posterior cruciate ligament with uniform low signal.

We measured the PCL width on sagittal images in 200 consecutive knee MR images and found 192 (96%) to be 6 mm or less (range, 4-7 mm), and then measured the PCL in 37 surgically confirmed torn PCLs. Thirty-five of 37 (94%) were 7 mm or greater (range, 4-15 mm). A PCL that has increased signal on T1 or proton density sequences and is thicker than 6 mm likely is torn.

Medial Collateral Ligament

The MCL originates on the medial aspect of the distal femur and inserts on the medial aspect of the proximal tibia. Its fibers are intimately interlaced with the joint capsule at the level of the joint, and the medial meniscus is attached directly to it. It is not an intrasynovial structure; it is not seen or repaired arthroscopically. Accuracy of MRI has not been established, but it is generally agreed that MRI is highly accurate in depicting the MCL.

The three grades of injury described clinically correspond to three appearances of the MCL seen with T2W coronal images. Grade 1, a sprain, shows high signal in the soft tissues medial to the MCL (Fig. 15-42). Grade 2, a severe sprain or partial tear, shows high signal in the soft tissues medial to the MCL, but also has high signal or partial disruption of the MCL itself (Fig. 15-43). Grade 3, or complete tear, shows disruption of the MCL (Fig. 15-44). The MCL is seldom repaired even if it is completely disrupted, unless multiple other ligaments are torn. Grade 1 and 2 sprains usually are treated conservatively with bracing and continuance of athletic activities as pain allows. High signal medial to the MCL may occur from causes unrelated to an MCL sprain, such as a radial tear of the meniscus or with osteoarthritis.[26]

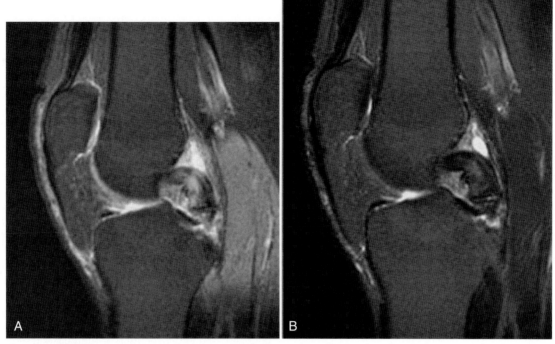

Figure 15-41   Torn posterior cruciate ligament. A, Sagittal proton density image through the intercondylar notch shows a posterior cruciate ligament that has torn off its insertion on the posterior tibia. The body of the posterior cruciate ligament is thicker than normal and has intermediate signal throughout. **B,** Fast spin echo–T2W image shows how the posterior cruciate ligament does not have increased signal even though it is torn.

A meniscocapsular separation is easily diagnosed on T2W coronal images by noting fluid between the MCL and the medial meniscus. This separation can be overlooked on T1W coronal images (Fig. 15-45). Because these patients present clinically in an identical manner to a patient with a sprained MCL, they often are allowed to continue their activities with a brace. This is unacceptable treatment for a meniscocapsular separation. The vascular interface between the MCL and the meniscus can become avascular with continued activity, resulting in a meniscus that does not heal to the capsule. These patients need either immobilization or surgical repair. If the meniscocapsular separation is isolated solely to the area of the MCL, it can be considered a partial tear of the deep fibers of the MCL. If the separation is over only a short portion of the meniscal attachment, it is unlikely to be significant. A meniscocapsular

Figure 15-42   Grade 1 medial collateral ligament sprain. Coronal gradient echo image in a patient with an injury to the medial collateral ligament (MCL) shows increased signal in the soft tissues medial to the MCL (*arrows*) with a normal-appearing MCL. This is a grade 1 MCL sprain.

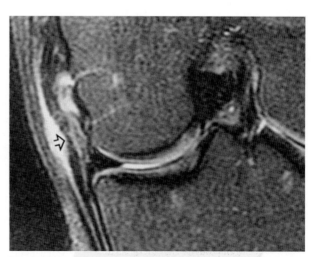

Figure 15-43   Grade 2 medial collateral ligament sprain. Coronal fast spin echo–T2W image shows increased signal in a thinned but otherwise intact medial collateral ligament (*arrow*)—a grade 2 sprain.

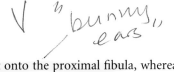

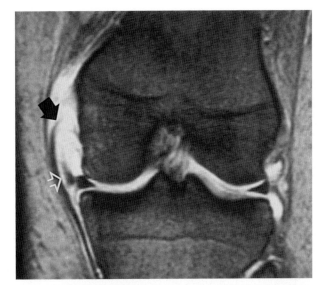

Figure 15-44 Torn medial collateral ligament and meniscocapsular separation. Coronal gradient echo image reveals a complete tear of the medial collateral ligament (*solid arrow*). Note also the fluid tracking between the medial collateral ligament and the meniscus (*open arrow*). This indicates a meniscocapsular separation because it could be seen on multiple adjacent images.

separation that extends posteriorly, involving the posterior oblique ligament (a thickening of the capsule at the joint line posterior to the MCL), seems to be more significant in terms of stability than one that is solely medial or anterior (Fig. 15-46).

Lateral Collateral Ligament

The lateral collateral ligament (LCL) complex is composed of many structures, but only three that are easily evaluated with MRI; posterior to anterior, they are the biceps femoris tendon, the fibulocollateral ligament (the true LCL) (Fig. 15-47A), and the iliotibial band. The biceps and the fibulo-

collateral ligament insert onto the proximal fibula, whereas the iliotibial band inserts onto Gerdy's tubercle on the anterior tibia. Tears of the lateral ligament (Fig. 15-47B) are not nearly as common as tears of the MCL. LCL tears often are associated with injury to other structures in the *posterolateral corner of the knee,* as this area is called.

Additional important structures in the posterolateral corner that can be seen on most, but not all, MRI studies include the arcuate ligament and the popliteofibular ligament. The arcuate ligament is Y-shaped and runs from the fibular styloid process to the lateral femoral condyle, with one limb inserting into the lateral joint capsule. Disruption of the capsule at the joint line is a reliable indicator of a tear of the arcuate ligament (Fig. 15-48).

The popliteofibular ligament is thought to be one of the strongest lateral stabilizers in the knee. It can be identified on most MRI studies by finding the lateral geniculate vessels on the coronal images and noting the ligament just beneath them (Fig. 15-49A). On sagittal images, it can be seen just superficial to the popliteus tendon and inserts onto the fibula (see Fig. 15-49B).

Injury to a component of the LCL in association with tears of the popliteus tendon, arcuate ligament, popliteofibular ligament, and either the ACL or the PCL is termed *posterolateral corner injury.* Such injury results in pain and instability with knee hyperextension if not surgically corrected. It is one of the few knee injuries that many surgeons consider a near-emergency. Failure to treat a posterolateral corner injury surgically in 10 to 14 days is said to have a high incidence of a poor result.[27] These knees are often operated on without delay.

The popliteus tendon can tear as an isolated injury, but usually tears in conjunction with other structures, as in posterolateral corner injuries or complete knee dislocations. A popliteus tear usually occurs at the musculotendinous junction and results in a large amount of fluid in the popliteus tendon sheath, a lax popliteus tendon, and high signal in or around the popliteus muscle (Fig. 15-50).[28]

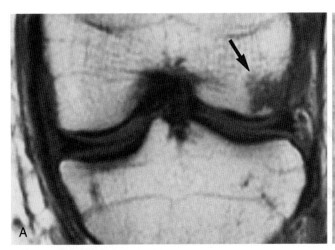

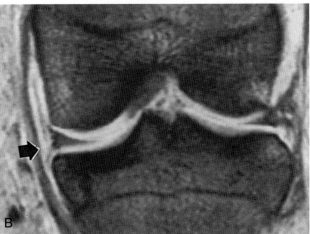

Figure 15-45 Meniscocapsular separation. **A,** Coronal T1W image in a patient with a blow to the lateral side of the knee shows a contusion on the lateral femoral condyle (*arrow*). **B,** Coronal gradient echo image shows fluid tracking between the medial meniscus and the medial collateral ligament (*arrow*), which indicates a meniscocapsular separation. In **A,** a meniscocapsular separation cannot be diagnosed.

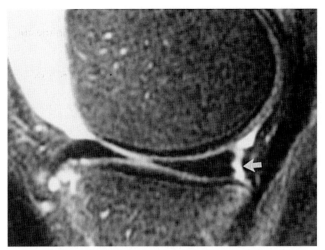

Figure 15-46 **Meniscocapsular separation.** Sagittal fast spin echo–T2W image through the medial meniscus shows fluid between the posterior horn attachment and the capsule (*arrow*). This indicates a meniscocapsular separation.

Pain in the anterolateral knee often is found in runners because of the iliotibial band rubbing on the lateral femoral condyle. This entity is called *iliotibial band friction syndrome* or *iliotibial band syndrome.*[29] It is easily diagnosed on MRI by noting fluid on both sides of the iliotibial band (Fig. 15-51). In the earlier stages, there may be only fluid or edema deep to the iliotibial band; this can be very difficult, if not impossible, to distinguish from fluid in the joint that has extended posterolaterally. If there is no joint fluid present, edema between the iliotibial band and the femur is a reliable indicator of iliotibial band syndrome (Fig. 15-52). It is seen most easily on axial images. The iliotibial band may have thickening or high signal within its fibers, but in our experience it usually has high signal around it. Iliotibial band syndrome can be confused clinically with a lateral meniscus tear, and imaging can play a vital role in avoiding unnecessary surgery.

PATELLA

Dislocation of the patella frequently is diagnosed with MRI, to the surprise of the referring physician. Because the dislocated patella often rapidly reduces on its own, only about half of patients with patella dislocations are aware of what really occurred. They get referred for imaging with the nebulous "rule out internal derangement" history. The MRI examination usually is easily interpreted as a patella dislocation.[30] A contusion characteristically occurs on the anterior lateral femoral condyle (Fig. 15-53A). The contusion is from the impaction of the patella as it either dislocates or reduces. There may or may not be a kissing contusion on the medial side of the patella. The medial retinaculum is always injured, although a frank tear can be difficult to appreciate. The key finding is the patellar cartilage. If a piece of cartilage is missing, it usually means an arthroscopic procedure is necessary (see Fig. 15-53B), whereas if the cartilage is normal, the patient usually is treated conservatively. The main role of the radiologist is to examine the patellar cartilage

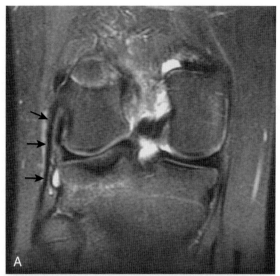

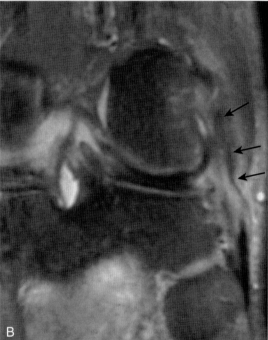

Figure 15-47 **Normal and torn fibulocollateral ligament. A,** Coronal T2W image shows a normal fibulocollateral ligament (*arrows*). **B,** This coronal fast spin echo–T2W image shows a torn fibulocollateral ligament (*arrows*).

carefully. One also should evaluate the depth of the trochlear notch, which often is hypoplastic in patients with dislocating patellae and is a predisposing factor to subsequent dislocations.

SYNOVIAL PLICAE

A thin, fibrous band frequently is seen on axial images that extends from the medial joint capsule toward the medial facet of the patella (Fig. 15-54). This is a normal structure, the medial patella plica, which is a remnant of the embryologic development of the knee.[31] Embryologically, the knee is divided into compartments by superior, inferior, and medial patella plicae. More than half of all normal knees

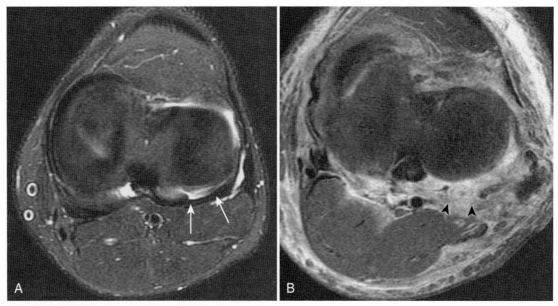

Figure 15-48 **Normal and torn arcuate ligament. A,** Axial image at the joint line shows the normal posterior capsule (*arrows*) which indicates the arcuate ligament is intact. **B,** Axial image through the joint line in another patient shows a large gap in the posterior capsule (*arrowheads*) which indicates that the arcuate ligament is torn.

show one or more of the plicae on MRI. The medial patella plica can become thickened, stiff, and trapped between the patella and the femur, causing pain, clicking, and locking, similar to a torn meniscus. No measurements are used to diagnose a thickened medial patellar plica. With experience, it becomes obvious when the plica appears to be too thick (Fig. 15-55). An axial T2W image and joint fluid are required to visualize the medial plica. An inflamed plica is easily removed at arthroscopy, but plica syndrome is an uncommon diagnosis.

The other plicae found in the knee are the suprapatellar plica and the infrapatellar plica. They commonly are seen on MR images. The suprapatellar plica can be imperforate and divide the suprapatellar pouch into a separate compartment. Rarely, pigmented villonodular synovitis, synovial chromatosis, or even a loculated effusion in this space can manifest as a mass in the anterior thigh that is mistaken for a tumor.

The infrapatellar plica originates in the inferior pole of the patella and extends through Hoffa's fat pad to the transverse

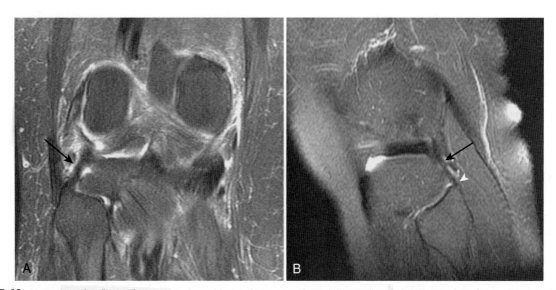

Figure 15-49 **Normal popliteofibular ligament. A,** Coronal image shows a prominent, intact popliteofibular ligament (*arrow*) extending from the popliteus tendon to the fibular styloid process. The lateral geniculate artery is just beneath the tip of the *arrow*. **B,** Sagittal image depicts the popliteofibular ligament (*arrow*) inserting on the fibular styloid process (*arrowhead*).

[handwritten annotation at top: "4 Medial bursae — popliteal (Baker's, pes anserinus, Semi-membranosus-tibial collateral, Tibial collateral)"]

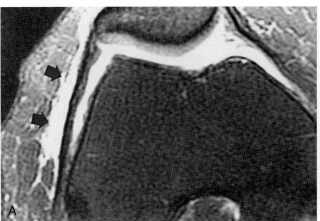

Figure 15-50 **Torn popliteus tendon.** Sagittal fast spin echo–T2W image shows a marked amount of fluid around the popliteus tendon. The tendon is wavy and lax, rather than taut (*arrow*). These findings are typical for a torn popliteus tendon.

ligament. It has a small artery that accompanies it and can often be seen on MRI as it curves through the fat pad. The infrapatellar plica usually ends at the transverse ligament, but occasionally can be seen extending beyond, anterior to the ACL, and inserts onto the roof of the intercondylar notch (Fig. 15-56). The infrapatellar plica can become thickened and irritated owing to chronic stress in some athletes resulting in anterior knee pain. This is commonly seen with MRI as abnormal increased T2 signal along its course in Hoffa's fat pad (Fig. 15-57). It is easily resected arthroscopically with pain relief.[32]

PATELLAR TENDON

Pain in the inferior patella region in athletes, so-called jumper's knee, is often seen on MRI as thickening of the proximal patellar tendon with high signal in and around it on T2W images (Fig. 15-58).[33] Jumper's knee can be a debilitating condition for athletes and can require surgery to remove the focus of myxoid degeneration in the tendon.

Fat Pad Impingement

A common source of patellofemoral pain is fat pad impingement. This is seen on MRI as increased T2 signal in Hoffa's fat pad just inferior to the patella (Fig. 15-59), or in the suprapatellar fat pad (Fig. 15-60). It is secondary to impingement of the fat pads on the femoral condyle by the patella tendon or the quadriceps tendon during flexion and has been reported to be present in 12% of cases.[34]

BURSAE

Several bursae are present around the knee that can become inflamed and cause symptoms that, in some cases, can mimic intra-articular pathology and result in inappropriate therapy, including surgery. It is important to recognize these and correctly report their occurrence so that the orthopedic surgeon can institute the appropriate treatment.

Popliteal (Baker's Cyst)

The most common knee bursa is a popliteal bursa, or Baker's cyst, which extends from the knee joint posteriorly between the tendons of the medial head of the gastrocnemius and the semimembranosus. It can contain a small amount of fluid in normal individuals, but any more than 5 to 10 mL of fluid should be mentioned because it could be a source of symptoms. These bursae can get quite large and cause a compartment syndrome. They can extend far down the leg in some patients. They can rupture and cause inflammation to the surrounding musculature, which can be very symptomatic. They often mimic deep vein thrombosis clinically.

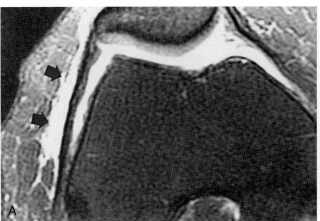
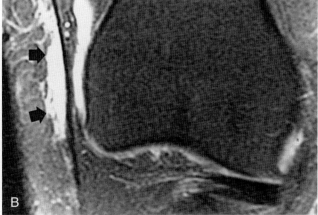

Figure 15-51 **Iliotibial band syndrome. A,** This axial fast spin echo–T2W image in a patient with lateral knee pain shows fluid around the iliotibial band (*arrows*), indicative of iliotibial band syndrome. **B,** Coronal fast spin echo–T2W image shows fluid around the iliotibial band (*arrows*).

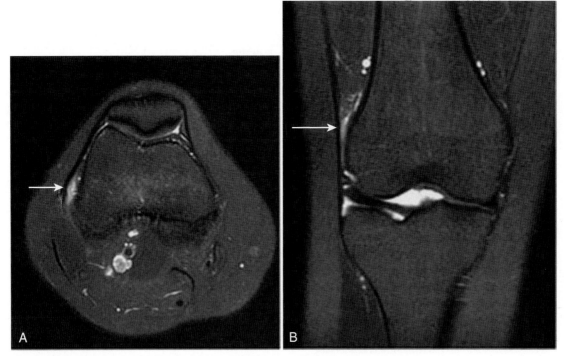

Figure 15-52 **Iliotibial band syndrome. A,** Axial image in a patient with lateral knee pain shows edema between the iliotibial band and the lateral femoral condyle (*arrow*). **B,** Coronal image shows the edema (*arrow*). This is characteristic for iliotibial band syndrome.

Prepatellar Bursa

Prepatellar bursitis is a common cause of anterior knee pain. It is caused from repetitive trauma from kneeling—it has been termed *housemaid's knee* in the older, less politically correct literature. Because it is an easy clinical diagnosis, we do not usually see prepatellar bursitis as an isolated finding, but often we see it in addition to other abnormalities. On MRI, it is seen as a fluid collection superficial to the patella (Fig. 15-61).

Pes Anserinus Bursa

A bursa that occurs on the anteromedial tibia, just below the joint line, is the pes anserinus bursa. *Pes anserinus* means "goose's foot" in Latin and refers to the configuration of the

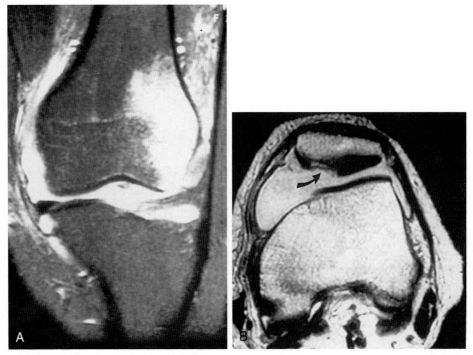

Figure 15-53 **Patellar dislocation. A,** Coronal fast spin echo–T2W image shows a large contusion on the anterior lateral femoral condyle. **B,** Axial fast spin echo–T2W image through the patella shows a large defect in the patellar cartilage (*arrow*). Although the contusion pattern seen in **A** is virtually diagnostic of a patellar dislocation, the cartilage defect usually means this is a surgical case.

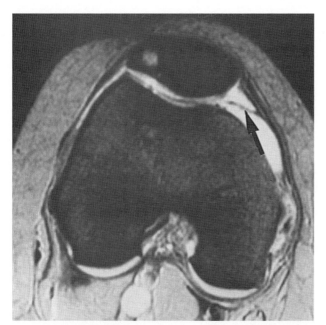

Figure 15-54 **Medial patellar plica.** Axial gradient echo image through the patella shows a thin fibrous band extending off the medial capsule (*arrow*), which is a normal medial patellar plica.

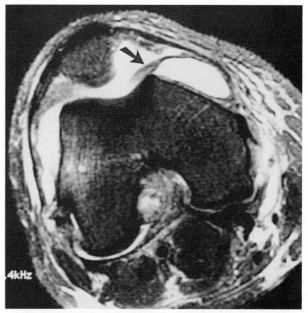

Figure 15-55 **Thickened medial patellar plica.** Axial fast spin echo–T2W image through the patella shows an enlarged, thickened medial patellar plica (*arrow*) trapped between the patella and femur that extends well posterior to the patella.

insertion of the pes tendons onto the tibia—it has a webbed foot appearance (it takes a little imagination). The pes tendons are the gracilis, sartorius, and semitendinosus. The pes bursa lies beneath the tendons and, when inflamed, extends proximally toward the joint (Fig. 15-62).[35] We have seen several patients who had arthroscopy for a clicking, popping, painful knee that was thought to be a meniscus tear but was simply a pes anserinus bursitis. Bursae around the knee are not seen at arthroscopy; it is imperative that MRI or physical diagnosis pick them up.

Semimembranosus–Tibial Collateral Ligament Bursa

Another bursa around the knee that can mimic an internal derangement is the semimembranosus–tibial collateral ligament bursa.[36] This commonly inflamed bursa has a characteristic appearance that makes it easily recognized with MRI. It occurs right on the joint line and drapes over the

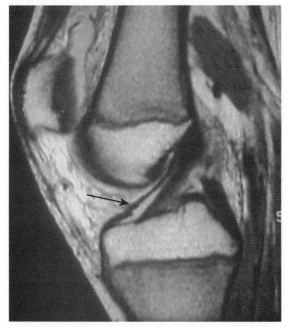

Figure 15-56 **Infrapatellar plica.** Sagittal image through the knee shows a linear structure (*arrow*) just anterior to the anterior cruciate ligament, which is an infrapatellar plica. It more commonly extends through Hoffa's fat pad and ends at the transverse ligament.

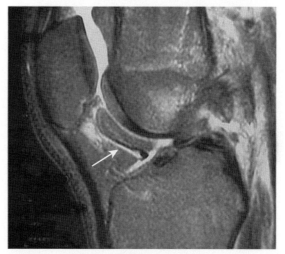

Figure 15-57 **Irritated infrapatellar plica.** Sagittal image shows increased signal along the infrapatellar plica in Hoffa's fat pad (*arrow*). This patient was an athlete with anterior knee pain; the plica was removed arthroscopically, with resolution of his symptoms.

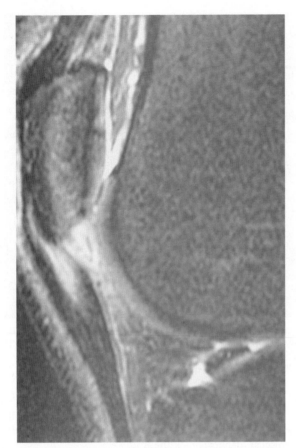

Figure 15-58   Jumper's knee. Sagittal fast spin echo–T2W image through the patellar tendon shows a thickened proximal portion of the tendon with high signal. This is diagnostic of jumper's knee.

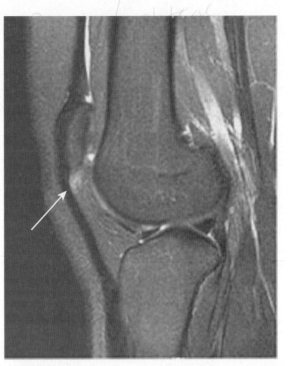

Figure 15-59   Hoffa's fat pad impingement. Edema is seen in Hoffa's fat pad just inferior to the patella in this patient with anterior knee pain. This is due to fat pad impingement.

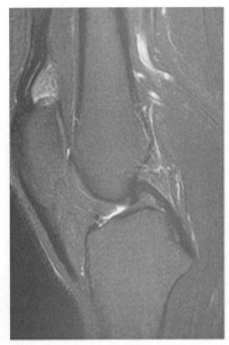

Figure 15-60   Suprapatellar fat pad impingement. Edema is seen in the suprapatellar fat pad in this patient with anterior knee pain secondary to fat pad impingement.

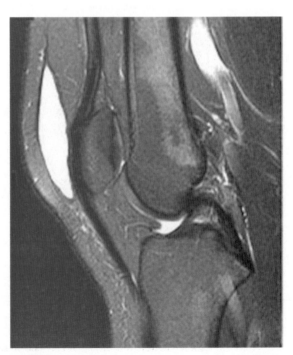

Figure 15-61   Prepatellar bursitis. Sagittal fast spin echo–T2W image through the knee shows a well-contained fluid collection anterior to the patella. This is prepatellar bursitis.

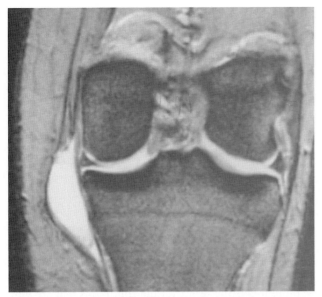

Figure 15-62   Pes anserinus bursitis. Coronal gradient echo image shows a fluid collection medially, just inferior to the joint line. This is pes anserinus bursitis.

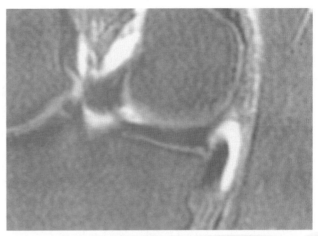

Figure 15-63   Semimembranosus–tibial collateral ligament bursitis. Coronal fast spin echo–T2W image shows a fluid collection at the medial joint line that is adjacent to the medial meniscus and is draped over the semimembranosus tendon. This is the appearance of a semimembranosus–tibial collateral ligament bursa.

semimembranosus tendon like a horseshoe (Fig. 15-63). On coronal and sagittal images (Fig. 15-64), it appears to arise at the meniscus and extend inferiorly, making the diagnosis of a meniscal cyst attractive. No connection to a meniscus is found, however.

Tibial Collateral Ligament Bursa

An uncommonly seen bursa is the tibial collateral ligament bursa. It lies just deep to the MCL and extends vertically above and below the joint line (Fig. 15-65). It can be confused for a meniscocapsular separation, but, in contrast to a traumatic separation, the fluid is well contained and cystlike, rather than diffusely distributed.

The four bursae described here all occur medially and are located in distinctly different locations (Fig. 15-66). Occasionally, a bursa is so distended that it overlaps an area usually reserved for another bursa, and it can be difficult to determine which bursa is present. Axial images usually allow for easy differentiation of each bursa. The actual name of the bursa is not as important as recognizing that there is a bursa and letting the surgeon know about it.

BONES

Bone contusions, seen as amorphous, subarticular high signal on T2W images, are commonly encountered on knee

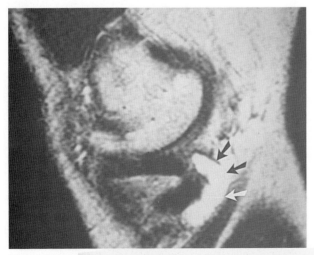

Figure 15-64   Semimembranosus–tibial collateral ligament bursitis. Sagittal fast spin echo–T2W image shows the semimembranosus–tibial collateral ligament bursa (*arrows*) at the level of the medial meniscus and draping over the semimembranosus tendon.

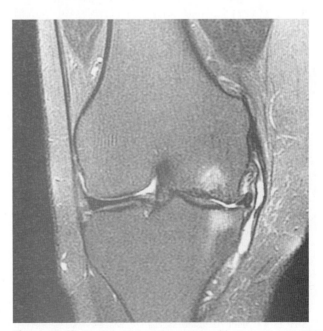

Figure 15-65   Medial collateral ligament bursitis. Fast spin echo–T2W image shows a fluid collection just deep to the medial collateral ligament, which is a medial collateral ligament bursitis.

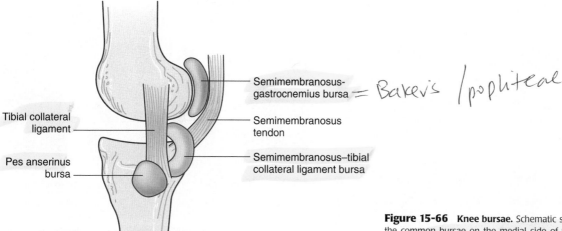

Figure 15-66 **Knee bursae.** Schematic shows the location of the common bursae on the medial side of the knee. Semimembranosus-gastrocnemius bursa is also known as Baker's cyst.

MRI. They have significance in that they can be the sole source of pain, they can precede a focal area of bone necrosis (osteochondritis dissecans), and they can indicate additional internal derangements when they have a specific pattern. Bone contusions are basically microfractures. They invariably heal with rest, as would any fracture. If they are not protected, however, there is at least the potential that they can progress to osteochondritis dissecans. This is thought to

be more frequently seen with the contusions that are more geographic in appearance (Fig. 15-67), as opposed to the reticular appearance of most contusions.[37]

A contusion pattern that is fairly specific for an ACL tear is one that involves the posterolateral aspect of the tibial plateau (Fig. 15-68). When the ACL tears, the tibia internally rotates on the femur, allowing the lateral femoral condyle to impact on the posterolateral tibial plateau. This has been termed the *pivot-shift phenomenon*. There is often a kissing contusion on the central to anterior lateral femoral condyle above the anterior horn of the lateral meniscus. This

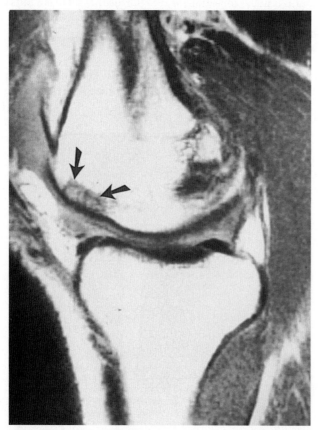

Figure 15-67 **Bone contusion.** Sagittal T1W image shows a well-defined, geographic contusion on the femoral condyle (*arrows*). This type of contusion is thought to be more likely to develop into osteochondritis dissecans compared with an ill-defined, reticular contusion.

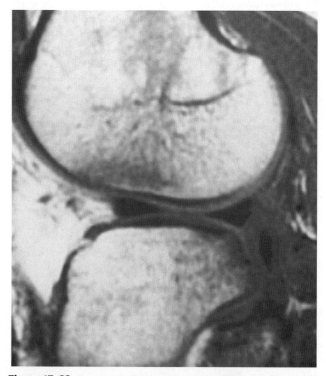

Figure 15-68 **Bone contusion.** Sagittal T1W image through the lateral side of the knee in a patient with a torn anterior cruciate ligament shows reticular contusions in the posterior tibial plateau and centrally in the femoral condyle. This pattern typically is seen with an anterior cruciate ligament tear.

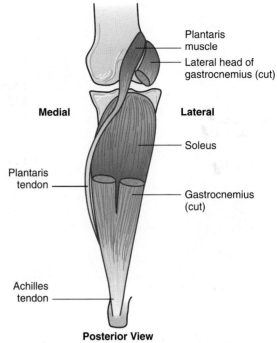

Plantaris
muscle

Lateral head of
gastrocnemius (cut)

Medial   **Lateral**

Soleus

Plantaris
tendon

Gastrocnemius
(cut)

Achilles
tendon

Posterior View

Figure 15-69 **Plantaris muscle and tendon.** Schematic shows the plantaris muscle and tendon from a posterior view.

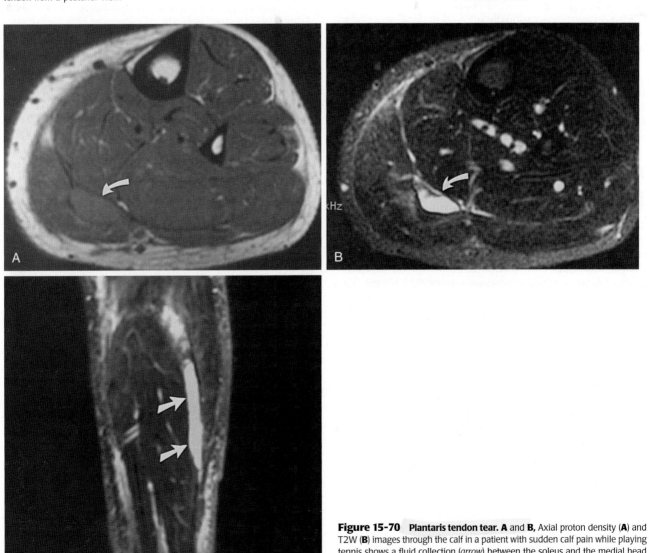

Figure 15-70 **Plantaris tendon tear. A** and **B,** Axial proton density (**A**) and T2W (**B**) images through the calf in a patient with sudden calf pain while playing tennis shows a fluid collection (*arrow*) between the soleus and the medial head of the gastrocnemius muscle. **C,** Sagittal T2W image shows a tubular fluid collection (*arrows*) just deep to the medial head of the gastrocnemius. This is characteristic of a torn plantaris tendon.

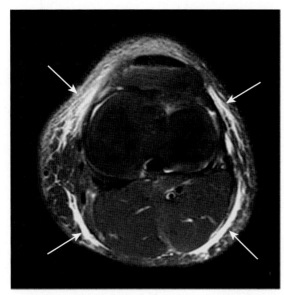

Figure 15-71   **Soft tissue twisting injury.** Fluid has collected at the subcutaneous fat–fascia interface (*arrows*) in this patient who sustained a twisting injury to the knee.

contusion pattern occasionally is found in the absence of an ACL tear in children who have stretched the ACL, but their increased flexibility protects it from tearing.

Another contusion that frequently is seen with an ACL tear is found on the posteromedial tibial plateau and sometimes the medial femoral condyle just posterior to the MCL. Kaplan and coworkers[38] found this contusion in 25 of 215 knees (12%). All had an ACL tear, and 24 of 25 had meniscocapsular injuries, which they termed *contrecoup injuries.*

SOFT TISSUES

Tears of the plantaris tendon have been termed *tennis leg* because of the frequent association with that activity. The patient presents with acute calf pain and occasionally displays swelling with purplish skin discoloration caused by the hemorrhage. It can clinically resemble a torn medial head of the gastrocnemius (which requires different treatment than a torn plantaris tendon) or deep venous thrombosis. The plantaris muscle arises on the lateral femoral condyle and runs distally just deep to the lateral head of the gastrocnemius and superficial to the soleus muscle. Its tendon begins in the upper part of the lower leg and courses medially deep to the medial head of the gastrocnemius and continues adjacent to the medial aspect of the Achilles tendon to the calcaneus (Fig. 15-69). MRI through the calf shows a focal fluid collection between the soleus and the medial head of the gastrocnemius (Fig. 15-70). A torn, retracted tendon sometimes may be seen. The fluid collection is often very tubular in configuration. An association between an injured plantaris muscle and a torn ACL has been noted.[39]

It is common to see fluid at the subcutaneous fat–fascia interface (Fig. 15-71), especially in obese individuals who sustain a twisting injury. This fluid is due to a degloving injury caused by the sudden arrest of the twisting motion by the bones and muscles while the subcutaneous fat continues to twist. The fat shears off of its attachment to the fascia, and

fluid accumulates in the injured tissue. This can result in pain localized to the damaged tissue.[40]

REFERENCES

1. Escobedo EM, Hunter JC, Zinkbrody GC, et al. Usefulness of turbo spin-echo MR imaging in the evaluation of meniscal tears—comparison with a conventional spin-echo sequence. *AJR Am J Roentgenol* 1996; 167:1223-1227.
2. Cheung L, Li K, Hollett M, et al. Meniscal tears of the knee: accuracy of detection with fast spin-echo MR imaging and arthroscopic correlation in 293 patients. *Radiology* 1997; 203:508-512.
3. Rubin D, Kneeland J, Listerud J, et al. MR diagnosis of meniscal tears of the knee: value of fast spin-echo vs conventional spin-echo pulse sequences. *AJR Am J Roentgenol* 1994; 162:1131-1136.
4. Anderson M, Raghavan N, Seidenwurm D, et al. Evaluation of meniscal tears: fast spin-echo versus conventional spin-echo MR imaging. *Acad Radiol* 1995; 2:209-214.
5. Blackmon GB, Major NM, Helms CA. Comparison of fast spin-echo versus conventional spin-echo MRI for evaluating meniscal tears. *AJR Am J Roentgenol* 2005; 184:1740-1743.
6. De Smet A, Norris M, Yandow D, et al. MR diagnosis of meniscal tears of the knee: importance of high signal in the meniscus that extends to the surface. *AJR Am J Roentgenol* 1993; 161:101-107.
7. Kaplan PA, Nelson NL, Garvin KL, Brown DE. MR of the knee: the significance of high signal in the meniscus that does not clearly extend to the surface. *AJR Am J Roentgenol* 1991; 156:333-336.
8. De Smet AA, Tuite MJ. Use of the "two-slice-touch" rule for the MRI diagnosis of meniscal tears. *AJR Am J Roentgenol* 2006; 187:911-914.
9. De Smet A, Graf B. Meniscal tears missed on MR imaging: relationship to meniscal tear patterns and anterior cruciate ligament tears. *AJR Am J Roentgenol* 1994; 162:905-911.
10. Helms CA, Laorr A, Cannon WD. The absent bow tie sign in bucket-handle tears of the menisci in the knee. *AJR Am J Roentgenol* 1998; 170:57-61.
11. Dorsay TA, Helms CA. Bucket-handle meniscal tears of the knee: sensitivity and specificity of MRI signs. *Skeletal Radiol* 2003; 32:266-272.
12. Watt AJ, Halliday T, Raby N, et al. The value of the absent bow tie sign in MRI of bucket-handle tears. *Clin Radiol* 2000; 55:622-626.
13. Harper KW, Helms CA, Lambert S, Higgins LD. Radial meniscal tears: significance, incidence, and MR appearance. *AJR Am J Roentgenol* 2005; 185:1429-1434.
14. Lecas L, Helms C, Kosarek F, Garrett W. Inferiorly displaced flap tears of the medial meniscus: MR appearance and clinical significance. *AJR Am J Roentgenol* 2000; 174:161-164.
15. Pedowitz R, Feagin J, Rajagopalan S. A surgical algorithm for treatment of cystic degeneration of the meniscus. *Arthroscopy* 1996; 12:209-216.
16. Silverman J, Mink J, Deutsch A. Discoid menisci of the knee: MR imaging appearance. *Radiology* 1989; 173:351-354.
17. Singh K, Helms CA, Jacobs MT, Higgins LD. MRI appearance of Wrisberg variant of discoid lateral meniscus. *AJR Am J Roentgenol* 2006; 187:384-387.
18. Shankman S, Beltran J, Melamed E, Rosenberg ZS. Anterior horn of the lateral meniscus—another potential pitfall in MR imaging of the knee. *Radiology* 1997; 204:181-184.
19. Peterfy C, Janzen D, Tirman P, et al. "Magic-angle" phenomenon: a cause of increased signal in the normal lateral meniscus on short-TE MR images of the knee. *Radiology* 1994; 163:149-154.
20. Erickson S, Cox I, Hyde J, et al. Effect of tendon orientation on MR imaging signal intensity: a manifestation of the "magic angle" phenomenon. *Radiology* 1991; 181:389-392.
21. Ha T, Li K, Beaulieu CF, et al. Anterior cruciate ligament injury—fast spin-echo MR imaging with arthroscopic correlation in 217 examinations. *AJR Am J Roentgenol* 1998; 170:1215-1219.
22. Mink J, Levy T, Crues JI. Tears of the anterior cruciate ligament and menisci of the knee: MR imaging evaluation. *Radiology* 1988; 167:769-774.
23. Lee J, Yao L, Phelps C, et al. Anterior cruciate ligament tears: MR imaging compared with arthroscopy and clinical tests. *Radiology* 1988; 166:861-864.
24. Kumar A, Bickerstaff DR, Grimwood JS, Suvarna SK. Mucoid cystic degeneration of the cruciate ligament. *J Bone Joint Surg [Br]* 1999; 81:304-305.

25. Recht MP, Piraino DW, Cohen MA, et al. Localized anterior arthrofibrosis (cyclops lesion) after reconstruction of the anterior cruciate ligament: MR imaging findings. *AJR Am J Roentgenol* 1995; 165:383-385.
26. Bergin D, Keogh C, O'Connell M, et al. Atraumatic medial collateral ligament oedema in medial compartment knee osteoarthritis. *Skeletal Radiol* 2002; 31:14-18.
27. Veltri D, Warren R. Posterolateral instability of the knee. *J Bone Joint Surg [Am]* 1994; 76:460-472.
28. Brown T, Quinn S, Wensel J, et al. Diagnosis of popliteus injuries with MR imaging. *Skeletal Radiol* 1995; 24:511-514.
29. Murphy B, Hechtman K, Uribe J, et al. Iliotibial band friction syndrome: MR imaging findings. *Radiology* 1992; 185:569-571.
30. Virolainen H, Visuri T, Kuusela T. Acute dislocation of the patella: MR findings. *Radiology* 1993; 189:243-246.
31. Deutsch AL, Resnick D, Dalinka MK, et al. Synovial plicae of the knee. *Radiology* 1981; 141:627-634.
32. Cothran RL, McGuire PM, Helms CA, et al. MR imaging of infrapatellar plica injury. *AJR Am J Roentgenol* 2003; 180:1443-1447.
33. Yu JS, Popp JE, Kaeding CC, Lucas J. Correlation of MR imaging and pathologic findings in athletes undergoing surgery for chronic patellar tendinitis. *AJR Am J Roentgenol* 1995; 165:115-118.
34. Roth C, Jacobson J, Jamadar D, et al. Quadriceps fat pad signal intensity and enlargement on MRI: prevalence and associated findings. *AJR Am J Roentgenol* 2004; 182:1383-1387.
35. Forbes JR, Helms CA, Janzen DL. Acute pes anserine bursitis: MR imaging. *Radiology* 1995; 194:525-527.
36. Rothstein CP, Laorr A, Helms CA, Tirman P. Semimembranosus-tibial collateral ligament bursitis—MR imaging findings. *AJR Am J Roentgenol* 1996; 166:875-877.
37. Vellet A, Marks P, Fowler P, Munro T. Occult posttraumatic osteochondral lesions of the knee: prevalence, classification, and short-term sequelae evaluated with MR imaging. *Radiology* 1991; 178:271-276.
38. Kaplan PA, Gehl RH, Dussault RG, et al. Bone contusions of the posterior lip of the medial tibial plateau (contrecoup injury) and associated internal derangements of the knee at MR imaging. *Radiology* 1999; 211:747-753.
39. Helms CA, Fritz RC, Garvin GJ. Plantaris muscle injury: evaluation with MR imaging. *Radiology* 1995; 195:201-203.
40. Magee T, Shapiro M. Soft tissue twisting injuries of the knee. *Skeletal Radiol* 2001; 30:460-463.

Knee Protocols

This is one set of suggested protocols; there are many variations that would work equally well.

DEDICATED KNEE MRI

Sequence No.	1	2	3	4
Sequence Type	Proton density with fat saturation	FSE with fat saturation	FSE with fat saturation	FSE with fat saturation
Orientation	Sagittal	Sagittal	Coronal	Axial
Field of View (cm)	14-16	14-16	14-16	14-16
Slice Thickness (mm)	4	4	4	4
Contrast	No	No	No	No

SAMPLE STANDARD REPORT

Clinical Information

Protocol

The examination was done using the routine knee protocol.

Discussion

1. **Joint effusion:** None; no evidence of a popliteal cyst
2. **Menisci:** Medial and lateral—no evidence of a tear
3. **Anterior and posterior cruciate ligaments:** Intact
4. **Medial and lateral collateral ligaments:** Intact
5. **Quadriceps and patellar tendons:** Normal
6. **Articular cartilage:** Normal; no focal defects, osteoarthritis, or other abnormalities
7. **Osseous structures:** Normal; no contusions, fractures, or other lesions
8. **Other abnormalities:** None

Opinion

Normal MRI of the (right/left) knee.

Foot and Ankle

How to Image the Foot and Ankle

See the protocols for foot and ankle MRI at the end of this chapter.

The foot and ankle are among the most difficult anatomic sites to image, simply because of the angle formed between the foot and ankle. Even the terminology for plane orientation in the foot and ankle is confusing and certainly not universal.

- *Coils and patient position:* Ideally, imaging of the ankle and foot should be done with the foot at right angles to the lower leg with the patient in a supine position. This positioning may require a support on the sole of the foot to maintain the alignment (special surface coils are now being made to accomplish this). A standard extremity coil generally is employed for the foot and ankle (the same one used for knee MRI), and such a precise position for the foot is not always possible to obtain or maintain. More importantly, the patient should be immobilized with padding and made comfortable to prevent movement that would degrade the images, and

the radiologist should know the anatomy well enough so that it is easily interpretable, regardless of slight variations in the angle of the foot with the ankle. How to angle MR images properly with the anatomic planes of the foot and ankle to obtain images that are reproducible and most easily understood is shown in the protocols of how to image the foot and ankle. The lower extremity externally rotates when a patient is in a relaxed supine position, and the planes of imaging must be oriented to the anatomy of the foot, rather than to the magnet. True sagittal images of the foot and ankle are mandatory to show the Achilles tendon accurately. If a slice cuts through the tendon obliquely, it gives the false impression of abnormal thickening of the tendon. Imaging the forefoot or toes often is done with the patient prone to allow the toes to be in a neutral position, more easily immobilized, and better centered in the coil. Some centers routinely image the foot and ankle in the prone position to decrease the magic angle effect.[1] Only the extremity with a suspected abnormality is imaged; the opposite normal side is never done

Foot and Ankle Structures to Evaluate in Different Planes

Sagittal

- Achilles tendon
- Sinus tarsi
- Plantar fascia
- Osseous structures (length of metatarsals)
- Ankle joint

Axial of Ankle and Long-Axis Axial (Coronal) of Foot

- Ankle tendons
- Sinus tarsi
- Tibiofibular ligaments
- Anterior and posterior talofibular ligaments
- Spring ligament
- Osseous structures (length of metatarsals)

Coronal of Ankle and Short-Axis Axial of Foot

- Deltoid ligaments, deep and superficial
- Calcaneofibular ligament
- Tarsal tunnel
- Sinus tarsi
- Ankle joint
- Osseous structures (metatarsals in cross section)
- Plantar fascia in cross section

simultaneously for comparison because it is unnecessary, and decreases the detail and resolution of the images owing to the larger field of view required. We try to employ a small field of view to increase resolution, so we divide the foot and ankle into one or the other and never scan both simultaneously. An ankle MRI does not include the toes and a forefoot examination does not include the ankle.

- *Image orientation (Box 16-1):* Planes of imaging in the ankle are standard and identical to elsewhere in the body. The foot is more complicated. For purposes of this chapter, we consider the images that run parallel with the long axis of the foot and appear similar to an anteroposterior foot radiograph as either long-axis axial or long-axis coronal images. Images obtained perpendicular to the long axis of the foot so that the metatarsals are seen as five circles of bone cut transversely are referred to as *short-axis axials.* Sagittal images are self-explanatory and standard.
- *Pulse sequences and regions of interest:* Different pulse sequences are used, based on the clinical indications. Generally, we do a combination of T1 and some type of T2 sequences in all three orthogonal planes to show the different anatomic structures and pathologic entities well. The pulse sequences are chosen by selecting one of the following clinical categories:
  1. "Routine" (pain, trauma)
  2. Infection/mass
  3. Morton's neuroma
  We select from three anatomic regions for imaging:
  1. Ankle/hindfoot/midfoot
  2. Forefoot/toes
  3. Entire foot
- *Contrast:* Gadolinium is used only in cases of suspected infection or for differentiating a solid from a cystic mass.

Normal and Abnormal

TENDONS

Tendon abnormalities affecting the foot and, particularly, the ankle are common because of the many tendons that are present and their close relationship to adjacent osseous structures that may cause irritation, and the frequent stresses and trauma affecting this anatomic location. Tendons generally are best evaluated on short axis axial images of the foot or axial images of the ankle where the tendons are depicted in cross section. Other imaging planes may help to substantiate findings in tendons, but do not show the tendons to greatest advantage because the tendons, with the exception of the Achilles tendon, run obliquely to these planes.

The general principles regarding the MRI appearance of normal and abnormal tendons are discussed in Chapter 3. As a brief review, the abnormalities that may affect tendons are tenosynovitis, tendon degeneration, partial or complete tendon tears, subluxation or dislocation of certain tendons from their normal locations, xanthomas from hyperlipidemia, calcific tendinitis, uric acid tophi from gout, and, rarely, tumors. Tendons may tear as the result of chronic repetitive microtrauma; acute major trauma; and weakening secondary to myxoid degeneration, rheumatoid arthritis, chronic renal failure, diabetes, gout, steroids, and other medications. Abnormalities on MRI consist of fluid completely surrounding a tendon (tenosynovitis), abnormal tendon size, intratendinous high signal intensity (from partial tears), abnormal position (from dislocation), or complete absence of a segment of tendon (complete tear). Tendons of the ankle are conveniently divided into four groups, based on their location in the ankle: anterior, posterior, medial, and lateral (Fig. 16-1).

POSTERIOR ANKLE TENDONS

Achilles and Plantaris (Box 16-2)

The Achilles tendon is located in the midline of the posterior ankle and is the largest tendon in the body, formed by the confluence of tendons from the gastrocnemius and the soleus muscles (Fig. 16-2). The Achilles tendon is normally low signal intensity diffusely; however, there is a vertically oriented line of high signal intensity in many Achilles tendons that probably represents a normal interface between the two components of the tendon (gastrocnemius and soleus) or else small vessels within the tendon. The Achilles does not have a tendon sheath because it does not come into close

Achilles Tendon

- No sheath, but a posterior paratenon
- Xanthomas
- Tears at midpoint, and proximal or distal extremes
- Plantaris medially may simulate tear
- "Pump bumps" or Haglund's deformity
- Retrocalcaneal bursitis
- Achilles tendon bursitis
- Thickened distal Achilles

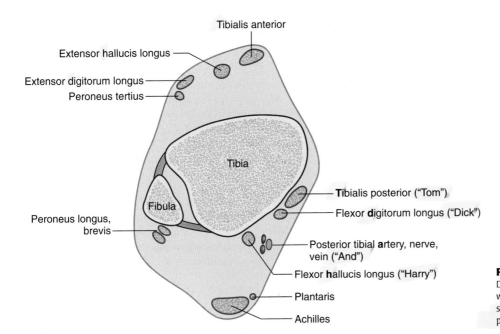

Figure 16-1 Normal ankle tendons. Diagram of tendons around the ankle, which are divided into the anterior extensors, medial flexors, posterior Achilles and plantaris, and lateral peroneals.

contact with other structures along its length; it cannot have changes of tenosynovitis, but only of paratendinitis. There is a paratenon present on the dorsal, medial, and lateral aspects of the Achilles tendon that allows smooth gliding of the tendon in lieu of a tendon sheath. This may be seen on axial images as a thin line of intermediate signal intensity paralleling the posterior tendon. Anterior to the Achilles tendon is a triangular fat pad called *Kager's triangle.*

The Achilles tendon usually has a flat or concave anterior margin on axial images (see Fig. 16-2); if it becomes diffusely convex, an abnormally thickened tendon exists.[2] The anterior margin of the Achilles tendon normally may have a focal

convexity that starts on the lateral side of the proximal tendon and shifts to the medial aspect of the distal tendon. This focal anterior contour convexity is caused by the fibers of the soleus merging with those of the gastrocnemius in a spiral configuration as they extend to insert on the calcaneus. The posterior margin of the Achilles has a convex contour. The normal tendon measures about 7 mm in the anteroposterior dimension, and the anterior and posterior margins are parallel on true sagittal images through the tendon.

Ninety percent of individuals have a small plantaris tendon lying anteromedial to the Achilles tendon, which inserts onto the Achilles tendon, or to the posterior calcaneus, or to

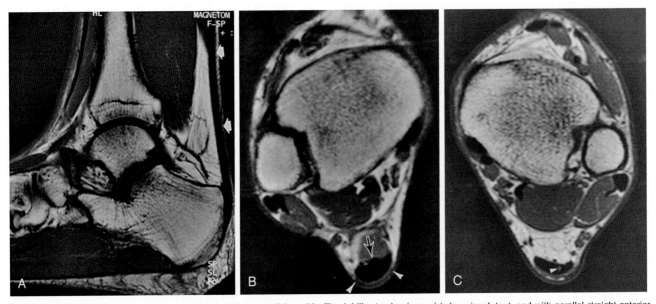

Figure 16-2 Achilles tendon: normal. A, T1W sagittal image of the ankle. The Achilles tendon (*arrows*) is low signal, taut, and with parallel straight anterior and posterior margins. **B,** T1W axial image of the ankle. The Achilles tendon has a flat or concave anterior margin, but a focal convexity (*arrow*) is a normal finding in many individuals. The paratenon is shown posterior to the tendon (*arrowheads*) as intermediate signal. **C,** T1W axial image of the ankle. The Achilles tendon is thin, has a concave anterior margin, and has a focus of high signal (*arrowhead*) in the substance.

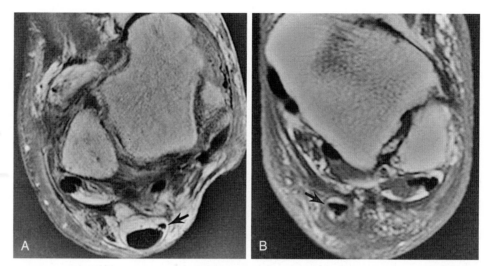

Figure 16-3 Plantaris tendon. A, T1W axial image of the ankle. The small plantaris tendon (*arrow*) is located medial to the Achilles tendon and may mimic a partial tear of the Achilles tendon. **B,** T1W axial image of the ankle (different patient than in **A**). The Achilles tendon is completely ruptured, and no fibers are evident on this cut. The plantaris tendon (*arrow*) should not be mistaken for a partially intact Achilles tendon.

the flexor retinaculum (Fig. 16-3). The high signal intensity plane between the plantaris and the Achilles tendons can be mistaken for a partially torn Achilles when none exists, or a completely torn Achilles may mistakenly be considered to have some remaining intact medial fibers, which are merely the fibers of the intact plantaris tendon. Evaluation of adjacent axial images distinguishes between a normal plantaris tendon and an abnormal Achilles tendon.

Degeneration and partial or complete tears of the Achilles tendon usually occur about 4 cm above its calcaneal insertion (Fig. 16-4), but may exist anywhere along the length of the tendon. Tears also may occur at the musculotendinous junction (Fig. 16-5), and the field of view must be large enough to include this region on sagittal images to look for hemorrhage and edema in the acute state, or muscle atrophy in the chronic setting.

Unconditioned, middle-aged athletes ("weekend athletes") are most commonly affected with Achilles tendon abnormalities. Complete tears are usually easy to diagnose clinically, but some clinicians believe that there is still a valuable role for imaging in these patients to evaluate how close the tendon fragments are to one another and the condition

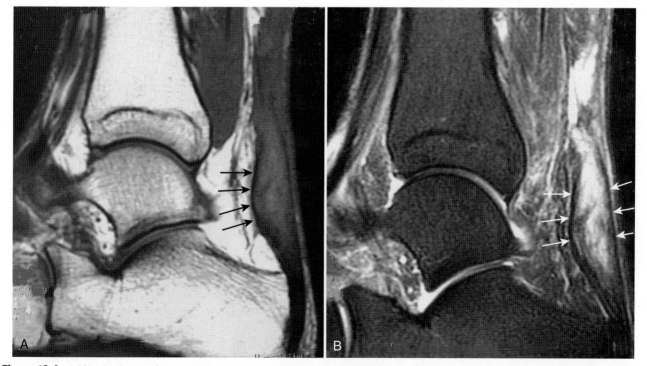

Figure 16-4   Achilles tendon: partial tears. A, T1W sagittal image of the ankle. The tendon has a fusiform thickening (*arrows*) with a convex anterior margin in its midsubstance, approximately 4 cm above the calcaneal insertion. The increased signal throughout the Achilles tendon could be tendinosis (myxoid degeneration) or partial tears. **B,** FSE-T2W sagittal image of the ankle. The tendon is thickened in the anteroposterior direction (*arrows*) and has increased signal, which indicates a partial tear. Tendinosis does not get fluid-bright on T2W sequences.

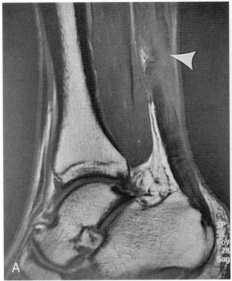
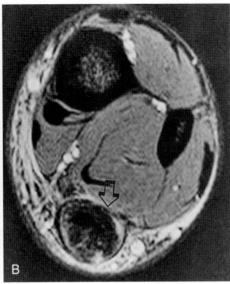

Figure 16-5 Achilles tendon: full-thickness tear. **A**, T1W sagittal image of the ankle. There is a full-thickness tear of the Achilles tendon at the myotendinous junction (*arrowhead*). The entire tendon is thickened and has abnormal high signal within it from partial tears as well. **B**, T2*W axial image of the ankle. A cut through the torn tendon (*arrow*) shows the tendon to be markedly thick, with a diffusely convex anterior margin. There is a stippled appearance as the result of hemorrhage and edema separating the low signal collagen fibers in the tendon.

of the tendon. Imaging may be done with a cast in place, which serves to hold the ankle in plantar flexion and cause increased apposition of tendon fragments. If there is a large gap between fragments, many orthopedists perform surgery to repair the tendon, whereas close apposition of tendon fragments can be treated with casting only. As with all things orthopedic, there is debate regarding the ideal method of treating these injuries.

Xanthomas occur from familial hyperlipidemia types II and III (hypercholesterolemia and hypertriglyceridemia) and have a predilection for the Achilles tendon (and the extensor tendons of the hands). Infiltration between the low signal intensity tendon fibers by intermediate signal intensity, lipid-laden foamy histiocytes causes a stippled pattern and either focal or diffuse enlargement of the tendon (Fig. 16-6). The findings often are bilateral and cannot be distinguished from partial tendon tears on MRI.[3] This must be remembered among the differential diagnostic possibilities for an abnormal Achilles tendon because the first manifestation of this deadly disease may be that of an Achilles xanthoma. The diagnosis may be proved with laboratory work-up.

Two bursae relate to the distal attachment of the Achilles tendon: the retrocalcaneal bursa and bursa of the Achilles tendon. The retrocalcaneal bursa is a teardrop-shaped structure that is normally located between the tendon and the posterior aspect of the upper calcaneus; it has little or no fluid within it when not inflamed. The bursa of the Achilles

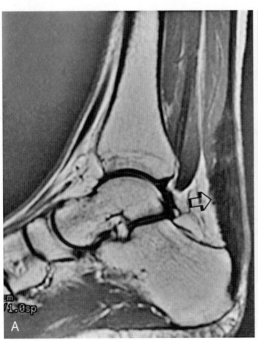
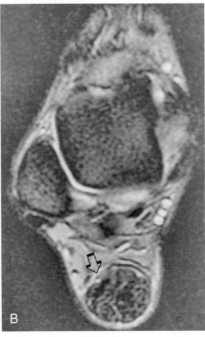

Figure 16-6 Achilles tendon: xanthoma. **A**, T1W sagittal image of the ankle. The Achilles tendon (*arrow*) is diffusely thickened, with linear areas of high signal in the substance. **B**, T2*W axial image of the ankle. The Achilles tendon (*arrow*) has a stippled appearance, with the focal low signal regions representing collagen fibers, and the higher signal being xanthoma from hyperlipidemia. The appearance on MRI is indistinguishable from the much more common tendon tear.

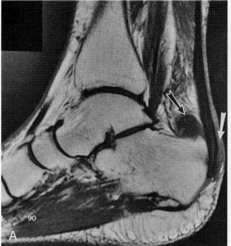
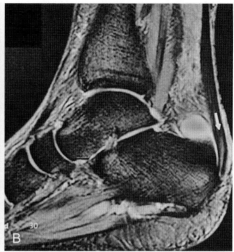

Figure 16-7 Haglund's deformity. A, T1W sagittal image of the ankle. The Achilles tendon is mildly thickened and has high signal in it from partial tears. Anterior to the tendon is a rounded mass (*black arrow*), representing the enlarged and inflamed retrocalcaneal bursa. Posterior to the tendon is an inflamed bursa of the Achilles tendon (*white arrow*). **B,** T2*W sagittal image of the ankle. The triad of Haglund's deformity is evident as high signal in the retrocalcaneal and Achilles tendon bursae, and in the partially torn Achilles tendon (*arrow*).

tendon (retro-Achilles) is an acquired or adventitious bursa, located just posterior to the distal Achilles tendon in the subcutaneous fat. Distention of these bursae with fluid or inflammatory thickening of the synovial linings indicates bursitis. If these bursae become inflamed, they may be a source of heel pain. Inflammation occurs with chronic overuse, especially from ill-fitting footwear, and from inflammatory arthropathies. The triad of retro-Achilles bursitis, retrocalcaneal bursitis, and thickening of the distal Achilles tendon is known as Haglund's deformity, or as "pump bumps," because wearing high-heeled or ill-fitting shoes is considered a predisposing factor (Fig. 16-7).[4]

MEDIAL ANKLE TENDONS

The flexor tendons are located on the medial side of the ankle (see Fig. 16-1). The position and names of these tendons can be easily remembered by using the mnemonic "**T**om, **D**ick, **A**nd **H**arry" to represent the structures running from medial to lateral. "**T**om" represents the posterior **t**ibial tendon; "**D**ick" is the flexor **d**igitorum longus tendon; "**A**nd" is the posterior tibial **a**rtery, nerve, and vein; and "**H**arry" is the flexor **h**allucis longus tendon. The tendons are surrounded by separate tendon sheaths, and they pass through the tarsal tunnel, discussed subsequently.

Posterior Tibial Tendon (Box 16-3)

The posterior tibial tendon is the largest of the three medial flexor tendons. It has an oval shape and is approximately twice as large as the adjacent round flexor digitorum and flexor hallucis longus tendons. The posterior tibial tendon passes beneath the medial malleolus, which it uses as a

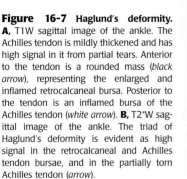

BOX 16-3

Posterior Tibial Tendon

- Most commonly abnormal medial tendon
- May tear or dislocate
- Tears lead to flat foot
- Tears associated with sinus tarsi syndrome
- Tears more common with accessory navicular

pulley, and attaches to the medial navicular bone, the three cuneiforms, and the bases of the first to fourth metatarsals. The attachment to the navicular bone is generally the only portion of the attachment identified by MRI. Because of the orientation of the tendinous attachment and the multiple tendon slips that attach to the bone, the attachment often has the appearance of a thickened tendon with high signal intensity within it; this normal appearance must not be confused with a partial tendon tear.

Most posterior tibial tendon tears occur at the level of the medial malleolus, rather than more distally. Generally, we disregard high signal in this tendon at its attachment site to the navicular because it typically is seen as a normal variant. High signal intensity or tendon thickening elsewhere in the length of the tendon is considered pathologic (Fig. 16-8). A longitudinal split tear of this tendon is commonly seen, in which case the axial images appear to show two posterior tibial tendons (Fig. 16-9). Fluid-bright T2 signal in the posterior tibial tendon, as in any tendon, indicates a partial tear (Fig. 16-10), as does thinning or attenuation of the tendon (Fig. 16-11).

The posterior tibial tendon is the most common abnormal tendon on the medial side of the ankle. This tendon provides a significant amount of support to the arch of the foot, and tears of the tendon can cause loss of the longitudinal arch, resulting in a flatfoot deformity. Middle-aged or older women and rheumatoid arthritis patients often have this abnormality.

There is a much higher incidence of posterior tibial tendon tears in individuals with accessory navicular bones or individuals with large medial tubercles of the navicular bone (the cornuate process), which result in altered stresses and premature tendon degeneration.[5] Three types of accessory naviculars have been described. Type I is a small sesamoid bone within the posterior tibial tendon near its insertion onto the navicular. No increased incidence of tendon pathology is associated with a type I accessory navicular. Type II is a large secondary ossification center that is present in about 10% of the population and normally has a fibrous or cartilaginous attachment to the navicular. With trauma (either overt trauma or repeated microtrauma), it can separate and

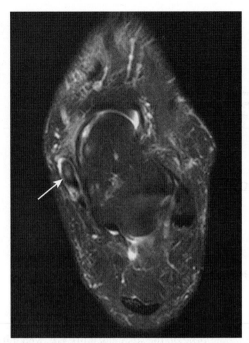

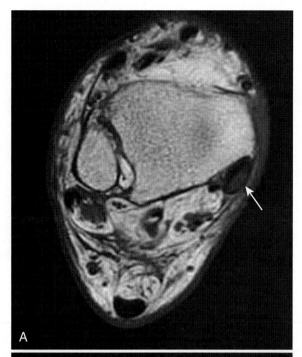

Figure 16-8 **Posterior tibial tendon: tendinosis.** FSE-T2W axial image of the ankle. The posterior tibial tendon is markedly enlarged (*arrow*) and has abnormal high signal within it. It is more than twice the size of the adjacent flexor digitorum and flexor hallucis tendons. The increased signal is not fluid-bright—hence this is tendinosis rather than a partial tear.

become painful.[6] Bony edema and high T2 signal can be seen between the os naviculare and the navicular bone (Fig. 16-12). A Kidner procedure is a common surgical procedure often performed to remove the os naviculare and reattach the posterior tibial tendon to the navicular bone.

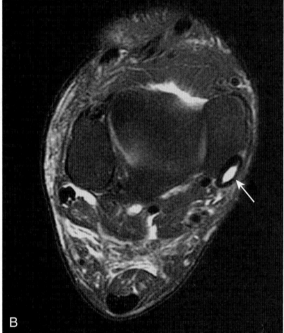

Figure 16-10 **Posterior tibial tendon: partial tear. A,** T1W axial image of the ankle. The posterior tibial tendon is markedly enlarged (*arrow*) and has increased signal within. **B,** FSE-T2W axial image of the ankle. The intermediate signal in the posterior tibial tendon seen on the T1W image in **A** is fluid-bright on the T2W image (*arrow*), indicating that this is a partial tear.

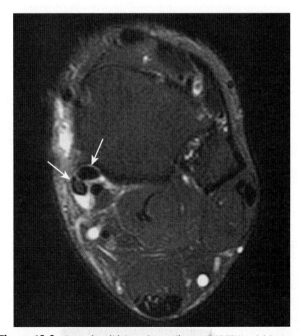

Figure 16-9 **Posterior tibial tendon: split tear.** FSE-T2W axial image of the ankle. The posterior tibial tendon is split into two (*arrows*) indicating a split tear. A longitudinal split tear has the same clinical significance as a complete tear.

Secondary signs of a posterior tibial tendon tear have been reported and include loss of the longitudinal arch of the foot and a small spur or periosteal reaction along the posterior aspect of the medial malleolus.[7] Tears of this tendon also are associated with the sinus tarsi syndrome and degenerative joint disease of the posterior subtalar joint, which may serve as sources of pain.

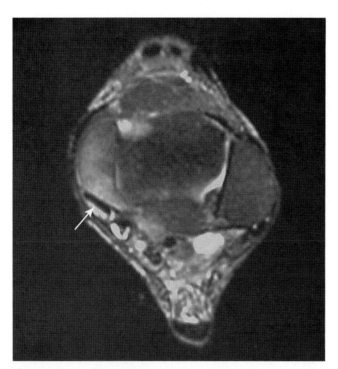

Figure 16-11   **Posterior tibial tendon: partial tear.** FSE-T2W axial image of the ankle. The posterior tibial tendon is thinned (*arrow*), indicating a partial tear. Note the adjacent edema in the medial malleolus, which is often seen with adjacent tendon abnormalities.

A high percentage of patients with a torn posterior tibial tendon have an abnormal spring ligament, which lies just deep to the posterior tibial tendon and contributes to supporting the longitudinal arch of the foot. The spring ligament is discussed in the section on medial ligaments. The posterior tibial tendon rarely can sublux or dislocate in a medial and anterior direction relative to the medial malleolus.

Flexor Digitorum Longus

The flexor digitorum longus tendon is rarely involved with abnormalities. It passes just lateral to the posterior tibial tendon and divides to send insertions to the plantar aspects of the distal phalanges of the second through fifth toes.

Flexor Hallucis Longus (Box 16-4)

The flexor hallucis longus tendon is the most lateral of the three medial flexor tendons (see Fig. 16-1). It passes in a groove on the medial side of the posterior process of the talus, and then beneath the sustentaculum tali, which it uses as a pulley. It passes along the plantar aspect of the foot, between the hallux sesamoids at the head of the first metatarsal, to attach to the base of the distal phalanx of the great toe.[8] The flexor hallucis longus synovial tendon sheath is in communication with the ankle joint in 20% of individuals; fluid surrounding the tendon is common and may have no significance if an ankle joint effusion also is present (Fig. 16-13). This tendon tends normally to have more fluid in its sheath than do the adjacent two tendons.

Focal, asymmetric pooling of fluid within the tendon sheath is indicative of stenosing tenosynovitis, which occurs as the result of focal areas of synovitis or fibrosis within the tendon sheath, interrupting normal synovial fluid flow (Fig.

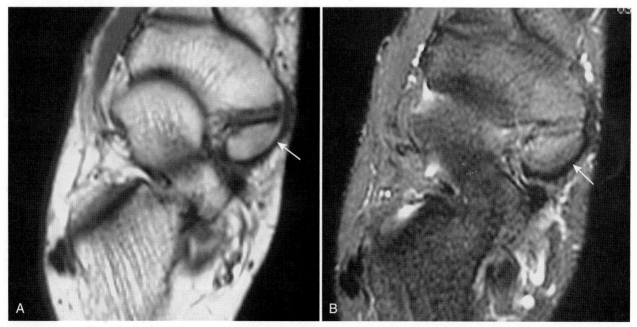

Figure 16-12   **Os naviculare. A,** T1W axial image of the ankle. An accessory navicular, called an *os naviculare,* is present (*arrow*). **B,** FSE-T2W axial image of the ankle. The os naviculare (*arrow*) and the adjacent navicular have increased signal, which is typically present in a painful os naviculare.

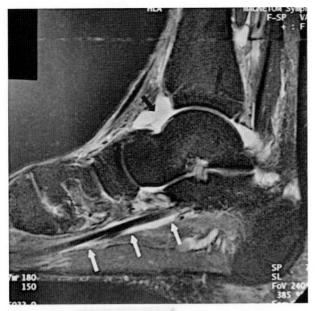

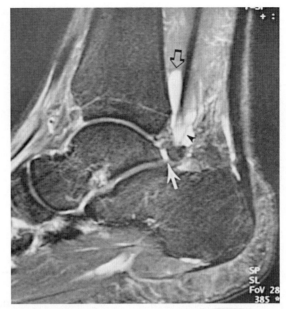

Figure 16-13 Flexor hallucis longus tendon: communication between ankle and tendon sheath. STIR sagittal image of the ankle. A large ankle joint effusion (*black arrow*) is present. Also, fluid surrounds the flexor hallucis longus tendon (*white arrows*), which runs beneath the sustentaculum tali. Fluid in this tendon sheath has no significance and cannot be called *tenosynovitis* when an ankle joint effusion is present because the two structures communicate in about 20% of individuals.

Figure 16-14 Flexor hallucis longus tendon: stenosing tenosynovitis and os trigonum syndrome. STIR sagittal image of the ankle. The tendon sheath of the flexor hallucis is distended with fluid proximally (*open arrow*). There is a septation in the fluid (*arrowhead*), indicating this is a stenosing tenosynovitis. There also is very high signal between the os trigonum and the talus (*white arrow*) because of disruption of the normal synchondrosis between the two structures (posterior impingement syndrome), which often is associated with stenosing tenosynovitis of the flexor hallucis.

16-14). Stenosing tenosynovitis of the flexor hallucis longus often is associated with the os trigonum syndrome, which occurs with extreme plantar flexion and causes the os trigonum and the flexor hallucis longus tendon to be trapped between the posterior malleolus of the tibia and the calcaneus.[9] Tears of the flexor hallucis longus tendon at the level of the ankle are rare, and tenosynovitis is far more common. Repeated plantar flexion of the ankle and foot, as occurs in ballet dancers and basketball players, results in inflammatory changes to the sheath of this tendon.

The distal end of the flexor hallucis longus tendon may be partially torn or may develop tenosynovitis where it passes through the confined space between the hallux sesamoid bones (Fig. 16-15). These distal tendon injuries are common in runners and in ballet dancers who dance en pointe.

LATERAL ANKLE TENDONS

Peroneal Tendons (Boxes 16-5 and 16-6)

The peroneus brevis and longus tendons are located on the posterolateral aspect of the ankle and serve as the major everters of the foot (see Fig. 16-1). These tendons pass

posterior and inferior to the lateral malleolus, which they use as a pulley. The tendons share a common tendon sheath proximally, but have separate sheaths distally. The brevis usually is located anterior to the longus (although the brevis sometimes may lie medial to the longus) and runs in a shallow retromalleolar groove on the back of the lateral

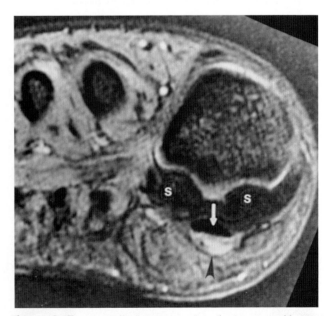

Figure 16-15 Flexor hallucis longus tendon: distal tenosynovitis. T2*W axial image of the forefoot. The distal flexor hallucis longus tendon (*arrow*) is positioned between the hallux sesamoids (S) beneath the first metatarsal head. There is high signal fluid (*arrowhead*) from tenosynovitis in this long-distance runner with pain.

BOX 16-5

Peroneus Tendons

- Brevis anterior or medial to longus
- Brevis: Flat or oval is normal; curved (boomerang shape) is abnormal
- Tear or dislocate laterally
- Calcaneal fractures cause entrapment, displacement, and tenosynovitis

malleolus (Fig. 16-16). The peroneal tendons are held in place relative to the lateral malleolus by the superior peroneal retinaculum. The tendons often are separated by the small peroneal tubercle on the lateral aspect of the calcaneus, with the brevis passing anterior to the tubercle (see Fig. 16-16), or both tendons may pass anterior to the peroneal tubercle. The brevis eventually attaches to the base of the fifth metatarsal. The longus has a broad-based insertion on the plantar surface of the base of the first metatarsal and medial cuneiform, after traversing the plantar aspect of the foot.

The peroneus brevis and longus tendons may be difficult to distinguish as separate structures at the level of the lateral malleolus on MRI. The brevis generally is much flatter and broader than the longus, which has a more rounded appearance (see Fig. 16-16). Flat is acceptable (for many things), but if the brevis becomes C-shaped, it is considered abnormal.

Calcaneal fractures can be associated with peroneal tendon abnormalities, including entrapment of the peroneal tendons between bone fragments, tendon tears, tendon displacement, or impingement on tendons by fracture fragments.[10] Complete and partial tears also occur in the absence of calcaneal fractures.[11,12]

Peroneus brevis splits is a term used for longitudinal or vertical tears of the peroneus brevis tendon that can occur in all ages and in athletes (Fig. 16-17). Tears occurring in the elderly may be asymptomatic, whereas younger patients usually have pain and swelling along the lateral malleolus and the course of the peroneal tendons. A history of recurrent inversion injuries and ankle sprains is common. The lateral collateral ligaments have a high association of tears with split tears of the peroneus brevis. The diagnosis is difficult or impossible clinically and overlaps with chronic ankle instability symptoms. Patients who do not respond to conservative management may benefit from surgery with anastomosis of fragments or tenodesis to the peroneus longus tendon.

Peroneus brevis longitudinal tears occur during dorsiflexion, when the brevis tendon is wedged between the lateral malleolus and the peroneus longus tendon. The tear originates at the distal tip of the lateral malleolus, but may propagate variable distances proximally and distally. The peroneus longus tendon also is partially torn in about 30% of individuals with a brevis tear because it becomes directly exposed to the lateral malleolus and subjected to abnormal stresses. A sharp posterolateral fibular spur may be seen

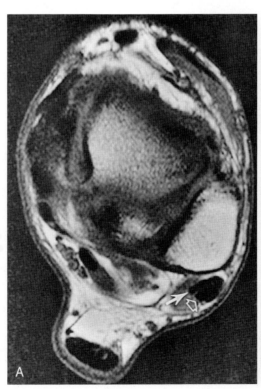

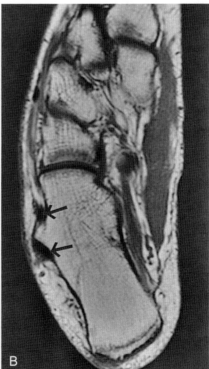

Figure 16-16 Peroneal tendons: normal. A, T1W axial image of the ankle. The peroneus brevis tendon (*solid arrow*) is flat and sandwiched between the posterior aspect of the lateral malleolus and the peroneus longus tendon (*open arrow*). The longus is more round than the brevis and located posteriorly. The intermediate signal muscle adjacent to the tendons is the peroneal muscle. **B,** T1W long axis coronal image of the foot. The peroneus brevis and longus tendons (*arrows*) are typically located anterior and posterior to the peroneal tubercle of the calcaneus, respectively, but can lie either anterior or posterior to the tubercle.

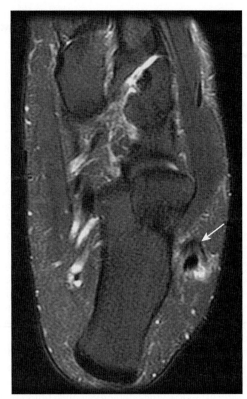

Figure 16-17   Peroneus brevis split tear.   FSE-T2W axial image of the ankle. There is a longitudinal tear or split of the peroneus brevis (*arrow*). A chevron shape to the brevis, as in this figure, is characteristic for a split tear.

with the peroneus brevis splits, representing a reactive periostitis.[12,13]

Certain conditions are associated with peroneus brevis longitudinal tears. Anything that causes compression or subluxation of the peroneal tendons may predispose to this abnormality by causing increased wear and tear on the tendons. Such conditions include a torn or lax superior peroneal retinaculum, a flat or convex (rather than normal concave) posterior aspect of the lateral malleolus, low-lying peroneus brevis muscle belly (extending to the tip of the lateral malleolus), and the presence of an accessory muscle called the *peroneus quartus.*

The diagnosis of a longitudinal split of the peroneus brevis tendon may be simulated by the presence of a bifurcated distal peroneus brevis tendon or by the peroneus quartus accessory muscle and tendon (Fig. 16-18). A brevis tendon tear can be distinguished from these two muscle variants, owing to the fact that separate muscle bellies surround each of the tendon slips in the case of a bifurcate brevis tendon, and a muscle belly separate from the peroneus brevis muscle is seen when a peroneus quartus is present. With a peroneus brevis split, there is one muscle belly and two tendons coming from it.[14]

The peroneal tendons are among the few tendons that can sublux or dislocate; this occurs when the superior retinaculum has been disrupted. The retinaculum becomes disrupted from a forced inversion injury with plantar flexion, typically occurring in skiing, basketball, or soccer injuries. The diagnosis is made on MRI if the tendons are located lateral to the distal fibula, instead of posterior to it, or if the torn retinaculum is identified (Fig. 16-19). A shallow or hypoplastic retromalleolar groove of the fibula may predispose to subluxation of the peroneal tendons.

The peroneus longus tendon has a sesamoid bone, the os peroneus, in about 10% of cases. This bone can serve as a stress riser with pain and eventual tendon disruption. This has been called *painful os peroneus syndrome.*[15] Edema can be seen on MRI in the os peroneus just before the peroneus longus tendon enters the cuboid tunnel (Fig. 16-20). Before the advent of MRI, a torn peroneus longus could be diag-

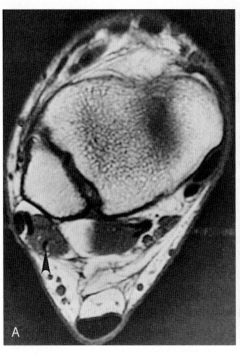

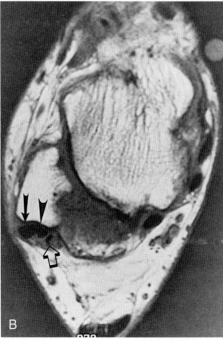

Figure 16-18   Accessory peroneus quartus. A, T1W axial image of the ankle. There are three tendons posterior to the lateral malleolus. The peroneus longus and brevis are the two most lateral tendons. The most posteromedial tendon (*arrowhead*) is surrounded by muscle, and this is the peroneus quartus accessory muscle and tendon. The peroneal retinaculum is stretched because of the increased volume in the confined space, and this may predispose to peroneus brevis splits. **B,** T1W axial image of the ankle (different patient than in **A**). Three tendons are posterior to the lateral malleolus: peroneus longus (*solid arrow*), peroneus brevis (*arrowhead*), and peroneus quartus (*open arrow*), which is the most medial tendon. The peroneus quartus simulates the appearance of a split peroneus brevis tendon. Each tendon has its own muscle belly on more proximal cuts, allowing differentiation.

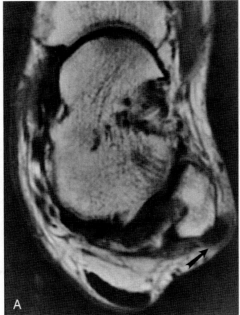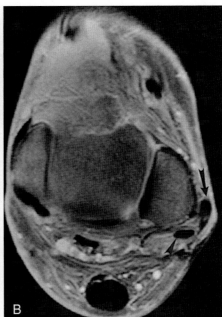

Figure 16-19 Peroneal tendons: dislocation. **A,** T1W axial image of the ankle. Both peroneal tendons are dislocated laterally (*arrow*). The flexor retinaculum is not evident. **B,** T1W axial image of the ankle with contrast enhancement and fat suppression. One of the peroneal tendons is dislocated laterally (*arrow*), whereas the other remains in normal position posterior to the lateral malleolus (*arrowhead*). The Achilles tendon is thickened and convex anteriorly from partial tears.

nosed with plain films by noting proximal migration of an os peroneus compared with prior films (like we might notice that). With MRI, painful os peroneus syndrome can be diagnosed before the tendon ruptures, which facilitates surgical treatment.

ANTERIOR ANKLE TENDONS

Four tendons can be found anterior to the ankle (see Fig. 16-1). From medial to lateral these are the anterior tibial, extensor hallucis longus, extensor digitorum longus, and peroneus tertius tendons. These tendons dorsiflex the ankle and foot. These tendons seldom are affected with pathology compared with the flexor tendons, so little attention is paid to these structures.

Anterior Tibial Tendon (Box 16-7)

The anterior tibial tendon is the most likely of all of the anterior tendons to be abnormal. This tendon is the most medial and the largest of the anterior tendons. Tears are uncommon, but may be seen with increasing age and in individuals who run on hills. Occasionally, patients with a partial or complete tear of this tendon present with a mass suspected to be a tumor, rather than with symptoms of a tendon abnormality (Fig. 16-21),[16,17] but most are diagnosed clinically before imaging. Imaging is done to see how much tendon retraction is present.

BOX 16-7

Anterior Tibial Tendon

- Most commonly abnormal anterior tendon
- Tears occur from age or running hills
- Tears often present as a mass

ANKLE LIGAMENTS

MRI is not routinely used to diagnose ligamentous injuries because they usually can be easily and less expensively diagnosed by clinical examination. In patients who have persistent pain, or who may be imaged for seemingly unrelated reasons, the ligaments need to be evaluated and well understood because abnormalities can be identified and may have clinical significance.[18-21] Also, it is becoming apparent that many ligament abnormalities are associated with other causes of chronic ankle pain (eg, sinus tarsi syndrome). One must be able to identify ligament pathology on MRI. Generally, the ligaments are thin, taut, low signal intensity structures; however, the thick bands of collagen may predictably create a striated appearance in certain ligaments, including the anterior tibiofibular, the posterior talofibular, and the deep (tibiotalar) and superficial (tibiocalcaneal) layers of the deltoid. The striated appearance in these ligaments must not be confused with partial tears.

Medial Ankle Ligaments

The medial collateral ligamentous complex (deltoid ligament) lies deep to the medial flexor tendons. It has several components—tibiotalar, tibiocalcaneal, talonavicular, and the spring ligament (between the sustentaculum of the calcaneus and navicular bone); the first two of these components routinely are seen well on coronal MR images (Fig. 16-22). The deep tibiotalar portion of the deltoid ligament is seen as a striated structure coursing obliquely between the medial malleolus and the talus on coronal and axial images, usually best on the coronal images. The tibiocalcaneal component of the deltoid runs vertically, just deep to the flexor retinaculum and superficial to the tibiotalar component of the ligament.[22] The deltoid ligament is only infrequently injured compared with the lateral ankle ligaments.

The MRI appearance of a deltoid ligament injury depends on which components were injured and to what extent

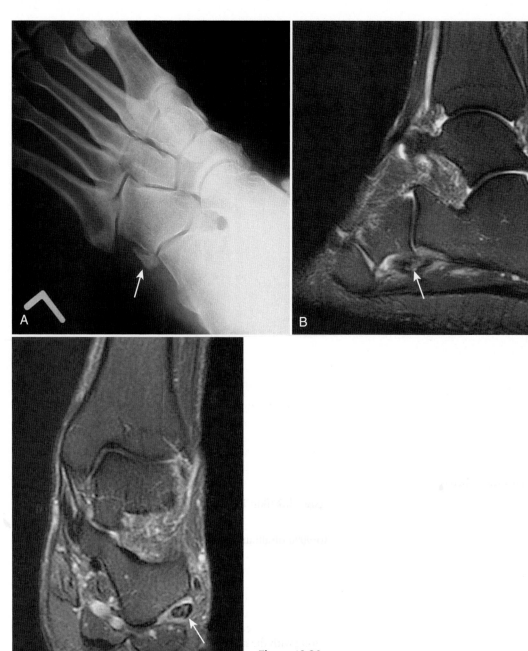

Figure 16-20 **Painful os peroneus syndrome. A,** Plain film of the midfoot shows an irregular, enlarged os peroneus (*arrow*). **B,** FSE-T2W sagittal image of the ankle. Increased signal is present in the os peroneus (*arrow*) just before the peroneus longus tendon courses beneath the cuboid. **C,** FSE-T2W coronal image of the ankle. The os peroneus (*arrow*) is has increased signal within and some surrounding increased signal. This is characteristic for painful os peroneus syndrome.

(Fig. 16-23). The tibiotalar component often loses its striated appearance and shows high signal intensity on T1W and T2W images. This appearance may indicate either a contusion or a tear of the ligament. The tibiocalcaneal portion may be discontinuous and have high signal intensity hemorrhage and edema acutely; a chronic tear may appear as a thickened or discontinuous ligament.

The spring ligament, also called the *tibio-spring ligament,* arises from the medial malleolus as the medialmost portion of the deltoid. It extends inferiorly just deep to the posterior tibial tendon and then curves medially to support the head

of the talus and inserts onto the sustentaculum tali (Fig. 16-24). Although we simplistically think of the spring ligament as having a J shape and supporting the head of the talus like a sling or a hammock, it is more complex than that.[23] Three portions of the spring ligament have been described,[23] but we typically do not identify each portion separately on MRI.

An abnormal spring ligament is often associated with a torn posterior tibial tendon.[24] The posterior tibial tendon and the spring ligament help support the longitudinal arch, and when the posterior tibial tendon fails to hold its share

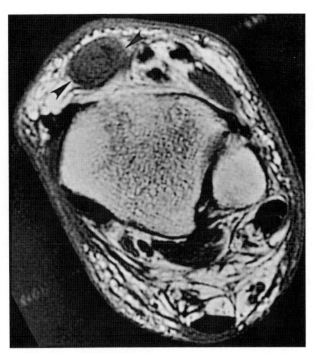

Figure 16-21 **Anterior tibial tendon: tear.** T1W axial image of the ankle. There is a large, round intermediate signal structure (*arrowheads*) anterior to the ankle from a complete tear of the tibialis anterior tendon.

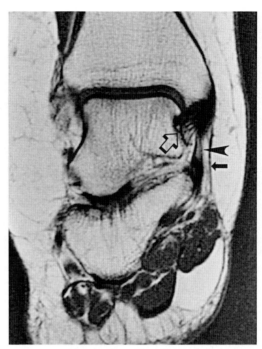

Figure 16-22 **Medial ankle ligaments: normal.** T1W coronal image of the ankle. Two layers of the deltoid (medial) ligament are seen on routine MRI. The deep tibiotalar ligament is striated (*open arrow*). The more superficial tibiocalcaneal ligament (*arrowhead*) may have vertical striations also. The thin, vertical, low signal structure superficial to the tibiocalcaneal ligament is the flexor retinaculum (*solid arrow*).

of the load, the spring ligament cannot support the arch by itself, so it too fails. An abnormal spring ligament is identified with MRI if it is unusually thickened or has intermediate signal within it on T1W or T2W sequences (Fig. 16-25). A

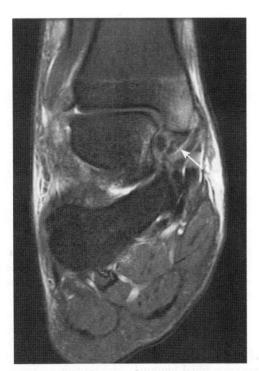

Figure 16-23 **Medial ankle ligaments: tears.** FSE-T2W coronal image of the ankle. The deep tibiotalar ligament (*arrow*) has lost its striated appearance and is enlarged secondary to a tear with some retraction of the tendon.

torn spring ligament is identified by noting a gap in the tendon (Fig. 16-26).[25]

Lateral Ankle Ligaments (Box 16-8)

The lateral collateral ligamentous complex is affected in 80% to 90% of all ankle ligament injuries. Generally, these ligaments are best evaluated on axial images. The superiorly located lateral ligaments include the anterior and posterior tibiofibular ligaments, which are located just above the tibiotalar joint (Fig. 16-27). These ligaments course superiorly from the fibula to the tibia (or inferiorly from the tibia to the fibula). The anterior and posterior tibiofibular ligaments, along with the interosseous membrane between the tibia and fibula, compose the syndesmosis. These ligaments are seen well on axial images and often are seen on coronal images also (see Fig. 16-27). These ligaments often are best identified on an axial cut that passes through the dome of the talus; this should not cause confusion in thinking that the cut is too distal to be the tibiofibular ligaments. On sagittal images through the ankle, the posterior tibiofibular ligament cut in cross section may resemble an intra-articular loose body in the ankle because it is surrounded by ankle joint fluid (see Fig. 16-27D). Following the structure on adjacent cuts and its predictable location at the level of the tibiotalar joint makes the differentiation between pathology and normal anatomy possible.[18] The tibiofibular ligaments can be torn, and this is recognized by discontinuity of the low signal structures on axial MR images (Fig. 16-28).

The second set of lateral ligaments is located just distal to the tibiotalar joint. This inferior set of ligaments is made of the anterior talofibular, calcaneofibular, and poste-

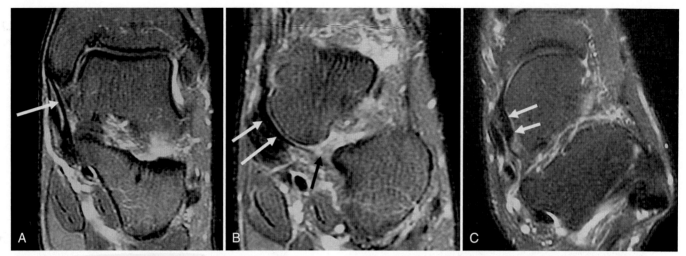

Figure 16-24   Spring ligament: normal. A, FSE-T2W coronal image of the ankle. The spring ligament (*arrow*) is visible as an extension of the medialmost part of the deltoid ligament, arising from the medial malleolus and inserting onto the sustentaculum tali. **B,** FSE-T2W coronal image of the ankle (anterior to **A**). The spring ligament (*white arrows*) can be seen supporting the head of the talus. Note the increased signal where it inserts onto the talus (*black arrow*). This is the normal appearance and should not be interpreted as a tear. **C,** FSE-T2W axial image of the ankle. The spring ligament (*arrows*) is seen adjacent to the talus and just deep to the posterior tibial tendon.

rior talofibular ligaments, from anterior to posterior (Fig. 16-29). The anterior and posterior talofibular ligaments are seen best on axial images just below the tibiotalar joint at the level of the concavity in the medial aspect of the lateral malleolus, called the *malleolar fossa* (Fig. 16-30). The calcaneofibular ligament is the most difficult ligament to identify routinely and may be best seen on coronal images (see Fig. 16-30).[18]

The anterior talofibular ligament is the most commonly torn of the ankle ligaments. It usually is an isolated tear, but if the traumatic forces are great enough, the other ligaments may tear in a sequential fashion. That is, after the anterior talofibular ligament tears, the calcaneofibular ligament tears, followed, only rarely, by the posterior talofibular ligament. The anterior talofibular ligament is a thickening of the ankle joint capsule. An acute ligament tear results in a capsular tear with leakage of fluid into the soft tissues around the ligament

(Fig. 16-31). An acute tear is seen as a discontinuous ligament with surrounding edema/hemorrhage. A chronic tear may show discontinuity of the ligament, but often scarring forms so that the ligament appears intact but irregular, with thickening, thinning, or detachment from the associated osseous structures (see Fig. 16-31D).[19,20]

Approximately 15% of ankle sprains result in instability, either mechanical (objective instability on physical examination) or functional (subjective feeling that the ankle is giving

---

BOX 16-8

Lateral Ankle Ligaments

Superior Group
- Anterior and posterior tibiofibular ligaments
  - Seen at top of ankle joint on axial images
  - Posterior tibiofibular ligament mimics ankle loose body on sagittal images

Inferior Group
- Anterior to posterior: Anterior talofibular, calcaneofibular, posterior talofibular
  - Calcaneofibular: Best seen on coronal images, but seen inconsistently
  - Anterior and posterior talofibular: Seen on axial images at level of malleolar fossa of fibula
- Usually tear in sequence from anterior to posterior
- Tears associated with
  Osteochondral fractures
  Long-term instability
  Sinus tarsi syndrome

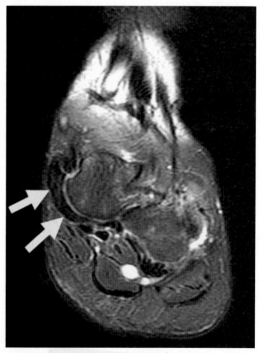

Figure 16-25   Spring ligament: thickened. FSE-T2W coronal image of the ankle. The spring ligament (*arrows*) is markedly thickened and has increased signal. At surgery, this was described as a thickened, fibrotic spring ligament.

way). Several entities have an association with lateral ankle ligament tears, including sinus tarsi syndrome, anterolateral impingement syndrome, and longitudinal split tears of the peroneus brevis tendon. Finally, bone contusions and osteochondral fractures of the talar dome are common complicating features, often impossible to identify by conventional radiography, but easily identified on MRI.

MISCELLANEOUS INFLAMMATORY CONDITIONS

Anterolateral Impingement Syndrome in the Ankle (Box 16-9)

Anterolateral impingement syndrome in the ankle is produced by entrapment of abnormal soft tissue in the anterolateral gutter of the ankle. The gutter is the space bounded by the anterior tibiofibular and anterior talofibular ligaments anteriorly, by the talus medially, and by the fibula laterally. The space extends superiorly to the tibial plafond and tibiofibular syndesmosis, and distally to the calcaneofibular ligament (Fig. 16-32).[26,27] This also is a common location for intra-articular loose bodies to lodge.

Patients with the impingement syndrome have anterolateral ankle pain, swelling, and limited dorsiflexion that is clinically indistinguishable from symptoms caused by several other abnormalities. The soft tissue lesions that may cause the problems are hypertrophic synovium, fibrotic scar, or an accessory fascicle of the anterior tibiofibular ligament. Most cases result from trauma or surgery, and the lesion can be removed arthroscopically. Patients often give a history of an inversion injury, and there is probably an injury to the anterior tibiofibular and talofibular ligaments at the time of the injury that leads to synovitis and scarring with resultant

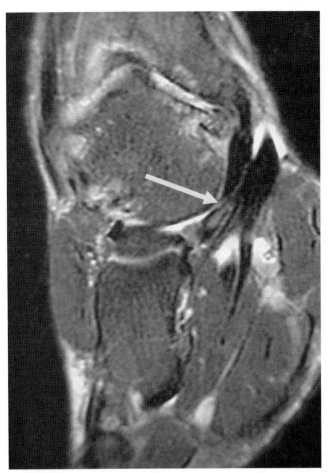

Figure 16-26   Spring ligament: torn. FSE-T2W coronal image of the ankle. The proximal part of the spring ligament is thickened with a gap (*arrow*) seen in the midportion. The distal spring ligament has increased signal within. At surgery, this was found to be a torn spring ligament.

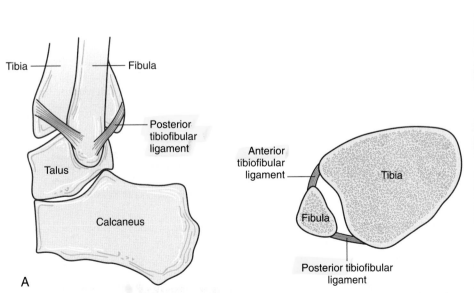
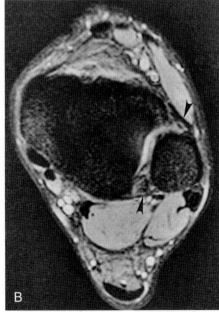

Figure 16-27   Tibiofibular ligaments: normal. A, Diagram of the anterior and posterior tibiofibular ligaments from sagittal and axial perspectives. These ligaments run inferiorly from the tibia to the fibula. **B,** T2*W axial image of the ankle. Intact anterior and posterior tibiofibular ligaments (*arrowheads*) are present.

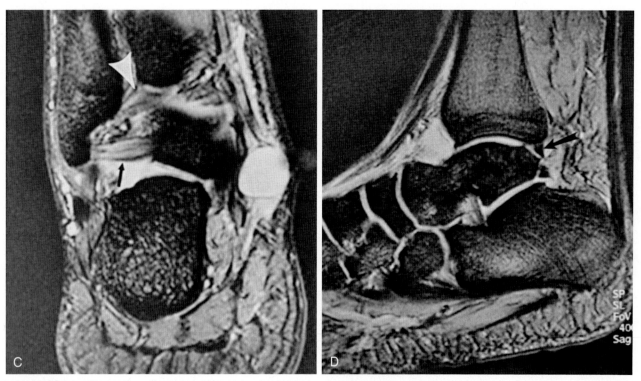

C   D

Figure 16-27, cont'd   C, T2*W coronal image of the ankle. The posterior tibiofibular ligament (*arrowhead*) and the posterior talofibular ligament (*arrow*) are seen as striated structures on this image. There is a ganglion cyst medially. **D,** T2*W sagittal image of the ankle. The posterior tibiofibular ligament is seen in cross section (*arrow*) at the ankle joint line. This ligament must not be confused with an intra-articular loose body. There is an os trigonum below the ligament with a similar size and appearance.

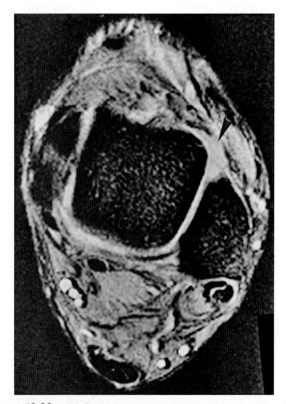

Figure 16-28   Tibiofibular ligament: tear. T2*W axial image of the ankle. The anterior tibiofibular ligament is absent (*arrowhead*), and there is high signal edema in the region.

anterolateral joint line tenderness and the sensation of the ankle giving way.

The diagnosis is made on MRI by identifying soft tissue deep to the anterior tibiofibular or anterior talofibular ligament where normally none is present (Fig. 16-33). A joint effusion can aid in the recognition of the soft tissue mass in this region. Instability related to a disrupted ligament can cause clinical features identical to those of anterior impingement syndrome.[26]

Sinus Tarsi Syndrome (Box 16-10)

The sinus tarsi, or tarsal sinus, is a cone-shaped space formed between the calcaneus and talus (Figs. 16-34 and 16-35). The narrow end of the cone is located medially, whereas the large

---

BOX 16-9

Anterolateral Impingement Syndrome

Clinical
- Anterolateral pain, swelling, limited dorsiflexion

Etiology
- Post-traumatic (inversion)

Pathology
- Synovitis, fibrosis in anterolateral gutter

MRI
- Low signal soft tissue mass deep to anterior tibiofibular and talofibular ligaments

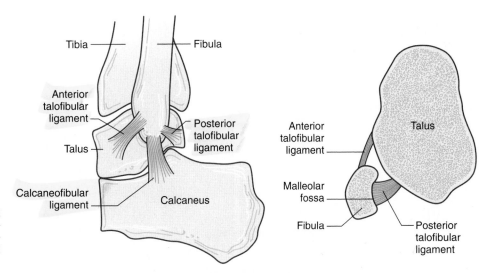

Figure 16-29 **Inferior set of lateral ankle ligaments.** Diagram of anterior talofibular, calcaneofibular, and posterior talofibular ligaments from sagittal and axial perspectives.

end is located laterally, beneath the lateral malleolus. The sinus tarsi contains fat, several ligaments, neurovascular structures, and portions of the joint capsule of the posterior subtalar joint. Nerve endings in the sinus tarsi are important for proprioception of the hindfoot. Hindfoot stability is partially maintained by the talocalcaneal ligaments located within the sinus tarsi. The most lateral of the ligaments are slips from the lateral extensor retinaculum; medial to these slips are the cervical ligament, and most medial is the interosseous ligament.[28-30]

The sinus tarsi syndrome is a pain syndrome characterized by lateral foot pain and the subjective feeling of hindfoot instability. There may be tenderness over the area on physical examination. Pathologically, the sinus tarsi is found to contain inflammatory tissue or fibrosis, depending on the chronicity of the changes. Disruption of the interosseous and cervical ligaments also is often found. The major cause of this syndrome (70%) is related to trauma, with lateral injuries and tears of the anterior talofibular and calcaneofibular ligaments usually present. The cervical and interosseous ligaments of the sinus tarsi are injured by an inversion injury, along with the lateral ankle ligaments. Eighty percent of patients with sinus tarsi syndrome may have a torn lateral ligament.[30] Disruption of the ligaments in the sinus tarsi and injury to the proprioceptive nerve fibers are thought to account for the sensation of instability.

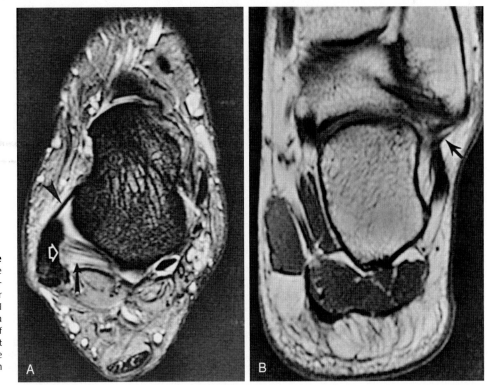

Figure 16-30 **Inferior lateral ankle ligaments: normal. A,** T2*W axial image of the ankle. The anterior talofibular ligament (*arrowhead*) and striated posterior talofibular ligament (*solid arrow*) are well seen at the level of the malleolar fossa (*open arrow*). **B,** T1W coronal image of the ankle. The calcaneofibular ligament (*arrow*) is best seen on this view. The posterior talofibular ligament is seen above it.

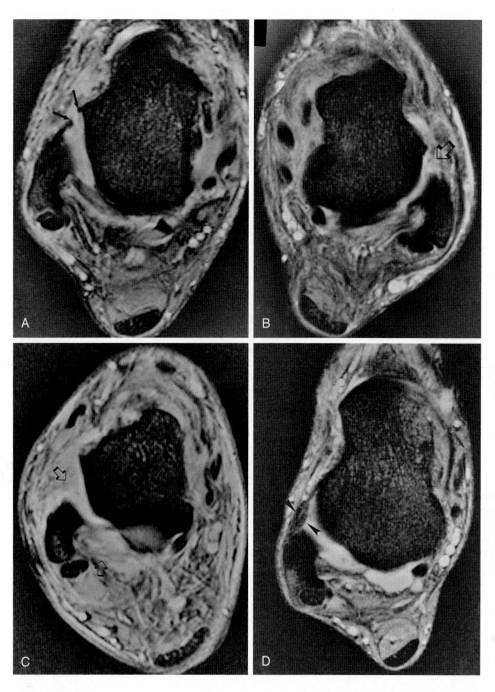

Figure 16-31 Talofibular ligaments: tears. A, T2*W axial image of the ankle. Torn fragments of the anterior talofibular ligament are seen (*arrows*), with hemorrhage/edema leaking from the ankle joint into the soft tissues. The striated posterior talofibular ligament remains intact. **B,** T2*W axial image of the ankle (different patient than in **A**). The *arrow* points to edema in the soft tissues, but no anterior talofibular ligament is evident because of a tear. The posterior ligament is not torn. **C,** T2*W axial image of the ankle (different patient). The anterior and the posterior talofibular ligaments (*arrows*) are not identified, indicating they are torn. By definition, the intervening calcaneofibular ligament also must be torn. The space between the talus and fibula is widened. **D,** T2*W axial image of the ankle (different patient). The lateral aspect of the anterior talofibular ligament is markedly thickened (*arrowheads*) and low signal. This indicates a previous rupture with scarring and fibrosis that mimics an intact ligament.

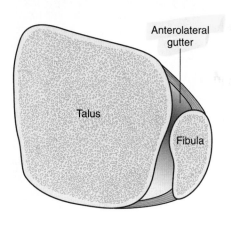

Boundaries

Anterior: Anterior tibiofibular and talofibular ligaments

Medial: Talus

Lateral: Fibula

Superior: Tibial plafond, syndesmosis

Inferior: Calcaneofibular ligament

Figure 16-32 Anterolateral impingement: anatomy. Diagram of the boundaries of the anterolateral gutter of the ankle. Soft tissue in the *shaded area* of the anterolateral gutter may be a source of pain.

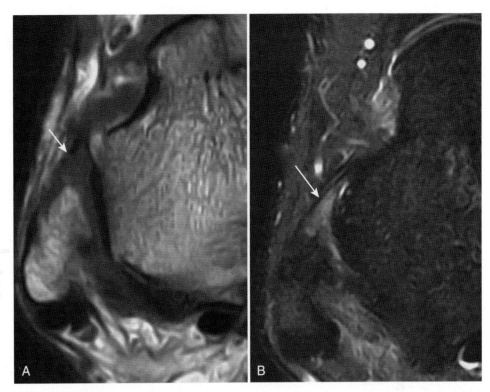

Figure 16-33 Anterolateral impingement syndrome. **A,** T1W axial image of the ankle. There is abnormal low signal (*arrow*) deep to the anterior talofibular ligament in the anterolateral gutter, compatible with either a joint effusion or scar tissue. **B,** FSE-T2W axial image of the ankle. No joint effusion is present. Scar tissue indicative of anterolateral impingement is seen in the joint (*arrow*). The anterior talofibular ligament is thin and attenuated.

Other conditions are related to this syndrome besides ligamentous injury from trauma. Inflammatory arthropathies with extension of pannus from the subtalar joint and chronic posterior tibial tendon tears also are associated with the syndrome in about 30% of cases.

MRI does not consistently show the ligaments of the sinus tarsi even when they are present and intact, so not identifying these ligaments has no significance. Abnormalities of the sinus tarsi on MRI include obliteration of the fat by low signal intensity material on T1W images and either high or low signal intensity (or a combination) on T2W images (Fig. 16-36). Acute abnormalities have inflammatory tissue that

is high signal intensity on T2W images, whereas chronic lesions have fibrosis that is often low signal intensity on T2W images. People with symptoms of sinus tarsi syndrome usually have obliteration of all of the fat in the sinus tarsi. If only part of the fat has been replaced, it is unlikely to be associated with the sinus tarsi syndrome. Associated findings of lateral ligament tears, inflammatory arthritis, and posterior tibial tendon tears should be searched for.[28] One must not confuse a large joint effusion of the ankle or subtalar joint extending into the sinus tarsi as evidence of an abnormal sinus tarsi. The fat in the sinus tarsi can be obscured by fluid or hemorrhage in acute ankle sprains; a diagnosis of sinus tarsi syndrome should not be made in the setting of acute trauma.

Abnormalities of the fat in the sinus tarsi on MRI do not always correlate with clinical features of the sinus tarsi syndrome. It is important to describe the abnormalities seen on MRI and state that this may indicate the patient has symptoms of the sinus tarsi syndrome, rather than making the dogmatic diagnosis of sinus tarsi syndrome based on the MRI features only. This syndrome can be treated by steroid injection, reconstruction of the ligaments of the sinus tarsi, surgical débridement, and, rarely, triple arthrodesis.

Plantar Fasciitis (Box 16-11)

The plantar fascia or aponeurosis is a longitudinal fibrous condensation that originates from the plantar aspect of the calcaneal tuberosity. It is composed of a thick, cordlike central portion and thinner, membrane-like lateral and medial expansions. The central cord of the fascia arises from the medial aspect of the calcaneus and attaches distally to the plantar surfaces of the phalanges and superficially into the skin. It is normally a low signal intensity structure on all

---

BOX 16-10

Sinus Tarsi Syndrome

Clinical
- Lateral foot pain, relieved by anesthetic injection
- Subjective hindfoot instability

Etiology
- Inflammatory arthritis (30%)
- Trauma from inversion (70%)
  - Torn lateral ankle and sinus tarsi ligaments
  - Disruption of proprioceptive nerves

Pathology
- Inflammatory tissue leads to fibrosis
- Disrupted ankle and sinus tarsi ligaments
- Posterior tibial tendon tears associated

MRI
- Obliteration of sinus tarsi fat
  - Low signal on T1W
  - High or low signal on T2W (inflammatory versus fibrosis)
- Tears of calcaneofibular and anterior talofibular ligaments, and of posterior tibial tendon associated

pulse sequences that should not measure more than 4 mm in thickness at its thickest proximal attachment to the calcaneus (Fig. 16-37).

Plantar fasciitis is an inflammatory condition of the plantar fascia that causes pain and tenderness, usually near its attachment to the anteromedial calcaneal tuberosity. The two groups most commonly affected by this condition are running athletes and obese, middle-aged women because of chronic repetitive microtrauma and overuse. Patients with seronegative spondyloarthropathies have a high incidence of plantar fasciitis as well, and it usually is bilateral in these patients. The clinical diagnosis of plantar fasciitis is often straightforward, without the necessity for performing MRI, but this is not always the case, especially if conservative management fails. Rarely, the plantar fascia can rupture completely, which is usually the result of forced dorsiflexion of the foot. This condition is clinically difficult to diagnose, but can be well seen on MRI.

BOX 16-11

Plantar Fasciitis and Rupture

Fasciitis

Clinical
- Obese women, runners, or patients with seronegative arthritis with heel pain

Etiology
- Chronic, repetitive stresses or inflammation

Pathology
- Tears, myxoid degeneration, inflammation

MRI
- Thickened with high signal (T1W, T2W) at calcaneal attachment
- Perifasciitis (edema around thickened fascia)
- Marrow edema/erosions, plantar aspect of calcaneal tuberosity

Rupture

Clinical
- Forced dorsiflexion
- Thickened, disruption in mid-portion (distal to calcaneal attachment)

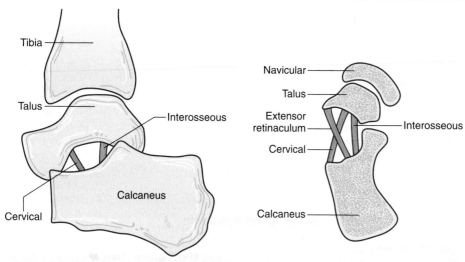

Figure 16-34 Sinus tarsi: anatomy. Diagram of the sinus tarsi (tarsal sinus) between the talus and calcaneus from sagittal and axial perspectives. The different talocalcaneal ligaments are shown.

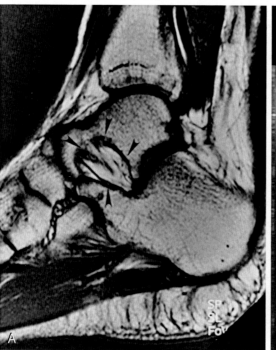 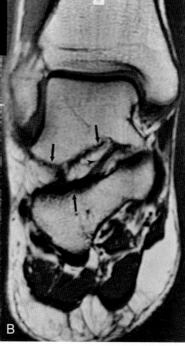

Figure 16-35 Sinus tarsi: normal. **A,** T1W sagittal image of the ankle. The sinus tarsi (*arrowheads*) is filled with high signal fat except for the linear low signal talocalcaneal ligaments coursing through it. **B,** T1W coronal image of the ankle. Another perspective of the fat-filled space between the talus and calcaneus (*arrows*) with a talocalcaneal ligament (*arrowhead*) passing through it.

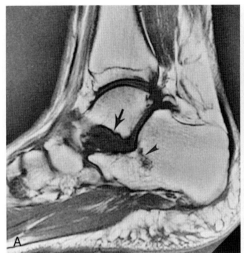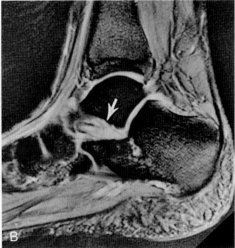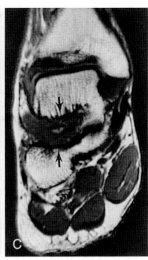

Figure 16-36   Sinus tarsi: abnormal. **A,** T1W sagittal image of the ankle. The fat in the sinus tarsi is obliterated with intermediate signal material (*arrow*). There is a vascular remnant in the calcaneus (*arrowhead*). **B,** T2*W sagittal image of the ankle. The sinus tarsi is high signal, indicating inflammatory tissue that has not yet become fibrotic (*arrow*). **C,** T1W coronal image of the ankle. Sinus tarsi fat obliteration (*arrows*) between the talus and calcaneus from another perspective.

MRI of plantar fasciitis shows thickening of the fascia, usually near the attachment to the calcaneus, with intermediate signal on T1W and high signal on T2W images. Edema often is seen surrounding the fascia, and adjacent bone marrow edema or erosions are common in the plantar aspect of the calcaneal tuberosity (Fig. 16-38). Plantar fascia rupture usually occurs in the midportion of the fascia, distal to the typical location of fasciitis at the calcaneal attachment (see Fig. 16-34). A ruptured fascia appears as discontinuity of the fascia with surrounding high signal in the soft tissues on T2W images, secondary to the hemorrhage and edema (Fig. 16-39).[31,32]

Plantar fasciitis is treated conservatively with rest, modified footwear, nonsteroidal anti-inflammatory drugs, and sometimes steroid injections. Surgery only rarely is performed for purposes of a fascial release or excision of damaged fascia.

NERVE ABNORMALITIES

Tarsal Tunnel Syndrome (Boxes 16-12 and 16-13)

The tarsal tunnel is a fibro-osseous tunnel located on the medial side of the ankle and hindfoot, extending from the medial malleolus to the navicular bone. The talus and calcaneus, including the sustentaculum tali, form the lateral side of the tunnel, whereas the medial side is bordered by the flexor retinaculum and abductor hallucis muscle. Within the confines of these structures is the tunnel, which contains the posterior tibial nerve and its divisions, the posterior tibial artery and vein, posterior tibial tendon, flexor digitorum longus tendon, and flexor hallucis longus tendon (Fig. 16-40).[33]

Tarsal tunnel syndrome consists of a constellation of symptoms that are secondary to compression of the poste-

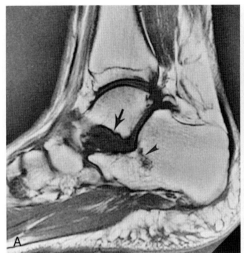

Figure 16-37   Plantar fascia: normal. STIR sagittal image of the ankle. The low signal plantar fascia (*arrows*) attaches to the calcaneal tuberosity proximally and gradually tapers as it extends distally. It originates medially (note the flexor hallucis longus tendon passing beneath the sustentaculum tali, indicating the medial side of the foot).

BOX 16-12

Tarsal Tunnel Anatomy

Confines

- Craniocaudal: Medial malleolus to navicular
- Lateral: Talus and calcaneus
- Medial: Flexor retinaculum, abductor hallucis muscle

Contents

- Posterior tibial, flexor hallucis longus, flexor digitorum longus tendons
- Posterior tibial nerve, artery, and veins

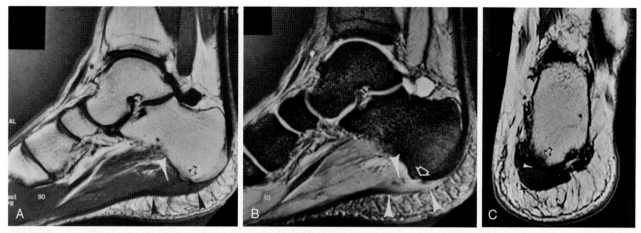

Figure 16-38 Plantar fasciitis. A, T1W sagittal image of the hindfoot. The proximal plantar fascia is thickened and high signal (between *arrowheads*). There is an erosion of the adjacent calcaneal tuberosity (*arrow*). **B,** T2*W sagittal image of the hindfoot. The same findings are seen as in **A,** but the signal in the fascia is higher, and the abnormality is easier to identify. **C,** T1W coronal image of the hindfoot. The calcaneal erosion and marrow edema are evident (*arrow*). The plantar fascia on the medial side of the calcaneus is about four times its normal thickness (between *arrowheads*) and higher signal than normal.

rior tibial nerve or its branches. The precise location of the compression determines exactly what the symptoms are because different nerve branches are affected. The symptoms consist of burning and paresthesias along the sole of the foot and to the toes, often worse with activity. Motor symptoms usually are absent until late.

Tarsal tunnel syndrome may arise from abnormalities intrinsic or extrinsic to the tunnel that cause compression of the nerves in the tunnel. Among the most common causes are ganglion cysts and nerve sheath tumors arising within the tunnel (Figs. 16-41 and 16-42). Other reported causes of the syndrome are tenosynovitis of the flexor hallucis longus tendon, tarsal coalition with bone hypertrophy of the middle facet of the subtalar joint, anomalous muscles (either the accessory soleus or the flexor digitorum longus), venous varices, pannus, hemangioma, and post-traumatic fibrosis, among others (Fig. 16-43).

MRI is valuable in showing the presence and precise location of the abnormality responsible for the compressive neuropathy. Ganglion cysts and nerve sheath tumors are the two most common causes of this syndrome seen on MRI; these masses can look identical with very homogeneous low signal on T1W images and high signal intensity on T2W images. This is a good indication for contrast administration to differentiate between the two entities because surgery for each is significantly different. Even if MRI shows no abnormality affecting the tarsal tunnel, it is valuable because it means that surgery is not indicated and would not benefit the patient. In the latter situation, the nerve generally is affected by scarring and fibrosis, which MRI cannot detect.

Morton's Neuroma (Box 16-14)

Morton's neuroma, or interdigital neuroma, previously was believed to represent a neoplastic process of the nerve, but now is thought to be secondary to chronic nerve entrapment

---

BOX 16-13

Tarsal Tunnel Syndrome

Clinical

- Burning, paresthesias in sole and into toes

Etiology/Pathology

- Compression of posterior tibial nerve or its branches from
  - Ganglion cyst
  - Nerve sheath tumors
  - Tenosynovitis
  - Varices
  - Pannus
  - Hemangioma
  - Tarsal coalition
  - Fibrosis

MRI

- Shows presence of a mass (or not), which determines surgery (or not)
- MRI features depend on underlying pathology

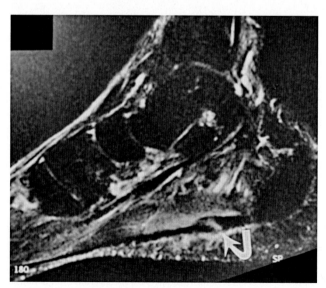

Figure 16-39 Plantar fascia: rupture. STIR sagittal image of the hindfoot. There is disruption of the plantar fascia (*arrow*) about 2 cm from its origin on the calcaneus. There is surrounding high signal edema/hemorrhage.

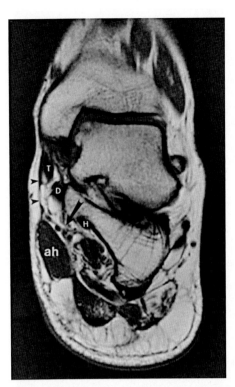

Figure 16-40   Tarsal tunnel: normal. T1W coronal image of the hindfoot. The tarsal tunnel is located between the flexor retinaculum (*arrowheads*) and the abductor hallucis muscle (ah) medially, and the osseous structures laterally. The flexor tendons are located in this tunnel. The posterior tibial nerve, artery, and vein (*arrow*) pass through the tunnel. D, flexor digitorum; H, flexor hallucis; T, tibialis posterior.

BOX 16-14

Morton's Neuroma

Clinical
- Pain in second or third web spaces, radiating to toes
- Women or others wearing high-heeled, poorly fitting shoes

Etiology/Pathology
- Chronic plantar digital nerve entrapment leading to perineural fibrosis, neural degeneration, adjacent intermetatarsal bursitis

MRI
- Teardrop-shaped soft tissue mass between and plantar to metatarsal heads
- T1W: Low signal
- T2W: High or low signal, depending on quantity of fibrosis
- Gadolinium: Enhances but unnecessary
- Fluid in adjacent intermetatarsal bursa and surrounding soft tissue edema is common (low signal on T1W; high signal on T2W)

---

with subsequent perineural fibrosis, neural degeneration, and often adjacent intermetatarsal bursitis. The usual location is around the plantar digital nerve of the second or third intermetatarsal space (Fig. 16-44).

Symptoms include pain, often electrical in nature, and throbbing in the affected web space, radiating to the toes. Young and middle-aged women most commonly are affected; this may be due to chronic trauma to the nerve from wearing high-heeled shoes. Morton's neuromas and intermetatarsal bursitis may be present on MRI in patients who are asymptomatic.[34,35]

Some clinicians advocate performing only T1W short-axis axial images through the metatarsal heads to screen

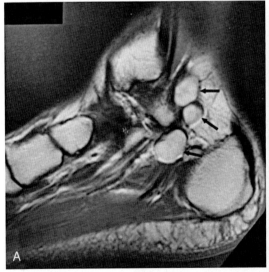

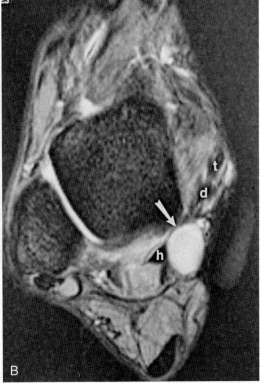

Figure 16-41   Tarsal tunnel syndrome: from schwannomas. A, T1W contrast-enhanced sagittal image of the hindfoot. Three round masses (*arrows*) that show enhancement are running through the tarsal tunnel. **B,** T2*W axial image of the hindfoot. One of the schwannomas is shown as a high signal mass (*arrow*) in the space normally occupied by the posterior tibial nerve, artery, and vein. d, flexor digitorum tendon; h, flexor hallucis tendon; t, tibialis posterior tendon.

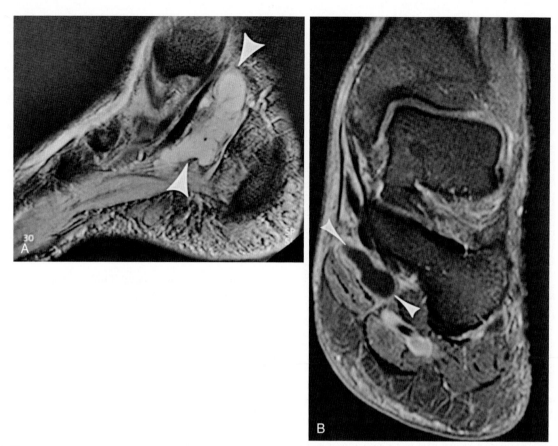

Figure 16-42 **Tarsal tunnel syndrome: from ganglion cyst. A,** T2*W sagittal image of the hindfoot. There is a long, septated mass (*arrowheads*) posterior to the flexor digitorum tendon in the tarsal tunnel. **B,** T1W coronal image of the hindfoot with contrast enhancement and fat suppression. The mass in the tarsal tunnel (*arrowheads*) shows enhancement only at its periphery, indicating this is a cystic lesion. The ganglion cyst lies adjacent to the posterior tibial nerve in the tunnel.

for Morton's neuroma. This approach presumes that the diagnosis is clear-cut clinically. That is not our experience, so we do a routine examination with all imaging planes, including T1W and T2W sequences. Although some clinicians believe T1W images do not show Morton's neuromas with the conspicuity of contrast-enhanced images,[36] we have not found giving gadolinium to be helpful in

distinguishing a Morton's neuroma, which is low signal on T2W sequences, from an intermetatarsal bursa, which is high signal on T2W sequences. The MRI appearance is of a teardrop-shaped soft tissue mass between the metatarsal heads that projects inferiorly into the plantar subcutaneous fat (Figs. 16-45 and 16-46). The signal intensity is intermediate on T1W and usually low signal

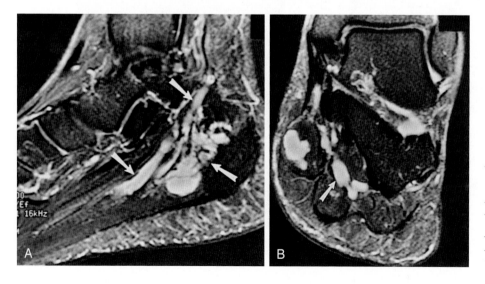

Figure 16-43 **Tarsal tunnel syndrome: from hemangioma. A,** Fast-T2W sagittal image of the hindfoot with fat suppression. High signal linear structures (*arrows*) course through the tarsal tunnel. These are vessels from a hemangioma. **B,** Fast-T2W coronal image of the hindfoot with fat suppression. The tortuous vessels are evident in the tarsal tunnel (*arrow*) and within the abductor hallucis muscle.

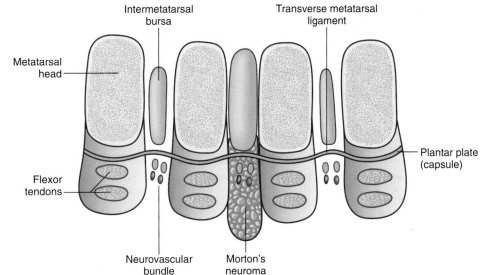

Figure 16-44 Morton's neuroma: anatomy. Diagram of the forefoot in cross section. The plantar digital nerves are located deep to the transverse metatarsal ligament between metatarsal heads. Above the nerves are the intermetatarsal bursae. Entrapment of the plantar digital nerve may lead to perineural fibrosis and neural degeneration (Morton's neuroma). Intermetatarsal bursitis is a common accompaniment.

intensity on T2W images because of the abundant fibrosis present. Fluid in the adjacent intermetatarsal bursa secondary to inflammation often is present as well (Fig. 16-47). The intermetatarsal bursa runs in a vertical direction between (not beneath) metatarsal heads; bursitis shows low signal intensity on T1W images and high signal intensity on T2W images. Treatment may consist of modification of footwear, percutaneous neurolysis, surgical release by dividing the transverse metatarsal ligament, or excision.

BONE ABNORMALITIES

Tarsal Coalition

Tarsal coalition is a common abnormality, occurring in about 6% of the population, and is thought to represent a failure of proper segmentation of the tarsal bones; it also can be acquired secondary to rheumatoid arthritis or trauma. Males are affected approximately four times more frequently than females, and it is bilateral in about 50% of individuals.

The two most common types are calcaneonavicular (which often is asymptomatic and diagnosed on medial oblique foot films rather than MRI) and talocalcaneal, which usually occurs between the sustentaculum tali process of the calcaneus and the adjacent talus at the middle facet of the subtalar joint.

Symptoms generally occur because of limited motion in the subtalar joint, which places increased stresses elsewhere in the tarsus, leading to spasm of the peroneals and extensors, with an associated flatfoot deformity. Coalitions may be osseous, fibrous, cartilaginous, or a combination.

MRI can be used to show the presence of the coalition, which type, and how extensive it is (Figs. 16-48 to 16-50). In addition, MRI can assess surrounding structures for impingement by the hypertrophic bony mass, such as displacement of the tibialis posterior and flexor hallucis longus tendons in the tarsal tunnel. Secondary degenerative joint disease in the posterior subtalar joint is common and can be documented with MRI. MRI shows narrowing and irregularity, or osseous fusion, of the middle facet of the subtalar joint. The angle of this joint is often abnormal, with a coalition being directed inferiorly.

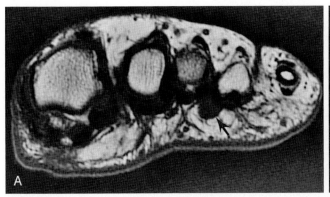
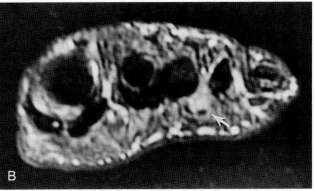

Figure 16-45 Morton's neuroma. **A,** T1W short-axis axial image of the forefoot. A low signal, teardrop-shaped mass (*arrow*) from Morton's neuroma is seen below the metatarsal heads in the third web space. **B,** STIR short-axis axial image of the forefoot. Morton's neuroma (*arrow*) becomes high signal, but is more difficult to see than on the T1W image.

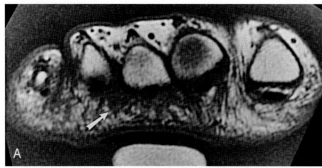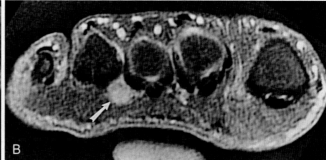

Figure 16-46   Morton's neuroma. **A,** T1W short-axis axial image of the forefoot. There is a mass (*arrow*) in the third web space beneath the metatarsal heads that is difficult to detect on this sequence. **B,** T1W short-axis axial image of the forefoot with contrast enhancement and fat suppression. The mass enhances diffusely (*arrow*) and is an easy diagnosis on this image.

Accessory Bones and Sesamoids (Box 16-15)

Accessory ossicles may result in painful syndromes and associated soft tissue abnormalities. The most common syndromes in the foot are the os trigonum syndrome and abnormalities associated with an accessory navicular bone or the hallux sesamoids.

Os Trigonum Syndrome. The os trigonum syndrome (also known as the posterior ankle impingement syndrome) occurs when the trigonal process of the talus or the os trigonum is compressed between the posterior tibia and the posterior calcaneus during forced plantar flexion, resulting in posterior ankle pain. Recurrent plantar flexion of the foot is required in ballet, running down hills, and kicking a football. Posterior talar compression can result in a stress reaction with marrow edema in the trigonal process or os trigonum (Fig. 16-51), an acute fracture or a chronic stress fracture of the trigonal process of the talus, or fracture through the synchondrosis that normally exists between the talus and the os trigonum. Disruption of the synchondrosis appears as high signal intensity fluid between the os trigonum and the rest of the talus on T2W images, where cartilage normally exists (see Fig. 16-14).[9] Compression of the flexor hallucis longus tendon, which lies immediately adjacent to the medial side of the os trigonum, may cause irritation, inflam-

mation, tenosynovitis, and stenosing tenosynovitis with abnormal high signal intensity within the tendon or surrounding it (see Fig. 16-14). Loose bodies may be seen in the ankle joint secondary to the bone impaction and fragmentation.

Accessory Navicular. The accessory navicular bone or prominent medial tuberosity of the navicular bone was discussed in the section on the posterior tibial tendon. It can cause pain for several reasons. Painful degenerative changes

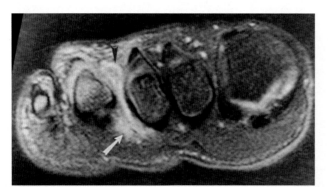

Figure 16-47   Morton's neuroma. T1W short-axis axial image of the forefoot with contrast enhancement and fat suppression. A teardrop-shaped mass (*arrow*) is diagnostic of Morton's neuroma in the third web space. The lining of the inflamed intermetatarsal bursa also enhances (*arrowhead*) between the metatarsal heads.

BOX 16-15

Accessory Ossicles

Os Trigonum Syndrome (Posterior Impingement Syndrome)

Clinical
- Repetitive plantar flexion (ballet, basketball, kicking football, running on hills)

Etiology
- Os trigonum/trigonal process and flexor hallucis tendon trapped between calcaneus and tibia

Pathology
- Marrow edema/fracture of trigonal process or synchondrosis of os trigonum; flexor hallucis longus irritation (stenosing tenosynovitis)

MRI
- T1W
  - Low signal in marrow of posterior talus
- T2W
  - High signal marrow in talus
  - High signal fracture of synchondrosis, os trigonum
  - Focal, loculated high signal fluid around flexor hallucis (stenosing tenosynovitis)

Navicular Bone
- Large cornuate process of navicular or accessory navicular bone
- Marrow edema, overlying bursitis, degenerative joint disease between accessory bone and navicular, associated posterior tibial tendon tears
- T2W MRI shows high signal of all abnormalities

Hallux Sesamoids
- Located in flexor hallucis brevis tendons at first metatarsal head
- Abnormalities: Acute or stress fractures, osteonecrosis, infection, sesamoiditis (inflammation), dislocation, participate in inflammatory and degenerative joint disease
- MRI is sensitive, but nonspecific; low signal on medial sesamoid more likely to be traumatic in origin; lateral sesamoid is more likely osteonecrosis

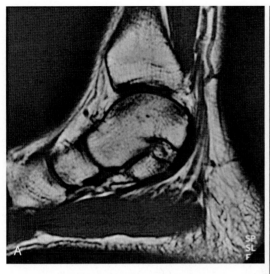

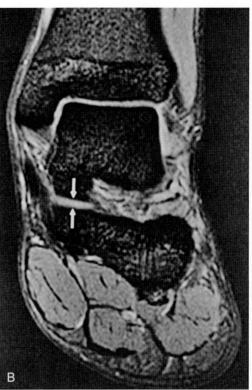

Figure 16-48 **Middle facet of the subtalar joint: normal. A,** T1W sagittal image of the hindfoot. The joint between the sustentaculum tali and talus is straight and uniform, without features of coalition. **B,** T2*W coronal image of the hindfoot. Uniform high signal cartilage is present in the middle facet of the subtalar joint (between *arrows*).

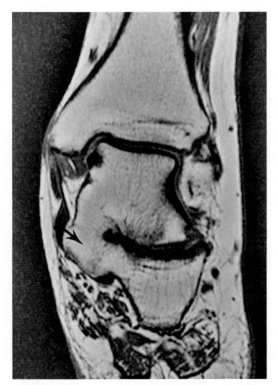

Figure 16-49 **Tarsal coalition: osseous.** T1W coronal image of the hind-foot. There is complete osseous ankylosis with no joint in the expected location (*arrow*) for the middle facet. This hypertrophic bone mass placed pressure on the adjacent posterior tibial nerve; the patient presented with tarsal tunnel syndrome.

between the accessory ossicle and the navicular can occur with marrow edema within the ossicle, a painful bursa can develop in the soft tissues superficial to the navicular prominence, and there is a much higher incidence of posterior tibial tendon tears in the presence of an accessory navicular bone, caused by altered stresses.[6]

Hallux Sesamoids. The medial and lateral hallux sesamoids, which are located in the flexor hallucis brevis tendons at the level of the first metatarsal head, provide mechanical advantage during flexion of the great toe and serve to reduce friction. They may be abnormal for several reasons, including acute fractures, stress fractures, osteonecrosis, infection, sesamoiditis, and dislocation, and they participate in degenerative and inflammatory arthritides. Generally, the medial sesamoid is more likely to be involved with traumatic abnormalities, whereas the lateral sesamoid more commonly is affected by ischemic changes with osteonecrosis (Fig. 16-52).

The MRI appearance of all of these varied abnormalities of the sesamoids is usually identical, regardless of the underlying pathology.[37] A differential diagnosis is necessary in most instances because the findings are nonspecific. If a fracture line is evident, however, or if subchondral bone lesions are seen in a sesamoid and the adjacent metatarsal head, a specific diagnosis of fracture or arthritis can be made (see Fig. 16-52).

The most common soft tissue abnormality to occur in the region of the hallux sesamoids is turf toe. Turf toe is the

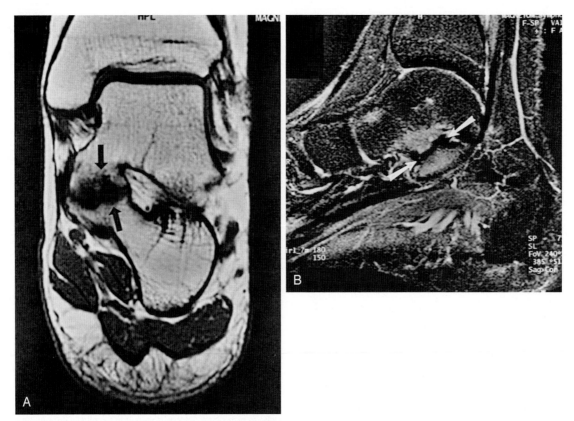

Figure 16-50 Tarsal coalition: fibrocartilaginous. **A,** T1W coronal image of the hindfoot. The joint between the sustentaculum tali and the talus is narrowed and irregular (between *arrows*). **B,** STIR sagittal image of the hindfoot. The joint of the middle facet is irregular and narrowed from fibrocartilaginous coalition (*arrows*). There is high signal bone marrow edema on both sides of the abnormal joint.

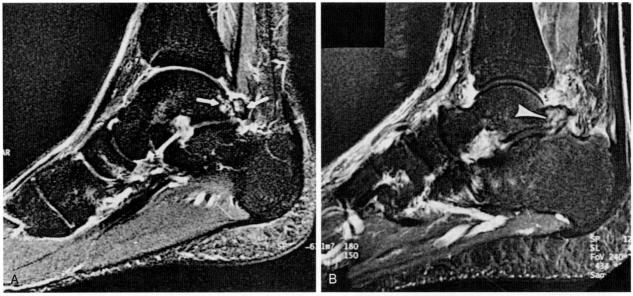

Figure 16-51 Os trigonum syndrome (posterior impingement syndrome). **A,** STIR sagittal image of the hindfoot. There is high signal marrow edema in the os trigonum and the adjacent posterior talus (*arrows*). **B,** STIR sagittal image of the hindfoot (different patient than in **A**). There is no os trigonum in this patient; instead, there is a trigonal process of the posterior talus that has abnormal high signal marrow edema (*arrowhead*) from impingement during repeated plantar flexion.

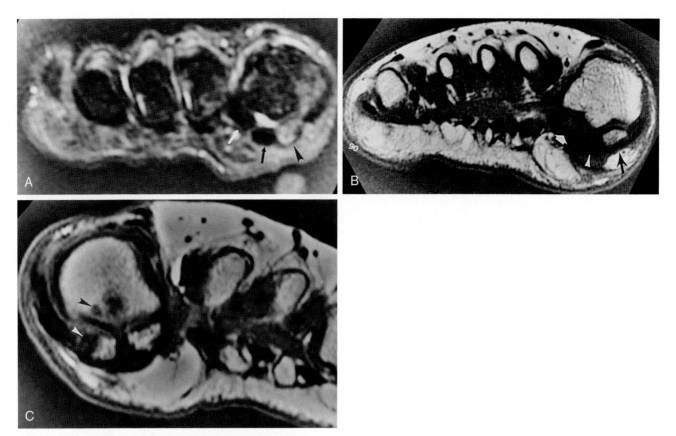

Figure 16-52   Hallux sesamoids. **A,** STIR short-axis axial image of the forefoot. There is abnormal high signal in the medial hallux sesamoid (*arrowhead*). This patient was a runner, and this image most likely shows a stress reaction. The normal lateral hallux sesamoid is shown with a *white arrow*; it is low signal because of fat suppression. The flexor hallucis longus tendon (*black arrow*) runs between the sesamoids. **B,** T1W short-axis axial image of the forefoot (different patient than in **A**). There is low signal throughout the lateral sesamoid (*white arrow*). This is in contrast to the high signal fat in the normal medial sesamoid (*black arrow*). The flexor hallucis tendon is shown with an *arrowhead*. An abnormal lateral sesamoid is more likely to be the result of ischemia than other causes. **C,** T1W short-axis axial image of the forefoot (different patient). There is focal low signal in the medial hallux sesamoid (*white arrowhead*). Similar focal low signal areas are seen in the adjacent first metatarsal head (*black arrowhead*), which makes the diagnosis of degenerative joint disease.

result of hyperdorsiflexion of the first metatarsophalangeal joint with disruption of the plantar capsular tissues. Sesamoid dislocation or subluxation may occur in conjunction with turf toe.

FRACTURES

MRI generally is used to diagnose fractures only when conventional radiographs are normal or inconclusive. The ability of MRI to show fractures is exquisite and is particularly useful for osteochondral fractures of the talar dome and stress and insufficiency fractures throughout the foot and ankle. Any soft tissue abnormalities also are evident.

Bone contusions or osteochondral fractures usually are seen with inversion or eversion injuries of the ankle; associated ligamentous injury virtually is always present. The term *osteochondritis dissecans* (which has been renamed *osteochondral lesion*) has been used for this same entity, suggesting spontaneous osteonecrosis as the cause, but osteochondral fracture is probably the most accurate reflection of the pathology. The medial or lateral aspects of the dome of the talus are affected with equal frequency by these fractures. The fractures may be mere bone contusions or true linear fractures, either with or without overlying cartilaginous

involvement. Sometimes a crack in the cartilage can lead to intrusion of joint fluid with development of large subchondral cysts in the talar dome that may resemble a bone tumor.

MRI of osteochondral fractures (Box 16-16) is useful to show their presence and to show if the fragment is loose (unstable) or not. MRI features to indicate a loose osteochondral fragment are high signal surrounding the fragment on T2W images, large subchondral cysts deep to the fragment, cracks in the overlying cartilage, or absence of the fragment with or without an intra-articular loose body seen

---

BOX 16-16

Osteochondral Fractures (Osteochondritis Dissecans, Osteochondral Lesions)

- Dome of talus affected from injury as talus impacts against tibia; medial or lateral aspect of talar dome involved
- Ligamentous injuries commonly are associated
- MRI shows whether fragment is unstable (loose)
  - High signal surrounding fragment on T2W
  - Absent or displaced fragment
  - Crack in overlying cartilage
  - Large subchondral cysts deep to fragment

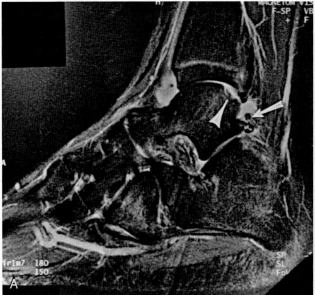
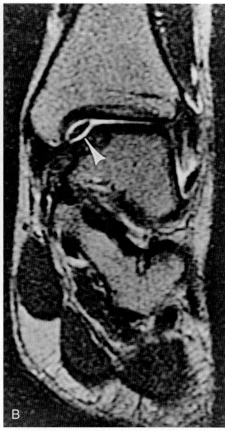

Figure 16-53   **Osteochondral injuries of the talus. A,** STIR sagittal image of the ankle. There is a focal osteochondral defect in the dome of the talus (*arrow-head*), with no fragment in the defect. The fragment has become loose and is an intra-articular loose body (*arrow*) in the posterior ankle. **B,** Spin echo–T2W coronal image of the ankle (different patient than in **A**). There is an osteochondral fracture of the medial dome of the talus. The fragment remains in the bed of the defect. The high signal between the fragment and the talus (*arrowhead*) indicates that this is an unstable fragment.

(Fig. 16-53). Commonly associated ligamentous injuries also can be identified.

Stress fractures are seen on MRI as linear areas of low signal intensity on T1W images with high or low signal intensity on T2W images. The fractures generally run perpendicular to the long axis of the affected bone; however, stress fractures of the medial malleolus usually are vertically oriented (Fig. 16-54). The findings on MRI are specific, in contrast to bone scans done for the same indications. Just as anywhere else in the skeleton, traumatic fractures can be found in any of the bones of the foot and ankle with great sensitivity by MRI when conventional radiographs are negative and bone scans are negative or nonspecific.

Osteonecrosis of the Foot and Ankle (Box 16-17)

Osteonecrosis may occur anywhere in the foot and ankle if the patient is taking steroids or has other predisposing systemic risk factors; however, the most common locations for osteonecrosis secondary to trauma include the following:

1. Navicular bone, which may have an unrecognized fracture, causing the bone fragments to develop osteonecrosis
2. Heads of the metatarsals, especially the second, in individuals who wear high-heeled shoes (Freiberg's infraction)
3. Lateral hallux sesamoid at the level of the head of the first metatarsal

4. Osteonecrosis of the dome of the talus, a well-known sequela of a previous talar neck fracture with disruption of the blood supply to the proximal portion of the bone (Fig. 16-55)[31,38]

The MRI appearance of osteonecrosis in the foot and ankle is identical to other bones in the skeleton: serpiginous low signal intensity lines creating a geographic pattern, or diffuse low signal on T1W images that may or may not become higher signal on T2W images. The differential diagnosis for the marrow changes in osteonecrosis, other than the pathognomonic serpiginous lines, include occult fractures, abnormal increased stresses, osteomyelitis, and regional migratory osteoporosis with bone marrow edema.

Osseous Tumors (Box 16-18)

A few tumors of bone have a predilection for the foot and ankle, but malignant primary and metastatic lesions are rare

---

BOX 16-17

Osteonecrosis in the Foot

- Navicular (unrecognized fracture)
- Metatarsal heads, especially second and third (repetitive stresses, high-heeled shoes)
- Talar dome (talar neck fracture)
- Lateral hallux sesamoid
- Anywhere else (steroids)

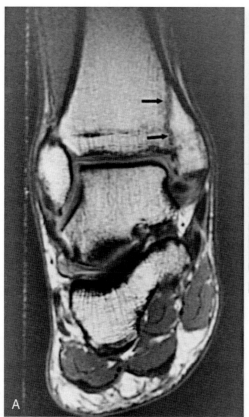
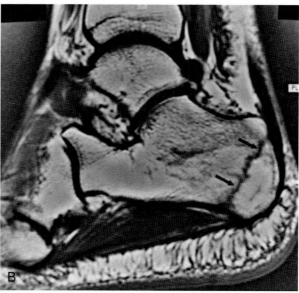

Figure 16-54 Fractures. **A,** T1W coronal image of the ankle. There is a vertical stress fracture (*arrows*) of the medial malleolus in a college basketball player with pain. Radiographs were normal. **B,** T1W sagittal image of the hindfoot (different patient than in **A**). There is a low signal linear stress fracture (*arrows*) in the posterior calcaneal tuberosity, running perpendicular to the long axis of the bone. This was not evident on radiographs.

in the foot and ankle. MRI generally does not add to our ability to make the diagnosis, but is useful for showing the extent of disease within the bone and for assessing for any soft tissue component. The distal tibia and fibula most commonly may be affected by nonossifying fibromas, aneurysmal bone cysts, and giant cell tumors.

The calcaneus is a common site for simple bone cysts (unicameral bone cyst), occurring in the midportion or neck of the calcaneus. This portion of the calcaneus has sparse trabeculae, caused by a paucity of stresses in this area, and normally often is filled with fat. Although some authors have

said intraosseous lipomas occur in the same location in the calcaneus and have an identical plain film appearance, it never made sense to us that two different tumors would look exactly the same. Most authors now believe these are simple bone cysts, which, as they resolve, can have some fatty elements that, when imaged with MRI or when biopsied, compel one to call them lipomas. Many fibro-osseous lesions that spontaneously resolve can have fatty elements during part of their evolution, but should not be considered intraosseous lipomas (Fig. 16-56). Other lesions that have a predilection for the calcaneus include chondroblastoma,

Figure 16-55 Osteonecrosis. **A,** T1W sagittal image of the hindfoot. There is diffuse low signal throughout the navicular bone (*arrows*) from osteonecrosis. This patient was a former basketball player with pain. **B,** T1W long-axis coronal image of the forefoot. Focal areas of low signal (*arrows*) are evident in the second and third metatarsal heads from osteonecrosis (Freiberg's infraction).

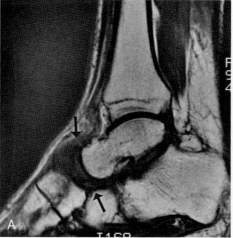
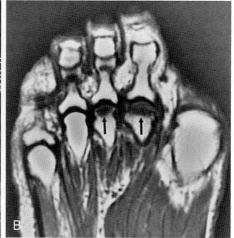

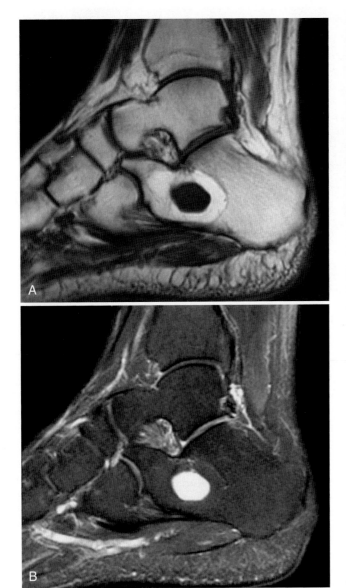

Figure 16-56 Unicameral bone cyst. **A,** T1W sagittal image of the hind-foot. There is a round, high signal fat mass in the neck of the calcaneus that is well circumscribed. In the center of this fatty mass is a focus of low signal. **B,** FSE-T2W sagittal image of the hindfoot. The low signal focus on T1W is fluid-bright on T2W and represents the remaining fluid in a resolving unicameral bone cyst. The periphery has resolved into normal marrow. Most clinicians believe that fat fills in around the periphery of preexisting simple bone cysts in the calcaneus as they resolve.

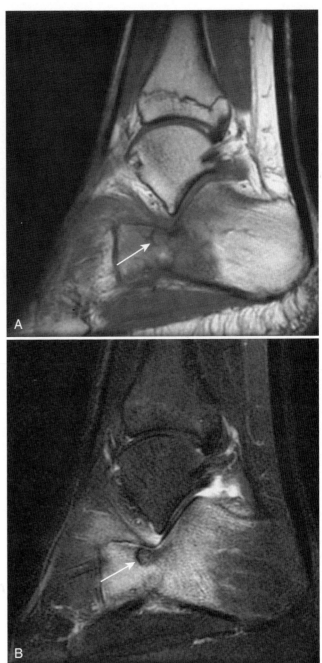

Figure 16-57 Osteoid osteoma. **A,** T1W sagittal image of the ankle. There is a large amount of low signal in the anterior half of the calcaneus, which is edema from an osteoid osteoma. The nidus is seen adjacent to the sinus tarsi (*arrow*). **B,** FSE-T2W sagittal image of the ankle. The edema in the calcaneus is seen as increased signal, and the nidus of the osteoid osteoma is low signal (*arrow*).

aneurysmal bone cyst, and giant cell tumors, all of which usually are located posteriorly in the apophysis of the calcaneal tuberosity.

The talus and calcaneus are sites of predilection for osteoid osteomas, which produce periosteal reaction and may show extensive bone marrow edema and edema in the surrounding soft tissues on MRI (Fig. 16-57). Two lesions often mistaken for bone tumors are intraosseous ganglion cyst, which is common in the medial malleolus, and post-traumatic subchondral cysts in the dome of the talus (Fig. 16-58); these lesions may grow to be quite large. MRI may document the diagnosis of a subchondral cyst by showing its communication to the articular surface.

An entity that can mimic a lesion (which we have been asked to biopsy on several occasions) is seen in the calcaneus adjacent to the sinus tarsi (Fig. 16-59; see Fig. 16-36). This represents vascular remnants and sometimes can be quite large. They are incidental and asymptomatic. We found them in 75% of a series of ankle MR images; they were described by one of our former fellows, Jake Fleming, so we refer to them as "Jake's lakes."[39]

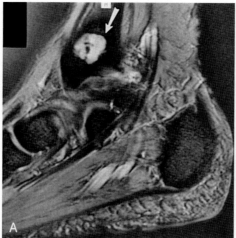
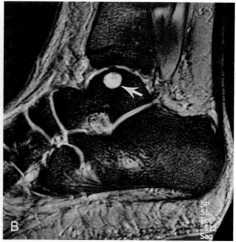

Figure 16-58 Bone tumor mimickers. **A,** T2*W sagittal image of the ankle. The lobulated, high signal lesion in the medial malleolus (*arrow*) was an intraosseous ganglion cyst at biopsy. This is a typical location for this lesion. **B,** T2*W sagittal image of the ankle. There is a large, round, high signal lesion in the dome of the talus (*arrow*). These may mimic tumors when large, but this is a subchondral cyst related to previous osteochondral injury. An abnormal low signal focus in the cartilage overlying the cyst can be seen, which helps to make the diagnosis.

BOX 16-18

Common Bone Tumors of the Foot and Ankle

Distal Tibia and Fibula
- Nonossifying fibroma, giant cell tumor, aneurysmal bone cyst

Calcaneus
- Neck: Simple bone cyst, lipoma
- Tuberosity: Aneurysmal bone cyst, chondroblastoma, giant cell tumor

Talus
- Osteoid osteoma

Bone Tumor Mimickers
- Medial malleolus: Intraosseous ganglion cyst
- Talar dome: Post-traumatic large subchondral cyst

BONE MARROW EDEMA SYNDROME

Patchy increased T2 signal is often seen scattered about multiple bones in the foot and ankle in patients with generalized pain not attributable to any source (Fig. 16-60). This has been termed *bone marrow edema syndrome*. It has been convincingly shown that it does not represent Sudeck's atrophy (now called *chronic regional pain syndrome*),[40,41] but its etiology is unknown. It affects all ages, but we tend to see it more frequently in young patients. It is often bilateral. It is self-limiting, but can last for many months or a year. We liken it to the painful edema syndromes such as idiopathic transient osteoporosis of the hip and regional migratory osteoporosis. Whatever it is, it does not need a biopsy. It is treated conservatively for symptoms.

SOFT TISSUE TUMORS (Box 16-19)

Benign

Benign soft tissue tumors of the foot that occur frequently include ganglion cysts, hemangiomas, lipomas, nerve sheath tumors, plantar fibromatosis, soft tissue chondroma (extra-articular synovial osteochondromatosis), and giant cell tumor of the tendon sheath (extra-articular pigmented villonodular synovitis).[42,43] MRI is useful to confirm the presence and extent of a soft tissue mass, and to determine the precise anatomic location, which aids in surgery; in some cases, the appearance is specific for a particular lesion. The MRI features of all but one of the above-listed entities are the same in the foot and ankle as elsewhere in the body and are not discussed in detail here. Plantar fibromatosis is unique to the foot and is discussed.

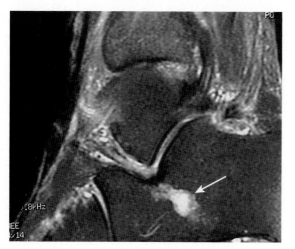

Figure 16-59 Vascular remnant. FSE-T2W sagittal image of the ankle. A focus of high signal is seen in the calcaneus (*arrow*), which is a normal variant seen in many ankles and is a vascular remnant.

BOX 16-19

Common Soft Tissue Tumors of the Foot and Ankle

Benign
- Ganglion cyst, hemangioma, lipoma, nerve sheath tumors, giant cell tumor of tendon sheath, soft tissue chondroma, plantar fibromatosis

Malignant
- Synovial sarcoma

Soft Tissue Tumor Mimickers
- Accessory muscles
  - Accessory soleus
  - Peroneus quartus
- Pressure lesions

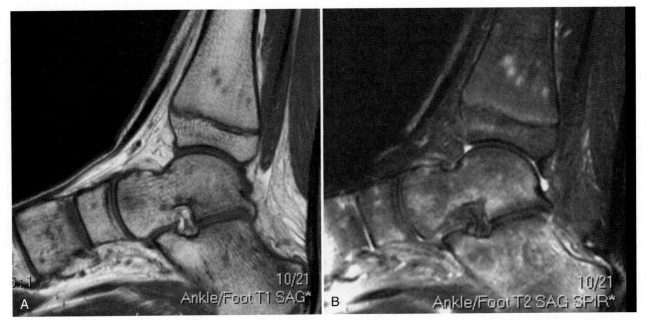

Figure 16-60 Bone marrow edema syndrome. **A** and **B**, T1W (**A**) and FSE-T2W (**B**) sagittal images of the ankle. Patchy or spotted high signal is seen scattered throughout the ankle and distal tibia in this young patient with generalized ankle pain. This is bone marrow edema as seen in bone marrow edema syndrome.

Plantar Fibromatosis. Plantar fibromatosis is a benign proliferation of fibrous tissue along the plantar aspect of the foot, arising in the plantar fascia. It manifests as a nodule on the sole of the foot, usually medial in location, and is usually, although not always, painless. It develops as either a single or multiple small nodular thickenings of the plantar fascia that appear as low to intermediate signal intensity on T1W and T2W sequences (Fig. 16-61). These lesions often, although not invariably, enhance with intravenous gadolinium. The upper margin may be infiltrative and can grow into the deeper compartments of the foot, whereas the lower margin usually is well defined and outlined by the subcutaneous fat.[44] As long as the MRI signal characteristics and anatomic location are typical of plantar fibromatosis, the lesions often are not biopsied or surgically removed, unless they are large.

Malignant

Synovial Sarcoma. The most common malignant soft tissue tumor of the foot is the synovial sarcoma. It is an extra-articular soft tissue mass, which, on conventional radiographs, may show scattered calcifications in approximately 20% of affected individuals. It usually affects young adults. It may be infiltrative and destroy adjacent bone, but also can appear well defined and benign by imaging criteria, sometimes creating a pressure erosion on adjacent bone. Necrosis and hemorrhage may be present and cause a heterogeneous appearance after gadolinium administration. There is essen-

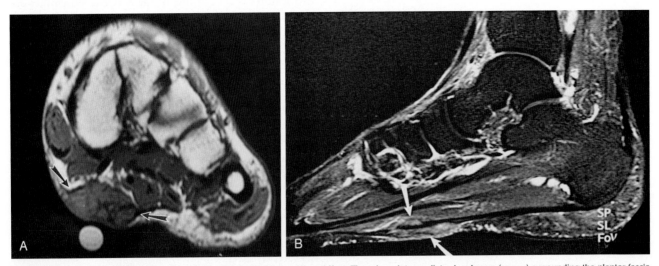

Figure 16-61 Plantar fibromatosis. **A,** T1W short-axis axial image of the midfoot. There is an intermediate signal mass (*arrows*) surrounding the plantar fascia. **B,** STIR sagittal image of the foot. The mass (*arrows*) is heterogeneous, but generally remains low signal. The plantar fascia courses through the center of the mass.

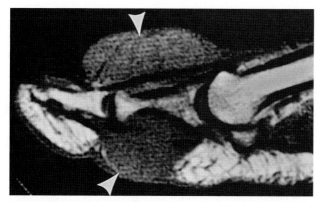

Figure 16-62 **Synovial sarcoma.** T1W sagittal image of the great toe. A large, intermediate signal mass (*arrowheads*) surrounds the great toe. This is a nonspecific MRI appearance, but was found to be a synovial sarcoma at surgery.

tially nothing specific about the appearance of this lesion, and one must be certain to include this in the differential diagnosis of a nondescript foot mass in a young patient (Fig. 16-62).[42]

Other Sarcomas. Liposarcoma and malignant fibrous histiocytoma are rare below the knee, but if they do occur in the foot/ankle region, they tend to be present at the ankle.

Soft Tissue Tumor Mimickers

Some masses in the foot and ankle are not the result of neoplasm, and MRI can easily differentiate neoplasm from these other entities. Accessory muscles and tears of the anterior tibial tendon are two entities that often manifest with a mass suspicious for neoplasm based on clinical examination.

Accessory Muscles. Anomalous or accessory muscles in the foot or ankle are common. The accessory soleus and peroneus quartus muscles are the most common accessory muscles encountered in this region. The MRI appearance is diagnostic because the signal and appearance are identical to other muscle on all pulse sequences.[45-47]

The accessory soleus muscle is an anatomic normal variant of the calf musculature that manifests as a mass on the medial aspect of the ankle, may be the source of pain secondary to ischemia that occurs during exercise as a form of a localized compartment syndrome, or may compress the posterior tibial nerve in the tarsal tunnel, resulting in tarsal tunnel syndrome. On MRI, it is located medial to the Achilles tendon and has a tendon of its own that inserts either into the Achilles tendon or to the calcaneus (Fig. 16-63).

The peroneus quartus accessory muscle also lies in the posterior ankle, just anterior and lateral to the Achilles tendon (see Fig. 16-18). Similar to the accessory soleus muscle, the peroneus quartus may manifest as a mass or be an incidental finding on MRI. Peroneus quartus accessory muscles occur in 13% to 25% of individuals. They often are asymptomatic, but have been considered responsible for lateral ankle pain and ankle joint instability. The accessory muscle may predispose to subluxation of the peroneal tendons because of its mass effect within the confined space created by the peroneal retinaculum and subsequent stretching and laxity of the retinaculum. The peroneus quartus runs posteromedial to the peroneus longus and brevis tendons and usually attaches to the retrotrochlear eminence on the calcaneus, which is located posterior to the peroneal tubercle.

The accessory flexor digitorum longus muscle may cause a compressive neuropathy of the posterior tibial nerve in the tarsal tunnel. The tendon from another accessory muscle, the peroneocalcaneus internus, runs parallel to a portion of

Figure 16-63 **Accessory muscle: soleus. A,** T1W sagittal image of the ankle. An accessory soleus muscle is seen on the medial side of the ankle between the Achilles tendon and the osseous structures (*arrows*). It attaches to the top of the posterior calcaneus. **B,** T1W axial image of the ankle. The accessory soleus (*open arrows*) is evident medially adjacent to the posterior tibial nerve, artery, and vein.

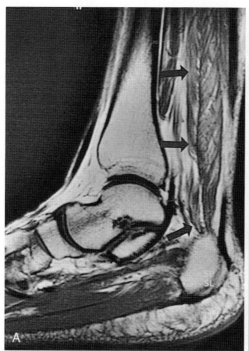
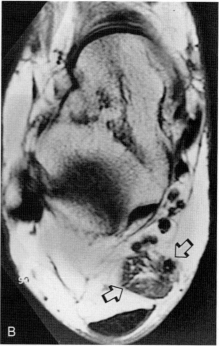

the flexor hallucis longus tendon and may simulate a longitudinal split of that tendon.

Pressure Lesions (Box 16-20). Increased stresses on certain musculoskeletal structures can cause changes in those structures that may be confused with pathology, but are of minimal or no significance. Marrow edema that occurs as a response to increased stresses on bones is an example and may be difficult to differentiate from infection, early osteonecrosis, painful bone marrow edema syndrome, or other abnormalities by MRI alone.[48]

Another entity related to chronic stresses is a pressure lesion that may occur in subcutaneous fat at points of increased pressure and chronic repeated friction. Pressure lesions may develop cystic centers and are called *adventitious bursae*. These lesions may or may not be symptomatic. Adventitious bursae are bursae that do not initially exist in the body, but form as a response to pressures on the soft tissues. Pressure lesions may mimic a soft tissue tumor, especially before developing cystic changes.

Pressure lesions in the foot occur at pressure points, predictably on the plantar surface of the first or fifth metatarsal heads, which lie lower than the other metatarsal heads; medial to the first metatarsal head in patients with hallux valgus; plantar to the medial aspect of the calcaneal tuberosity; and posterior to the distal Achilles tendon (bursa of Achilles tendon) from ill-fitting shoes. Pressure lesions/adventitious bursae also may occur after surgery to the foot

BOX 16-20
Pressure Lesions in Foot

Clinical
- Usually asymptomatic, occasionally painful
- Probably related to adventitious bursa formation
- Common locations
  - Plantar to first and fifth metatarsal heads
  - Plantar to plantar fascia at calcaneal tuberosity
  - Posterior to distal Achilles (bursa of Achilles tendon)
  - Medial to metatarsal head in hallux valgus
- Histology: Fibrous and fatty tissue

MRI
- Low signal all sequences, usually
- Fat may be intermixed in mass
- Often not a true mass appearance on T2W
- May have cystic center (high signal on T2W)

that results in stresses being transferred to a new site, and these are often called *transfer lesions* by orthopedists. Feet that are deformed have pressure lesions occurring in atypical locations, where pressure is greatest.

The lesion is a rounded abnormality in the subcutaneous fat that is low to intermediate signal intensity on T1W images and becomes vague in appearance with areas of intermediate and high signal intensity on T2W images (Fig. 16-64). Because these pressure lesions appear as a soft tissue mass, they may be mistaken for significant pathology. The key to diagnosis is that the lesions occur in typical

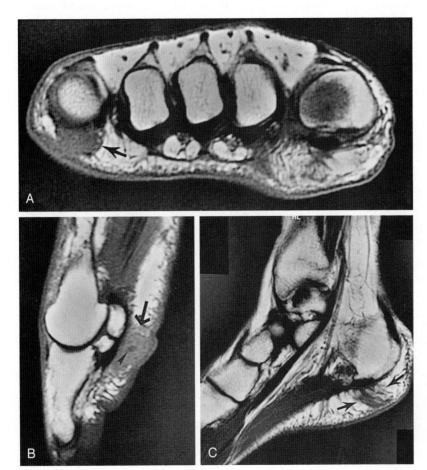

Figure 16-64 Pressure lesions. A, T1W short-axis axial image of the forefoot. There is a mass (*arrow*) beneath the fifth metatarsal head. **B,** T1W sagittal image of the forefoot (different patient than in **A**). An intermediate signal mass (*arrow*) is present directly beneath the first metatarsal head and sesamoids. There is a low signal center (*arrowhead*), indicating a cystic center; this is an adventitious bursa. **C,** T1W sagittal image of the hindfoot (different patient than in **A** and **B**). There is a pressure lesion with focal intermediate signal interspersed with fat beneath the medial calcaneal tuberosity.

BOX 16-21

Marrow Signal Abnormalities in Diabetic Foot

- High T1W (fat), low STIR (fat)
  - Normal
- High T1W (fat), high STIR
  - Reactive marrow edema from adjacent soft tissue inflammation
- Low T1W, low STIR
  - Neuropathic, chronic
- Low T1W, high STIR
  - Osteomyelitis most likely diagnosis if there is an overlying ulcer and located at a pressure point
  - Reactive marrow edema from adjacent inflammation cannot be excluded
  - Neuropathic acute changes most likely if a joint is involved, no overlying ulcer, or does not occur at pressure points

BOX 16-21

Marrow Signal Abnormalities in Diabetic Foot

- High T1W (fat), low STIR (fat)
  - Normal
- High T1W (fat), high STIR
  - Reactive marrow edema from adjacent soft tissue inflammation
- Low T1W, low STIR
  - Neuropathic, chronic
- Low T1W, high STIR
  - Osteomyelitis most likely diagnosis if there is an overlying ulcer and located at a pressure point
  - Reactive marrow edema from adjacent inflammation cannot be excluded
  - Neuropathic acute changes most likely if a joint is involved, no overlying ulcer, or does not occur at pressure points

BOX 16-22

Diabetic Foot

Osteomyelitis

- Marrow signal: Low T1W, high STIR
- Soft tissue ulcer adjacent to abnormal bone (>90%)
- Occurs at pressure points: First and fifth metatarsal heads, calcaneal tuberosity, distal toes, malleoli
- Nonspecific other possible findings: Cortical destruction, periosteal reaction, joint effusion, high signal in soft tissues on STIR from cellulitis/abscesses

Neuropathic Changes

- Marrow signal, low on T1W and either low or high signal (chronic or acute changes) on STIR
- Abnormalities are joint based; tarsometatarsal joints usually involved
- Bones have deformed shape (fragmentation, resorption)
- Muscles atrophied (high signal T1W and STIR)
- Nonspecific other possible findings: Periosteal reaction, cortical destruction, joint effusion

locations, the MRI characteristics are not entirely typical of a true mass lesion, and fat often is intermixed. If these are biopsied, fibrous and fatty tissue is found histologically.

DIABETIC FOOT (Boxes 16-21 and 16-22)

Problems in the feet of diabetics are common and often devastating. These problems have a multifactorial etiology, including small vessel ischemia, neuropathic arthropathy, fractures, and infections. Clinicians treating these patients usually are primarily interested in differentiating osteomyelitis from soft tissue infection because the patients usually have developed a soft tissue ulcer over a pressure area in the foot. Differentiation is difficult clinically, but is important and affects the therapy the patient receives, including the length of antibiotic treatment and the decision for surgical débridement. The role of imaging is not only to detect osteo-

myelitis or soft tissue abscesses, but also to assess the extent of these changes and be useful in the planning of any surgical procedure or biopsy.

Studies have shown MRI to be more cost-effective than the standard three-phase radionuclide bone scan and indium-labeled white blood cell scans for diabetic foot infections.[49] MRI is a faster examination to perform, and it shows other lesions important to clinical management, such as sinus tracts, cellulitis, abscesses, and tendon abnormalities.

MRI shows changes in the bone marrow from osteomyelitis, consisting of low signal intensity on T1W sequences, replacing the normal high signal fatty marrow, and high signal intensity on T2W or STIR images (Fig. 16-65).[50-54]

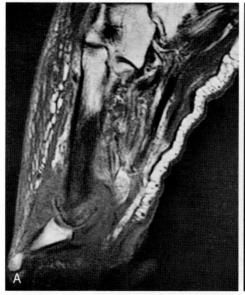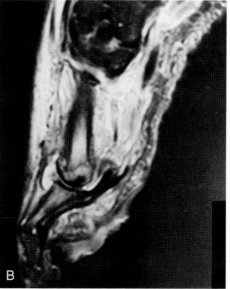

Figure 16-65 **Osteomyelitis.** **A,** T1W sagittal image of the first ray. There is an ulcer on the plantar aspect of the first metatarsophalangeal joint and abnormal low signal in the distal two thirds of the shaft of the first metatarsal. The proximal phalanx of the toe is normal fat signal. There is cellulitis involving the dorsal skin and subcutaneous fat. The muscles in the plantar aspect of the foot have fatty infiltration from ischemic or neuropathic changes (denervation). **B,** STIR sagittal image of the first ray. The first metatarsal is high signal, compatible with osteomyelitis. The proximal phalanx of the great toe that was normal on T1W is high signal on STIR, indicating reactive marrow edema, rather than osteomyelitis. The dorsal cellulitis and the plantar denervated muscle are diffusely high signal.

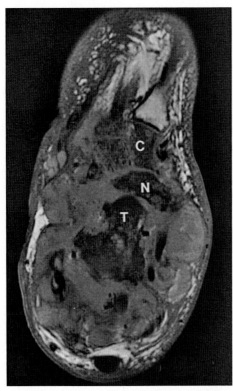

Figure 16-66 Neuropathic changes: chronic. T1W long-axis coronal image of the foot. The hindfoot and midfoot of this diabetic patient have disorganization and fragmentation of bones with surrounding soft tissue swelling. The talus (T), navicular (N), and cuneiforms (C) are very low signal and remained low signal on T2W images. The location of abnormalities in the midfoot, no overlying ulcers at pressure points, joints being affected, and low signal on all pulse sequences are typical of chronic neuropathic changes.

MRI is limited in much the same way as bone scans by the inability to differentiate true osteomyelitis from marrow edema secondary to adjacent soft tissue inflammatory changes ("sympathetic" or reactive edema) or from occult fractures with marrow edema, which are common in the neuropathic diabetic foot. Periosteal reaction and cortical destruction may occur with osteomyelitis and neuropathic changes. If there is normal fatty marrow signal on all pulse sequences, one can be certain there is no osteomyelitis. If marrow signal is abnormal on T1W and STIR images, it may be the result of osteomyelitis, reactive marrow edema from an adjacent soft tissue infection, or acute neuropathic changes. If there is an adjacent soft tissue ulcer or sinus tract, and the abnormalities of bone occur at a pressure point, the findings are almost certainly from osteomyelitis even without the presence of cortical destruction. If the T1W images are normal, but T2W or STIR images show high signal in marrow, it is almost certainly from reactive marrow edema and not osteomyelitis (see Fig. 16-65).

Location of bone abnormalities in the diabetic foot is useful for distinguishing neuropathic changes from osteomyelitis. Osteomyelitis occurs at predictable pressure points where soft tissue ulcers develop (plantar to the first and fifth metatarsal heads, calcaneal tuberosity, malleoli, and plantar aspect of distal toes). Patients with foot deformities or previous surgery may have pressure points in different locations than those just listed, so it is important to think about the biomechanics of the specific foot being evaluated to avoid making errors. Neuropathic changes generally are unrelated to soft tissue ulcers, always involve joints, and are most common at the tarsometatarsal joints.

Distinguishing neuropathic changes from osteomyelitis may be difficult with all imaging techniques, including MRI. Classically, MRI shows neuropathic changes as low signal intensity on T1W and T2W (STIR) sequences in bone marrow on both sides of a grossly disrupted joint space (Fig. 16-66). Aggressive and active neuropathic changes with bone fragmentation and joint destruction result in high signal intensity marrow edema and soft tissue swelling on T2W images, similar to osteomyelitis.[51] The location of the abnormal bone, the presence or absence of an overlying ulcer, joint involvement, and identification of fracture lines are the best means to differentiate osteomyelitis from neuropathic changes (Fig. 16-67). Infection superimposed on a neuropathic foot is impossible to distinguish in general and serves to keep us humble.

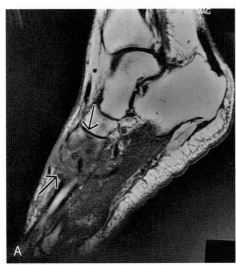
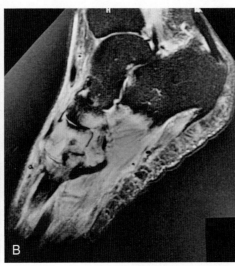

Figure 16-67 Neuropathic changes: acute. A, T1W sagittal image of the foot. Intermediate signal and bone fragmentation are present in the midfoot of this diabetic patient (*arrows*). **B,** STIR sagittal image of the foot. The osseous abnormalities all are high signal. Osteomyelitis could have the same MRI features, but this is much more likely to be neuropathic in origin because there is no overlying ulcer or pressure point. Also, the location in the midfoot with multiple joints involved is typical of neuropathic changes.

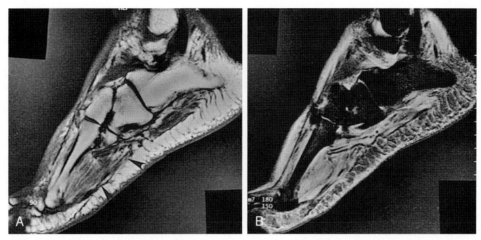

Figure 16-68   Diabetic muscle changes. **A,** T1W sagittal image of the foot. There is fatty infiltration of the plantar muscles (*arrowheads*) from denervation or ischemia. **B,** STIR sagittal image of the foot. The denervated muscle is high signal on this sequence, not to be confused with infection. There also is dorsal cellulitis that is diffusely high signal.

The presence of joint fluid does not make the diagnosis of a septic joint by MRI because reactive or sympathetic joint effusions are common. MRI aids, however, in directing which bones or joints should be biopsied or aspirated.

MRI is valuable in showing the extent of soft tissue abnormality and abscesses, and accuracy may improve with contrast administration. Cellulitis is seen as diffuse contrast enhancement, whereas abscesses show peripheral enhancement with a nonenhancing central portion that can be difficult or impossible to determine without gadolinium.

Other soft tissue abnormalities commonly seen in the feet of diabetics include fatty replacement and edema of the muscles (high signal muscle on T1W and high signal on T2W or STIR images), as the result of neuropathic and possibly ischemic changes (Fig. 16-68). High signal on the T2W or STIR images should not be misinterpreted as pyomyositis; fatty infiltration of the atrophied muscles on T1W sequences should allow the proper diagnosis of denervation from neuropathic changes to be made. The Achilles and posterior tibial tendons frequently are partially or completely torn in diabetics, probably from ischemia owing to microvascular disease.

FOREIGN BODIES

Foreign bodies are common in the foot because people inadvertently step on penetrating objects when barefoot. Most foreign bodies are not radiopaque and cannot be seen on radiographs. Small foreign bodies often migrate from the site of entry through the skin to a distant site. Most foreign bodies are linear and low signal intensity on T1W and T2W sequences (Fig. 16-69). Soft tissue edema or abscess often is seen surrounding the foreign body, reflecting the inflammatory response to it, and is high signal intensity on T2W sequences. The response to the foreign body is usually much more impressive than the foreign body, which may be easily overlooked.[55]

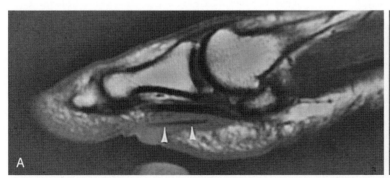
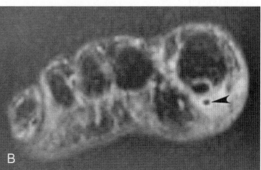

Figure 16-69   Foreign bodies. **A,** T1W sagittal image of the great toe. A linear, low signal structure (*arrowheads*) deep to the flexor hallucis tendon was a piece of wood at surgery. It is surrounded by intermediate signal from pus and granulation tissue. **B,** STIR short-axis axial image of the forefoot. The wood foreign body (*arrowhead*) remains low signal and is surrounded by high signal inflammatory tissue.

REFERENCES

1. Mengiardi B, Pfirrmann CW, Schöttle PB, et al. Magic angle effect in MR imaging of ankle tendons: influence of foot positioning on prevalence and site in asymptomatic subjects and cadaveric tendons. *Eur Radiol* 2006; 16:2197-2206.
2. Chandnani VP, Bradley YC. Achilles tendon and miscellaneous tendon lesions. *Magn Reson Imaging Clin N Am* 1994; 2:89-95.
3. Dussault RG, Kaplan PA, Roederer G. MR imaging of Achilles tendon in patients with familial hyperlipidemia: comparison with plain films, physical examination and patients with traumatic tendon lesions. *AJR Am J Roentgenol* 1995; 164:403-407.
4. Pavlov H, Heneghan MA, Hersh A, et al. Haglund's deformity: diagnosis and differential diagnosis of posterior heel pain. *Radiology* 1982; 144:83-87.
5. Schweitzer ME, Caccese R, Karasick D, et al. Posterior tibial tendon tears: utility of secondary signs for MR imaging diagnosis. *Radiology* 1993; 188:655-659.
6. Miller TT, Staron RB, Feldman F, et al. The symptomatic accessory tarsal navicular bone: assessment with MR imaging. *Radiology* 1995; 195:849-853.
7. Karasick D, Schweitzer ME. Tear of the posterior tibial tendon causing asymmetric flatfoot: radiologic findings. *AJR Am J Roentgenol* 1993; 161:1237-1240.
8. Cheung Y, Rosenberg ZS, Magee T, Chinitz L. Normal anatomy and pathologic conditions of ankle tendons: current imaging techniques. *RadioGraphics* 1992; 12:429-444.
9. Karasick D, Schweitzer M. The os trigonum syndrome: imaging features. *AJR Am J Roentgenol* 1996; 166:125-129.
10. Rosenberg ZS, Feldman F, Singson RD, et al. Peroneal tendon injury associated with calcaneal fractures: CT findings. *AJR Am J Roentgenol* 1987; 149:125-129.
11. Khoury NJ, El-Khoury GY, Saltzman CL, Kathol MH. Peroneus longus and brevis tendon tears: MR imaging evaluation. *Radiology* 1996; 200:833-841.
12. Tjin A, Ton ER, Schweitzer ME, Karasick D. MR imaging of peroneal tendon disorders. *AJR Am J Roentgenol* 1997; 168:135-140.
13. Schweitzer ME, Eid ME, Deely D, et al. Using MR imaging to differentiate peroneal splits from other peroneal disorders. *AJR Am J Roentgenol* 1997; 168:129-133.
14. Rosenberg ZS, Beltran J, Cheung YY. MR features of longitudinal tears of the peroneus brevis tendon. *AJR Am J Roentgenol* 1997; 168:141-147.
15. Wang XT, Rosenberg ZS, Mechlin MB, Schweitzer ME. Normal variants and diseases of the peroneal tendons and superior peroneal retinaculum: MR imaging features. *RadioGraphics* 2005; 25:587-602.
16. Dooley BJ, Kudelkapp P, Menelaus MB. Subcutaneous rupture of the tendon of tibialis anterior. *J Bone Joint Surg [Br]* 1980; 62:471-472.
17. Khoury NJ, El-Khoury GY, Saltman C, et al. Rupture of the anterior tibial tendon: diagnosis by MR imaging. *AJR Am J Roentgenol* 1996; 167:351-354.
18. Erickson SJ, Smith JW, Ruiz ME, et al. MR imaging of the lateral collateral ligament of the ankle. *AJR Am J Roentgenol* 1991; 156:131-136.
19. Schneck CD, Mesgarzadeh M, Bonakdarpour A, Ross GJ. MR imaging of the most commonly injured ankle ligaments, I: normal anatomy. *Radiology* 1992; 184:499-506.
20. Schneck CD, Mesgarzadeh M, Bonakdarpour A. MR imaging of the most commonly injured ankle ligaments, II: ligament injuries. *Radiology* 1992; 184:507-512.
21. Klein MA. MR imaging of the ankle: normal and abnormal findings in the medial collateral ligament. *AJR Am J Roentgenol* 1994; 162:377-383.
22. Mengiardi B, Pfirrmann CW, Vienne P, et al. Medial collateral ligament complex of the ankle: MR appearance in asymptomatic subjects. *Radiology* 2007; 242:817-824.
23. Mengiardi B, Zanetti M, Schöttle PB, et al. Spring ligament complex: MR imaging-anatomic correlation and findings in asymptomatic subjects. *Radiology* 2005; 237:242-249.
24. Balen PF, Helms CA: Association of posterior tibial tendon injury with spring ligament injury, sinus tarsi abnormality, and plantar fasciitis on MR imaging. *AJR Am J Roentgenol* 2001; 176:1137-1143.
25. Toye LR, Helms CA, Hoffman BD, et al. MRI of spring ligament tears. *AJR Am J Roentgenol* 2005; 184:1475-1480.
26. Rubin DA, Tishkoff NW, Britton CA, et al. Anterolateral soft-tissue impingement in the ankle: diagnosis using MR imaging. *AJR Am J Roentgenol* 1997; 169:829-835.
27. Jordan LK, Helms CA, Cooperman AE, Speer KP. Magnetic resonance imaging findings in anterolateral impingement of the ankle. *Skeletal Radiol* 2000; 29:34-39.
28. Taillard W, Meyer J-M, Garcia J, Blanc Y. The sinus tarsi syndrome. *Int Orthop* 1981; 5:117-130.
29. Beltran J, Munchow AM, Khabiri H, et al. Ligaments of the lateral aspect of the ankle and sinus tarsi: an MR imaging study. *Radiology* 1990; 177:455-458.
30. Klein M, Spreitzer A. MR imaging of the tarsal sinus and canal: normal anatomy, pathologic findings, and features of the sinus tarsi syndrome. *Radiology* 1993; 186:233-240.
31. Lucas P, Kaplan P, Dussault R, Hurwitz S. MRI of the foot and ankle. *Curr Probl Diagn Radiol* 1997; 26:209-268.
32. Berkowitz JF, Kier R, Rudicel S. Plantar fasciitis: MR imaging. *Radiology* 1991; 179:665-667.
33. Erickson SJ, Quinn SF, Kneeland JB, et al. MR imaging of the tarsal tunnel and related spaces: normal and abnormal findings with anatomic correlation. *AJR Am J Roentgenol* 1990; 155:323-328.
34. Zanetti M, Ledermann T, Zollinger H, Hodler J. Efficacy of MR imaging in patients suspected of having Morton's neuroma. *AJR Am J Roentgenol* 1997; 168:529-532.
35. Zanetti M, Strehle JK, Zollinger H, Hodler J. Morton neuroma and fluid in the intermetatarsal bursae on MR images of 70 asymptomatic volunteers. *Radiology* 1997; 203:516-520.
36. Terk MR, Kwong PK, Suthar M, et al. Morton neuroma: evaluation with MR imaging performed with contrast enhancement and fat suppression. *Radiology* 1992; 189:239-241.
37. Karasick D, Schweitzer ME. Disorders of the hallux sesamoid complex: MR features. *Skeletal Radiol* 1998; 27:411-418.
38. Haller J, Sartoris DJ, Resnick D, et al. Spontaneous osteonecrosis of the tarsal navicular in adults: imaging findings. *AJR Am J Roentgenol* 1988; 151:355-358.
39. Fleming JL 2nd, Dodd L, Helms CA. Prominent vascular remnants in the calcaneus simulating a lesion on MRI of the ankle: findings in 67 patients with cadaveric correlation. *AJR Am J Roentgenol* 2005; 185:1449-1452.
40. Zanetti M, Steiner CL, Seifert B, Hodler J, et al. Clinical outcome of edema-like bone marrow abnormalities of the foot. *Radiology* 2002; 222:184-188.
41. Fernandez-Canton G, Casado O, Capelastegui A, et al. Bone marrow edema syndrome of the foot: one year follow-up with MR imaging. *Skeletal Radiol* 2003; 32:273-278.
42. Wetzel LH, Levine E. Soft-tissue tumors of the foot: value of MR imaging for specific diagnosis. *AJR Am J Roentgenol* 1990; 155:1025-1030.
43. Llauger J, Palmer J, Monill JM, et al. MR imaging of benign soft-tissue masses of the foot and ankle. *RadioGraphics* 1998; 18:1481-1498.
44. Morrison WB, Schweitzer ME, Wapner KL, Lackman RD. Plantar fibromatosis: a benign aggressive neoplasm with a characteristic appearance on MR images. *Radiology* 1994; 193:841-845.
45. Mellado JM, Rosenberg ZS, Beltran J, Colon E. The peroneocalcaneus internus muscle: MR imaging features. *AJR Am J Roentgenol* 1997; 169:585-588.
46. Cheung YY, Rosenberg ZS, Ramsinghani R, et al. Peroneus quartus muscle: MR imaging features. *Radiology* 1997; 202:745-750.
47. Mellado J, Rosenberg ZS, Beltran J. Low incorporation of soleus tendon: a potential diagnostic pitfall on MR imaging. *Skeletal Radiol* 1998; 27:222-224.
48. Mizel MS, Yodlowski ML. Disorders of the lesser metatarsophalangeal joints. *J Am Acad Orthop Surg* 1995; 3:166-173.
49. Morrison WB, Schweitzer ME, Wapner KL, et al. Osteomyelitis in feet of diabetics: clinical accuracy, surgical utility and cost effectiveness of MR imaging. *Radiology* 1995; 196:557-564.
50. Yuh WT, Carson JD, Baraniewski H, et al. Osteomyelitis of the foot in diabetic patients: evaluation with plain film, TcMDP bone scintigraphy and MR imaging. *AJR Am J Roentgenol* 1989; 152:795-800.
51. Beltran J, Campanini DS, Knight C. The diabetic foot: magnetic resonance imaging evaluation. *Skeletal Radiol* 1990; 19:37-41.
52. Moore TE, Yuh WTC, Kathol MH, et al. Abnormalities of the foot in patients with diabetes mellitus: findings on MR imaging. *AJR Am J Roentgenol* 1991; 157:813-816.
53. Beltran J, Chandnani V, McGhee RA, et al. Gadopentetate dimeglumine-enhanced MR imaging of the musculoskeletal system. *AJR Am J Roentgenol* 1991; 156:457-461.
54. Craig JG, Amin MB, Wu K, et al. Osteomyelitis of the diabetic foot: MR imaging-pathologic correlation. *Radiology* 1997; 203:849-855.
55. Peterson JJ, Bancroft LW, Kransdorf MJ. Wooden foreign bodies: imaging appearance. *AJR Am J Roentgenol* 2002; 178:557-562.

Foot/Ankle Protocols

This is one set of suggested protocols; there are many variations that would work equally well.

ANKLE/HINDFOOT/MIDFOOT: ROUTINE (PAIN)

Sequence No.	1	2	3	4	5	6
Sequence Type	T1W	STIR	T1W	T2*W	T1W	T2*W
Orientation	Sagittal	Sagittal	Long-axis axial	Long-axis axial	Short-axis axial	Short-axis axial
Field of View (cm)	14	14	14	14	14	14
Slice Thickness (mm)	4	4	4	4	4	4
Contrast	No	No	No	No	No	No

ANKLE/HINDFOOT/MIDFOOT: INFECTION/MASS

Sequence No.	1	2	3	4	5	6
Sequence Type	T1W	STIR	T1W	STIR	T1W fat saturation	T1W fat saturation
Orientation	Sagittal	Sagittal	Long-axis axial	Short-axis axial	Long-axis axial	Sagittal
Field of View (cm)	14	14	14	14	14	14
Slice Thickness (mm)	4	4	4	4	4	4
Contrast	No	No	No	No	Yes	Yes

ENTIRE FOOT: INFECTION/MASS

Sequence No.	1	2	3	4	5	6
Sequence Type	T1W	T1W	STIR	STIR	T1W fat saturation	T1W fat saturation
Orientation	Long-axis axial	Sagittal	Sagittal	Short-axis axial	Sagittal	Long-axis axial
Field of View (cm)	14	14	14	14	14	14
Slice Thickness (mm)	4	4	4	4	4	4
Contrast	No	No	No	No	Yes	Yes

FOREFOOT/TOES: ROUTINE (PAIN)

Sequence No.	1	2	3	4	5	6
Sequence Type	T1W	STIR	T1W	STIR	T1W	T2*W
Orientation	Sagittal	Sagittal	Long-axis axial	Short-axis axial	Short-axis axial	Short-axis axial
Field of View (cm)	12	12	12	12	12	12
Slice Thickness (mm)	4	4	4	4	4	4
Contrast	No	No	No	No	No	No

FOREFOOT/TOES: INFECTION/MASS

Sequence No.	1	2	3	4	5	6
Sequence Type	T1W	T1W	STIR	T1W fat saturation	T1W fat saturation	
Orientation	Sagittal	Long-axis axial	Short-axis axial	Sagittal	Long-axis axial	
Field of View (cm)	12	12	12	12	12	
Slice Thickness (mm)	4	4	4	4	4	
Contrast	No	No	No	Yes	Yes	

FOREFOOT/TOES: MORTON'S NEUROMA

Sequence No.	1	2	3	4	5	6
Sequence Type	T1W	Turbo T2W	STIR	T1W fat saturation		
Orientation	Short-axis axial	Short-axis axial	Long-axis axial	Short-axis axial		
Field of View (cm)	12	12	12	12		
Slice Thickness (mm)	4	4	4	4		
Contrast				No		

Foot/Ankle Protocols (Continued)

This is one set of suggested protocols; there are many variations that would work equally well.

SAMPLE STANDARD REPORT

MRI of the Ankle

Clinical Indications

Protocol

The routine protocol with multiple sequences and planes of imaging was used.

Discussion

1. **Joint effusion, bursitis:** None

2. **Osseous structures:** Normal; without evidence of fracture or osteochondritis; no arthritis

3. **Tendons:** Flexor and extensor tendons of the ankle are normal in position, size, and signal

4. **Ligaments:** Medial collateral (deltoid) and spring (talocalcaneonavicular) ligaments are intact; anterior and posterior tibiofibular ligaments, anterior and posterior talofibular ligaments, and calcaneofibular ligament on the lateral side of the ankle are intact

5. **Plantar fascia:** Normal morphology and signal

6. **Tarsal tunnel and sinus tarsi:** Normal

7. **Other abnormalities:** None

Opinion

Normal MRI of the (right/left) ankle.

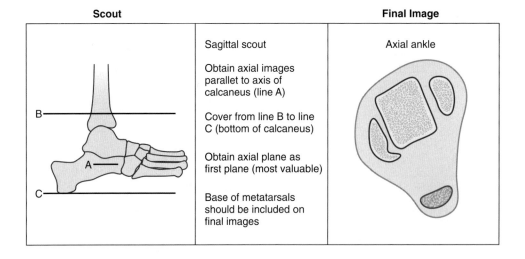

Scout

Final Image

Sagittal scout

Obtain axial images parallet to axis of calcaneus (line A)

Cover from line B to line C (bottom of calcaneus)

Obtain axial plane as first plane (most valuable)

Base of metatarsals should be included on final images

Axial ankle

Scout		Final Image
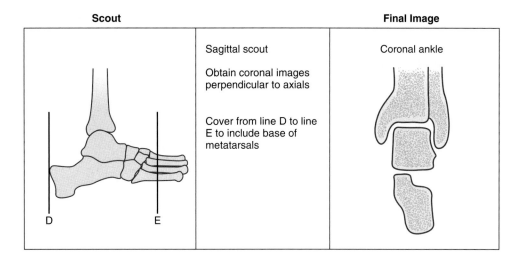	Sagittal scout Obtain coronal images perpendicular to axials Cover from line D to line E to include base of metatarsals	Coronal ankle

Scout		Final Image
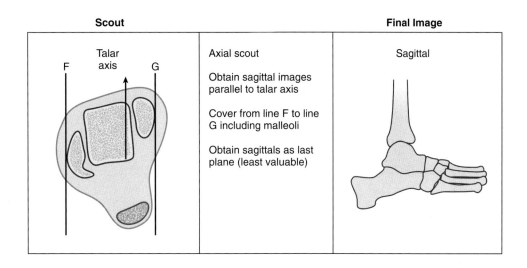	Axial scout Obtain sagittal images parallel to talar axis Cover from line F to line G including malleoli Obtain sagittals as last plane (least valuable)	Sagittal

Scout		Final Image
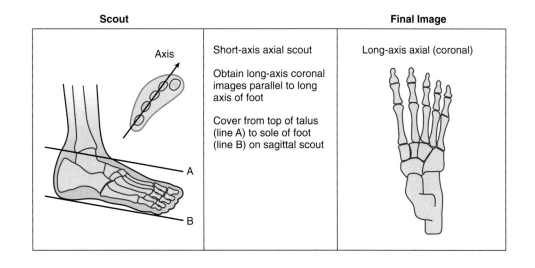	Short-axis axial scout Obtain long-axis coronal images parallel to long axis of foot Cover from top of talus (line A) to sole of foot (line B) on sagittal scout	Long-axis axial (coronal)

Scout		**Final Image**
	Long-axis coronal scout Obtain sagittal images parallel to long axis of foot Cover from line C to D	Sagittal

Scout		**Final Image**
	Sagittal scout Obtain short-axis axial images perpendicular to axis of metatarsals Cover entire foot from lines E to F	Short-axis axial

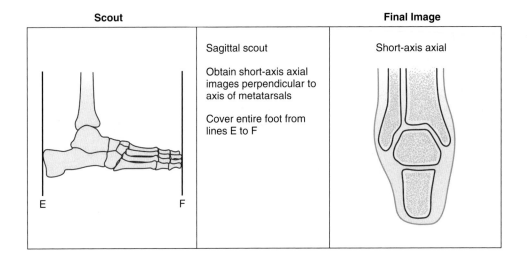

Scout		**Final Image**
	Short-axis axial scout of metatarsals Obtain sagittal images perpendicular to line roughly connecting metatarsals 2 through 5 (line A) Cover entire width of foot (lines B to C)*	Sagittal

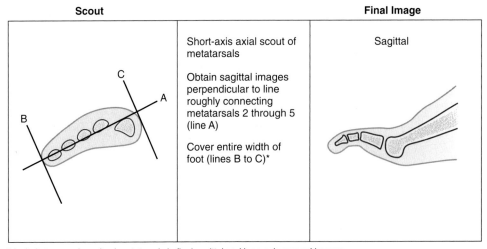

* Include toes and proximal metatarsals in final sagittal and long-axis coronal images

Scout		Final Image
	Short-axis axial scout Obtain long-axis coronal images parallel to line roughly connecting metatarsals 2 through 5 (line A) Cover entire foot from lines D to E*	Long-axis coronal

* Include toes and proximal metatarsals in final sagittal and long-axis coronal images

Scout		Final Image
	Sagittal scout Obtain short-axis axial images perpendicular to axis of metatarsal 2 or 3 Cover from proximal metatarsal line F through toes (line G) Final images should fill the frame	Short-axis axial

Index

Note: Page numbers followed by f refer to figures; page numbers followed by t refer to tables; page numbers followed by b refer to boxes.